PHARMACY PRACTICE
Social and
Behavioral Aspects

Third Edition

PHARMACY PRACTICE

Social and Behavioral Aspects

Third Edition

Edited by

ALBERT I. WERTHEIMER, Ph.D.
Department of Graduate Studies
   in Social and Administrative Pharmacy
College of Pharmacy
University of Minnesota
Minneapolis, Minnesota

MICKEY C. SMITH, Ph.D.
Department of Health Care Administration
School of Pharmacy
University of Mississippi
University, Mississippi

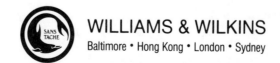

WILLIAMS & WILKINS
Baltimore • Hong Kong • London • Sydney

Editor: John P. Butler
Associate Editor: Linda Napora
Copy Editor: Susan Vaupel
Design: Alice Johnson
Illustration Planning: Lorraine Wrzosek
Production: Raymond E. Reter

Copyright © 1989
Williams & Wilkins
428 East Preston Street
Baltimore, Maryland 21202, USA

Accurate indications, adverse reactions, and dosage schedules for drugs are provided in this book, but it is possible that they may change. The reader is urged to review the package information data of the manufacturers of the medications mentioned.

Printed in the United States of America

First Edition 1974
Second Edition 1981

Library of Congress Cataloging in Publication Data
Pharmacy practice: social and behavioral aspects/edited by Albert I. Wertheimer, Mickey C. Smith.—3rd ed.
    p. cm.
Includes bibliographies and index.
ISBN 0-683-08932-3
1. Pharmacy—Social aspects.   2. Pharmacy management.
3. Pharmacist and patient.   I. Wertheimer, Albert I.   II. Smith, Mickey C.
  [DNLM: 1. Community Pharmacy Services. 2. Pharmacy. QV 704
P5453]
RS92.P48 1989
362.1′782—dc 19
DNLM/DLC
for Library of Congress
                                     88-17289
                                       CIP

90 91 92 93
4 5 6 7 8 9 10

Foreword

Although the social and behavioral sciences have been around for a long time, having been accorded academic legitimacy as early as the beginning of this century, their perceived usefulness to problems of everyday life has been slow. They began to be regarded as useful for various practitioners in the health field after World War II: nurses, physicians, dentists, medical social workers, and eventually pharmacists—the latter as illustrated in this useful book of readings. Still, it is necessary to recognize that the social and behavioral sciences by their very nature cannot be applied as specifically as the medical reductionist model to the ills of human beings.

The social and behavioral sciences are grounded in the life experiences of humankind; the physical and natural sciences are grounded in the seeming rationality and predictability of the natural order. The derivative disciplines of pharmacy and medicine continue to be in biochemistry, physics, and physiology, but the practice of pharmacy and medicine takes place in the everyday world of human beings—patients, clients, and customers—their feelings, fears, expectations, and interpretations. And because pharmacists and physicians are also social beings, their interactions with others must perforce transcend the seeming specificity of their base disciplines in order for them to function more effectively in their practitioner roles.

As a matter of necessity, physicians and pharmacists already practice more social behavior than they realize simply in order to relate to people at all. The articles in this book will help to sharpen their perceptions of themselves and other human beings as behaving entities in their social and psychological worlds. The fact that there are tremendous ranges of volume of prescribing medications by country and between physicians shows that there are many social and behavioral variables involved.

A usual dichotomy in pharmaceutical and medical practices has been defined as the biomedical and biopsychosocial models. The biomedical model assumes a specious precision in dealing with ill (and well) people, but the psychosocial model provides relatively little guidance in specifying relevant variables for individual patients. Nevertheless, the practitioner must draw on the biopsychosocial model to become sensitized to the complexity of human life, which has more order than is generally recognized. Even the simple recognition that human beings are products of cultures is a good start for practitioners to become aware of reasons for what they may perceive as irrational behavior but may be considered rational behavior among people from different backgrounds.

In sum, the faith of social and behavioral scientists is that if more and more people begin to perceive the world as we do, the persons in the street would make more rational decisions, or at least, realize why they made those they did, and health practitioners would become more understanding, compassionate, and efficient.

PROFESSOR ODIN W. ANDERSON, Ph.D.
Sociology Department
University of Wisconsin-Madison
Madison, Wisconsin
and
Graduate School of Business
and
Sociology Department
University of Chicago
Chicago, Illinois

v

Preface

When the first edition of this book appeared in 1974, we addressed a newly emerging discipline with a great deal of excitement, enthusiasm, and also uncertainty as the subject of social and behavioral pharmacy was in its infancy. We hoped that perhaps about 15 colleges might offer such an undergraduate course with the availability of a textbook. We saw our expectations met and exceeded during the following few years.

By the time of the publication of the second edition in 1981, we were pleased to learn that the course is offered at virtually all of the more than 70 colleges of pharmacy in the United States as well as at faculties in many other countries.

The second edition incorporated some changes that reflected the growth of scientific research in the relevant social science fields and also the inclusion of recommendations and suggestions made by your colleagues who used the first edition.

We are pleased to be able to report that this 1989, third edition contains the most radical changes to date. We find that the pharmacy students of this era are more exposed to the social and behavioral sciences than were their colleagues who matriculated only a decade ago. Therefore, we are able to eliminate some very basic material, permitting us more space for emerging areas not represented in the previous two editions. These include international issues and public health considerations, to list just two examples.

Once again, there is more available to us in the scientific and professional literature than ever before in the most relevant areas of social psychology, medical sociology, medical anthropology, and communications. In addition, the graduate programs at close to a dozen colleges are now producing an ever-greater number of faculty members who will be qualified to teach and conduct research in this area. Therefore, with these factors in mind we present our third edition. We hope that its improvements are seen as such. Much of the credit for this endeavor should be shared with John Butler at Williams & Wilkins, Sandy Dewing at the University of Minnesota, and Renate Lutz at the University of Mississippi. However, the final responsibility lies solely with us.

ALBERT I. WERTHEIMER, Ph.D.
Minneapolis, Minnesota

MICKEY C. SMITH, Ph.D.
University, Mississippi

Contributors

ROBERT A. BUERKI, Ph.D.
College of Pharmacy
Ohio State University
Columbus, Ohio

PATRICIA J. BUSH, Ph.D.
Department of Community Medicine
School of Medicine
Georgetown University
Washington, DC

CARMEN CATIZONE, R.Ph., M.S.
College of Pharmacy
University of Illinois at Chicago
Chicago, Illinois

DONNA DOLINSKY, Ph.D.
College of Pharmacy
University of Illinois at Chicago
Chicago, Illinois

JACK E. FINCHAM, Ph.D.
School of Pharmacy
Health Care Administration
University of Mississippi
University, Mississippi

TOMAS L. GRIEBLING, B.A.
Wartburg College
Waverly, Iowa

JEROME A. HALPERIN, V.P.
CIBA Consumer Pharmaceuticals
Edison, New Jersey

CHARLES D. HEPLER, Ph.D.
School of Pharmacy
Virginia Commonwealth University
MCV Campus
Richmond, Virginia

KEITH W. JOHNSON, Ph.D.
Rockville, Maryland

CAROLE L. KIMBERLIN
College of Pharmacy
University of Florida
Gainesville, Florida

HENRI R. MANASSE, JR., Ph.D., R.Ph.
College of Pharmacy
University of Illinois at Chicago
Chicago, Illinois

WILLIAM F. McGHAN, Pharm.D., Ph.D.
College of Pharmacy
University of Arizona
Tucson, Arizona

JEANINE K. MOUNT, Ph.D., R.Ph.
School of Pharmacy
University of Wisconsin-Madison
Madison, Wisconsin

ROBERT G. MRTEK, Ph.D., R.Ph.
College of Pharmacy
University of Illinois at Chicago
Chicago, Illinois

MICKEY C. SMITH, Ph.D.
Health Care Administration
School of Pharmacy
University of Mississippi
University, Mississippi

ELLIOTT M. SOGOL, Ph.D., R.Ph.
College of Pharmacy
University of Illinois at Chicago
Chicago, Illinois

BERNARD SOROFMAN, Ph.D., R.Ph.
College of Pharmacy
University of Iowa
Iowa City, Iowa

BONNIE L. SVARSTAD, Ph.D.
School of Pharmacy
University of Wisconsin-Madison
Madison, Wisconsin

LOUIS D. VOTTERO, M.S.
College of Pharmacy
Ohio Northern University
Ada, Ohio

ALBERT I. WERTHEIMER, Ph.D.
Social and Administrative Pharmacy
University of Minnesota
Minneapolis, Minnesota

Contents

1

Contributions of the Social Sciences

JEANINE K. MOUNT

> . . . (D)espite the enormous gains which have accrued from biomedical research, there is a growing
> uneasiness among the public as well as among physicians, and especially among the younger genera-
> tion, that health needs are not being met and that biomedical research is not having a sufficient impact
> in human terms. This is usually ascribed to the all too obvious inadequacies of existing health care
> delivery systems. But this is certainly not a complete explanation. . . . Medicine's unrest derives from a
> growing awareness among many physicians of the contradiction between the excellence of their bio-
> medical background on the one hand and the weakness of their qualifications in certain attributes
> essential for good patient care on the other. Many recognize that these cannot be improved by working
> within the biomedical model alone. (1)

With these words, George Engel, a prominent medical educator, describes the growing
sense of disillusionment with the dominant approach to health and health care provision.
Engel summarizes how the biomedical model underemphasizes the human aspects of patient care and neglects important psychosocial issues. His proposal is to adopt the biopsychosocial model as an alternate for understanding health and health care. What is new
about Engel's model is the explicit consideration of the social sciences, complements to the
physical and biological sciences that define the biomedical model.

Inclusion of the social sciences within this framework enables us to understand things
and events that are otherwise inaccessible. Furthermore, it offers a new agenda for research
and training in health care. In this chapter, we present an overview of the social sciences and
outline their major contributions to our understanding of pharmacy and health care. This
will set the stage for discussion of application of the social sciences to a specific area of
concern within pharmacy in subsequent chapters and selected readings in this book.

Why are we embarking on such a task? As we look at pharmacy practice in contemporary health care, we see a picture that is changing dramatically. The medications we distribute are potentially more effective—and potentially more harmful—than ever before, assuming increasing importance as components of overall treatment regimens (2). Large corporate
groups, including pharmaceutical manufacturers and governmental regulators, continue to
grow in size, complexity, and influence (3). Amid this state of flux, the pharmacist is called
upon to adopt new professional roles and patient care orientations (4). How are we to understand these changes? What elements underlie them? What will be their effects? The thread
common to these changes is their focus on *human* aspects of pharmacy and pharmacy practice. In situations such as these, the social sciences are able to provide us with needed,
unique insights.

PRELIMINARIES

Prior to discussing the contributions of the social sciences to pharmacy and pharmacy practice, we must address several preliminary points. To establish a common basis for understanding, we must clarify what is meant by the "social sciences." We next explore why we should consider the relevance of the social sciences. Thus, the stage will be set for identifying what the social sciences are able to bring to those of us involved in pharmacy.

What Are the "Social Sciences"?

We use the term social sciences frequently but without the precision we require here. The social sciences have a shared focus on understanding patterns and meaning of human behavior.[a] Typically, a wide variety of scientific disciplines are considered within this category. Many of these, such as anthropology, psychology, social psychology, sociology, political science, and geography, have names that are likely familiar to you. Other social science disciplines, such as demography, epidemiology, and health services research, although less familiar provide us with additional ways of understanding the world.

What *are* the social sciences, though? To answer this question, we must address a preliminary question: What is a science? Again, throughout this discussion, we use the term "science" frequently and need to define it precisely here. Four characteristics distinguish a science from a nonscience.[b] First, a science is theory based. A theory is a series of interrelated, testable propositions or assertions that describe how a set of facts are related to one another and under what conditions these relationships hold (8).

Perhaps we can better understand by discussing an example. The germ theory of disease is one of the more widely held theories in the biomedical sciences. Briefly summarized, it states that contagious disease in a host organism is caused by "germs" (microorganisms) that proliferate when certain favorable environmental conditions are present. Few people now question the accuracy of this theory. When originally proposed, however, it stood in radical opposition to widely held beliefs. Through a series of scientific experiments, the accuracy of the germ theory of disease was able to be tested and established. This illustrates the second characteristic of a science: It uses precise, highly systematized principles for investigation, which specify appropriate techniques for collecting and analyzing information or data.

Scientific investigators continually pursue new knowledge. As such knowledge develops, it may serve to support, refine, and/or refute existing theories or specific propositions posed within them. This leads to the third characteristic of a science: Its knowledge base is ever expanding and cumulative. Successive research efforts result in improved precision and, as advances take place, the final characteristic of a science becomes evident. Extensive, precise knowledge allows us to move beyond simply describing relationships among

---

[a] In this chapter, we will consider one particular group of social sciences. The administrative sciences (such as economics and management) are social sciences in that they, too, study patterns of human behavior. They differ, however, in that they specifically focus on human systems that are rationally planned, organized, and/or administered. Within the discipline of pharmacy administration, the administrative sciences have had a longer history and received greater attention than have other social sciences. They are not directly examined here (although much of what is discussed is pertinent to them). Rucker (5) provides an overview of the discipline of pharmacy administration.

Similarly, disciplines that are identified as "humanities" (such as history and literature) lie outside this discussion. Excellent specialty resources are available for further study; *Kremer and Urdang's History of Pharmacy* (6) is highly recommended as an introduction to this area.

[b] This discussion draws on Kuhn's *The Structure of Scientific Revolutions* (7).

discrete facts. A developed science identifies cause-effect relationships and, thus, is said to be predictive.

Let us now return to our original question: What are the social sciences? As described above, the social sciences attempt to identify and understand the patterns and meaning of human behavior. This focus distinguishes the social sciences from their physical and biological counterparts. Like their physical and biological counterparts, however, the social sciences are sciences: They are theory based, use systematic research techniques, are cumulative, and are predictive. Predictive accuracy is generally viewed as the weakest aspect of the social science disciplines. We can better understand why this is so by placing the social sciences within the historical context of their development. Compared to older physical and biological sciences (such as physics, chemistry, physiology), the social sciences are still at an early stage of development. It is likely that predictive ability will improve as our social scientific knowledge base improves in its depth and precision.

Systematic application of the physical and biological sciences to pharmacy- or drug-related questions like those examined in pharmaceutics, medicinal chemistry, and pharmacology has occurred primarily within the last 50 to 100 years. Pharmacy applications of the social sciences have an even more brief history, one encompassing perhaps 15 to 20 years.[c] This relative "newness" helps explain why social and behavioral pharmacy is not more widely recognized as an area of inquiry and why our knowledge base is quite restricted in many areas. In many respects, social and behavioral pharmacy is in its infancy. For this reason, as you explore topics considered in this book, be sensitive to questions that require further investigation.

About the Social Sciences

Before continuing, we should clarify some commonly held impressions of the social sciences. Let us briefly consider what the social sciences are and what they are not.

More so than the physical or biological sciences, the social sciences deal with phenomena that are part of our life-world. They are not, however, simply common sense or common knowledge. Certainly you know of instances in which logic or intuition does not lead to appropriate conclusions about everyday events. Although we sometimes see this in day-to-day situations, we oftentimes see it in social scientific research. For example, logic would argue that supplying more information about medications to patients, physicians, and/or pharmacists would result in improved medication use. Although this may result some of the time, it is not universally true. The social sciences help us sort out how and why such results vary.

People sometimes describe the social sciences as "soft" or "imprecise" sciences, reflecting the belief that it is impossible to measure or quantify sentiments or subjective experiences. Needless to say, social scientists do not share this belief. The social sciences can more accurately be described as interpretive sciences, highlighting their focus on the social world and individuals' understanding of it. Although the subjective nature of their subject matter makes it impossible for social scientists to be perfectly objective, social scientists strive to be neutral in their orientation.

---

[c] For background in the early application of social sciences to pharmacy, see presentations made at the 1969 Invitational Conference in Social Studies of Pharmacy (9). More recent statements regarding the scope of social and behavioral pharmacy are seen in Svarstad (10), Johnson and Wertheimer (11), and Dolinsky (12). Developments in the field are reflected in the evolution of this book, from its original (13) to the current edition.

Many would argue that to varying degrees all sciences are interpretive because all scientists engage in interpretive activity when collecting and organizing their data. Sophisticated machinery and complicated instruments do not guarantee scientific precision. Objectivity should not be taken for granted either. Physical and biological scientists, like their social science colleagues, expend significant time and energy establishing the reliability and validity of their techniques for data collection and verification. Compared to others, social scientists often must be more explicit in their recognition of the interpretive process and more deliberate in their efforts to control it.

Finally, although social scientists recognize and often explicitly analyze social values held within a society, social scientists are not "social engineers" trying to impose a particular social agenda or ideology. The social sciences do not contain a social action element or political stance, although their theories or findings may suggest such. We can distinguish between "basic" and "applied" aspects of the social sciences. Basic social science research seeks enhanced understanding and has the primary goal of discovery of knowledge for its own sake. For example, a basic science investigator in social and behavioral pharmacy may ask a research question such as: Does patient recall of information affect compliance with medication regimens? Other researchers focus on how we can apply knowledge about human behavior to address real concerns in real situations. An applied social and behavioral pharmacy research question might ask: What memory-enhancing technique(s) best improve patient compliance with medication regimens?

The Social Systems Approach

Health researchers' adoption of the biomedical model has resulted in tremendous growth in our understanding of the biological bases of disease and comparable advances in disease treatment. Engel's quotation at the opening of this chapter, however, reflects the fact that as we have continued to rely on the biomedical model, several significant weaknesses have become visible. The first weakness is evident precisely because of the success of the biomedical model: once the best of physical and biological science knowledge is applied to the treatment of diseases, a number of problems are not completely resolved. This is most obvious when we consider chronic diseases (e.g., arthritis) or diseases that are related to personal lifestyle (e.g., high blood pressure). A second weakness of the biomedical model is its tendency to consider patients as biologically active organisms and its frequent failure to consider patients as socially active participants in health care endeavors. As thinking, feeling beings, patients play active roles as health care decision makers. A final weakness of the biomedical model is its inability to address how the activities of health care providers and the health care system itself affect health-related outcomes.

These weaknesses are systematically addressed in Engel's biopsychosocial model, an adaptation of which is presented in column 1 of Figure 1.1. We can identify the central domain as encompassing the levels of organization that begin with the individual person, continue through the social groups of various size, and conclude with the biosphere. Thus, the social sciences allow us to view pharmacy and drugs within the human context in which they exist.

The biopsychosocial model provides a "systems approach" (14) to understanding the world. Looking at Figure 1.1, we can specify several important characteristics of this approach. The systems approach illustrates *relationships* among the physical, biological, and social sciences; how *levels* of phenomena are logically related to one another but are able to be separated for specific analyses; and a *holistic* orientation toward scientific understanding.

Looking back at Figure 1.1, we see how the systems approach can assist us in analyzing a variety of events relevant to pharmacy. Columns 2 through 5 describe a sequence of events related to an unfortunate, yet common occurrence, a patient experiencing an adverse drug reaction (ADR). In Column 2, we see that the initial event directly affects the patient's biological functioning. Immediate consequences at social levels are also evident, however, as the patient interprets the situation and reacts to it. Responding to this, the patient's spouse intervenes (column 3), clarifying that a problem exists and engaging in help-seeking behavior. We now see the reverse series of consequences: The social action of seeking and accepting help initiates changes in biological functioning. Detection of the adverse drug reaction (column 4) results in further activities for the patient (understanding, communication), for health professionals (pharmacist's report of the medication causing the ADR), and for the health care system (governmental monitoring of prescription medications). With resolution of the ADR (column 5), we see continuing social consequences intimately tied to an event having direct effects at biological levels. Thus, we see how a comprehensive approach to health and health care, one that considers both biomedical and social aspects, results in a more thorough understanding of such events.

CONTRIBUTIONS OF THE SOCIAL SCIENCES

What do the social sciences contribute to our understanding of pharmacy? I believe we can identify three specific areas in which the social sciences contribute to our understanding of pharmacy and pharmacy practice. The social sciences provide us with (*a*) approaches to asking questions in pharmacy, (*b*) conceptual and explanatory frameworks, and (*c*) research tools and techniques. Let us look at each of these in turn.

Contribution No. 1: Approaches to Analyzing Pharmacy

One of the most important contributions of the social sciences to pharmacy is their assistance in identifying questions and subjects that need to be addressed. That is, the social sciences help us identify the central problematics of social and behavioral pharmacy. Questions of central interest can be grouped into three general topics: (*a*) drugs and drug use, (*b*) pharmacy practice and services, and (*c*) pharmacy as a profession.

We use a variety of terms, including drug, medication, and medicine, to refer to substances that are biologically and/or psychologically active. Often we are concerned with their use in the prevention, diagnosis, treatment, or cure of disease. We recognize, however, that such substances also can be used for numerous nonmedical purposes. For this reason, we define the topic of "drug use" very broadly as focusing on the processes, attitudes, and beliefs related to the acquisition, consumption, and response to drug substances. Contributions by authors Svarstad (Chapter 7), Smith (Chapter 8), and Briebling and Sorofman (Chapter 9) provide further discussion of specific aspects of drugs and drug use.

In some situations, we are primarily interested in studying the drug use process and its interpretation by individuals. Several of the social science disciplines, notably psychology, social psychology, and anthropology, provide important insight into drug use at this more microsocial level. At other times, we are more interested in understanding drugs and drug use at a group level. Perspectives provided by more macrosocial disciplines complement those provided by the microsocial disciplines in such instances, as described in Table 1.1.

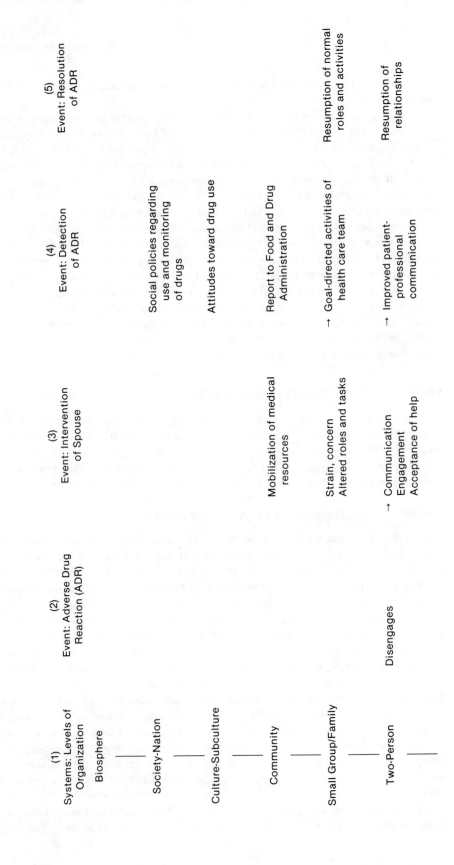

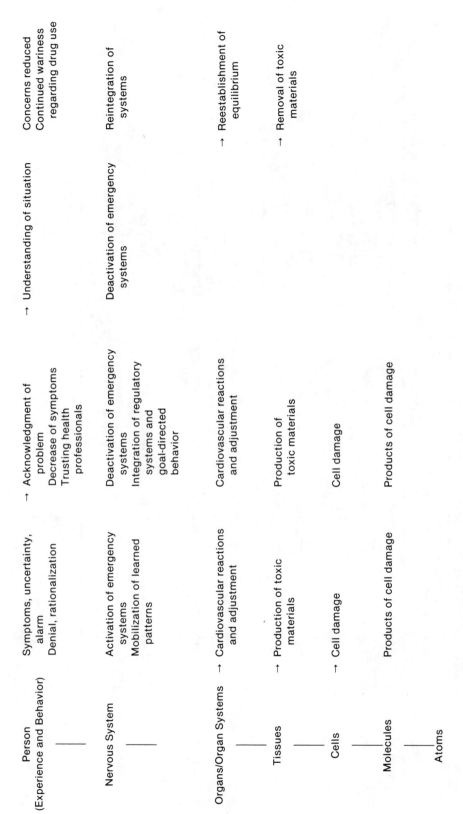

Figure 1.1. Hierarchy of natural systems and application to social and behavioral pharmacy. (Adapted from Engel GL: The clinical application of the biopsychosocial model. Am J Psychiatry 1977;137:535–544.

Table 1.1. Social science disciplines and their orientations.

Discipline	System Levels of Interest		Central Focus	Example of Application
	Lowest	Highest		
Psychology	Nervous System	2-Person System	Individual person	Patient learning styles Patient response to illness symptoms
Social Psychology	Single Person	Small Groups	Individual within group context	Patient-pharmacist communication Patient compliance with medication regimens
Sociology	Small Group	Society/Nation	Structure of social groups	Professional codes of ethics Interprofessional relationships
Political Science	Small Group	Society/Nation	Power in social groups	Dynamics of professionalization Regulation and drug policy formation
Health Services Research	Community	Society/Nation	Health care delivery system functioning	Channels for drug distribution Patterns of pharmacy services provision
Anthropology	Community	Biosphere	Human groups within the man-made environment	Societal attitudes toward drug use Value placed on existence of the health care system
Geography	Community	Biosphere	Physical environment of human groups	Effects of pharmacy location on access to health services Effects of climate-related health needs
Demography	Community	Biosphere	Dynamics of human populations	Maldistribution of health manpower Effects of population planning efforts
Epidemiology	Community	Biosphere	Patterns of human health and disease	Patterns of physican prescribing Impact of pharmacy services on the public's health

For example, sociology and political science can provide us with insight into the regulatory aspects of new drug development. Epidemiology and health services research may provide us with insight into aggregate patterns of medication consumption. This is described in Table 1.1.

The basic work of pharmacy is the second topic that the social sciences help us to understand (15, 16). We can distinguish two major, strongly interrelated aspects of this work. At the more microsocial level, we can describe pharmacy practice as the discrete activities and interactions carried out as part of pharmacists' day-to-day functioning. At a somewhat broader level, pharmacy services describe formally or informally organized sets or systems of pharmacists' work activities.

Our ability to differentiate aspects at the microsocial level from those at macrosocial levels (pharmacy practice and pharmacy services, respectively) again suggests that different social science disciplines will assist us in our understanding. As reflected in Table 1.2, contributions by McGhan (Chapter 4), Kimberlin (Chapter 6), Fincham (Chapter 10), and Bush and Johnson (Chapter 13) focus on the work of pharmacy. The utility of the perspectives provided by the various disciplines is demonstrated in their in-depth discussions.

The third topic informed by the social sciences focuses on the state and status of the pharmacy profession. In analyzing the pharmacy profession, contributors to this book again identify numerous micro- and macrosocial phenomena. Wertheimer's (Chapter 12) use of an international comparative approach to assessing the status of pharmacy exemplifies a truly macrosocial perspective. Mrtek and Catizone's (Chapter 2) sociohistorical overview of how occupational groups develop into professions again reflects a macrosocial application. When discussing how belonging to a profession affects individual members, they move to a microsocial level. This is also true as Sogol and Manasse (Chapter 3) and Buersi and Vottero (Chapter 11) consider specific aspects of professional training and ethical aspects of professional behavior.

Contribution No. 2: Conceptual and Explanatory Frameworks

As we have discussed, the social sciences assist us in identifying questions that we wish to investigate. We give order to thoughts related to those questions by constructing *models*. We can define a model as a pattern of interrelated concepts or ideas that is found to imitate, duplicate, or illustrate a pattern of relationships that one observes in the world.[d] Usually models are simplified versions of reality that allow us to analyze a well-focused question and a limited set of ideas related to it.

Model building is an important step in advancing our understanding. In addition to identifying concepts and specifying how they are interrelated, models can be tested empirically. That is, social scientific research methods can be used to examine the "correctness" of the model. (We will have more to say about this later.) The building and testing of models also accommodate a dynamic process orientation toward pharmacy-related developments. Thus, in addition to being able to pose and answer important questions, we are able to explore changes within the system of pharmacy and drug use.

Once we have specified a question relevant to the social aspects of pharmacy and constructed a model that captures the essence of the question, the social sciences assist with the next step in our inquiry by providing explanatory frameworks for interpreting our question

---

[d]There are numerous sources that provide background information regarding social science terminology and definitions. I have drawn primarily from *A Modern Dictionary of Sociology* by Theodorson and Theodorson (17).

Table 1.2.   Social Science Research Methods.

Research Method	Strengths	Weaknesses	Example of Application (and Chapter where employed)
Experiment	Good internal control Random assignment used	Situations often artificially structured	Educational interventions (Kimberlin, Ch. 6)
Survey Research	Random sampling can be used Good representation of population possible	Generally only cross-sectional data collected	Consumer surveys (McGhan, Ch. 4) Drug epidemiology (Smith, Ch. 8)
Field Research	Can study events in natural surroundings	Internal control very difficult to achieve	Observation of patient-professional interaction (Kimberlin, Ch. 6)
Content Analysis	Researcher has direct effect on subjects being studied	Problems with data completeness, accuracy, and verification	Analysis of professional curriculum (Sogol and Manasse, Ch. 3)
Existing Data Research	Same as Content Analysis	Same as Content Analysis	
Historical Research	Allows comparisons not possible at one point in time	Restrictions of types, amount, and quality of data available	Pharmacy records review (Smith, Ch. 8) Development of professional codes of ethics (Buerki and Vottero, Ch. 11)
Comparative Research	Allows comparisons not possible in any single community or society	Comparability of data difficult to assess (as is accuracy oftentimes)	State of pharmacy throughout the world (Werheimer, Ch. 12)
Evaluation Research	Determination of effects of interventions possible	Value biases and value conflict problems often arise	Evaluation of patient counseling techniques (Svarstad, Ch. 7)

and its answer(s). We generally refer to such an explanatory framework as a theory or a theoretical approach. Recall from our earlier discussion of what constitutes a science that the presence of a theory base distinguishes scientific investigation from casual inquiry.

Within the social sciences, dozens of specific theories have been advanced. Presenting even brief synopses of these theories is an overwhelming task and beyond our purposes here. You will be introduced to a variety of them as they are discussed within the contributed chapters and selected readings.

Several broad theoretical orientations serve as underpinnings to most of the specific theories that social scientists examine. We can describe a theoretical orientation as a basic set of assumptions regarding the factors that influence human behavior. I believe we can distinguish six basic theoretical orientations in the social sciences: psychological, social psychological, functional, political, cultural, and ecological. These differ in the extent to which they emphasize individual persons, social groups, or the environment of such groups as their points of focus. Generally, each of the social science disciplines has one or two of these orientations associated with it.

The psychological orientation emphasizes how personality and psychological processes (such as learning, feeling, thinking) affect behavior. Not surprisingly, this orientation dominates the discipline of psychology. The social psychological orientation shares some of the interests of the psychological but differs in that it gives comparable emphasis to how individual behavior is affected by social group membership.

The functional and political orientations both are associated with the disciplines of sociology, political science, and health services research. In attempting to explain patterns of human behavior, both of these orientations focus on the influences that result from the existence, organization, and operation of large social groups. These two orientations differ from one another in that the functional orientation assumes that consensus and agreement dominate these social groups while the political orientation assumes that conflict and competition dominate.

The cultural and ecological orientations are similar in the fact that they focus on social groups within their environmental context. They differ, though, with respect to what aspect of the environment is emphasized. The cultural orientation places greater emphasis on social/man-made environmental influences on human behaviors while the ecological orientation emphasizes physical/natural environmental influences. Anthropology most clearly adheres to a cultural orientation, just as geography adheres to an ecological orientation. In their diverse applications, demography and epidemiology may assume a more culture-dominant or more ecology-dominant orientation.

Contribution No. 3: Research Techniques and Tools

One of the central problems in any science is understanding how we know what we know. To address this problem, researchers continually investigate, develop, apply, and evaluate alternate procedures for conducting social science research. We refer to this systematic study of research procedures as research methodology.

There are three major components in the planning of a specific research project: research design, data collection, and data analysis (18). This is presented schematically in Figure 1.2. The research design can be thought of as a "blueprint" for a research project. It specifies how we are to conduct the research by outlining (a) relevant concepts, (b) measurement of variables, (c) methods for collecting data, and (d) the subjects of the research.

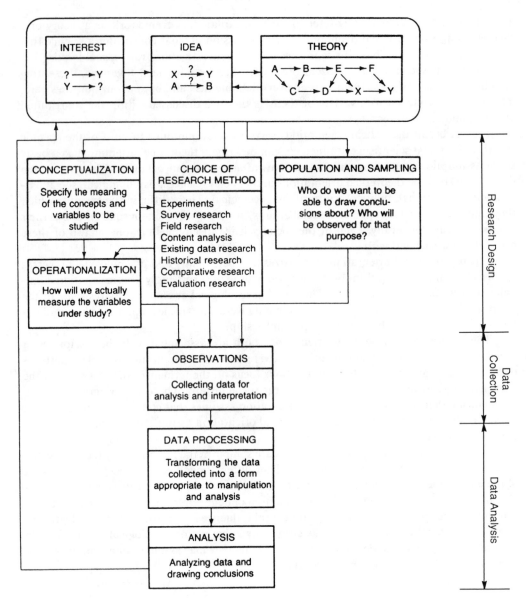

Figure 1.2.   Research process. (From Babbie E: The Practice of Social Research. Belmont, CA, Wadsworth Publishing, 1983.)

Decisions related to each component of the research design have important implications for the subsequent collection, analysis, and evaluation of data.

From the physical and biological sciences, you are familiar with the controlled experiment, the research method most commonly used in laboratory research. Although social science researchers sometimes conduct controlled experiments, many of the questions that they wish to investigate cannot be addressed using laboratory-oriented research procedures.

Because they study events occurring in everyday life, social scientists must often use nonexperimental research designs. Nonexperimental research designs allow social scientists to study human activities in their natural social contexts.

Some of the research methods described in Table 1.2 may have familiar names. You can see that each research method has its own set of strengths and weaknesses, making different methods more appropriate for analyzing different types of research questions.

Let us illustrate this with some examples related to the topic of drug use. Survey research, with its ability to study a sample of persons who are representative of a target population, can be used to accurately describe characteristics of that population (e.g., patients' level of satisfaction with the information they receive about medication) or to pose questions that require further study (e.g., suggesting types of information about medications needed by patients). Likewise, field research methods can be used for describing naturally occurring phenomena. For example, direct observation of pharmacists' counseling activities can be used to document the types of information that patients receive. The high degree of internal control seen in experimental research methods allows establishment of true cause-effect relationships. For example, experimental research methods can evaluate whether patients who are randomly assigned to an experimental group receiving medication information (versus a control group that receives no information) have better compliance with their medication regimens.

Collection of social science data takes a variety of forms, depending upon which research method is being used in a particular study. Methods of data collection include direct observation, review of written records, personal interviews, and paper-and-pencil surveys. Again, this diversity of techniques is necessitated by the diversity of research designs used in actual research circumstances. Multiple types of data collection techniques frequently are used within the same study. Use of multiple techniques allows us to gather different types of information and to verify the accuracy of information we collect. That is, we can cross-check the data we collect using differing techniques to assess its reliability or internal consistency.

Having designed and collected data as part of a social science research project, we now come to the data analysis stage. Approaches to analysis of social science data again differ somewhat from those of the physical and biological sciences. In part, this is due to the fact that the research methods and data collection procedures used by social scientists require specialized data analysis techniques. This is the case, for example, with analysis of data collected using survey research methods based on a sampling of the population. Specialized data analysis techniques are also necessary due to the nature of the phenomena that social scientists study. An important application of this is to address how broad social science concepts (which often must be measured using multiple questions or questioning techniques) can be incorporated into an overall measure or scale that is reliable and valid.

CONCLUSION

So what is it that the social sciences provide to our understanding of pharmacy? We can easily summarize the major contributions as (a) providing a unique perspective for enhanced understanding of contemporary pharmacy, (b) outlining of new questions for the pharmacy research and education agenda, and (c) supplying a set of approaches, tools, and techniques for addressing these questions. As you read this book, you will see how much has been accomplished in a short span of time. Be sensitive, as well, to how much work still remains.

REFERENCES

1. Engel GL. The clinical application of the biopsychosocial model. Am J Psychiatry 1977;137:535–544.
2. U.S. Department of Health and Human Services. National Ambulatory Medical Care Survey, 1981 Summary. Washington, DC: Government Printing Office, 1982.
3. Torrens PR. Historical evolution and overview of health services in the United States. In Williams SJ, Torrens PR (eds), Introduction to Health Services. New York: John Wiley and Sons, 1984.
4. Standards of Practice for the Profession of Pharmacy. American Pharmacy. NS 19:21ff, 1979.
5. Rucker TD. Pharmacy administration as an academic discipline, Am J Pharm Educ 1984;48:385–388.
6. Sonnedecker G. Kremer and Urdang's History of Pharmacy. Philadelphia: Lippincott, 1976.
7. Kuhn TS. The Structure of Scientific Revolutions. Chicago: University of Chicago Press, 1962.
8. Turner JH. The Structure of Sociological Theory. Homewood, IL: Dorsey Press, 1978.
9. Sonnedecker G. Social Studies in Pharmacy: A symposium in Print. Am J Pharm Educ 1970;34:529–586.
10. Svarstad BL. Pharmaceutical sociology: Issues in research, education and service, Am J Pharm Educ 1979;43:252–257.
11. Johnson C, Wertheimer A and AI. Behavioral pharmacy, Am J Pharm Educ 1979;43:257–261.
12. Dolinsky D. Pharmaceutical psychology, Am J Pharm Educ 1979;43:261–266.
13. Wertheimer AI, Smith MC (eds): Pharmacy Practice: Social and Behavioral Aspects. Baltimore: University Park Press, 1974.
14. Olsen ME. The Process of Social Organization. New York: Holt, Rinehart and Winston, 1978.
15. Hall RH. Dimensions of Work. Beverly Hills, CA: Sage Publications, 1986.
16. Strauss A, Fagerhaugh S, Suczek B, Wiener C. Social Organization of Medical Work. Chicago: University of Chicago Press, 1985.
17. Theodorson GA, Theodorson AG. A Modern Dictionary of Sociology. New York: Harper and Row, 1969.
18. Babbie E. The Practice of Social Research. Belmont, CA: Wadsworth Publishing, 1983.

SUGGESTED READINGS

Application of the Social Sciences to Health-Related Topics

1. Angrosino MV. A Health Practitioner's Guide to the Social and Behavioral Sciences. Dover, MA: Auburn House Publishing. (Accessible and highly recommended as an introduction) 1987.
2. Giovannini MJ, Brownlee AT. The contribution of social science to international health training. Social Science and Medicine 1982;16:957–964.
3. Ibrahim MA. Epidemiology and Health Policy. Rockville, MD: Aspen Systems Corp, 1985.
4. Mechanic D, Aiken LH. Social science, medicine and health policy. In Aiken LH, Mechanic D (eds). Applications of Social Science to Clinical Medicine and Health Policy. New Brunswick, NJ: Rutgers University Press, 1986.

Introduction to Social Science Research

1. Babbie E. The Practice of Social Research. Belmont, CA: Wadsworth Publishing, 1983.
2. Blalock HH Jr. Social Statistics. New York: McGraw-Hill, 1979.
3. Blalock HH Jr. Conceptualization and Measurement in the Social Sciences. Beverly Hills: Sage, 1982.
4. Campbell DT, Stanley JC. Experimental and Quasi-experimental Designs for Research. Chicago: Rand McNally, 1963.

Journals in the Area: There are numerous journals dedicated to social science resarch on health-related topics. Several "top" journals (and their disciplinary orientations) include:

1. Social Science and Medicine (Multidisciplinary)
2. Journal of Social and Administrative Pharmacy (Multidisciplinary)
3. Health Psychology (Psychology, Social Psychology)
4. Journal of Health and Social Behavior (Social Psychology, Sociology)
5. Sociology of Health and Illness (Social Psychology, Sociology)

SELECTED READINGS

SOCIAL SCIENCE APPROACHES TO HEALTH SERVICES RESEARCH[e]

Thomas Choi
Jay N. Greenberg

In each of six chapters a distinguished social scientist(s) was asked to present an overview of the concepts, methods and contributions that his/her respective field of inquiry has contributed to health services research. To make comparisons as easy as possible, each author or set of authors was asked to respond to the following common set of questions:

1. What theoretical framework or model of behavior underpins the empirical work of your discipline? Is there more than one dominant framework or model?
2. What are the critical shared assumptions that underpin the theoretical and empirical work of your discipline? What are the consequences of these assumptions?
3. What methods of data gathering are most often used by your discipline? Which methods are most often advocated?
4. What types of research design and empirical analysis are typically used? What are some of the limits that result from such methods?
5. What impact have the findings from your discipline had on policy or on the policy debate?

Thus, in each chapter the author(s) attempts to highlight four important dimensions: methods, discovery, explanation and evaluation.

SOCIOLOGY

Shortell suggests that in sociology there is not one, but a host of competing theories and paradigms which govern research. He delineates these competing theories and paradigms into three major perspectives: structural-functional, conflict, and symbolic interaction. Each of these approaches spawns the following paradigms: the social facts paradigm (emphasis on how social structure and institutions shape human behavior), the social definition paradigm (emphasis on human meaning), and the social behavior paradigm (emphasis on interaction between individual and environment).

Shortell sees the impact made by sociologists primarily through the social behaviorist paradigm which encompasses work related to the incentives and disincentives that shape human behavior. He sees sociology as having relevance and policy impact in implementation of policies to competing and conflicting interest groups. The values and expectations of these different interest groups and their social structure are obstacles which need to be reckoned with. He also sees the emphasis on open systems in sociology as an important contribu-

---

´Edited with permission from Choi T, Greenberg JN (eds): *Social Science Approaches to Health Services Research*. Ann Arbor, MI, Health Administration Press, 1982, pp. 14–18.

tion to understanding the interdependence of health care organizations. The nature of these interdependencies should lend itself to more enlightened health policy. Methodologically, Shortell sees sociology as contributing to the development of important independent variables such as culture, social norm, social sanction, and organizational structure.

POLITICAL SCIENCE

Political science is similar to sociology in that there is no one overall theory or paradigm, though there are some principles and assumptions which underlie the large domain of political science. Marmor maintains that political science is the study of how men are governed. The focus is on social choices concerning the distribution of benefits and burdens within society. The benefits and burdens of interest are not just material but symbolic and psychological as well, involving power and status.

Marmor and Dunham shy away from identifying a distinct area called the politics of health in large measure because the health industry faces the same governmental arrangements as do most other industries. From a political science perspective, the health industry faces the same mixing and balancing between public and private responsibility, the same "marbled cake" of local, state and federal authorities, the same voting alignments and party systems, the same federal legislature representing local interests and divided into contained committees, the same political culture, social structure and so on.

While Marmor and Dunham acknowledge that there is no single politics of health (but politics throughout the health industry instead), they are quick to point out that the nature of these politics differ markedly depending on the political system: redistributive, regulatory or distributive. It is clear from their chapter that there is no shared theory in political science. Political scientists are joined rather by a common object of inquiry: the differences among us and how we resolve them.

Marmor and Dunham's basic view of political science contributions concerns how diverse elements combine to produce public policy, a sort of multipolitics perspective that runs counter to some current fashions in the discipline which place more stress on the social structure and less on the individual public actor. Yet their perspective is an important one. They see multiple forces contributing to health policy, and by so doing they refuse to mechanize their discipline. Marmor and Dunham show how to use political science to illuminate and change health policy. Nothing they say allows one to think that there is a separate political science of health.

JURISPRUDENCE

From the perspective of jurisprudence, Schramm sees health services delivery intertwined with legislative initiatives. He sees health services research as being concerned with developing change in the way the health care system operates, and health policy impacting health services, especially in the area of organizational change. Schramm argues that unless the process of legal decision making is understood, research on organizational change is incomplete. His analysis of the legal perspective uncovers no clear theoretical approaches. However, the law operates by way of precedents and as such, norms guide legal behavior. The understanding of these norms and their contrast to prevailing models in other perspectives provide insights into the underpinnings of legal action and its impact on health services.

Schramm sees two current models prevalent in health services research. The first he labels the rational-patient model, which describes the patient as the one making medical choices in a way which optimizes his/her enjoyment of life within the context of limited resources (e.g., consumer choice plans). The second model is the scientific-provider model which views health providers doing the utmost to intervene in patient problems, regardless of efficiency and efficacy (e.g., kidney dialysis, CT scanners). The two models are antithetical: patient choice vs. provider choice. Both models are goal-oriented. The incompatibility of the two models results in looking to the legislature for resolution.

In contrast, the legal perspective is process-oriented and perceives all medical transactions like all other contractual transactions. The lawyer (or at least the more recent breed of lawyers) is seen as the policy maker who knows precisely how to deal within the boundaries of the law.

EPIDEMIOLOGY

In contrast to the legal perspective, epidemiology deals directly with the outcome of health services—namely, the health status of the population. Ibrahim defines epidemiology as the study of the distribution and determination of disease, disability, death, or health in population groups. Traditionally, epidemiology has been concerned with the understanding and ultimate control of communicable diseases. Thus, the emphasis was on the germ theory of disease. As such, epidemiology would not directly relate to the topic at hand. However, Ibrahim argues that many of man's modern plagues such as heart disease, hypertension, cancer, obesity and mental illness are such that the germ theory is insufficient to explain the occurrence of these conditions. Thus, modern epidemiology looks to the social and behavioral sciences as well as to the biological sciences for its explanation.

He sees epidemiology as having an impact on health services research in several ways: methodologically, epidemiology contributes to a way of thinking by the use of a set of techniques and methods established to answer certain questions. Techniques used include cohort study, historical cohort, cross-sectional analysis, case-control study, before—after design, experimental designs, and multivariate analysis. Substantively, epidemiology is seen as a perspective which contributes to clarifying the causes of the population's health status.

The several uses of epidemiology in health services research are discussed throughout the chapter. Many of these are illustrated by examples of health manpower.

DEMOGRAPHY

Verbrugge defines demography as the study of the structure and dynamics of human populations. It is composed of three major approaches. Social demography deals with the way demographic variables such as fertility and mortality affect health services utilization; population dynamics or mathematical demography deals with the impact of population changes on health planning; and technical demography, which she sees as a set of useful tools for health services researchers and planners. She also discusses a new branch called health demography which investigates the relationship between demographic variables and health status.

Demography is a particular way of asking scientific questions and of analyzing data. It takes characteristics such as age, sex, and marital status and provides a framework of reference as a set of independent variables to predict health services utilization. Verbrugge points out that unlike the other social sciences, demography treats these variables as central, not merely "control variables." Thus, its major theoretical contribution is in seeking explanations to population differentials rather than just acknowledging them.

Verbrugge sees demography's major methodological contribution as the development and refinement of survey research techniques. She presents several examples of their use throughout the chapter.

ECONOMICS

Berry and Feldman view economics as primarily a science of scarcity. As such, three predominant themes emerge in health care economics: (1) What goods and services will be produced? (2) How will they be produced? (3) How will they be distributed? The theoretical framework of economics, as the authors see it, deals with the choice and economic activities of health care providers and consumers in the health market. The underlying assumption is that each actor in the market, whether provider or consumer, wants to maximize gains subject to certain constraints. The basic model of the economist is the intersection of supply and demand in the health services marketplace. Demand comes from individual consumers or household units that are assumed to be maximizing their utility or satisfaction subject to an income constraint, and the prices given in the several markets for the various goods and services among which they may choose. On the supply side, producers are assumed to be maximizing their profit subject to the constraints imposed by the technology available, market demand and prices they face in hiring or purchasing inputs or resources. The market is the basic mechanism for allocating scarce resources. The authors go on to discuss the nature of the market for health services, the problems associated with that market, and the economic and policy implications of market imperfections and "nonstandard" provider behavior.

They present several examples of the types of empirical studies that health economists have conducted. These range from estimation of production processes to estimation of the impact that a price change would have on the quantity of a service demanded. The authors also suggest that economics has contributed rather significantly to the methodological sophistication of the field.

Berry and Feldman conclude with an interesting discussion of several areas of inquiry that lend themselves well to collaborative research among disciplines. These areas include the role of physicians as consumers' agents, theories of hospital behavior, and the effect of group practice on physicians' incentives.

SCIENCE, THE HUMAN CONDITION AND PHARMACY [f]

John H. Kilwein

Science exerts such a pervasive influence on the health professions that it is rather difficult to pause and critically analyse that influence. The task is further complicated by the enormous prestige that the physical and biological sciences enjoy in academic circles and in society at large. Yet, precisely because of that pervasiveness and prestige it behooves us to reflect for a moment on the limitations of science when applied to certain aspects of the human condition, aspects of importance to the health professions. We live in an age where health professionals are encouraged to consider the total patient, not just the disease process. Furthermore, the clinician, as healer, usually approaches the patient with a perspective that is broader than that of the scientist. The clinician often follows a case for an extended period of time, responds to both objective and subjective factors, and may have to deal with the social milieu in which the patient is situated. While science answers many questions on the biological level, it sheds much less light on the psychological and social dimensions of a case.

Nevertheless, because of the great success science has had in providing us with an understanding of the physical world, some retain the notion that science can, or some day will, illuminate all realms of existence. This is not so. To begin with, many of the pressing issues facing society and health professionals today, such as permitting or not permitting abortion, or providing health care to all citizens as a 'right', are issues of ethics and social philosophy, not science. Take the question of health care as a right. Science cannot tell us whether this is a worthwhile goal or not. The answer to this question is to be found in the values espoused by a particular society. Science may, however, be able to tell us whether a social goal is realistic in light of current knowledge, technology and resources.

Even where science can be applied to the study of human experience it does not always illuminate those aspects that are most relevant. Victor Weisskopf, former chairman of the Department of Physics at the Massachusetts Institute of Technology, believes that just as the quantum state is destroyed when observed with some sharp instrument, so too the significance of certain human experiences, especially relating to art, ethics and human relations, may be lost when subject to scientific analysis.[1] Weisskopf states, 'that in human relations a piece of art or a well-written novel could be much more meaningful than any scientific study. In many respects *Madam Bovary* is a piece of sociology—in fact, better sociology than much of what is done by aping the techniques and language of the natural sciences.'

The language, then, that is used to describe and explain those areas of reality that interest us is very important if our professional and scholarly efforts are to bear fruit. Interestingly, it has become common in recent years for social and behavioral scientists to appropriate the language and paradigms of the natural sciences and mathematics, e.g. systems theory and set theory, and incorporate them liberally in their own disciplines. Articles that now appear in social and behavioral science journals are often impressively embellished with mathematical notations. However, Murray Eden, a computer scientist, warns that when the theories and methods of the hard sciences and mathematics are applied to domains for

---

[f] Edited with permission from Kilwein J: Science, the human condition and pharmacy. Pharm Internatl 1982;12:202-204.

which they were not developed they frequently fail to illuminate, despite the impression of depth and precision provided.[2]

In a somewhat similar vein I have often thought that psychotherapy would be more productive if various theories incorporated more natural language, the language in which patients express their plight, and less scientific sounding terminology, e.g. psychological entropy and drive derivatives. Hilda Bruch, a teacher and practitioner of psychoanalysis, has criticized the tendency of many in her field to employ professional clichés instead of ordinary words.[3] She expresses concern about those therapists who, in trying to force a case into a theoretical mold, see only psychological bits and pieces, failing to maintain an open mind and concern for the total patient.

John Birtchnell asks whether we are not damaging our chances of getting a better understanding of human behavior and interpersonal relationships by adhering too closely to the natural sciences model in behavioral research.[4] His doubts are based on epidemiological investigations done on the relationship of family factors, such as the number of siblings and birth order to the development of mental illness. He believes that the often contradictory findings in such studies are due to restrictions imposed by the epidemiological method itself. Much of the appeal of variables like sibship size and birth order is due to the fact that they are readily and accurately measured and easily lend themselves to statistical analysis. Yet, it is the significance of these events to the individual that really matters, that contributes to mental health or mental illness, and this significance is difficult enough to express in 'words', let alone numbers. Thus, by selecting only those factors that can be easily expressed in numerical terms we often derive results that are superficial and unclear. Birtchnell concludes that for many of the more subjective aspects of man, careful observation, case studies, participant observation and literature still tell us more than findings from more complex and statistically sophisticated research.

However, even where sophisticated research design and data analysis are clearly the appropriate approach to investigating some particular aspect of the human condition we must repeatedly remind ourselves of what the resultant data mean in human terms. Computer printouts and statistics look very much the same whether they describe corn production or infant deaths in a particular region. At this point a saying comes to mind to the effect that one death is a tragedy, 100,000 deaths are a statistic. To present relevant data and research results on health in emotionally neutral terms is fine, provided that in time this does not insidiously result in our becoming emotionally neutral towards that very humanity that we are to serve. It is here where I find art an excellent complement to data. Poverty, for example, takes on very different dimensions when approached through scientifically derived statistics or through a moving literary work such as Steinbeck's *The Grapes of Wrath*. Finally, since science often provides us with valuable knowledge of people in their generality, we must be careful not to relate to individuals and their problems only in terms of general categories.[5] We must be able and willing to individualize.

What has all this to do with pharmacy? To begin, there is increasing concern today about humanizing the health care system, about treating people not just disease. The concept of clinical pharmacy, with its greater patient orientation, has come of age. This in turn requires pharmacists with a better understanding of psychological and social forces and with better skills in human relations which are not acquired in traditional pharmaceutical science courses. Because of these developments about one-quarter of U.S.A. pharmacy schools now include courses dealing with the social and behavioral aspects of the profession. While this trend is to be welcomed, I do hope that these new courses do not stress the science of behavior to the neglect of humanistic considerations.

In sum, I am in no way advocating that science be removed from the study of human affairs. However, health professionals, with their extensive training in the natural and biological sciences, should be aware that as they move from the physical and biological to the psychological and social realms the explanatory power and usefulness of science weakens. Nevertheless, patients continue to come to health professionals not just with problems that can be dealt with by science, but also with problems related to love, despair and the purpose of life—problems at the very core of human existence. As health professionals we must be sensitive to these problems and respond to them. I say respond to them, not necessarily solve them, for many times all we can do is provide a simple, but compassionate understanding of the patient's plight, and often this will suffice. If the health care system is to be humanized, health professionals must broaden their perspective and develop more diverse ways of comprehending and relating to the world and its inhabitants. Above all, they must not allow the spectacular successes of science to blind them to its limitations and to alternative ways of understanding their patients, themselves, and society.

REFERENCES

1. Weisskopf VF. Am Sci 1977;65:405–411.
2. Eden M. The Sciences 1977;17:22–23.
3. Bruch H. Learning Psychotherapy, Harvard University Press, Cambridge, Massachusetts, 1974.
4. Birtchnell J. Soc Sci Med 1974;8:335–350.
5. Downie RS, Telfer E. Caring and Curing, Methuen, London, 1980.

2
Pharmacy and the Professions*a*

ROBERT G. MRTEK
CARMEN CATIZONE

The butcher, the baker, and the candlestick maker all have different jobs. So do artists, lawyers, plumbers, physicians, and pharmacists. Sociologists, in particular, have categorized the work that people do into various groupings. Some are called skilled labor, others semiskilled; some are labeled as crafts, arts, and technical trades, and others are known broadly as professions.

PROFESSIONS

Society accords privileges to working members in part from the relative difficulty with which ordinary citizens evaluate the products and services provided by the workers. Those workers who exhibit great skill and creativity in delivering a service or product ordinarily are highly compensated for their work. For the baker the proof of the pudding truly is in the eating. Other workers, although they may not receive high compensation for their products, may achieve relatively higher status in the social structure of occupations because their efforts cannot be so readily evaluated by the majority of people to whom they provide goods and services (1).

The differentiation is usually made when an occupation becomes defined as a profession and its members as professionals. Lewis and Maude reviewed the accepted definition of a profession in 1952 and decided it would be to the best advantage to list those characteristics that differentiated professions from other occupations:

1. Registration or state certification embodying standards of training and practice in some statutory form;
2. A fiduciary practitioner-client relationship;
3. An ethical code;
4. A ban on the advertising of services; and
5. Independence from external control.

Goode provided a list of basic or "generating traits" that he considered the core of the learned or traditional professions: (*a*) advanced training in a highly specialized body of knowledge; and (*b*) the use of that knowledge in the service of mankind (2).

---

*a*This chapter is dedicated to the memory of Juanita and Robert Fischelis.

A profession is defined by all of these characteristics, which can be simplified into two interrelated groupings.

Body of Knowledge	Use of the Knowledge to Serve Mankind
Formal organization	Enduring ideals
Autonomy	Altruistic attitude
Ethics	

The service or products provided by a profession are usually elevated in proportion to the degree of impact or danger they may have on the individual person or the collective group who make up the citizenry. This includes the amount of judgment and interpretation that the professional must exert for the client and the extent to which coworkers in the same or related occupations acknowledge the expertise of the profession, thereby making it more legitimate. Most important, the differentiation of professions from other occupations rests on the level of blind faith that members of society must ultimately place on the work performance of the professional (3, 4).

Work of Professionals

In their practices, professionals use a variety of observable techniques, tangible goods, and intangible skills, knowledge, and previous experience that often go unrecognized by members of the public. The end results take the form of products, services, advice, opinion, and even a physical presence on behalf of another person or group. They also may be represented in forms not readily recognized for their full value even among coworkers. Examples might include continuing education programming, adherence to strict standards of care, or fidelity to professional ethics. Professionals, therefore, may practice their professions in a variety of settings.

Mere observations of professionals at work can be misleading. An observer may see nothing more than a person sitting quietly, reading, thinking, or talking in what appears to be a casual manner with a client or professional colleague. Frequently there is nothing at all present in the observable behavior of the professionals to hint at the inherent difficulty of the work or the dangers implicit in the judgments they routinely make. Observation may even suggest that the tasks are mundane, better suited to the skills of a lower status worker.

Observations notwithstanding, the activities a professional engages in to satisfy a societal need are always more complex than the mechanical functions being observed. There are decisions involved that may be aimed at helping one specific client about whom much may be known. On the other hand, efforts may be directed toward other professionals who need the services, goods, or interpreted knowledge and advice in order to advance the case or the problem to the next step toward a solution. It is not unusual for the professional to practice in relative isolation from the routines of daily life and provide services in abstract ways to society itself.

What emerges is a changing, complicated, and sometimes confusing picture of occupations deemed special by society and called the professions. These are occupations carefully defined by the professionals themselves who are given the unusual authority to determine who may be permitted to practice and under what conditions. Professionals define the kinds of activities allowed, what privileges members may claim, and what kinds of controls guarantee that the social privileges are not abused. Whatever else a profession is, it represents a kind of work that men and women do for a living. In the presence of expanding scientific and technical knowledge needed to serve professions, much of modern professionalism has been interpreted as a logical extension of the quest to make life more rational (5, 6).

Societal Need for Professions

It is possible to trace most of the old professions such as law, medicine, pharmacy, and theology back to the dawn of civilization. Their formal designation as professions distinguished from other occupational groups is a result of the emergence of complex urban societies that grew up in Europe and North America toward the end of the last century. Since that time the professions have developed as integral parts of society and increased dramatically in numbers after 1900. This is simply because life in general, but especially life in congested urban environments, is just too complex for the majority of the populace to live with success and grace completely without the benefit of expert consultation and services.

Conversely there has been a steady decline in the number of farm workers, a rise and then a decline in the number of blue collar (semiskilled) workers, and a consequential rise in the categories known as managers and technical workers. Among the work groups of society, only the crafts (skilled blue-collar workers) have remained constant as a proportion of the labor force in this century (7). This constancy reflects the needs of society in the postindustrial era, a time in which greater value is placed on the production and utilization of knowledge and services than on the manufacture of goods (8).

Sociologists have attributed the power professionals exercise among themselves and in relation to other occupational groups to the services provided and the environments in which they practice. Studies have been conducted to learn the ways that professionals affect their status by using and transforming a formal knowledge base that is at the heart of each profession (9).

Formal Knowledge and Expertise

In the post-Civil War period, the modern group of credentialed professions began an uninterrupted ascent in society. Quite continuously from the time since their emergence as organized occupational endeavors, they have been the subject of intense scrutiny and study by researchers on both sides of the Atlantic ocean. Trends in fashion regarding the definition of what the professions are and how they serve society have moved from purely descriptive studies through functional accounts beyond a period of intense social criticism, including the outcry of abolitionists and critical evaluation of the impacts that their privileged class has had on modern society (10).

What may be drawn as a consensus from all of the research efforts is that each profession does indeed have some unique formal knowledge base. This is expanded mostly by the efforts of research and through the creative contributions and abstract reasoning by academics. It is sometimes referred to as the elite foundation of the profession and is not usually found as part of the everyday commonsense knowledge held by the citizenry. Formal knowledge is an important "first distinction" between the profession and the laity.

The services provided by professionals emanate from the application of formal knowledge, sometimes in highly modified form, to complex tasks and problems of immediate importance to clients. Those who are not members of the profession nevertheless try to use and benefit from the services of the profession, even though they will not understand or be able to use directly the formal knowledge base of the profession. They may not even be aware of the existence of the specialized knowledge. However, expertise in a profession is connoted beyond knowledge to include skills, judgments, and experiences necessary to practice the profession at competent levels determined by academics, regulators, and the public. For this reason expertise is sometimes equated with the power to control and master the formal knowledge base of the profession.

This knowledge is gained by practitioners from the professional curriculum that is the foundation of its expertise. The curriculum is a dynamic fabric of educational units designed to permit the maximal absorption of the extant knowledge. It usually is mastered only through a protracted period of intense full-time college-level study, defined by the profession and lasting 4 or more years.

Formal education and professional socialization both are accomplished by a variety of learning methods including the provision of clerkship mentoring experiences for students, independent study opportunities, and limited examples of case studies in which the student is given an opportunity to "learn by doing" (11). It is for this reason that the processes of professional socialization are undertaken concurrently with the more formal period of didactic study. Professional socialization is always more subtle than the various pedagogical methods of encouraging mastery learning within the curriculum, but nonetheless, students do learn about the unwritten codes and rules of behavior that exert a more gentle yet undeniable force on the arduous process of joining a profession (12, 13). The problem for educators is that sometimes the student learns attitudes and values with which the academician does not necessarily agree. Then arises the question of whether the classroom professor is an appropriate role model for the aspiring practitioner (14).

Within highly differentiated professions, especially in health care, there may be further postgraduate didactic experiences and residencies as well as additional credentials to be secured in order to receive the opportunity to practice within a recognized specialty. "Expertise in a complex society is inseparable from some forms of credentialism, for there is too much to know to be able to know it directly; one has no alternative but to rely on indicators like credentials" (15). These added credentials may be essential to secure local privileges wholly controlled within the employing institutions according to standards set by semiofficial bodies that accredit the institutions themselves (16, 17).

Credentials as Societal Protection

Attaining a university degree, which essentially attests to satisfactory completion of all curricular requirements, is the beginning of the entrance into a profession. It is followed in nearly all professions by some form of public credential awarded in a separate process outside the control of the academic institution. Most often the credential is a license given in recognition of satisfactory performance on a strictly controlled, standardized examination. Usually some department of state government "registers" or lists those persons holding credentials that qualify them to enter the practice of the profession.

Credentials are awarded after proof of the completion of all requirements in order to protect society from incompetence and individuals practicing below the minimum of required standards set by contemporary norms (18). The system of professional licensure is viewed by some social critics as a kind of monopoly that has the effect of becoming an exclusionary, restrictive, and elitist instrument that ultimately protects the profession more than the society that grants the licenses. It has also been argued that the license itself serves as a positive influence upon its holder to remain committed to the profession.[b] The argument is understandable because credentials are intended to offer a degree of economic shelter to credentialed professionals by assuring them employment potential in professional practice. For pharmacy, the licensing of professionals occurs after successful completion of a standardized written practice examination (NABPLEX), which *sets* minimal criteria as defined by law and implemented by the authority of an examining and regulating Board of Pharmacy in each state.[c] Despite the stringent and arduous mechanisms established by state boards, it is not clear whether the promulgation of rules and regulations affects the actual quality of services provided by professionals (19).

It should be obvious that entry into professions is by no means an easy or certain process. The steps, hurdles, and layers of challenge seem to the neophyte to be more forbidding than the 12 great labors of Hercules. Yet for all of the tradition and apparent opportunities for failure, there is a high success rate among the aspirants who possess the initial university degree and seek to become fully credentialed. Society, after all, must be assured of adequate numbers of qualified professionals to carry out the work that others with less training cannot undertake with safety.

Having once been admitted to the full rights and privileges of a profession, the holder of the license and other credentials must periodically renew them, demonstrating anew that competence has been maintained. The measures for assuring continuing competence among practitioners are less well developed than is the original process of admission to the profession. Usually all that is needed is some form of affidavit that approved programs of self-study or continuing education have been undertaken (20).

Professional Discretion, Authority, and Autonomy

It is generally acknowledged among investigators who study the practice by professionals that society must necessarily relax supervisory controls over day-to-day work performed by professionals. In the professions, the knowledge and skills needed in daily practice are so esoteric and the tasks are so complex, requiring such high levels of judgment experience and individual interpretation as to warrant no external interference.

Society grants to each profession varying amounts of discretionary powers and self-supervision based on the goods and services provided by the profession. The more central to the values of society these goods and services are, the more discretionary power the profession is able to carve out. Discretionary power is a privilege that once given, is very difficult for society to revoke. Furthermore, society has difficulty in controlling or limiting discretionary power even when it is determined that the power has grown beyond the bounds of the best interests of citizens.

Those researchers who have written critically about professions, especially in the 1960s, have frequently cited the unsanctioned expansion of discretionary powers of the professions as examples of what they term flagrant disregard of the social contract. Some haved claimed that social privileges have been distorted and abused beyond even the most liberal interpretations of internal control and self-discipline (21). The discretion thus accorded to profes-

---

[b]For a more thorough discussion on various aspects of the social impacts of credentialing, see Ref. 7, pp 16–24.

[c]It is important to recognize that individuals are usually hired into occupational practice of the professions based almost exclusively on the possession of the credential itself. It is not possible to find work as a pharmacist without producing evidence that a valid pharmacy license is held at the time of hire and continuously thereafter throughout employment.

sions represents evidence of a social contract made on behalf of the public in order to receive professional services of adequate quality and quantity in return for fair compensation and the privileges of internal control. Professional discretion, like wealth, may be increased by careful and clever manipulation within and among the professions themselves.

To be sure, the health professions have received their share of criticism on this matter. Medicine, in particular, is the most frequently mentioned example of a profession that has husbanded its discretionary powers into a kind of professional authority, and then expanded them even further into what has been described as professional autonomy—a condition in which society itself is prone to falling victim to an all but unlimited exercise of power (22). Not far behind medicine is the legal profession, which has been accused of being above the law in too many documented examples.[d]

There can be little doubt that while society is willing to defer to judgments within the legitimate expertise of professionals, it is quite reluctant to permit any profession to raise its own discretionary powers up to the level of professional autonomy. Such autonomy would provide professionals with a mechanism to define, control, and monopolize the services of other interdependent professions. The question then becomes at what point does society intervene? A profession must have sufficient philosophic direction to define the nature of its services to society. However, if it also seeks to control the need of society for those services and attempts to limit the general availability and conditions under which services and goods are provided, it destroys the purpose of professions as service-oriented helping occupations that hold limited privileges and powers for the good of society. When society determines that intolerable excesses have occurred, there ensues pressure of the severest kind, with the issues themselves sometimes requiring tests based on constitutional law.

A Differentiated Working Class

The social status of job holders in the professions has always been of interest to historians and sociologists. If the employed labor force is considered as a hierarchy without any distinctions being drawn as to the specific nature of the work being done, an upper tier may be differentiated within the primary labor market of fully employed persons.[e]

Practitioners of professions are full-time lifelong specialists whose jobs fit all of the characteristics of the upper tier of the primary labor market. Some acknowledgement must be given to the fact that the tier also contains workers not considered professionals: man-

---

[d]CBS: "Sixty Minutes," Weekly Electronic News Magazine. December 27, 1987. (Also see Galanter, M, Chapt. 7, "Mega-Law and Mega-Lawyering in the Contemporary United States," in Ref. 1, and Halliday TC: "Beyond Monopoly: Lawyers, State Crises, and Professional Empowerment." Chicago IL, University of Chicago Press, 1987 for discussion of the law profession.)

[e]The professions are found within that group, but they alone do not constitute the upper labor market tier. Employees in this large group share some common job-related characteristics. They have steady employment, certain job rights, some job protection offered by their credentials, and life tenure or "bumping" rights according to seniority. Their occupations are characterized by lifetimes of relatively secure and stable work in identifiable careers. In addition, individual workers enjoy high job mobility even during periods of moderate economic difficulty. They work with relatively little supervision, some have substantial discretion in the conduct of their jobs, and they frequently work autonomously without direct requirements for intraday reporting to superiors. Where there is any supervision, it may be in the form of a "team leader" who is a colleague peer, in many cases selected by those to be supervised and who agrees to accept the administrative privilege usually for a fixed period of time from a few weeks to several years, depending on the nature of the projects or the organization of the department.

agers, technicians, and those who work in the crafts (23). Although they share important similarities with professionals, the differences are significant.*

Regardless of the differences, usually in employment privileges or educational requirements, society acknowledges the expertise of virtually all workers in the top tier of the primary labor market. The jobs are routinely ranked among the most desirous and prestigious. The group has been separated further into strata, one of which includes the general-technical group, which is itself internally differentiated into a hierarchy with the top being the creative scientists, academics and intellectuals, practicing professionals, semiprofessionals, and technicians at the bottom. The most influential factor that increases the prestige of jobs is the ability of the occupation to control its work and regulate itself (24).

It is apparent that the prestigious professions are populated by full-time specialist workers who are committed to their work as a means for making a living. They discharge their responsibilities with great skill. They are not "amateurish" in their approach to the work, nor are they part-time dabblers in the pursuit of their practice. Professionals accept the responsibility of difficult and dangerous work that is not easily evaluated, and in return they expect the compensation and privileges that society accords to those whose services are considered indispensable.

PROFESSIONAL STATUS OF PHARMACY

Changing Social Roles in Pharmacy

Pharmacy is among the oldest of the health professions. Together with medicine it provides services of fundamental value to society. These professions have been found whenever humans have lived together in socialized groups.

During the late 19th century, American pharmacy began to undergo a remarkable set of changes. It permanently moved away from the ancient path that had characterized it since the earliest times. That path centered around the pharmacist's knowledge of and skills needed to compound a drug product. It required an expertise that could as well be learned through practical experience as by formal university study. With the broad scale develop-

---

*The *crafts* rely on highly skilled workers who have acquired their skills through practical, on-the-job training or through secondary or vocational trade schools. Craft workers have little or no contact with higher education. Persons in these occupations are usually credentialed and have lifetime careers in their work. Often they are as mobile in the workforce as are the professionals. The crafts are frequently entered via a long period of apprenticeship after which journeyman or master status is achieved. The crafts are sometimes associated with artistic content, in which case there may be another long period of time to achieve independence, artistic maturity, and individual style. Before reaching artistic autonomy, the person engaged in a craft may live with the shadow of a self-imposed requirement to demonstrate mastery of the best of all styles that have come before.

Technicians are practitioners without the responsibility for policy determination. They have limited 2-year training or 4-year college education, which tends to emphasize technical or concrete subjects at the expense of a general liberal education that is augmented by intense study of the foundations through abstract generalizations and theory. Sometimes technicians work in conjunction with professionals, but they do not have the discretion to interpret their work results in the larger context. Also, they do not have professional authority although some groups of technician occupations are credentialed.

Managers perform work in which specialized education and credentialing are not necessary. Many managers have completed a general college education. Some have also acquired the Masters of Business Administration degree, which is helpful in expanding an understanding of the techniques of management, but the degree is not required to be hired. Managers frequently obtain their positions by being promoted along a vertical career ladder extending up from lower level white-collar work. For years managers have claimed professional status on their own but without much recognition from society.

ment of pharmaceutical manufacturing in the United States, the primary function of the pharmacist—the ability to compound—no longer was necessary, or even desirable. The development of the American pharmaceutical industry retired the need for every American pharmacist to also be a part-time drug manufacturer (25). The mechanized processes of industry leading to standardized dosage forms of uniform quality and wide availability made obsolete the back room compounding laboratories of most corner drugstores. Furthermore, the emergence of new drugs in the 20th century from laboratories designed specifically for pharmaceutical research placed the complexity of drug preparation far beyond the reach of the average pharmacist in a small drugstore.

High speed manufacture of dosage forms brought with it the need to understand the synthesis of new chemical drug compounds through intensive study of the complex sciences of chemistry and biology. The proud and timeless role of the pharmacist's art, represented by skill in compounding the drugs into pills, syrups, elixirs, and other elegant dosage forms, all crafted by hand, slipped away. With each new pharmaceutical catalog introduced by manufacturers, more and more products in potent standardized forms replaced the old galenicals that were the pride of previous generations of pharmacists.

Even the old roles of procuring and storing crude drugs were now taken over, virtually 100%, by the large manufacturers. They relied on world markets rather than local wholesale druggists for the raw materials needed to make 20th century medicinals. No longer was the quality and purity of crude drug starting materials based on the personal knowledge and reputation of the supplier but rather on the sophisticated laboratory testing prescribed in the rubrics of the official compendia.

The pharmacist was forced to change historical practices and develop a more technologically advanced role in quality assurance. Because drugs are inherently dangerous substances and the pharmacist's knowledge about their proper preparation, storage, and handling is greater than any other professional group, the quality assurance aspects of drug use are assigned to pharmacy. The function, as defined by society and the profession, is to ensure that the drugs provided to patients are safely and accurately dispensed, thereby upholding the public trust that pharmacy has earned over many generations.

The close relationship between pharmacists and physicians that had existed for so many generations was eroded. Pharmaceutical manufacturers printed glossy catalogs promenading their products and employed, often from within the ranks of the profession, sales representatives whose primary role was to promote the products of their company to physicians. Their personal attention and distribution of free professional samples did much to diminish the role of the pharmacist as expert and counsel to physicians. It also reduced the deference physicians gave to their sister professional whose "office" was the friendly corner drugstore.

In the span of about 50 years, the profession lost no less than three of the four functions that had been the mainstay of the work of pharmacists since at least the 8th century! The old mysteries of the art of the apothecary, drug procurement, storage, and compounding, had vanished. The loss of such deeply rooted functions endangered the identity of the entire profession. By the mid-20th century, the work of the pharmacist was defined by the dispensing task. The only mystery remaining was in the myriad of endless trade names that bewildered physician and pharmacist alike. The language of the profession had changed along with everything else that was familiar. The shock to pharmacy could not have been sharper (26, 27).

Dispensing: a Dubious Remainder

By midcentury one fact was apparent, although it was often too painful to be acknowledged by pharmacy practitioners themselves. The changes in practice had left a limited role for community pharmacists, the simple dispensing of drugs on order of the prescriber, with its associated monetary transactions. Everything else had been swept aside by "progress."

Hospital pharmacy, too, was primarily an extension of the drug distribution system then in use in the community pharmacy. Especially in small community hospitals, those who tended to the drug needs of hospitalized patients did so on a part-time basis. Some used their community pharmacies as wholesaling points for the needs of the hospital that they serviced as a vendor under contract. However, there remained considerably more compounding and manufacturing of custom drug products in hospitals than in the community pharmacy. The situation changed abruptly when large manufacturers entered the hospital drug supply market with unit dose packaging and disposable large volume fluids for the administration of drugs by the parenteral route.

Observers noted changes in the work of pharmacists and labeled them as signs that pharmacy had irretrievably lost status as a profession (28–30). It was not difficult to see that the majority of the time formerly spent in compounding medicines was now given over to tasks related to the management of the expanded front-end merchandising of goods that were either not related to health care or only peripherally so (31, 32). As far as some were concerned, the professional functions of the pharmacist had shrunk to only those tasks associated with selling a product.

Dilemma of the Business of Community Practice

The dispensing of drugs with its related transactions by small business operators who purchased at wholesale and sold repackaged quantities at retail called up again the painful question of whether pharmacy was anymore being practiced as a profession (33, 34).

Pharmacists knew that their professional practices had always been closely associated with the front-end merchandising of unrelated goods, at least throughout the history of pharmacy in the United States. The sale of general merchandise in drugstores was necessary in order to build an adequate cash volume to permit pharmacists to continue to operate their pharmacies (35). Having other items available in the pharmacy besides drugs also helped to establish the corner drugstore as a place in the community where people could obtain needed health goods, sundries, and convenience items both in times of health and during illness. The presence of expanded departments outside the prescription counter therefore was not seen as a particularly deprofessionalizing dilemma for pharmacists when compounding was still an important daily activity. Pharmacist-owners and their clients who appreciated the one-stop shopping convenience that became important to the American way of life after the Second World War welcomed the added lines of merchandise.

Pharmacists who clung to the old mystery of the art of compounding assured themselves that the dispensing process involved much more than could be observed. It included checking for prescribing errors, counseling of patients and family members regarding proper use of drugs, and establishing longstanding relationships with families (35). These trusted family relationships made the pharmacist the most accessible and most frequently consulted health professional (36). Continuous contact with whole families gave the community pharmacist a better picture of the health status and drugs used by each member than could ever be pieced together from the various records kept by individual prescribers including dentists, obstetricians, dermatologists, and psychiatrists. The importance of this record to the family could be easily appreciated simply by asking any pharmacist about the numbers of families who requested copies of their pharmaceutical histories as they prepared to move to a different town or state.

Nevertheless, the erosion of confidence caused by the loss of such a large portion of the traditional functions of pharmacy took its toll on the self-esteem of the profession itself and, in particular, appeared with unrelenting frequency in the pages of the journals aimed at practitioners (37). This fact alone coupled with the fueling of differences in opinions among national organizations representing segments of the profession magnified the disharmony. Contrasting philosophies arose out of the camps of practitioners in retail and hospital pharmacies, staff and owner pharmacists, chain and independent pharmacists, and academicians versus practitioners.

The appearance of drugstore chains (25) threatened the continued existence of the small independent pharmacy by undercutting the prices that supported the remaining dispensing function. Some pharmacies went out of business at alarming rates, and not because the chains were taking away all of the prescription volume. The annual count of prescriptions being filled continued to rise sharply, and chain drugstores dispensed less than half of all prescriptions written by prescribers (38).[g] What squeezed independently owned pharmacies out of existence was their own inability to compete successfully with the enormous buying power and skill in advertising that were the hallmarks of the chains. In many cases, the independent pharmacy put itself out of business by trying to beat the chains at their own unbeatable merchandising tactics (25).

Diminished Image: Losses and Gains

Events played out in the professional press from about the 1950s to the 1970s reveal an angst that can now be seen as important evidence that pharmacy was in an upheaval and was about to undergo a philosophic redefinition of its practice mission. It did not particularly matter that those whom the traditional corner drugstore served never lost faith nor doubted the value of the pharmacist's services amid the jumble of unrelated merchandise. Those who chose to patronize the large chain pharmacies openly acknowledged that they did so most often for convenience of the location of the chain store or for price reasons alone. Certainly the large chain drugstore presented an even more heterogeneous mix of non-drug-related merchandise than was usually found in the small independent pharmacy (25).

The perceived difference in image became important in the spilling-over of feelings that pharmacy had lost something essential. This was felt by the public and other professionals who viewed the pharmacist's work as simply "count and pour, lick and stick" and by some pharmacists who confined themselves behind enormous glass partitions in the prescription department, unable to practice their profession as they had learned it. It is not clear whether the shift in perception arose spontaneously or whether the perception of a vanquished profession was fostered from forces outside (39).

---

[g]In 1966 independent pharmacies accounted for 73.4% of the prescription market share. By then, chains had captured 20.3% [see NARD J 93:41-44. Dec, 1971]. However, in terms of total drug store retail volume, chains operated 26% of all stores and accounted for 51% share of sails in 1967. Figures available for 1977 show that chains had captured 70% of all volume while operating nearly 42% of all stores. [see "Annual Report of the Chain Drug Industry," Chain Store Age, April 1978, pp 79-199.]

The effect was threatening because it impacted on deference itself: the willingness of others, especially other professionals, to accept without question the intrinsic value of the knowledge and services provided by pharmacy. A profession may withstand the annealing effect of internal differences in philosophy and emerge more strongly unified and in sharper focus for having witnessed its own disharmony. But little else can plague a profession so thoroughly as a loss of its external credibility as advisor among the interdependent spheres of professions that make up the American system of health care. To diminish the deference which others accord a profession is to decimate it.

The diminishment of the image of pharmacy certainly worked to the advantage of drug manufacturers. With shrewd business sense, the drug manufacturers recognized that the point of sale for their products was the individual who wrote or telephoned a prescription order that could not be altered by the pharmacist. Therefore, it was in the best business interest of the manufacturers to intensify and continue the process of drug detailing at the point of sale. Pharmacists were thereby effectively excluded from influencing the selection of rational drug therapy by prescribers and not recognized for the contributions pharmacy could make regarding the evaluation and interpretation of drug-related information. Their arguments of scientific impartiality in evaluating the advantages and cost benefits among generically equivalent products prepared by a number of different manufacturers went, at least for a time, unheeded and vehemently opposed by the manufacturers.

In the 1960s, state after state passed antisubstitution laws to "protect the patient" from the dangers of what was described (but undocumented) as widespread drug counterfeiting operations. The reported intent of antisubstitution was to keep the public safe from forged look-alikes that could unintentionally end up in their medicine cabinets. The public would remain safe only so long as physicians wrote prescriptions for brand name drug products manufactured only by reputable companies that were committed to research and improving the public health. However, the plan would not work unless pharmacists were required to dispense the products as written on the prescription itself (40).

The profession viewed the attitude of the manufacturers as an attack on the professional stature of pharmacy. Pharmacy entrenched itself for a battle with the manufacturers of multisource prescription drug products. Pharmaceutical scientists and academicians rallied behind the new sciences of physical pharmacy, biopharmacy, pharmacokinetics, and others developed since World War II. The new sciences were coupled with the useful techniques of drug information analysis, biometrics, and a broad understanding of drug therapies, providing the profession with new ammunition for a battle that might very well determine the role of pharmacy for years to come. The profession argued for the repeal of the antisubstitution laws, maintaining that the performance of drugs in patients was far less dependent on the physician's clinical impressions than claimed. Indeed, drug performance was a predictable and quantifiable outcome that yielded to the rationality of science in the same way that most other parts of the drug use process had become scientifically understood during earlier decades of this century.

The arguments for repeal of antisubstitution laws stressed that the new skills of the pharmaceutical sciences would reveal clinically important differences among products where these existed. Insofar as no differences might be found among the clinical responses of generically equivalent products from a variety of manufacturers, this would be grounds for declaring the products to be therapeutically equivalent. Among equivalent drugs, other deciding factors, such as cost, could be used in impartial ways to select products for use by patients (41).

Clinical Paradigm for Pharmacy Practice

Finally, the newly developed pharmaceutical sciences proved beneficial in securing the pharmacist's right to select the drug product. At about the same time other scientific advancements related to the access and processing of patient-related drug information made possible important demonstrations of the value of nontraditional pharmacy services in clinical settings. By the 1970s there was no question that the profession had opened for itself a new clinical role in the area of consultation (42–49).

Pharmacists practiced in at least two new ways not defined in the majority of pharmacy practice acts. Initially they began providing useful information and services relating to the implementation of drug therapy decisions that had already been made. This part of clinical pharmacy practice at first appeared no different from the old patient advisory roles pharmacists had exercised in community pharmacies for years, including explaining the proper use of medications and warning against potential side effects or hazards. Although the pharmacist's "duty to warn" is not yet widely recognized legally, and there are recent court cases implying that the pharmacist has no obligation to provide any information or service other than that associated with accurate preparation and delivery of the prescribed drug to the patient,[h] standards of pharmacy practice and professional ethics suggest that the pharmacist fulfill a professional obligation to inform and warn about drug use when it is in the best interest of the patient.

Two features of the new clinical orientation made it something quite new. These are (a) the location of the practice setting and (b) legitimate free access to information never before made available to pharmacists. First, the clinical setting, for the most part, has been the hospital. The patients are nonambulatory, and the recipients of the nondispensing services of pharmacists are, most often, physicians and nurses.

The second feature that marks the clinical role as something new is the contribution pharmacists make in terms of assisting physicians and nurses *prospectively* with drug use aspects of therapeutic decisions not yet made. By the 1970s when the existence of the clinical practice role was already widely acknowledged, for the first time in modern American pharmacy practice, the pharmacist was close enough to the setting and the time when therapeutic decisions were made to influence the quality of the decisions in terms of rational drug therapy. The clinician pharmacist became truly a contributing partner in the decision process—a colleague whose participation is viewed as essential, by right of independent expertise, for planning rational and optimal drug usage for each patient.

Without this opportunity to participate when the decisions on therapy are being made, the pharmacist is forced into the difficult and less effective role of a person who must only react to decisions made by others (50). The pharmacist may react to lots of things, however, it is a professional constriction to be forced to do nothing more than react to decisions already made by others versus having an opportunity to influence the decision as it is being made. The reaction, which in most cases is initiated by some error in therapy or disagreement in judgment, is viewed negatively, and the pharmacist is regarded as one "who objects to what has already been decided." The respect as an independent expert is lost, as other professionals defend their prior decisions by questioning or minimizing the expertise of the pharmacist.

There are a number of reasons why the pharmacist's clinical role took root primarily in hospital settings and not in the community. It began in earnest during the mid-1960s and

---

[h]See *Rx Ipsa Loquitur* (a newsletter publication of the American Society for Pharmacy Law) Vol. 14 (4), April, 1987.

was first noted by the presence of pharmacists on patient care units in proximity with physicians and nurses. This created a natural opportunity for pharmacists to contribute their drug use knowledge and have it valued in drug-related clinical considerations (51). It was unimportant that the pharmacist's entrée to the patient care unit originally was for the purpose of reducing medication errors by the use of unit dose drug distribution (52–54). Once the pharmacist was on the patient care unit with the other professionals responsible for therapeutic decisions, recognition of the pharmacist's expertise in contributing quality drug information and opinion to decisions regarding drug therapy naturally emerged.

Second, the pharmacist obtained access to all of the information used by other health professionals in the clinical decision process. The importance of this new information cannot be overstated. At last the pharmacist could contribute intelligently to decisions as they were being made, in large part, because the latest information about the patient's health status was available to the pharmacist for the first time.

This single feature is so important that it may very well be the limiting constraint that will account for the success or failure of transferring the clinical role function to the community pharmacy setting. Wherever clinical pharmacy has failed to take hold, close examination of the conditions may well reveal that the pharmacist was limited by incomplete access to information essential to the clinical perspective.

What has emerged from the exercise of clinical judgment by the pharmacist is a new patient-oriented practice paradigm for pharmacy. Throughout this century, pharmacy practice has experienced a gradual shift away from the technical paradigm, emphasizing drug products and their preparation, toward a more disease- and patient-oriented approach to pharmaceutical decisions. In community practice settings, however, the paradigm shift in favor of more active involvement directly with patient care experienced severe difficulty in gaining acceptance by other health professionals.

When questioned prospectively, nurses and physicians are reluctant to permit pharmacists to interact with the patient in ways that are perceived as being threatening to the status quo (55, 56). However, the true measure of the value of clinical services rests not so much with the evaluation of pharmacists by physicians or nurses, but with outcome evaluations of the profession as a whole from programs of quality assurance: the value, accuracy, usefulness, impact, cost, and appropriateness of services performed by the pharmacist and pharmacy. Furthermore, clinical service outcomes relate directly to the quality and impact of the pharmacy clinician in terms of the *patient*. For this reason, the assessment of clinical services requires measurement of *outcomes*, as opposed to evaluations made on the process or structural organizations responsible for the delivery of services (57).

It is interesting to note that, once implemented, clinical pharmacy services are more readily accepted by nurses and physicians for their intrinsic value in improving the therapeutic decision. There is also the consideration that the pharmacist's presence reduces, or at least shares more widely, the risk of litigation to nurses and physicians from injuries due to improper drug usage. The hospital setting also allows the pharmacist an opportunity to engage in clinical consultation without posing a threat to the earning ability of other health professionals. Costs related to the provision of clinical pharmacy services are absorbed by per diem and drug dispensing charges.

Information and Peer Interactions: Prerequisites for Clinical Practice

Clinical service depends on direct access to the knowledge base relevant to the current health status of specific patients. Pharmacists in the community have very little current or relevant data about patients other than the information they themselves generate by questioning patients directly, or information learned secondhand by asking physicians or nurses about specific cases. Few, if any, community pharmacists make it a routine part of their in-store record augmentation to get current clinical impressions from physicians and nurses or note significant laboratory results each time the patient obtains a prescription.

Patients, too, have little useful or reliable information to volunteer to pharmacists simply because of the technical nature of the questions and their own lack of understanding of what the information is or why it is needed by the pharmacist. In general, close questioning of the patient by the pharmacist creates anxiety and alarm among patients who may feel that information of such apparent importance to the pharmacist should best be obtained directly from their physician. It also causes anxiety for the physician who may feel second-guessed or doubted.

Isolated as they are from an accurate and complete patient health status record, there is little that most community pharmacists can do to render clinical judgments that are central to drug therapy decisions. They do not benefit from the wealth of data and resources accessible to pharmacists practicing in inpatient institutional settings. Because they are not present when therapeutic decisions are made, comments offered after the fact are more likely to be rejected out of hand.

Four Practice-Setting Examples

If one considers only four of the many different settings available to pharmacists for practice, it may be seen that although the *process* of decision making and arriving at professional judgments is essentially the same, the *knowledge base* in each setting and its central relevance to the therapeutic decision varies enormously. Licensed pharmacists (with only the professional practice entry degree) are routinely found in such diverse environments as the pharmaceutical manufacturing laboratory, community drug stores, long-term care facilities, and inpatient hospitals.

1. In the manufacturing laboratory, the principal concern of the pharmacist is in producing products that meet or exceed current good manufacturing standards as well as conform to all quality control standards established for each specific product. This practice setting adheres exclusively to the technical paradigm, demanding accuracy and fidelity to the scientific and technical steps required to produce safe and effective drug products. In a practical sense a consideration of the patient does not enter into the routine work of the pharmacists except, of course, for the overriding philosophical commitment to manufacture products that are safe and effective in their use by patients.

2. The community pharmacy is the place where pharmacists are most visible to the general public. The routine work there involves the greatest care possible in fulfilling all of the safety and accuracy requirements in the drug dispensing process. The guiding paradigm is still largely technical, in that much of the pharmacist's attention must focus on the risks and outright dangers to patients resulting from dispensing errors, therapeutic incompatibilities, and incorrect use of medications by patients.

    It is true that pharmacists and patients (or members of their families) meet face to face more frequently in the community pharmacy than elsewhere. Therefore, one may be tempted to argue that these patient-pharmacist interactions are evidence that the clinical paradigm operates in the corner drugstore. This is infrequently the case.

Nearly all discussions with patients center around proper use of drug products or their prices. The therapeutic and clinical judgment involved in the determination of a need for the particular drug product was in the overwhelming majority of times made elsewhere, usually in a physician's office and without participation by the pharmacist (58). It is also true that the pharmacist may have the final choice in selecting which multisource drug product will be used by the patient. But even this function is an extension of the technical paradigm and limited by drug product selection laws to drugs that experts outside the pharmacy have considered to be therapeutic equivalents. The patient and the pharmacist simply are not professional peers: the patient neither understands nor possesses the formal knowledge or the specific clinical data regarding the circumstances of the decisions—even though these may relate to his own personal well-being.

In community pharmacies, there is some assistance provided to patients by the pharmacist in recommending nonprescription (OTC) products or in helping the patient to decide whether to seek the consultation of other health professionals. This function embodies the closest approximation that the community pharmacist enjoys to exercising any clinical judgment. Unfortunately, when scrutinized carefully, the recommendation of nonprescription drugs for self-diagnosed problems falls short of the rigid standards for information requirements used by pharmacists practicing in the clinical paradigm. With no access to the patient's complete health record and no objective information available about the current problem, the pharmacist who chooses to recommend OTC drug therapy does so almost exclusively on the anecdotal strength of the patient's own description of symptoms, duration, and severity. This may be helpful to the patient who leaves the drugstore with a palliative remedy but it hardly qualifies the pharmacist to claim the experience as a significant therapeutic encounter. As the minimum, online access must be obtained in the community pharmacy to a computer record containing the current health status of each patient including progress notes and the most recent laboratory findings.

Presently the clinical paradigm for pharmacy has a real chance to operate only in those settings where access to health status information is provided to the pharmacist and where other health professionals are at hand with whom the pharmacist may interact as a respected peer. The situations in long-term care facilities and hospitals fulfill these requirements more completely than do community practice settings.

3. In nursing homes, the pharmacist finds, in addition to nurse and physician peers, health status records regarding each resident and the elements of prospective decision making mandated by state departments of public health. Here, care is given over a long period of time, therapeutic plans and goals are established, and there are significant opportunities for pharmacists to exercise clinical judgment.

    The provision of pharmaceutical services to nursing homes has been the usual way that community pharmacists are introduced to the concept of the clinical paradigm. Some faced the challenge head on and obtained the necessary drug information resources and relevant experiences needed to interpret health status data and expanded their knowledge base to include topics in drug therapy for long-term treatment of chronic degenerative conditions (59-61). Other pharmacists recognized that although the decisions required in these settings might be familiar to them, acquiring the extended formal knowledge essential to making clinical decisions was more than they were able to undertake, given the usual constraints of midcareer obligations. In these instances, additional pharmacists were hired who possessed the augmented formal knowledge or a consulting firm representing pharmacy clinicians was retained in order to meet the expectations of the new practice setting and the clinical paradigm. In the latter case, in which clinical expertise is hired, the community pharmacist serving as vendor to the long-term care facility continued the traditional relationship with the nursing home substantially unaltered. The technical paradigm was the underlying philosophy for the provision of drugs and distributive services. The clinical aspects of the drug use process were left to others who possessed the necessary formal knowledge base.

4. In the hospitals, of course, the situation of the pharmacy clinician is nearly ideal insofar as meeting the conditions necessary to participate in meaningful ways in the therapeutic judgment. Other health professionals are in relatively continuous contact with the pharmacist, the facilities for obtaining laboratory data are at hand, and the patient is nearly always available. It is in the best interests of all concerned to obtain the widest possible consultation as decisions are formulated, and for the most part the impact of clinical decisions may be monitored closely as the patient's condition changes.

With regard to clinical pharmacy services, it is not surprising, then, to find the clinical paradigm receives its most favored status in the hospital environment. The pharmacy clinician, however, interacts directly with the patient relatively infrequently except for the routine observations that are part of the clinical rounds. Even here pharmacy finds its clinical role, aimed at improving the patient's health condition, flourishing without significant participation directly from the patient.

At first it may seem unusual that the patient appears so necessary to the clinical role function of pharmacy, and yet when the patient is continuously available, as in hospitals and other kinds of institutionalized settings, there is only tangential interaction between the patient and the pharmacist. What is far more critical to the function of the clinical role is the presence of other professionals with whom the pharmacist may interact in meaningful ways, all of whom serve as agents of the patient—the truest mark of the services of the health professions.

CONCLUSION

The ability to render judgmental decisions based on acknowledged expertise represents the essential skill of every clinical professional—a service contribution that is not likely to be performed as well by computers, technicians, or other professionals who have different areas of expertise. The use of drug therapy-related information with the greatest exercise of professional skill and judgment gives the pharmacy clinician unique value to the modern health care system. When decisions are made by groups of colleagues functioning together harmoniously, unimpeded by the biased influences of outside commercial interests, the nucleus of a truly functional health care *system* emerges. Through technical innovations, costs may be reduced to their achievable minimums consistent with good patient care.

The goal of achieving better patient care at lower costs requires the optimization of drug use based on the expertise of those prepared to contribute to the determination of rational therapy. To attain this level of medical enlightenment in the late 20th century requires that the skills of all qualified health professional colleagues be used at the highest level permitted by their training and experience. Only with the fullest collegial participation among all health professionals will the best decisions be made to enhance the quality of patient care.

Where the clinical role has emerged in practice, pharmacists now enjoy a more central function in contributing to the decisions made about patient drug therapy. Furthermore, the clinical role as it has been described should be achievable in any health care setting, provided that the two foundation principles are permitted to operate: access to complete information and the achievement of peer relationships among clinical practitioners.

Acknowledgments

The authors appreciate the valued critical analysis of various drafts of this chapter by colleagues Paul G. Grussing, Ph.D., Associate Professor of Pharmacy Administration at the University of Illinois, and Marsha Bedford-Mrtek, Ph.D., Coordinator of Pharmacy Quality Assurance and Education at Michael Reese Hospital and Medical Center in Chicago.

REFERENCES

1.   Freidson E. The theory of professions: state of the art. In: Dingwall R, Lewis P, eds. The Sociology of the Professions: Lawyers, Doctors and Others. New York, St Martin's Press, 1983, p 25.
2.   Ladinsky J. The professions, In: Wertheimer AI, Smith, MC, eds. Pharmacy practice: social and behavioral aspects. 2nd ed. Baltimore MD, University Park Press, 1981, pp 2-3.
3.   Dingwall R, Lewis P, eds. The sociology of the professions: lawyers, doctors and others. New York, St Martin's Press, 1983, p 25.
4.   Horobin G. Professional Mystery: the maintenance of charisma in general medical practice. In: Dingwall R, Lewis P, eds. The sociology of the professions: laywers, doctors and others. New York, St Martin's Press, 1983, pp 100-101.
5.   Cullen JB. The structure of professionalism: a quantitative examination. New York, 1978, pp 3-5.
6.   Bledstein B. The culture of professionalism: the middle class and the development of higher education in America. New York, WW Norton & Co., 1976, p x, 94-95.
7.   Freidson E. Are professions necessary? In: Haskell TL, ed. The authority of experts: studies in history and theory, Bloomington IN, Indiana University Press, 1984, p 6.
8.   Haskell TL, ed. The authority of experts: studies in history and theory. Bloomington IN, Indiana University Press, 1984, p 12.
9.   Freidson E. Professional powers, a study of the institutionalization of formal knowledge. Chicago IL, Univ. of Chicago Press, 1986, see especially p xi, chapt 1 and 10.
10. Freidson E. Are professions necessary? In: Haskell TL, ed. The authority of experts: studies in history and theory. Bloomington IN, Indiana University Press, 1984, pp 4-5, 12-13.
11. Mahaffey FT, et al. (1980). In: The internship experience, Grussing PA ed. Chicago IL, National Association of Boards of Pharmacy, 1980, pp 1-9.
12. Atkinson P. The reproduction of the professional community. In: Dingwall R, Lewis P, eds. The sociology of the professions: laywers, doctors and others. New York, St Martin's Press, 1983, pp 228-232, 238-239.
13. Chalmers RK, et al. The need for a new way of thinking in pharmaceutical education: the 1986 Argus Commission Report. Am J Pharm Educ 1986;50:382-385.
14. Francke DE. Models for professional practitioners (editorial). Drug Intell Clin Pharm 1973; 7:201.
15. Freidson E. Are professions necessary? In: Haskell TL, ed. The authority of experts: studies in history and theory. Bloomington IN, Indiana University Press, 1984, p 16.
16. Gross S J. Of foxes and hen houses: licensing in the health professions. Westport CT, Quorum Books, 1984, pp 88-89.

17. Belsheim DJ, et al. The design and evaluation of a clinical clerkship for hospital pharmacists. Am J Pharm Educ 1986;50:139–145.
18. Gross SJ. Of foxes and hen houses: licensing in the health professions. Westport CT, Quorum Books, 1984, pp 82–83.
19. Jackson RA, et al. The quality of pharmaceutical services: structure, process and state board requirements, Drugs Health Care, 1975;2:39–48.
20. Gross SJ. Of foxes and hen houses: licensing in the health professions. Westport CT, Quorum books, 1984, pp 84–85.
21. Geison GL. Professions and professional ideologies in America. Geison, GL, ed. Chapel Hill NC, University of North Carolina Press, 1983, p 5.
22. Geison GL, ed. Professions and professional ideologies in America. Chapel Hill NC, University of North Carolina Press, 1983, p 7.
23. Freidson E. Are professions necessary? In: Haskell TL, ed. The authority of experts: studies in history and theory. Bloomington IN, Indiana University Press, 1984, pp 7–9.
24. Freidson E. Are professions necessary? In: Haskell TL, ed. The authority of experts: studies in history and theory. Bloomington IN, Indiana University Press, 1984, p 10.
25. Fletcher FM. Market restraints in the retail drug industry, Philadelphia, University of Pennsylvania Press, 1967, p 24.
26. Mrtek RG. Pharmaceutical education in these United States — an interpretive historical of the twentieth century, Am J Pharm Educ 1976;40:339–365 (see especially p 360).
27. Sonnedecker G. Kremers and Urdang's history of pharmacy, 4th ed. Philadelphia, JB Lippincott & Co., 1976, pp 27–28, 29T, 314–15, 329–330.
28. Sanazaro PJ. Medicine and pharmacy: our once and future status as professions. Am J Hosp Pharm 1987;44:521–524.
29. Fletcher FM. Market restraints in the retail drug industry. Philadelphia, University of Pennsylvania Press, 1967, pp 24–25.
30. Peterson AF. What difference does it make? Am J Pharm Educ 1971;35:267–274.
31. Parness H. Big ticket merchandise can be the fillip for greater up front profits, NARD J 1963;85(1):22–23, 32, 40–41.
32. McDermott CB. Intelligent commercialism and professionalism: co-partners in renaissance of pharmacy, NARD J 1963;85(18):23–24, 43–44.
33. Francke DE. Let's separate pharmacies and drugstores, Am J Pharm 1969;141:161–176.
34. Ladinsky J. Research on pharmacy: retrospect and prospect, Am J Pharm Educ 1970;34:550–559.
35. Catizone C. and Mrtek R. Office-based pharmacy in the United States, Am Pharm 1984;NS24:76–84.
36. Simmons WB. Accessibility and service: two potent weapons of the retail pharmacist for overcoming discounters' pricing tactics, NARD J 1963;85(10):22–23, 32, 34.
37. Fischelis RP. Pharmacists' professional conduct represents drug industry in public's mind. NARD J 1961;83(24):18–23, 26–27, 42.
38. Anonymous. Independent pharmacists can win over statistical projections. NARD J 1977;99:(13)7–8, 12–13. (July, 1977. N.B.: error in masthead numbering of issue).
39. Elliott EC. The general report of the pharmaceutical survey, 1946–49, Washington DC, American Council on Education, 1950, p 4.
40. Burton T, et al. A history of antisubstitution laws and their replacement by drug product substitution laws. In: Generic drug laws: a decade of trial—a prescription for progress. Goldberg T, DeVito CA, Raskin IE, eds. Natl Ctr for Health Services Res, Dept HHS, Rockville MD. 1986, pp 125–135.
41. Masson A, Steiner RL. Generic substitution and prescription drug prices: economic effects of state drug product selection laws. Washington DC, Bureau of Economics, Federal Trade Commission, 1985, pp 2–7.
42. Brodie DC. Drug use control—keystone to pharmaceutical service. Drug Intell Clin Pharm 1967;1:63–65.
43. Francke GN. Evolvement of clinical pharmacy. In Francke DE, Whitney HAK Jr, eds. Perspectives in clinical pharmacy. Hamilton IL, Drug Intell Publ 1972, pp 26–36.
44. Walton CA. Clinical pharmacy practice and education—the concept and its implementation, Am J Pharm 141:186–197.

45. Brodie DC and Benson RA. The evolution of the clinical pharmacy concept, Drug Intell Clin Pharm 1976;10:506–510.
46. Francke DE. Establishing a model for clinical practitioners (editorial). Drug Intell Clin Pharm 1976;7:251.
47. Francke DE. Levels of pharmacy practice. Drug Intell Clin Pharm 1976;10:534–535.
48. Francke DE. Roles for pharmacy practice. Drug Intell Clin Pharm 1976;10:593–595.
49. McLeod DC. Clinical pharmacy: the past, present and future. Am J Hosp Pharm 1981;38:1893–96.
50. Brodie DC. The decisions pharmacists make, Am J Pharm Educ 1980;44:40–43.
51. Kern SM. New ideas about drug systems, Am J Nurs 1968;68(6):1251–53.
52. Barker KN. How to detect medication errors, Mod Hosp July 1962;99(1):95–98, ff.
53. Pellegrino ED. Drug information services and the clinician, Am J Hosp Pharm 1965;22:39–41.
54. Pellegrino ED. The unit dose system (editorial). JAMA 1968;205:585.
55. Ritchey FJ and Raney MR. Medical role-task boundary maintenance: physicians opinions on clinical pharmacy, Medical Care 1981;19:90–103.
56. Adamcik BA, et al. New clinical roles for pharmacists: a study of role expansion, Soc Sci Med, 1986;23:1187–1200.
57. Hynniman CE. Quality assurance and performance standards. In Brown TR, Smith MC (eds): Handbook of institutional pharmacy practice, 2nd ed. Baltimore, Williams & Wilkins, 1986, pp 632–645.
58. Smith MC. General practice in the U.K. and U.S.: some comparisons and contrasts, Pharm J 1973;210:9–12.
59. Cheung A and Kayne R. An application of clinical pharmacy services for extended care facilities, Calif Pharm 1975;23:22.
60. Strandberg LR et al. Drug utilization of pharmacy services in the long term care facility: an eight year study, Am J Hosp Pharm 1980;37:92–94.
61. Anon. Special Section: Nursing homes: opportunities for pharmacy, NARD J 1981;103(3):12–20.

SELECTED READINGS

THE PROFESSIONS AND SOCIETAL NEEDS[i]

William K. Selden

PHARMACY IS DIRECTLY AFFECTED BY SOCIETAL FORCES

To an analyst of the professions it is interesting to observe how they both stimulate change in society and are in turn themselves affected by social changes. Without describing any of these forces I will merely enumerate ten of those that are directly affecting the profession of pharmacy:

1. increased life expectancy and decrease in infant mortality;
2. expansion of population,
3. development of influential political pressure groups;
4. recognition of rights of women and of minority groups for opportunities in the professions,
5. expanding governmental financial support and regulation;
6. growing institutionalization and decreasing personal professional relationships,
7. larger organizations and capital requirements in development, manufacture, distribution and dispensing of pharmaceutical agents,
8. greater public use of pharmaceuticals and drugs of all kinds,
9. increasing demands for public and social accountability and assurance to the public that is prerogatives are not usurped by any special interest group;
10. growing recognition and attention to economic and social benefits to be gained from preventive health care.

PHARMACY IS AFFECTED BY THE ERA OF POLITICAL UNCERTAINTY

All organizations, not merely the profession of pharmacy, are being affected by what we may call this era of political uncertainty. Each of us as individuals, through our emotional and cognitive reactions, is sensitive to the lack of political and social direction of western society during the decade of the '70s.

Several characteristics of the period may be noted. We have expressed a repeated demand for more freedom at the same time that we have desired more order, especially the latter for others. We have bemoaned the benefits accorded to special interest groups, but participate in such groups ourselves and have been unwilling to support changes in the structure of our political system that would limit the influence of these groups. We know that one does not get something for nothing, but have collectively acted on the assumption that we can have what we want now and someone else will pay later.

---

[i]Edited with permission from Selden WK: The professions and societal needs. *Am J Pharm Educ* 44:359–361, 1980.

The sad but true commentary has been made by Professor Walter Laquer of Georgetown University that in democratic societies, national consensus is usually achieved for any length of time only during a period of war or similar threat of such magnitude, as an economic depression or widespread natural disaster (1).

We must appreciate that the development of pharmacy occurs not in a vacuum but within this larger sphere of broad political uncertainty.

PHARMACY IS AFFECTED BY THE ASPIRATIONS OF ITS MEMBERS

All professions manifest aspirations for greater responsibilities, larger incomes and enhanced status for their members. They do so in different ways: (*i*) by expanding educational requirements; (*ii*) by extending their areas of service, not infrequently into the areas of other professional service, or developing new areas of service: (*iii*) by encouraging the development of auxiliary or supporting personnel and then endeavoring to control the education and functions of this technical personnel: (*iv*) by seeking governmental sanctions through tightly controlled licensure; and (*v*) by developing quasi-governmental controls and certification of specialties.

Each of these activities is legitimate and generally accepted as part of the panoply of methods employed by professions in their endeavors to provide services to meet public demands. It is the abuse of these functions that arouses the ire of those whose welfare may be harmed by the excesses of execution.

Relating these observations to the profession of pharmacy I will quote Alvin L. Morris, immediate past Executive Director of the Association of Academic Health Centers. He had commented on the lack of consensus as to how and in what areas pharmacists should be educated, and then stated that pharmacists regard themselves as the most poorly used health professionals in the light of their extensive education. He continued: "Those in leadership positions in academic pharmacy recognize that their profession's upward mobility in the academic pecking order is related to more direct involvement of pharmacists in patient care" (2).

REFERENCES

1. Laquer W. Europe astray: part I—but will it come on course in the 1980s? Europe: Magazine of the European Community, January-February, 1980.
2. Morris AL. Inter-school relationships in academic health centers, in the organization and governance of academic health centers, Volume 3, Association of Academic Health Centers, Washington DC (1980), p 180.

PHARMACY AS A CLINICAL PROFESSION*

Charles D. Hepler

Everyone, it seems, wants to be a "professional." Real estate agents want to be professionals. Automobile repairmen want to be professionals. In a recent television commercial, a

---

Edited with permission from Hepler CD: Pharmacy as a clinical profession. *Am J Hosp Pharm* 42:1298–1306, 1985.

service manager, wearing a clean white shirt, reassures a bride-to-be that the groom will arrive at the church on time. That's a lot of concern to show a mere customer. There are many senses of the word professional, some invested with quite different connotations. There is the world's oldest profession, the professional athlete, the professional soldier, the "real pro," and the health professional.

In the early days, sociologist identified a need to clarify the senses of the word, and they produced definitions that would discriminate between occupations usually thought to be professions and those thought not to be. A good example, one that appeared eventually in the *American Journal of Pharmaceutical Education,* was in Thorner's 1942 essay on pharmacy.[1] His essay included the following list of characteristics defining a profession:

- A specific and socially necessary function, the performance of which requires
- A special technique that rests upon
- A body of knowledge, mastery of which requires theoretic study; and
- A traditional and generally accepted ethic subordinating immediate private interests to the most effective performance of the function; and
- A formal association fostering the ethic.

Many other definitions of profession have been proposed by sociologists and others over the past 50-100 years. In my opinion, most agree reasonably well in their general outline, although they have different emphases and details. Today, the question of whether an occupation is a profession or not is viewed as meaningless. Everett Hughes[2] pointed out some years ago that an occupational group, especially a clearly defined group, is a reality that can be observed with the senses, while the concept of a profession is just that—a concept. A concept of a profession, therefore, is useful only as an ideal or standard.

Let me use an engineering example to illustrate this point. If we happened to be interested in making ball bearings, the mathematical equation defining a sphere might be quite helpful, despite our expecting never to find a perfect sphere in nature. As we tried to make ball bearings, the concept would help us communicate the idea of a sphere precisely to others and to decide whether our efforts were taking us in the desired direction.

These are likewise the uses of a well-developed definition of a profession. Rather than speaking of profession as a static concept, most sociologists prefer to speak of professionalization or deprofessionalization, meaning occupational movement over time. Some pharmacists, however, want to know whether pharmacy is a profession or not. If they read the sociological literature, they usually find a catalog of pharmacy's shortcomings. The feelings of disappointment this engenders result in part from unfamiliarity with the methods and objectives of sociology and are to that extent unwarranted. I suggest that we should be more concerned with those elements of pharmacy that can move it toward or away from the ideal rather than how close it already is or whether it will ever become perfect.

Most pharmacists already have conceptions of what a profession is or ideally should be, and in this paper I wish to clarify, to make explicit, and to build upon those concepts rather than try to change them. I will use concepts and models of professions that are reasonably well accepted,[a] and I think these will each contribute to our overall understanding of pharmacy as a clinical profession.

In this paper, I will first explore the social purpose of professions in a historical context, clarifying why professions were created. Then I will examine a profession's relationship to society—its manner of providing services. Third, I will discuss the concept of professional authority and examine the need for professional consensus to obtain authority. Finally, I will identify characteristics of clinical pharmacy's client, paying particular attention to the possible industrialization of health care services. Some of this material is the result of empirical research, but some is at the level of plausible but untested hypotheses.

SOCIAL ROLE OF CLINICAL PHARMACY

According to Larsen,[4] modern professions in England and the United States developed about the same time as the industrial revolution. In response to social upheavals such as widespread migration to the cities, many people were faced with problems of buying and selling services. Industrialization, despite its intrusion into all aspects of society, was built around changes in the production of goods, not services. When people moved from the rural villages in which their families had lived for generations to cities so that they could find jobs making cloth or steam engines or whatever, they left behind midwives, herbalists, bonesetters, and other service providers they knew and trusted. When the new city dwellers needed those services, they had to find a stranger to provide them. Larsen says in effect that services with three characteristics became the objects of the developing professional service market:

- They were closely linked to major human values (e.g., health or property);
- They required a degree of knowledge, skill, and understanding beyond those possessed by ordinary people of the day and beyond a layman's ability to evaluate (e.g., the accuracy of a diagnosis or the purity of a prescription); and
- They were inherently personal or individualized in nature, meaning that they could not be readily standardized or mass-produced.

Such services require "trust between strangers," an idea I will develop later in this paper. Certainly medicine, surgery, and law met these criteria in those days. The services of the apothecaries of that day apparently met them also. The point is that professions developed in response to social needs. It is also interesting that those social needs resulted from rapid socioeconomic change such as our society is experiencing now.

Role of Pharmacy in General

With that brief background, let me turn to the analysis of modern pharmacy that it suggests. First, consider the criterion that the service must closely relate to basic human values. Of course, health is a major value, perhaps the most important value. Similarly, most people tend to recognize, perhaps even to overestimate, the importance of drugs in preserving or restoring health. I think the issue for pharmacy here is society's perception of pharmacy's role in drug therapy. I will return to this point later.

The second criterion concerns complexity, knowledge, and skill beyond a layman's understanding. For convenience, we can call this the "complexity" criterion, although it refers as much to the competence needed to provide the service. People are able to evaluate many services that once were beyond their capacities because of higher educational levels and access to information once considered esoteric. This increased sophistication of the population may explain in part the diminishing prestige of all professions, but it seems to have affected pharmacy more than others. Many people are not away of any pharmaceutical services beyond the basic services that one would expect from any merchant, and they usually feel qualified to evaluate those. I can symbolize this problem with the cliche, "Why does it take so long to take my pills out of a big bottle and put them in a little one?" According to this analysis, pharmacy can professionalize in the eyes of the patient by increasing or more effectively communicating the complexity of pharmaceutical services and the knowledge and skill required to provide them.

Larsen's third criterion distinguishes professional services from the world of mass-produced materials or standardized services. Her point is that the professions were not needed for readily standardized services or goods that could be mass-produced and resold in normal mercantile channels of distribution.

Early pharmacy practice involved the compounding of highly individualized prescriptions. We are all too familiar with the standardization that accompanied the industrialization of drug products and the perhaps not coincidental rise of large, bureaucratic pharmaceutical service corporations, such as chain drugstores. I believe that bureaucratic pharmacy attempts to standardize pharmaceutical services just as the manufacturing industry has attempted to standardize pharmaceutical products. Such bureaucracies tend to ignore services that cannot be standardized. I am struck by chain pharmacy's apparent avoidance of drug interaction and allergy-checking services until they became available as computerized, that is to say standardized, products. Unfortunately, many pharmaceutical services that are most closely related to health and that involve the most knowledge, skill, and complexity also are the hardest to standardize. Such services tend to be ignored by bureaucratic pharmacy corporations. This seems an important source of deprofessionalization to the extent that patients believe that pharmacy is represented by chain drugstores and other bureaucracies (Including, of course, some bureaucratically organized institutional pharmacies).

The obvious competitive strategy of nonbureaucratic ("independent") pharmacists would be to provide highly personalized service, but this seems to have been unsuccessful. Many advisory services were discouraged or prohibited by the APhA Code of Ethics until 1969.[5] Perhaps chains were able to shift the basis of competition to price because independent pharmacies were unable or unwilling to publicly offer such services. It is possible, albeit tragic, that some independent pharmacists thought of themselves as merchants and accepted price as a basis of competition, unfavorable a basis as it may have been.

Many hospital pharmacists have escaped this source of deprofessionalization, but some have not. It is useful to recognize that many hospital pharmacy departments are bureaucratic to a greater or lesser degree. Bureaucratic departments may tend to discourage pharmaceutical services that cannot be made routine outputs of a production process, such as services requiring judgment in using patient-specific information. Such services are extremely difficult to supervise by usual bureaucratic methods. A dilemma results because some hospital pharmacy managers claim a right, perhaps even a duty, to supervise all of the work in their departments but think only of bureaucratic methods of supervision. This problem has retarded or even reversed professionalization in some pharmacy departments.

Distinguishing Roles of Clinical and Distributive Pharmacy?

This same kind of analysis can be applied to the important issue of "clinical" services vis-à-vis the distribution of drug products in hospitals. This issue expresses the central question of clinical pharmacy's social purpose.

Some pharmacists argue for the separation of so-called distributive functions from clinical functions, while others argue for their integration. In the framework of Larsen's analysis, distributive functions appear as the highly standardized, mass-produced services that were left outside the professional system. In contrast, primarily informative and advisory functions, like therapeutic monitoring and pharmacokinetic analyses, appear as the highly personalized nontransferable services for which the professional system was developed.

Many pharmacists have devoted years of education and practice to performing informative functions. The term *clinical* became attached to *pharmacy* to distinguish these functions and these pharmacists from other pharmacists who had not developed in this way. It is common for clinically oriented pharmacists to avoid performing standardized, mass-produced services like drug distribution.

By emphasizing personal service, informative functions meet Larsen's third criterion. Because informative services usually are complex and require substantial competence, they meet the second criterion as well. We must, however, address concerns about the first criterion, the one that involves a service's closeness to primary human values. What services should constitute the core of clinical pharmacy? Two dimensions of this issue are (1) whether clinical pharmacy should be defined in terms of functions or in terms of responsibilities, and (2) whether these functions or responsibilities should include both drug products and information about the use of drugs or just the information.

My general impression as a pharmacy educator is that most people refer only to informative functions when they use the term *clinical pharmacy*. A good example of such use occurs in the "ASHP Statement on Clinical Functions in Institutional Pharmacy Practice,"[6] The statement virtually defines clinical pharmacy in terms of informative functions, except that it does include control of drug distribution and administration as one of 10 clinical functions. (Controlling drug distribution and administration involves managerial functions which some practitioners may not wish to perform nor be capable of performing well, so this item is as confusing as it is helpful.)

In the context of Larsen's criteria for professional services, such a definition of clinical pharmaceutical services does not convey clinical pharmacy's maximum value to society. Professions exist to meet social needs, not to perform isolated functions. Performing informative functions alone seems less valuable to society—to have less apparent impact on health—than acceptance of responsibility for the appropriate use of drugs in patients, including providing the drug products themselves.

Defining clinical pharmacy in terms of responsibilities instead of functions is clear and unequivocal. It clearly suggests the social value of clinical pharmaceutical services. It also allows clinical pharmacists to accept responsibility for certain technical functions without having to imply that they personally should perform them. This is Brodie's concept of drug-use control expressed as a responsibility.[7] As he pointed out, technique alone will not make us professionals. It is a good thing for clinical pharmacists to claim authority over drug use—to claim that they are drug experts. It is a much better thing, however, to accept a share of responsibility for drug use.

This is certainly not a finished idea, for as it stands it has some serious problems. For one thing, I think that we have a dilemma because this definition is really a definition of the role of pharmacy practice itself. It excludes many more pharmacists than it includes, so perhaps it is a goal rather than a definition. On the other hand, I doubt that further definitions in terms of functions will advance the professionalization of clinical pharmacy. I leave this dilemma to conference participants to resolve.

The second problem with defining clinical pharmacy in terms of responsibility for drug-use control is that pharmacists do not currently have legal responsibility for drug use in patients. This does not prevent clinical pharmacy from offering to take such responsibility, but the reality is that today we could have at most only shared responsibility for drug use.

This analysis of the reason for the existence of professions suggests that we define clinical pharmacy in terms of responsibilities rather than functions and in terms of a complete set of drug-use goods and services.

Manner of Providing Professional Service

I now wish to extend this examination of professional services a bit further. Obviously, if you needed to purchase a service that was of vital importance to you and that was unique and beyond your ability to evaluate, you would want the provider to be trustworthy. You would be at a terrible disadvantage; you simply could not protect your interests as you would in a normal business dealing. The professions' response to this need is sometimes called professional altruism, but this term is often quite misleading. I prefer to explain that society entered into a covenant with the professions to protect itself in these circumstances.[8]

The word covenant is unfamiliar to many people. It seems to have only two common uses today. One refers to real estate or partnership agreements and has nothing whatever to do with my use of the word. The other use is religious. Both Jews and Christians describe their relationship to God as covenantal. God offered Abraham, and later Moses, to make the people of Israel His chosen people and to take care of them. In return, He asked the people of Israel to love Him and obey His commandments. Christians believe that Jesus renewed that covenant.

Regardless of one's religious beliefs or disbeliefs, that relationship between God and His people is a good metaphor for the covenant that I believe exists between society and a profession. (My use of this metaphor is not intended to suggest that religious motives are necessary for professionalization.) Society asks a profession to obey certain rules in providing very valuable, complex, and personalized services. The effect of these rules is to ensure that the profession will serve society.

For example, every profession accepts a duty to protect the long-term interest of its clients and never to take advantage of a client's dependency or weakness. Each profession promises to maintain its members in number, knowledge, skill, and attitude. In return, society promises to give the profession authority. This occurs through a long process of exchange in which the would-be profession demonstrates its value and commitment while society grants a bit of authority.

It can also work the other way, as a disillusioned society gradually withdraws authority from a profession. For example, pharmacy, medicine, and law have lost substantial amounts of authority over the past few years. Prominent examples are loss of the internal control made possible by prohibitions of advertising and partial loss of control of professional school admissions. This process may continue at a relatively rapid rate for medicine as the market for health-care services is restructured and industrialized.

Now we have an answer to the question, "What does a professional profess?" Every professional primarily professes his side of the convenant: a commitment to the welfare of a client. In addition, a professional professes competence and a belief that his techniques are safe and effective. But professionals are expected to show such competence and effectiveness objectively, not merely to profess them. As outlined in the next section, the ability to show effectiveness is an important prerequisite for professional authority.

Professional Authority

In return for its commitment, society gives the professional authority—legitimate power to influence behavior. At first, that may not sound like much, but it multiplies rapidly and lasts as long as the covenant with society, just as Abraham's descendants multiplied and endured.

A profession can use authority to gain wealth, and many do just that. The professional covenant, even as a lofty ideal, in no way asks the professional to live in poverty. This is, however, a common misunderstanding of the concept of professions, probably a result of using the word altruism to describe this idea. In his book, *The Social Transformation of American Medicine,* Starr[9] explains,

> The historical success of a profession rests fundamentally on the growth of its . . . authority. Acknowledged skills and cultural authority are to the professional classes what land and capital are to the propertied. They are the means of securing income and power.

Starr emphasizes that a professional's knowledge and competence must have been validated by a community of peers.[10] This implies, of course, that the peer group is collegiately organized, hence the need for a professional association. Note, however, the emphasis on an organization that actively validates competence, not one that merely accumulates members. We in pharmacy desire consensus, but seldom achieve it. Our organizations may sometimes confuse membership numbers with organizational strength. Starr seems to be suggesting that a professional's authority could be increased by membership in an organization that is generally recognized as being selective on the basis of consensually valid and professionally relevant competence criteria. Such an organization might have its own continuing competence criteria as does, for example, the American Academy of Family Physicians.

Starr's second point regarding authority is that the profession's consensually validated knowledge and competence must rest on rational scientific grounds.[10] To gain professional authority we must have research into the bases and methods of clinical pharmaceutical services. It is often difficult (although by no means impossible) to find support from the sources that support most health-services research. The money available from the ASHP Research and Education Foundation and other sources is helpful, although the amounts available do not support enough research. The shortage of money is aggravated from the profession's viewpoint because the money is seldom directed into areas that the profession has agreed will help it or the public.

I believe that money funneled through the Foundation would do more good for the professionalization of clinical pharmacy if it were targeted on selected problems, perhaps as a part of the ongoing ASHP strategic planning process. I also think that the recognition awards of the Foundation could encourage research in targeted areas by recognizing the best projects on a selected topic. This might achieve the greatest effect for the fewest dollars, given most people's thirst for peer recognition. Finally, I want to stress that the valid studies of the effectiveness of clinical pharmacy do exist but seem to get little attention. I will mention studies led by Smith,[11] Herfindal,[12] Helling,[13] Bootman,[14] and Avorn[15] as examples. These and other studies lend support to clinical pharmacy's claim to authority over the drug-use process.

Starr distinguishes two types of authority.[16] The first and most familiar type is social authority, the probability that someone will obey a command or follow a suggestion, for example. Cultural authority is the legitimate power to interpret facts, to define what is real, and to impose values. Medical diagnosis is a good example of cultural authority. A syndrome becomes labeled and eventually becomes a disease through the cultural authority of medicine. Legionnaires' disease is a recent example. Many more examples are available in psychiatry.

A clinical pharmacist uses cultural authority when he defines a set of symptoms as an adverse drug reaction. To a large degree, this assertion is true only because he says it is true: It would rarely if every be empirically tested in the clinical setting. If his authority were accepted, the drug would be discontinued and treatment would continue without it. The more adverse drug reactions, inappropriate therapies, and so forth there are, the more important pharmacists are to society. Once an occupation gains social and cultural authority, then, it is allowed to define the client's need for its services and is on its way to control of its own market. This is why authority is much more valuable than money. It confers professional autonomy, fruitfulness, and virtual immortality, but only as long as the profession's convenant with society lasts.

The Professional versus the Businessman

Pharmacists seem perpetually confused about their so-called dual roles as professionals and businessmen.

Business does not rely on a covenant but rather uses a more concrete, legally enforceable agreement, the contract. There is a contract within every professional covenant, and, when a convenant is washed away by breaches of faith, what remains is a businessman's contract. Society gives cultural authority to business only reluctantly and gives social authority only over an employee. That is, business has no basis to tell customers what products to buy. Correspondingly, business makes no promise to guard the interests of the customer. Its doctrine is *caveat emptor:* Let the buyer beware.

In my view, a business relationship is a limited, special case of a professional relationship, not a separate and distinctly different type of relationship. Mixing business with a professional relationship, therefore, narrows and limits the professional relationship. A businessman's aspiration to become professional to gain cultural authority over the client is not so much immoral as it is misguided. Society grants authority slowly and only in proportion to demonstrated social value and commitment to the interests of clients. Society is not stupid. A professional covenant with society leads to professional authority, while a business relationship does not. These rather philosophical lines of demarcation can be made quite concrete by putting them in terms of an occupation's acceptance of responsibility, its standards of conduct, its recognition of exemplary practitioners, and its rejection of the unfit.

A practical example of the difference between a business and a professional concerns the issue of whether we should charge separately for clinical services, what I have been calling informative services. To address this question, it seems that we need to know whether the pharmacist accepts responsibility for the clinical use of drugs and claims at least shared authority to decide what services are to be provided to a patient. If one adopts the position that informative services are separable from the drug products involved and especially if the services are considered optional extras that the patient or his physician may select, then it seems logical to charge for them separately. However, it is not logical to separately bill for goods and services if the pharmacist decides what is needed.

Sometimes this question is asked in an entirely differently context, such as, "Why should pharmacists give away their services?" I think this question is insidiously misleading, and people who take it seriously should know better. This question can only be asked in a business environment, and it forces a businesslike answer. A businessman has a right to request payment for everything he sells to his customer, unless he chooses to give it away for goodwill. In contrast, a professional takes responsibility for a package of goods and services. His services should be distinctive and valuable enough so that he can set his fees to compensate for the occasional client who costs more than the fee covers. It seems unnecessary to tack on charge for the routine elements that are needed to meet those responsibilities. You may have heard the joke about the patient who tried to get a discount on a vasectomy by only having one side done. Pricing is always a game, and I do not want to appear dogmatic about this. My point is that there is a difference between a businessman's price and a professional's fee. The professional takes care of his client and the businessman takes care of his business.

Professionalization as a Social Project

I began this paper with a discussion of society's needs during the industrial revolution, as England and America converted from agriculture to industry. Now, for a moment, we should turn our attention to the service provider in the rapidly growing cities during this period. The midwife, bonesetter, herbalist, or apothecary: Each would have a very tenuous hold on the market for his or her services. The industrial city would be flooded with people offering services. Many would be charlatans. The problem of the would-be profession was, in essence, to create a basis for the sale of services to strangers in a climate of extreme competitiveness. According to Larsen,[4] this required the would-be professions to organize themselves along the following lines:

- To develop exclusive education, training, and standards so that the services provided by the would-be professionals were distinct and recognizable by the public;
- To persuade recruits to forego income long enough to complete their training, so that a sufficient number of providers were available to meet the claims of the professions; and
- To seek governmental license to eliminate competing occupations.

These three elements depend upon and influence each other.

This was a somewhat tightly constrained project for a large group of free people. They had to define and agree on apparently distinctive services that met the criteria of value, complexity, and specificity, and they had to recruit and train new disciples. Starr[17] emphasizes the importance of consensus in the development of a professional market. If the members of the would-be professional cannot agree at least on the education and training required to enter the occupation and cannot agree on the basic nature and content of their services, the other steps may well be impossible to complete.

CONCLUSION

In a free society, the people ultimately will have their way. They created the health professions and were served well, except from a fiscal viewpoint. Now society will try a mixture of corporate, professional, and market mechanisms to serve its needs. Pharmacy will prosper most by serving the needs of society best.

REFERENCES

1. Thorner I: Pharmacy: the functional significance of an institutional pattern. *Soc Forces,* 1942;20:321–8. Reprinted in *Am J Pharm Educ.* 1942; 6:305–19.
2. Hughes EC. Men and their work. Glencoe, IL: The Free Press; 1958.

3.   Hepler CD: Professions in modern society: contract vs. covenant. *Pharm Manage.* 1979; 151:102-4.
4.   Larsen MS: The rise of professionalism. Berkeley, CA: University of California Press; 1977.
5.   American Pharmaceutical Association. Code of ethics. *J Am Pharm Assoc.* 1963; NS3:72.
6.   American Society of Hospital Pharmacists. ASHP statement on clinical functions in institutional pharmacy practice. *Am J Hosp Pharm.* 1983; 40:1385-6.
7.   Brodie DC: Pharmacy's societal purpose. *Am J Hosp Pharm.* 1981; 38:1893-6.
8.   May WF: Code and covenant or philanthropy and contract? *Hastings Cent Rep.* 1975; 5:29-38.
9.   Starr P. The Social transformation of american medicine. New York: Basic Books; 1982:79-80.
10. Ibid. p. 15.
11. Smith WE. The economic feasibility of clinical pharmacy in the hospital setting: personnel costs. Springfield, VA: National Technical Information Service; 1973.
12. Herfindal ET, Bernstein LR, Kishi, DT: Effect of clinical pharmacy services on prescribing on an orthopedic unit. *Am J Hosp Pharm.* 1983; 40:1945-51.
13. Helling DK, Hepler CD, Jones ME: Effect of direct clinical pharmaceutical services on patients' perceptions of health care quality. *Am J Hosp Pharm.* 1979; 36:325-9.
14. Bootman JL, Wertheimer AL, Zaske D et al: Individualizing gentamicin dosage regimens in burn patients with gram-negative septicemia: a cost-benefit analysis. *J Pharm Sci.* 1979; 68:267-72.
15. Avorn J, Soumerai SB. Improving drug therapy decisions through educational outreach. *N Engl J Med.* 1983; 308:1457-63.
16. Starr P. Op. cit. p. 13.
17. Ibid. p. 80.

PHARMACY'S SOCIETAL PURPOSE[k]

Donald C. Brodie

PROFESSIONS SERVE

The professions exist to serve society. They serve in ways defined by the scope of the knowledge and skills that they command, and the needs of society for that knowledge and those skills. At the risk of oversimplification, permit me to suggest that the professions serve in two ways. First, they serve through the practice of a technique—the technique of pharmacy, law, medicine, and theology. When we use the term "practice of technique," we refer to the minimum standard of professional behavior. Sometimes we see professionals performing a set of routine skills with little visible concern for those follow-up services that the client may need as a consequence of the "technique." Here we see the pharmacist dispensing medicine, the physician conducting a routine office visit and finishing it with a written prescription for medicine, and the dentist probing the patient's mouth and examining the teeth. In each case, the practice of technique seems to be an end unto itself, and the encounter often terminates with a flurry of hastily given and poorly comprehended last-minute instructions. We may see the practitioner in a pattern of behavior that suggests self-interest and a concern for the rewards of practice. All too often certain inner, basic needs of the patient are not fulfilled. This is one of the reasons why the professions today are in such trouble. The practice of technique has dominated professional behavior and commitment.

The second way the professions serve is by practicing what they profess. Palmer[1] sees a professional as one who professes, testifies, or bears witness to some sort of faith and

[k]Edited with permission from Brodie DC: Pharmacy's societal purpose. *Am J Hosp Pharm* 38:1893-1896, 1981.

" . . . it was only because he did so that he merited being called "professional." The ideology of the professions is based on their profession—the statement of the faith that they profess. The true professional weaves what he professes into the practice of his technique resulting in a fabric of professional behavior that embodies both ideas—technique and profession or commitment. His life is the epitome of a professional ideology. This profession ideology for the classical professions of theology, medicine, and law has been highly visible to society from the earliest times. It has created a pattern worthy of emulation by other occupational groups seeking professional status. But even the images of these historical professions have been tarnished by the changes brought about by the scientific and industrial revolutions, expansion of knowledge and technology, growth of materialism, and the dominance of the practice of technique over client concerns and needs. The public has lost much of the confidence it once held for the commitment of professionals, often seeing them as shallow and self-serving practitioners seeking financial rewards, status, and social and political influence. Palmer[1] continues:

> My definition of professional—as one who professes a faith—is anathema to the engineer, the chemist, the business manager, the academic. They see themselves not as bearers of a faith or of proclaimers of a confidence but as practitioners of technique . . . pure, empirical, pragmatic marketable technique. And the world of technique admits of no ambiguity, no tragedy, no demons; that is, technique admits of no need of faith.

We must remember that our profession lends itself exceptionally well to the practice of technique. Some would say that we are victims of our own technique. It is common knowledge that consumers often see only a bottle of pills. Many of our practitioners see the boundaries of their professional responsibility circumscribed by the practice of technique—the dispensing of medicines. The mission of clinical pharmacy is to move that boundary toward the patient. There is controversy today in the field of pharmaceutical education about where that boundary should be. The boundary is a dynamic one—it is ever changing and will continue to be so as new knowledge and new technology evolve and our understanding of human health behavior increases. We must realize that we will always be seeking to interface with a boundary that actually is never there. We are left agonizing with the fact that we are not in complete command of that knowledge that is uniquely ours. As professionals, we are forced into a pattern of life-long learning as a condition of our survival. We help determine where that boundary is for our profession. The decision hinges on the answer to the questions "What do I profess?" and "What do we profess?" After these questions, "What is our professional ideology?"

SOCIETAL PURPOSE

The ideal of a service role identifies one of the generic purposes of the professions. To this we might add a pattern of professional behavior that assures continuity of concern for client's welfare, accountability, integrity, reliability, and a commitment to the common good. Most people will associate "societal purpose" with the stereotyped pattern of professional practice that they have observed and experienced. They associate medicine with healing, theology with salvation, and law with justice, and "purpose" is seen in light of these associations. The perceived needs that society has developed for the services of each of these professions provide the basis for the societal purpose to which each is committed. But the needs of society change, and they have and are changing markedly in our time because of the enormous advances in knowledge and technology. In his *Uses of the University*,[2] Clark Kerr said:

> The production, distribution, and consumption of "knowledge" in all its forms is said to account for 29% of gross national product (figures credited to F. Machlup), and "knowledge production" is growing at about twice the rate of the rest of the economy. Knowledge has certainly never in history been so central to the conduct of an entire society. What the railroads did for the second half of the last century and the automobile did for the first half of this century may be done for the second half of this century by the knowledge industry: that is, to serve as the focal point for national growth.

Or consider a more recent statement by Dr. Donald S. Fredrickson,[3] then Director of the National Institutes of Health. He was delivering a paper entitled, "Biomedical Research in the 1980s," before the Royal College of Physicians in London and introduced his address with the thought that the present state of the biological sciences is one of "revolution." He went on to say:

> The current revolution . . . is not a simple, linear projection of the growth curve in knowledge for the past century. A striking perturbation of that growth has occurred, amounting to a geometric progression of available information. Achievements of research in chemistry, physics, and many allied disciplines . . . have led to new technologies contributing to a flood of discovery in biochemistry, physiology, and medicine. Our ignorance is still vast, but we are on the threshold of some unusual transformations in health practices, agriculture, and industry.

Using the above statements to focus our attention on knowledge, we can ask what impact the knowledge explosion of the twentieth century has or will have first, on needs for the services of health-care providers, and second, on the purpose or purposes for which the health professions exist. Let us consider the biomedical and pharmaceutical knowledge and the resultant technology that has evolved during the past 50 years. This takes us back to the 1930s in France when the golden age of therapeutics started with the discovery that sulfanilamide (para-aminobenzenesulfonamide) had remarkable antibacterial action against both gram-positive and gram-negative organisms. Penicillin was discovered in the 1940s, followed by many other antibiotics, and, in succession came the corticosteroids, anticoagulants, tranquilizers, oral diuretics, oral contraceptives, poliovirus vaccine, and others. Add to this list of drugs the biomedical discoveries such as organ transplantation, open heart surgery, and successful drug treatment of hypertension, elucidation of the structure of DNA and, now, genetic engineering. During this relatively short period, infectious disease came under control for the first time in history because of the availability of antiinfective drugs, and ". . . today, only 1% of people who die before age 75 in the United States die from infectious diseases."[4]

IMPACT ON SOCIETAL PURPOSE

Has this period of spectacular biomedical and pharmaceutical accomplishments modified, changed, or even increased pharmacy's societal purpose? Has it added a new dimension to our respective societal purpose? I suspect that with the classical professions of theology, medicine, and law, one might argue that societal purpose remains constant in relationship to time. The reason for their existence—healing, salvation, and justice—in each case is so all-encompassing that new knowledge and new skills can be accommodated within the traditional boundaries of perceived purpose. But in the case of pharmacy, our perceived purpose, by comparison, is "narrow" and "specific" and will not accommodate the expansion of the knowledge base without a conscious recognition that our purpose is or may be changing, however small or subtle the changes may be.

In a historical sense, the societal purpose of pharmacy has been one of making drugs and medicines "available." Available meant two things: first, the actual making or preparing of medicines, and second, distributing medicines to consumers at community practice sites. Although both forms were the pattern well into the twentieth century, the industrialization of pharmacy since World War I has minimized the pharmacist's role in making medicine. For all practical purposes, this role of making medications available means dispensing and distributing medicines and health supplies in community and institutional settings. Within the context of societal purpose, this function remains central to pharmacy's reasons (purpose) for existence, and there is no reason to believe it will change, although the process of distribution will be subject to changing technology and innovation.

While the core of pharmacy's societal purpose remains unchanged, the scope of the profession's purpose appears to have broadened, and now, in my opinion, may be visualized as consisting of three parts. The first responds to the need for all health professionals to serve a dual role—the role of a health generalist and the role of a health specialist, the specific role for which each is trained. In their role as health generalists, physicians, nurses, dentists, and pharmacists share actively in the responsibility for directing people into the health-care system. This is a broad public-health function, and it includes offering advice on community and personal health matters, counseling to increase compliance with drug and other therapeutic regimens, referral to sources of treatment including public health clinics, and participation in community planning for health education and allocation of resources. Although pharmacists have performed many public-health functions in the past, they have not been particularly visible in this role, nor has the profession promoted it with any apparent conviction. Certainly, pharmacy education has not designated a great deal of time in the curriculum to this role, a point underscored by Bush and Johnson.[5] In 1980, however, the American Public Health Association[6] adopted a position paper that recognized pharmacy as a profession with major responsibilities for public health. It defined the pharmacist's role broadly in a set of five public-health functions:

1. Planning for health care for wide geographic areas or communities;
2. Managing, administering, and evaluating health-care programs, systems, and facilities;
3. Providing direct personal health care service (including health education, maternal, and child health, etc.) and environmental health;
4. Developing and promoting legislation, and deriving regulations pertaining to the public's health; and
5. Training health-care workers needed to carry out these functions.

The second part of pharmacy's purpose is making medicines and selected health supplies available to consumers and other providers of health care. Today, it is much more than the traditional dispensing function—the practice of technique. It includes developing and managing systems of drug distribution that provide access points to consumers and assure drug safety and compliance with legal and professional standards. These new responsibilities have required pharmacists to acquire expertise in the storage of data, distribution, and inventory-control functions, and the management of data for drug histories, patient records, quality-assurance programs, and drug information services. Included in this area are the personnel to carry on the historic purpose of the profession in an age of changing technology. This means pharmacists and support personnel who are qualified to perform the physical and scientific aspects of drug distribution and control must also be competent in handling the interpersonal relationships required at the interface of the pharmacy system and the ultimate consumer—patient, physician, nurse, or public official. And under the title of "unmet needs" are a number of health services that are broadening the scope of pharmacy's societal purpose. Many of these needs, including kidney dialysis and parenteral nutrition services, can be provided by pharmacists. Certain classes of patients are finding that pharmacists are uniquely qualified to care for their needs, which previously have been unmet. These patients include the disabled who are in wheelchairs or confined to nursing and convalescent homes, as well as those with impaired hearing and vision. Lastly, there are those patients who need prosthetic and other fitted devices for maintaining their normal level of health.

The third part of pharmacy's purpose is an extension of the second; in fact, it can be argued that it is an integral part of the second purpose. It consists of services that have their basis in the knowledge and skills a pharmacist should have at his command. The pharmacist is unique among health care providers. He is the only one who has knowledge of the physical and chemical properties of drugs in addition to their pharmacologic and therapeutic properties. The modern pharmacist should be qualified to work with the physician in planning and monitoring drug therapy. When necessary, he can rely on his background in the physical sciences as a special adjunct in solving difficult clinical problems. By understanding the pathways by which drugs are metabolized and the rates at which they are biotransformed in the body, he has a special role as pharmacokineticist in planning and adjusting dosage regimens. As biologist, chemist, pharmacokineticist, and pharmacist, he must be prepared to be spokesman for select portions of the scientific literature. This literature represents a dynamic knowledge system from which he gathers the information he uses daily in consulting with physicians, patients, and other pharmacists. This knowledge system has had somewhat traditional boundaries for many years, but as we approach the era of genetic engineering and molecular biology, the system will increase in specificity and complexity, and the boundaries will be extended. As we anticipate advances in immunology and new drugs for control of cardiovascular disease, hypertension, cancer, and arthritis, the service component of pharmacy's societal purpose assumes larger proportions. The Study Commission on Pharmacy certainly recognized the need for a service component when it defined pharmacy as:

> a knowledge system that renders a health service by concerning itself with understanding drugs and their effects upon people and animals.

The Commission's report continued:

> Pharmacy is a generally excellent system for generating knowledge, for translating knowledge into a product, for distributing the product, and for dispensing the product; but it is far from an excellent system for transmitting knowledge and information, particularly to the ultimate consumer—the patient.

And then, as if to reinforce its earlier statement, the Commission repeats:

> . . . the greatest failing of pharmacy is its inadequacy as an information transmitting system.

The deficiency in the existing health-care system is at the point where the pharmacist interacts with the patient or client. The report, in turning to clinical pharmacy, said:

. . . it is clear that there is one common idea which is present in all of the manifestations (of clinical pharmacy); that idea is an emphasis upon *drugs* as they are *utilized* by and in the patient. It is the joining of *drug* and *patient* which is the inseparable and continuing concern of the evolving pharmacist.

These three points—that pharmacy is a knowledge system; that the transmission of information is its greatest weakness; and that the joining of drug and patient is the concern of the evolving pharmacist—provide a conceptual basis for the service component that must complement and supplement our ability to practice our technique. And the ingredient that binds these three together is knowledge—knowledge of the biomedical, pharmaceutical, and behavioral sciences: knowledge of drugs, knowledge of people.

REFERENCES

1. Palmer PJ. Profession in the seventies. Church society for college work. 1973; 31:2-6.
2. Kerr C. The uses of the University. Cambridge MA, Harvard University Press; 1963.
3. Fredrickson DS. Biomedical research in the 1980s. *N Engl J Med* 1981; 304:509-17.
4. Healthy people. The surgeon general's report on health promotion and disease prevention. U.S. Department of Health, Education, and Welfare, 1979. (DHEW publication no. (PHS)79-55071).
5. Bush PJ, Johnson KW. Where is the public health pharmacist? *Am J Pharm Educ* 1979; 43:249-52.
6. The American Public Health Association. Policy statements adopted by the governing council. The role of the pharmacist in public health. *Am J Public Health* 1981; 71:213-6.
7. The American Association of Colleges of Pharmacy. Pharmacists for the future: The report of the Study Commission on Pharmacy. Ann Arbor: Health Administration Press, 1975.

3
The Pharmacist

ELLIOTT M. SOGOL
HENRI R. MANASSE, JR.

The process one uses to define the term pharmacist is, at best, a difficult task to undertake. Should one include the necessary requisites to becoming a pharmacist? Is a pharmacist someone who practices pharmacy? Is a pharmacist someone who is licensed to practice? Is the definition shaped by the socialization, professionalization, and education of the individual? Is it possible to define the pharmacist in terms of occupational role, job tasks, job specification, environment, or setting? These questions give some insight into the difficulties that have been evidenced over the years in developing an encompassing yet comprehensive definition of the pharmacist.

For the purposes of furthering this analysis, it may be beneficial to utilize the following definition: A pharmacist is an individual who has acquired the formal knowledge of the profession. This definition is admittedly oversimplified as it does not delineate (a) the different types of pharmacists, (b) their employment status, (c) the environment in which they practice, (d) their licensure as a Registered Pharmacist (R.Ph.), (e) their educational background, (f) their sex, (g) their age, or (h) their status within the profession. However, it is a basis from which one may gain insight into the population of pharmacists in the United States.[a] As one utilizes this definition of the pharmacist, one must examine (a) how the formal knowledge base is acquired by the pharmacist, (b) how this knowledge is disseminated through professional services, and (c) how this knowledge affects the practice of pharmacy.

ROLE OF PHARMACY

The role of pharmacy can be defined to include professional pharmacy services that promote and assure rational drug therapy in order to maximize patient benefits and minimize patient risk. Of utmost importance is the role that the pharmacist plays in maximizing patient benefits by practicing in a patient-oriented behavior utilizing a formal theoretical knowledge base. In this manner, the pharmacist is considered an integral part of the provision of primary health care services for the patient is placed as the foremost concern over the product or disease state. This example indicates how the pharmacist becomes an active copractitioner or collaborator in the overall care of the patient with primary responsibilities for patient care (1). As this occurs, rational drug therapy can be accomplished by providing the

---

[a] This definition can be further delineated to include practitioners and nonpractitioners. However, for discussion purposes of this chapter, this definition will pertain to those practitioners actively involved with the profession of pharmacy.

right drug for the right patient in the right amount at the right time with due regard to relative cost and intended therapeutic outcomes. The patient can be expected to be placed on a rational drug regimen with the greatest therapeutic efficacy and lowest potential risk through clinically applied pharmacy services.

The above definitions attempt to include aspects of pharmacy practice regardless of practice setting, environment, or style of practice. The definitions also imply that the profession of pharmacy, by definition, is clinical (2). In other words, to be a practitioner within the pharmacy profession one must perform clinical pharmacy activities and thus be responsible and accountable for therapeutic appropriateness.

PHARMACY EVOLUTION

> The direction and nature of evolutionary changes in a profession are the outcome of a complex interplay between the professional educational curriculum, societal needs, public policy, and the aspirations and activities of new graduates.
>
> Gehard Levy

The profession of pharmacy has evolved as a clinical profession with the strongest development occurring in the last decade (3, 4). This evolution has been observed throughout the profession as the clinical practice of pharmacy has moved toward functions that seemed remote just 10 to 15 years ago. The clinical evolution process continues today as pharmacists now participate in (a) the selection of drug entities to treat different disease states, (b) drug information centers as resources for other health care providers, (c) monitoring therapeutic outcomes, and (d) direct patient care through suggestions of alternative therapeutic approaches for individual patients (5, 6).

The evolution of the pharmacy profession also has been observed as pharmacists use their expertise in moving from the selection of a brand versus a generic product (drug product selection) to the selection of a drug entity within a therapeutic class of drugs (therapeutic interchange).

Along with these changing functions, pharmacists are increasing services through the implementation of total drug use control, another mainstream issue in the development of a clinical profession (7). As this occurs, the management of drug utilization review and drug regimen review also enter into the responsibility of the pharmacist and thus, the evolutionary process continues to mature.

Today, pharmacists are continuing to establish their commitment to being drug information experts. In this role, pharmacists obtain information from a variety of sources, interpret and evaluate data, and then disseminate information to the broader community (8). As pharmacists continue to expand these functions, recognition is found for their contributions to health care providers, patients, and the community as a whole. This recognition occurs regardless of the environment in which the individual is employed or the style of the individual practitioner.

PROFESSIONAL STRATIFICATION

As the role of the pharmacist continues to expand, several levels of classifications have been delineated (9). The classifications listed in Table 3.1 describe the role individual practitioners play in the pharmacy profession. Although five distinct classifications were delineated in the mid-1970s, pharmacists continue to play key roles through a continuum of functions and services provided based on individual and professional initiatives.

More than a decade later, it is possible to argue that the pharmacy profession itself is and has emerged as a clinical profession. The definitions presented earlier indicate that this delineation is based on role performance, functional specialization, educational background, qualifications, and responsibilities of an occupational environment. In other words, the clinical frontier established over a decade ago is not solely based on a specialized educational training process provided by the colleges of pharmacy but, moreover, is related to the variety of functional characteristics, educational backgrounds, environmental effects, and role performance and responsibilities of the individual pharmacist. An example noted is the M. D. Anderson Hospital and Tumor Institute where the hospital pharmacy operations department is now a clinical division equal in rank to medicine, nursing, and surgery (10). This example reinforces the functional characteristics of clinical pharmacy.

Within the abovementioned framework, professional and social stratification issues relative to class, status, power, and occupational environment need to be addressed. However, given that professional status is but one feasible single indicator, problems remain in defining stratification and deciding on the most valid way to rank order them (11). Perhaps further investigation into pharmacy curriculum, professionalization, and lifelong learning will help to delineate the stratification in pharmacy.

CURRICULUM: FROM NOVICE TO EXPERT

> While it may or may not be true that the most important changes in the learner are those which may be described as cognitive, (i.e., knowledge, problem-solving, higher mental process, etc.), it is true that these are the types of changes educators seek to bring out.
>
> Benjamin Bloom

Table 3.1.   Levels of Pharmacy Practice [a]

Clinical pharmacists
1. Clinical scientists
2. Clinical pharmacy specialists
   a. Pharmacotherapeutic specialist of applied pharmacologist
   b. Clinical radiopharmacist specialist
   c. Drug information specialist
   d. Pediatric clinical pharmacy specialist
   e. Others
3. Clinical pharmacy generalists

Generic pharmacists
4. Generic pharmacists involved in a high percentage of professional activities perform clinical functions and have numerous patient-physician contacts daily.

Generic pharmacists—pharmacy technologists
5. Generic pharmacists involved in a low percentage of professional activity perform little or no clinical functions and have little contact with patients or physicians. Ninety percent of trained pharmacy technologists could perform 90% of what these generic pharmacists do.

[a]Reprinted with permission from Francke DE. Levels of pharmacy practice. Drug Intell Clin Pharm 1976;10:534–535.

Any planned educational program that is evaluated for continued improvement must have a conception of the goals and aspirations that are to be reached (12). Within the pharmacy curriculum, the theoretical framework consists of an intellectual system based on empirical information, attitudinal information, and skills that are composed of concepts and other abstract ideas brought together to form the ideal state (13). This theoretical framework must be able to incorporate the stated goals and develop an evaluation process from the formation and knowledge presented in the basic coursework to completion of a given curriculum.

Although many pharmaceutical science educators talk of the starting point in a pharmacy student's educational endeavor as being entrance into the pharmacy curriculum itself, this thinking omits the influence of the prepharmacy curriculum beginning with high school science education. Admission policies of the respective schools and colleges of pharmacy establish those courses that must be taken before one enters the professional school. These policies affect the high schools by tracking students into a science knowledge background. As this process occurs, the moving from novice to expert can be divided into three basic categories: (a) prepharmacy education (education up to pharmacy school); (b) pharmacy education (education starting in pharmacy school); and (c) postpharmacy education (continuing professional education).

It is difficult to analyze prepharmacy curriculum effects on becoming a pharmacist as this knowledge base is used for numerous health professionals and is not specific to pharmacy. Prepharmacy education serves a basic level on which students build for the theoretical base in pharmacy education. The use of knowledge presented in the sciences (i.e., biology, organic chemistry, math, physics, etc.) and the humanities (i.e., economics, English, health education, sociology, etc.) is critical to the pharmacy student because the theoretical framework for the profession lies in an understanding of this knowledge. Pharmacy educators can then build upon this knowledge to a higher scholarly level of acquisition, utilization, and application.

An examination of the pharmacy curriculum through an analytical framework includes four levels of difficulty and complexity. These four levels are defined as (a) basic courses—those courses that build upon the knowledge acquired before entrance into the pharmacy model; (b) intermediate courses—those courses that build on the basic courses before the pharmacy curriculum and those courses in the basic model; (c) advanced level courses—those courses that tie together the theoretical framework of earlier coursework; and (d) experiential courses—those courses that encourage the application and utilization of acquired knowledge to the practice of pharmacy under the supervision of faculty members.

In looking at the coursework offerings for students in pharmacy, four functional groupings exist for which knowledge and skills are particularly intertwined. Figure 3.1 illustrates that all four of these categories build upon prepharmacy courses and, ultimately, to the final phases of the program that include experiential courses. The analytical framework listed in Table 3.2 considers the curriculum as being composed of a series of horizontal tracks that take the student from the basic beginnings of science to the eventual expertise required to provide pharmaceutical services brought out in the experiential component of the curriculum. It should be noted that the table lists categories of courses that may differ in title from college to college.

The five functional areas include:

1. Drug disease/technical knowledge—a categorization that is comprised of the disease state process, pharmacology, therapeutics, pharmaceutics, and the associated

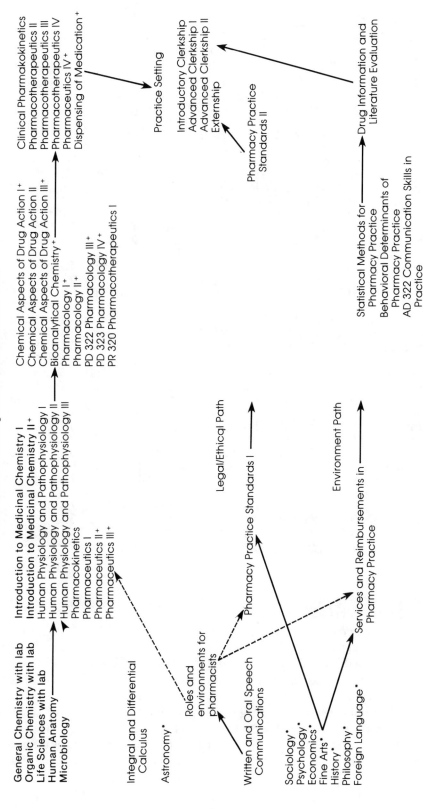

Drug Disease Knowledge and Technical Skills[+] Path[a]

Figure 3.1.   Curriculum guide for colleges of pharmacy.

[a]Unpublished data expanded on original work by Bruce Seiker. *, general education coursework; [+], associated lab to advance technical skills.

Table 3.2. Honesty and Ethical Standards Ratings of 25 Occupations [a]

| | Honesty and Ethical Standards | | | | | | | | | | | |
| | Very High, High, | | | Average | | | Low, Very Low | | | No Opinion | | |
	'85	'83	'81	'85	'83	'81	'85	'83	'81	'85	'83	'81
Clergymen.........	67%	64%	63%	26%	27%	28%	4%	4%	6%	3%	5%	3%
Druggists, pharmacists......	65%	61%	59%	30%	33%	33%	3%	4%	5%	2%	2%	3%
Medical doctors	58%	52%	50%	33%	35%	38%	8%	11%	10%	1%	2%	2%
Dentists.............	56%	51%	52%	37%	41%	38%	5%	5%	7%	2%	3%	3%
College teachers....	54%	47%	45%	35%	38%	36%	5%	5%	8%	6%	10%	11%
Engineers..........	53%	45%	48%	37%	39%	35%	3%	3%	5%	7%	13%	12%
Policemen	47%	41%	44%	41%	45%	41%	10%	11%	13%	2%	3%	2%
Bankers............	37%	38%	39%	51%	49%	47%	9%	9%	10%	3%	4%	4%
TV reporters, commentators	33%	33%	36%	48%	47%	45%	15%	15%	15%	4%	5%	4%
Funeral directors	31%	29%	30%	45%	43%	41%	15%	19%	19%	9%	9%	10%
Journalists..........	31%	28%	32%	47%	47%	44%	17%	17%	15%	5%	8%	9%
Newspaper reporters.........	29%	26%	30%	52%	52%	49%	16%	16%	16%	3%	6%	5%
Lawyers	27%	24%	25%	40%	43%	41%	30%	27%	27%	3%	6%	7%
Business executives ..	23%	18%	19%	54%	55%	53%	18%	20%	19%	5%	7%	9%
Senators...........	23%	16%	20%	53%	48%	50%	21%	30%	25%	3%	6%	5%
Building contractors..	20%	18%	19%	53%	53%	48%	21%	23%	27%	6%	6%	6%
Congressmen.......	20%	14%	15%	49%	43%	47%	27%	38%	32%	4%	5%	6%
Stockbrokers........	20%	19%	21%	51%	45%	46%	10%	11%	7%	19%	25%	26%
Local political officeholders......	18%	16%	14%	53%	49%	51%	24%	29%	30%	5%	6%	5%
State political officeholders......	15%	13%	12%	55%	49%	50%	24%	31%	30%	6%	7%	8%
Realtors	15%	13%	14%	49%	52%	48%	31%	28%	30%	5%	7%	8%
Labor union leaders .	13%	12%	14%	35%	35%	29%	45%	44%	48%	7%	9%	9%
Advertising practitioners......	12%	9%	9%	42%	42%	41%	39%	39%	38%	7%	10%	12%
Insurance salesmen..	10%	13%	11%	49%	49%	49%	38%	34%	36%	3%	4%	4%
Car salesmen.......	5%	6%	6%	32%	34%	33%	59%	55%	55%	4%	5%	6%

[a]Reprinted with permission from *Pharm Times* 1985;51(10):1.

technical and manipulative skills from drug preparation to drug dispensing (both macro and micro levels).

2. Legal/ethical knowledge—a categorization that is comprised of legal and ethical issues. The legal aspects take into consideration the state and federal laws that are associated with the practice of pharmacy. Ethical considerations are manifested in all areas of the practice of pharmacy from basic scientific research decisions to practice decisions.

3. Sociobehavioral knowledge—a categorization that is comprised of issues related to society and the behavior and attitudes of society and the profession. This track brings to the knowledge base a different type of technical skill needed by the health professional. The ability to communicate information, advise patients, and evalu-

ate psychological and social characteristics of the patient and other health care providers are elements of this area.
4. Administrative/environmental knowledge—a categorization that is comprised of information related to financial, managerial, administrative, and clinical principles relevant to the profession. Drug literature evaluation, statistical methodology, and financial systems play key roles in this track.
5. Practice knowledge settings—a categorization that is comprised of experiential learning through established clerkships. Actual practice setting experience and education leading up to the culmination of the individual student becoming a professional are included in this category.

The above functional areas overlap in many instances and build upon each other through the educational process. As an example, it must be kept in mind that a course in ethics will overlap with each of the five categories presented. The teaching of ethical decision-making skills through theoretical and practical components to recognize and resolve ethical dilemmas (14) will also be applicable to the functional groups.

Students' perceptions relative to the five functional areas outlined will vary dependent on the individual curriculum at a given school or college and the emphasis of its educators. Traditionally it has been difficult for students and educators to achieve a balance between the scientific aspects of disease and the humanistic aspects of patient care. In a 1983 survey of medical students, between 35 and 60% of the graduates from three schools believed there was not enough time set aside in the curriculum for the management of patients' socioeconomic, educational, and emotional problems (15). As education shifts toward the drug use process and patient care, it is the responsibility of curriculum committees to understand the needs of all of the parties involved including students, educators, practitioners, and consumers.

Finally, it is important for the pharmacy student to understand the sequential grouping of courses offered. One must note that specific courses play unique roles in the educational system. They act as an integral point to "begin" and "exit" the system. To begin the system, basic coursework introducing the student to the pharmacy curriculum provides a plan for continuation through the curriculum. The examination of drug disease state issues, legal/ethical issues, sociobehavioral issues, administrative/environmental issues, and practice issues gives the student an understanding of the educational structure that he or she is about to experience.

PROFESSIONS AND PROFESSIONALISM

A profession can be defined as having three service-related characteristics: (a) being closely linked to human values; (b) possessing a specific knowledge base and technical skill understanding beyond that of the individual layperson; and (c) offering personal individualized services not readily standardized or mass produced (16).

Professionalism, on the other hand, is a concept that develops around a given profession. At the basic level, professionalism is composed of four multivariate aspects: (a) the psychological aspect; (b) the social aspect; (c) the sociological aspect; and (d) the legal/ethical aspect.

The psychological aspect is comprised of the individual's personal sense of worth, the notion of what an individual wants to be, his or her own self-esteem and self-concept. It is then the challenge of the educator, the individual, and the employer to continue developing professionalism. In a 1982 survey of the University of California at San Francisco graduates (1970–1981), 94% were fairly satisfied to very satisfied relative to the pharmacy profession and life in general (17), or as an indication of personal self-worth.

The social aspect is comprised of how professionals evolve socially for a specific purpose. The pharmacist acquires a given theoretical knowledge base, a power, that others do not have. The professional's power (authority) is based on the acknowledged technical expertise that is maintained (18). This in turn leads to a variety of special privileges that society as a whole is willing to give to the profession. Public trust and public perception are key elements to this component of a profession. In a 1981 Gallup Poll, the pharmacy profession was ranked second in a list of 25 professions and occupations relative to honesty and ethical standards. The public's perception of the pharmacy profession was very high relative to the above-mentioned standards. This trend continued in 1983 and 1985 as the pharmacy profession again ranked second in public perception of ethics and honesty relative to a list of 25 occupations and professions as noted in Table 3.2 (19).

One also must look at the relationship of other health professionals to pharmacy. Table 3.3 outlines the results of a corresponding 1981 survey of physicians' opinions on clinical pharmacy (20, 21). The physicians' opinions tend to be split on the acceptance of clinical functions of hospital pharmacists. Unlike the Gallup Poll findings, a wider range of results were found relative to physicians as is noted in Table 3.3. This may help to explain the problems that sociologists and others have had in defining pharmacy as a profession because available data tends to suggest a split between the consumers' and other health professionals' acceptance of the clinical role. This inconsistent socialization process may have been caused by a nonuniformity or lack of agreement about the idealized model for pharmacy from both the consumer and health professional perspective (22). Perhaps in a decade from now this inconsistency may decrease as younger health professionals in pharmacy and other related health care fields begin to view the interdisciplinary strengths of health care.

The sociological aspects of professionalism center on the professional model, the code of ethics, and the theoretical knowledge base drawn from the educational requirements. In this regard, a significant challenge to the pharmacy profession has arisen as new developments in science, technology, social organization, and financing have entered the health care market. From a structural/functional perspective, an occupation becomes a profession when granted autonomy and recognition from society for possessing a technical knowledge base, demonstrating effective performance, developing lengthy and superior education, and espousing ethical commitments to the common good (23). The pharmacy profession has evolved based on these perspectives regarding the educational curriculum discussed earlier and the components of professionalism being outlined. The profession has undergone an almost constant evolution that leads to reprofessionalization as both society and the profession change relative to structural/functional perspectives. Along with this constant change, there needs to be an emphasis on communicating the ideas, problems, descriptions, and solutions brought out by the educational systems (21). The profession has moved rapidly to secure a theoretical knowledge base that establishes the base for a professional (24). The professional status of pharmacy, although questioned at times as being a profession or a trade/business, rests on the claims of a theoretical knowledge base, autonomy, service, and licensure (25).

The legal/ethical aspects of professionalism include those laws relevant to a given profession. For example, the pharmacy profession follows a Pharmacy Practice Act, as well as

Table 3.3. Physicians' Acceptance and Resistance to Clinical Pharmacy [a]

Attitudes Toward Pharmacists Performing Specific Tasks		
Task Generally Accepted by Physicians	Tasks Gaining Acceptance	Tasks Generally Rejected by Physicians
Pharmacists maintaining patient drug profiles; type of task: clerical	Pharmacists counseling hospital patients on the use of physician-prescribed drugs; type of task: patient management	Pharmacists deciding on the frequency of use or dosage forms of physician prescribed drugs; type of task: technical-therapeutic decision making
Pharmacists monitoring prescribing patterns of physicians; type of task: clerical	Aid physician in selecting drugs; type of task: technical-therapeutic decision making	Pharmacist independently choosing drug to be prescribed based on the physician's diagnosis; type of task: technical-therapeutic decision making
	Adjunct Tasks	Autonomous Tasks

Characteristics of Physicians Most and Least Favorable to Clinical Pharmacy	
Physicians Most Favorable	Physicians Least Favorable
Those who spend a substantial part of their practice time in hospitals	Older physicians
Younger physicians (although they are especially opposed to pharmacists making technical decisions)	Those in high malpractice risk specialties
Those who have been exposed to clinical pharmacists or have used their services	Those who write large numbers of prescription

[a]Adapted from data of Ritchey FJ, Raney MR. Medical role-task boundary maintenance: physicians' opinions on clinical pharmacy. Med Care 1981;19:90–110.

local, state, and federal regulations pertaining to the profession of pharmacy. Even with the number of laws regulating the pharmacy profession, the legal profession view of pharmacy is mixed (26). Some rulings on the laws have been favorable to pharmacy as a clinical profession by delineating the pharmacist's role as a part of the health care team with a duty to warn patients about their medications. In contrast, other rulings have been unfavorable relative to pharmacists' expanding roles. Examples are noted where the judge's ruling implied that the pharmacist does not have a duty to warn the patient about his or her therapy and is in fact merely a technician who serves as a conduit between the physician and the patient (26). In other words, the pharmacist is not to be considered as an integral component in the health care team. Such a discrepancy in the interpretation of the pharmacist's role may begin to decrease as the pharmacist's expanded role emphasizes a service versus product orientation.

Finally, the ethical component is comprised of those issues related to the public good such as professional standards, counseling, advising, and other aspects of practice that require moral judgment. A concern has been raised relative to increasing ethical and moral educational aspects of the pharmacy curriculum (14). This concern for increased education in the ethical area needs to be addressed from the individual pharmacy student level to the national professional organization level.

PROFESSIONALIZATION

The process of becoming a professional begins at the college level with admission to a professional school as students are exposed to a variety of educational materials and problem solving skills that will enable them to function within the current standards of the profession. This professional development (socialization) occurs throughout the educational process and is influenced by the individual pharmacy student, the pharmacy faculty, and the practitioners with whom the students interact. This socialization process also can be differentiated across the educational timeline from prepharmacy to postpharmacy educational experiences (27). It does not suffice to say that the professionalization process is based solely on the education that the student receives. Encouragement to participate in professional activities, involvement in legislative issues, joining professional student organizations on and off campus, and a sense of worth are essential starting points for the professionalization process. Once the student begins to understand his or her role in a professional field, the process will continue throughout the educational experience.

However, it is also noted that individual students also may proceed through the system in spite of understanding that there are established ways of behaving—the so-called norms values and standards of practice that are to be met (5, 28). To foster the professional development process, students should be given the opportunity to understand the socialization process that is occurring. This should be accomplished through a curricular approach while in the educational institution.

Enhancing and maintaining professional development then becomes a major focus for the pharmacist once entrance into the profession has been completed. Table 3.4 outlines the unique characteristics of professional development career stages (29). The four stages outline the role of the professional and can be adapted to pharmacy if stage one is considered as the time when a newly licensed pharmacist enters the profession. General concern over job specifications and the contributions that can be made are brought to the forefront of development. Stage two leads to the concerns of independent work and recognition. If professionals are not learning, growing, and gaining greater competence, they can become bored, frustrated, and complacent (29). Stages three and four indicate the satisfaction that can occur from the professional role itself.

Career planning is important to all individuals regardless of their work environment. Planning can be based on promotional aspects, lateral movement, and/or increased responsibilities in which the individual may wish to engage. These aspects of career planning should be dealt with when the pharmacy student begins his career choice and continue while a person is in the work force.

The challenge for the professional is to assume responsibility, obtain career development information, develop a career plan, evaluate the plan, and follow through. It may be difficult for individuals to proceed through this process unless a mainstream occupational function or a philosophy of pharmacy practice is utilized as the focal point for continued professionalism (13).

Table 3.4.   Characteristics of Career Stages [a]

Stage I	Stage II
Works under the supervision and direction of a more senior professional in the field	Goes into depth in one problem or technical area
Work is never entirely his or her own, but assignments are given that are a portion of a larger project or activity being overseen by a senior professional	Assumes responsibility for a definable portion of the project, process, or clients
Lacks experience and status in organization	Works independently and produces significant results
Is expected to willingly accept supervision and direction	Develops credibility and a reputation
Is expected to do most of the detailed and routine work on a project	Relies less on supervisor or mentor for answers, develops more of his or her own resources to solve problems
Is expected to exercise "directed" creativity and initiative	Increases in confidence and ability
Learns to perform well under pressure and accomplish a task within the time budgeted	

Stage III	Stage IV
Is involved enough in his or her own work to make significant technical contributions but begins working in more than one area	Provides direction for the organization by:
Greater breadth of technical skills and application of those skills	"Mapping" the organization's environment to highlight opportunities and dangers
Stimulates others through ideas and information	Focusing activities in areas of "distinctive competence"
Involved in developing people in one or more of the following ways:	Managing the process by which decisions are made
Acts as an idea leader for a small group	Exercises formal and informal power to:
Serves as a mentor to younger professionals	Initiate action and influence decisions
Assumes a formal supervisory position	Obtain resources and approvals
Deals with the outside to benefit others in organizations—i.e., works out relationships with client organizations, develops new business, etc.	Represents the organization:
	To individuals and groups at different levels inside the organization
	To individuals and institutions outside the organization
	Sponsors promising individuals to test and prepare them for key roles in the organization

[a]Reprinted with permission from Thompson PH, Baker RZ, Smallwood N. Improving professional development by applying the four-stage career model. Organ Dynamics 1986;49–62.

70   Pharmacy Practice

LIFELONG LEARNING: CONTINUED PROFESSIONALISM

> The aim of every advanced, subtle, and mature form of continuing education is to convey a complex attitude made up of a readiness to use the best ideas and techniques of the moment but also to expect that they will be modified or replaced. The new machine will soon be antiquated, the new drug outmoded, and the revolutionary approach will become first familiar and then old fashioned. Everyone must expect constant change and with it new goals to be achieved and new understanding and skill to be mastered.
>
> Cyril O. Houle

Continuing education may be defined in numerous ways. At the basic level, continuing professional education offers informal and formal opportunities to both individual practitioners and groups to continue the lifelong learning process within their chosen profession. Informal involvement in continuing education may include (a) reading of journals and promotional literature, (b) discussions with colleagues, (c) professional organization work, (d) informal cable television programs (i.e., those programs focusing on general health issues with no evaluation component), and (e) the everyday experiential learning that takes place in the work environment. Formal types of continuing education include such techniques as (a) lectures, (b) seminars, (c) workshops, (d) educational teleconference network programs, (e) correspondence courses, (f) slow scan television, (g) closed circuit television, and (h) formal cable television programs (i.e., those programs focusing on specific health issues utilizing formal evaluation components).

The overall purpose of continuing education efforts is to build upon the professional training and skills that the practitioner brings into the profession. Therefore, a basic goal is to "facilitate the successful performance of practitioners in the diverse practice characteristic of professional work (30).

The ultimate goal of continuing education would then be to ensure the establishment and maintenance of ethical, intellectual, social, and professional standards of practice (30). To achieve this goal, continuing education should serve more than just an episodic occurrence that provides the participant with a brief and cursory update or overview. Continuing education must go beyond this and, in addition to the above, not only provide in-depth knowledge of what is new, but also to prepare practitioners for future change.

The idea of a theoretical framework designed for lifelong learning and continued professionalism has begun to come to fruition in some places. College level coursework, applicable to the pharmacy profession, appears to be one example of a means to provide the practitioner with the required in-depth knowledge and preparedness for change. In this manner, well-developed external or extended degree programs will give individual practitioners the opportunity for advanced college level credentials.

REFERENCES

1. Emswiller CF. The pharmacist as a primary health care practitioner. Presented at the American Association for the Advancement of Science, New York, 1975.
2. Manasse HR Jr. The twenty-first century hospital: where is the pharmacist? Hosp Pharm 1987;22:16–26.
3. McLeod DA. Clinical pharmacy: the past, present and future. Am J Hosp Pharm 1976;33:29–37.
4. TIME, Oct. 12, 1981.

5. Penna RP. Don't call it prescribing. Am Pharm 1986;11:25-28.
6. Wolf HH. Personal conviction, commitment and choice: foundations for professional practice. Presented at The Kenneth L Water Lectures, 1986, University of Georgia College of Pharmacy.
7. Brodie DC. Drug use control: keystone to pharmaceutical service. Drug Intell 1967;1:63-65.
8. Schondelmeyer SW. Pharmacists, pharmaceuticals, and drug information in the 21st century. Drug Inf J 1985;19:185-193.
9. Francke DE. Levels of pharmacy practice. Drug Intell Clin Pharm 1976;10:534-535.
10. Zellmer WA. Progressive leadership. Am J Hosp Pharm 1986;43:2157.
11. Haug MR. Measurement in social stratification. Ann Rev Sociol 1977;3:51-77.
12. Tyler RW. Basic principles of curriculum and instruction. Chicago, University of Chicago Press, 1949, pp. 3-60.
13. Brodie DC. Need for a theoretical base for pharmacy practice. In Harvey AK Whitney Award Lecture 1950-1986. Am Soc Hosp Pharm 1986;251-259.
14. Miederhoff PA, Olin BR, LeFevre J. Ethics education for clinical pharmacy practice. Drug Intell Clin Pharm 1980;14:537-539.
15. Maheux B, Beland F. Students' perceptions of values emphasized in three medical schools. J Med Educ 1986;61:308-315.
16. Hepler CD. Pharmacy as a clinical profession. Am J Hosp Pharm 1985;42:1298-1306.
17. Koda-Kimble MA, et al. Practice patterns, attitudes, and activities of University of California Pharm D graduates. Am J Hosp Pharm 1985;42:2463-2471.
18. Bay JE, Bay C. Professionalism and the erosion of rationality in the health care field. Am J Orthopsych 1973;43:55-64.
19. Pharmacy Times 1985;51(10):1.
20. Ritchey FJ, Raney MR. Medical role-task boundary maintenance: physicians' opinions on clinical pharmacy. Med Care 1981;19:90-110.
21. Reilly MJ. Old dreams, young hopes. In Harvey AK Whitney Award Lecture 1950-1986. Am Soc Hosp Pharm 1986;305-314.
22. Manasse HR Jr, Stewart JE, Hall RH. Inconsistent socialization in pharmacy—a pattern in need of change. J Am Pharm Assoc 1975;15NS:616-621.
23. Birenbaum A. Reprofessionalization in pharmacy. Soc Sci Med 1982;16:871-878.
24. Quintrell N. Pharmacy: the push to professionalisation. Aust J Pharm 1981;680-681.
25. Shuval JT. The pharmacist, process of becoming. In Wertheimer and Smith ed., Pharmacy Practice, Baltimore, University Park Press, 1981, pp. 27-35.
26. Brushwood DB. Trends to watch in pharmacy practice liability. Drug Topics 1987;131:3.
27. Shuval JT. From "Boy" to "Colleague:" Processes of role transformation in professional socialization. Soc Sci Med 1975;9:413-420.
28. Olmstead AG, Paget A. Some theoretical issues in professional socialization. Soc Issues Prof Soc 1969;44:663-669.
29. Thompson PH, Baker RZ, Smallwood N. Improving professional development by applying the four-stage career model. Organ Dynamics 1986;49-62.
30. Houle CO. Continuing learning in the professions. San Francisco, Josey-Bass Publishers, 1981, p. 74.

SELECTED READINGS

LEVELS OF PHARMACY PRACTICE[b]

Donald E. Francke

One can identify several levels of practice in pharmacy and one such arbitrary classification is shown in Table 1. The criteria I used to judge the five levels of practice was whether 90 percent of one level could perform 90 percent of the responsibilities of the next higher level. If they could not then they are separate levels; if they could, I merged the levels. For example, I believe there is a significant difference between the levels of practice of what the Millis Commission called a generic pharmacist and what I call a clinical pharmacist generalist and that 90 percent of the present generic pharmacists cannot carry out 90 percent of the responsibilities of the clinical pharmacist generalist. In the same way, I believe that 90 percent of the clinical pharmacist generalists cannot carry out the responsibilities of 90 percent of the pharmacotherapeutic specialists or applied pharmacologists. However, until levels of competency are determined and applied, any graduate can continue to claim any level of competency in professional practice he chooses.

At present, an underdeveloped area of pharmacy practice is that performed by the *clinical scientist* who in the words of the Millis Commission is "equally at home at the patient's bedside or in the laboratory" (1). The use of the term laboratory has generated a great deal of confusion as to the nature of the clinical scientist and how he will be developed and I am now seeking clarification of this point. However, if we relate the clinical scientist in medicine to the clinical scientist in pharmacy what do we find? First that the large majority of physicians who are clinical scientists possess only their basic professional degree; a few also have a research degree. Second, physicians with this background perform significant research in such fields as lipid research, cancer research, hematology, hypertension and many others. Third, the research team is almost always multidisciplinary and numerous specialists contribute. Fourth, the physician, since he bears the chief responsibility for the patient, is the leader of the research team. It would be my judgment that clinical scientists in pharmacy will develop in somewhat the same manner. A number of those who receive good training in the basic sciences, who have the appropriate motivation, who possess excellent clinical training and who have a proper health care setting for research involvement will become clinical scientists without too much additional formalized effort.

A second level of practice is that which I would call areas of specialization as exemplified by the *pharmacotherapeutic specialist* or *applied pharmacologist*. In the early days of clinical pharmacy education, I attempted to conceptualize what a clinical pharmacist was and thought of him as an applied pharmacologist. I thought of the clinical pharmacist as being a person who, in addition to his basic pharmacology, had taken courses in pharmacology and therapeutics with medical students, courses in which he would receive a great deal of therapeutics. I thought of him as having graduate level courses in biostatistics, patho-

[b] Reprinted with permission from *Drug Intell Clin Pharm* 10:534–535, 1976.

Table 1.   Levels of Pharmacy Practice

Clinical pharmacists
  1. Clinical scientists
  2. Clinical pharmacy specialists
      a. Pharmacotherapeutic specialist or applied pharmacologist
      b. Clinical radiopharmacist specialist
      c. Drug information specialist
      d. Pediatric clinical pharmacy specialist
      e. Others
  3. Clinical pharmacy generalists

Generic pharmacists
  4. Generic pharmacists involved in a high percentage of professional activities, perform clinical functions and have numerous patient-physician contacts daily.

Generic pharmacists—pharmacy technologists
  5. Generic pharmacists involved in a low percentage of professional activity, perform little or no clinical functions and have little contact with patients or physicians. Ninety percent of trained pharmacy technologists could perform 90 percent of what these generic pharmacists do.

physiology, biopharmaceutics and pharmacokinetics, and the sociology of health care. These courses plus his general educational background in microbiology, pharmaceutics, formulation, etc., plus suitable clinical training such as a residency or clerkship would produce one of the most drug knowledgeable people on the health care team. Some people don't like calling the clinical pharmacist an applied pharmacologist because they think it might antagonize clinical pharmacologists. Thus, I also think of the clinical pharmacist as a pharmacotherapeutic specialist. The important considerations, I believe, are his knowledge of therapeutics and the actions of drugs in humans. In the preface to the first edition of *Applied Pharmacology* which the British physician, A. J. Clark, wrote more than fifty years ago, he said that his objective was "to give an account of the direct scientific evidence for the therapeutic action of the most important drugs, and to demonstrate the importance of this knowledge in the clinical application of drugs (2)." This is essentially the objective of the high level clinical pharmacist whether one calls him a pharmacotherapeutic specialist or an applied pharmacologist.

Of course a number of other specialists may eventually be approved after due consideration by the APhA's Board of Pharmaceutical Specialties (3). Some of these may be, for example, Clinical Radiopharmacist Specialist, Drug Information Specialist, Pediatric Clinical Pharmacy Specialist, Geriatric Clinical Pharmacist, and perhaps others. However, I would expect that the large umbrella for the areas of specialization would be the Pharmacotherapeutic Specialist or Applied Pharmacologist, or some similar designation. For example, I would expect this person's knowledge and experience would be such that he would be equally at home with patients and physicians in such specialties as medicine, surgery, obstetrics and gynecology, neurology, etc. The principal reason pediatric and geriatric clinical pharmacy may be eventually judged as specialties is because of the differences in metabolism of drugs in the very young and very old. Whether this difference warrants specialization remains to be seen.

A third level of pharmacy practice is exemplified by the *clinical pharmacy generalist*. As this title implies, this person is a generalist with a broad range of knowledge. This person is not as well grounded as the applied pharmacologist in pharmacology, therapeutics, biostatistics or pharmacokinetics and lacks his clinical training and experience. Still he has a sufficient background to be a most valuable member of the health care team.

A fourth level of practice is that exemplified by the hundreds of what the Millis Commission describes as *generic pharmacists* who practice in community and hospital pharmacies. Some of these are involved in a high percentage of professional activities and are engaged in daily patient-physician contacts and perform numerous important clinical services for patients and the health team. In due course, I anticipate that this level will merge with the clinical pharmacy generalist as the colleges improve their educational programs and decrease their student load.

In addition, there is a fifth level of practice carried out by generic pharmacists who are involved in a low percentage of professional activities and perform few if any clinical functions. These are the pharmacists who stand behind a counter all day repetitively filling and labeling prescriptions, turning the filled prescription over to a clerical person to transfer to the patient. In my opinion, this group of generic pharmacists should be merged with trained pharmacy technologists, technicians or dispensing assistants. These technical people could, in my opinion, competently perform 90 percent of what this group of pharmacists do.

I would like to see the profession recognize that it does not require the training a pharmacist receives to carry out the functions now performed by a large number of pharmacists. Once this was accepted, the number of pharmacists enrolled in schools of pharmacy could be greatly decreased. On the other hand, the importance and significance of the pharmacist would be greatly enhanced because they would be trained to perform tasks which are now neglected. Schools of pharmacy would have fewer pharmacy students but they would be superior students trained to an entirely different level than they are at present. The education and training of these students would be such that a professional doctoral degree would be entirely appropriate. Schools of pharmacy would be involved, directly or indirectly, in the training of technical personnel to the level required by the function they will be called upon to perform. I believe that this is the general pattern that will finally emerge and when it does, pharmacy will become a much stronger profession because of it.

REFERENCES

1. Millis JS. Pharmacists For The Future, Health Administration Press, Ann Arbor, Michigan. 1975.
2. Modell W, et al. Preface to Applied Pharmacology, American Edition, W. B. Saunders Co. 1976.
3. Board of Pharmaceutical Specialties: Petitioners Guide to Specialty Recognition, 6 page document available from the American Pharmaceutical Association, 2215 Constitution Avenue, Northwest, Washington, D.C. 20037.

SCENARIO OF THE HEALTH CARE SYSTEM IN THE YEAR 2010 [c]

Stephen W. Schondelmeyer

Expectations for the health care system and pharmacy in the year 2010 are capsulized in the following scenario. This scenario is presented as if it were a feature story being aired

[c]Edited and reprinted with permission from Schondelmeyer SW: Pharmacists, pharmaceuticals, and drug information in the 21st century. *Drug Inf J* 19:185–193, 1985.

on a network news program. So, while reading it, imagine that the date is September 18, 2010 and you are listening to the evening news.

. . . And finally this evening, we will close with an historical note from the health sector. The nation's pharmacists met this week to reflect upon "Changes in Pharmacy: 1980 to 2010."

Pharmacists at the conference observed that the self-care diagnostic aids and medications, which we routinely use today, were once controlled by physicians and pharmacists according to federal and state laws. Consumers now have direct access to these moderately effective symptomatic therapies which were the mainstay of medical therapy before the turn of the century.

Our 21st century pharmacists, in highlighting their current roles in society, took pride in the wide-spectrum of health-related products and services offered through many different practice settings. Counseling pharmacists in community pharmacies are easily accessible at our workplace, near our homes, or at other convenient sites throughout the community. Community pharmacies may be operated and managed by our employers, by regional or natonal health facility chains, or as part of a cooperative coalition of the formerly independent community pharmacies.

Information on most health products is widely available today through the computer services accessible by personal computers at work or at home. Despite direct access to these vast databases, the counseling pharmacist's advice is sought to provide interpretations and application of the information for the purpose of meeting an individual's particular health or wellness needs. These pharmacists maintain complete profiles on our individual health behavior and product consumption, they counsel us on the safe and effective use of self-care diagnostic aids and therapies, and they provide us with information and supplies for our longevity-enhancing lifestyles.

When our wellness declines significantly or an illness cannot be resolved by standard self-care methods, health care is sought from among specialized physicians and their ancillary services which are organized into community-wide mega-health systems. The broad based mega-health systems have streamlined the operation and effectiveness of health care delivery in contrast to the extremely inefficient aggregation of hospitals, nursing homes, and other health facilities for disease treatment found in the 1980s. Many services are provided directly at the workplace or at home; however, a few highly technical services are delivered by a specific provider at a particular health facility. Employer-provided longevity-enhancement plans cover the economic costs of both self-care and allopathic-directed health care.

Pharmacists within the mega-health system serve two roles in addition to the counseling pharmacist role. One group of pharmacy specialists are clinical scientists who use genetic engineering and biochemical synthesis methods to prepare patient-specific, high-tech pharmaceuticals such as immunomodulators or biochemical mediators. A second group of pharmacy specialists are clinical pharmacotherapists who customize, monitor, and adjust therapeutic modalities to assure effective patient outcomes. These pharmacists also advise physicians on the safe and effective use of highly toxic or dangerous medications which remain in the prescription only status.

This conference surveying change in pharmacy from 1980 to 2010 closed with a presentation on manpower utilization which suggested that the pharmacist's productivity and effectiveness have increased substantially over the past 30 years. The number of pharmacists increased less than 10% in this period while the nation's population increased more than 25%. Few pharmacy technicians are used today, in contrast to the latter part of the 20th century, due to high technology robotics and mechanization.

Pharmacists in the 21st century continue to make very significant contributions to the level of health and wellness which our society enjoys today. That concludes today's news from the health sector. Good day and be well.

REPROFESSIONALIZATION IN PHARMACY[d]

Arnold Birenbaum

There is a spectre haunting the profession of pharmacy, manifest in the fear of displacement and downgrading of the craft. This concern is strikingly similar to the fears expressed by English artisans in the late eighteenth century when faced with the rise of the factory system of production (1). The honorable craft of pharmacy is facing a loss of power or control over scarce resources, including the utilization of learned skills, and the loss of status or the social approval accorded by others.

Reprofessionalization is advocated by elites in pharmacy but it is met with resistance inside and outside the field. The goal of upgrading pharmacy into a clinical profession involves the acquisition of qualitatively different roles from those performed by members of the profession in the past. Simply to view pharmacy as smoothly changing from craft to profession ignores the new consciousness of those members of the profession who see themselves as clinicians—possessing knowledge which directly benefits patients, and services which deserve respect from both patients and physicians. A need for intervention for patients is brought about by universal recognition that adverse drug interactions can lead to death and is one of the ten leading causes of hospitalization. The pharmacist, by virtue of careful record keeping and knowledge of drug interactions, is able to warn patients and physicians when a drug therapy is prescribed which can adversely interact with a drug now being taken by a patient. A new practice has been created which goes far beyond filling a prescription; it is called clinical pharmacy.

The clinical pharmacy segment is seeking to change the knowledge, ability and motivation of pharmacists, and convince outsiders, e.g. physicians and hospital administrators, that pharmacists should be allowed to consult with patients and physicians. Having complete control over entry into the profession—physicians do not sit on the state pharmacy licensing boards—has been an insufficient basis for acquiring new responsibilities.

Medicine is not the only source of resistance. The clinically oriented members of the profession are also critical of the lack of unity in pharmacy. They note that community and hospital pharmacists have few common professional interests; that many older pharmacists have shown no interest in acquiring new knowledge and responsibilities; that there is a great deal of direct competition between community pharmacies. Further, the clinically oriented also find that physicians and patients do not give them enough respect, claiming that the entire profession is judged by the worst aspects of pharmacy, i.e. high prices, steering patients to over-the-counter drugs, lavish gifts to physicians and the filling of illegal prescriptions.

---

[d]Edited and reprinted with permission from Birenbaum A: Reprofessionalization in pharmacy. *Soc Sci Med* 16:871–878, 1982.

NEW BELIEFS AND REPROFESSIONALIZATION

Reprofessionalization represents both a problem (status and power loss) and an opportunity (new roles and recognition). Larson (2) considers professionalization a form of social mobility. The success of a profession's organizational efforts determines whether mobility is going to occur, and such an effort must be cooperative among those similarly situated.

> . . . the professional project of social mobility is considered as a *collective* project, because only through a joint organizational effort could roles be created—or redefined—that would bring the desired social position to their occupants (italics in the original) (3).

Unlike medicine or engineering, pharmacy is not seeking to enhance its status as much as it seeks to avoid being dispossessed. Moreover, reprofessionalization must be accomplished within a highly complex health care system. Given the structural changes discussed above, and the idiom by which status is expressed in the medically dominated health care field in the United States, the direction pharmacy is compelled to take is away from the technical and business components and toward the clinical service ideal. Redefinitions of technical functions as clinical services has occurred in the health care field in the past. The specialities of anesthesiology, radiology and pathology which were once outside of medicine, became defined as clinical services and increased their prestige by joining it. Pharmacy has no such goals at this time but does demand more responsibility.

The goals of the advocates of clinical pharmacy reflect confidence in pharmacists as professionals who can work directly with patients; they also are viewed as information specialists. The increased education of pharmacists has made them more knowledgeable about drugs and adverse drug interactions. They can now not only observe other health care practitioners make mistakes in prescribing or administering medications but also explain to them *why* these procedures are in error. Such encounters confirm beliefs among pharmacists that they are rightfully drug experts.

Pharmacists are aware of their contribution to health care but are also dismayed at the lack of recognition for what they do. An independently derived report urges reforms in education and practice of pharmacy to make pharmacists better able to communicate their skills as clinicians and providers of information. The American Association of Colleges of Pharmacy commissioned a study directed by a noted scholar, John Millis, to evaluate the state of practice and education in pharmacy. The American Foundation for Pharmaceutical Education, an offshoot of the APhA, helped to fund the commission (4). The director of the commission had performed a similar study on graduate education in medicine a few years earlier.

The Millis report, like the Flexner report on medicine 60 years ago, focuses on the need to remove the noted entrepreneurial character to the field. Moreover, the end of compounding is not considered as the removal of the technical basis of the craft but rather as a way of freeing the pharmacist to do more professional tasks. This theme has been echoed in various professional publications, pointing to the ". . . widespread and serious problems related to the use of therapeutic drugs . . ." (5). The advocates of reform argue that the pharmacist does not simply sell a product but provides an essential service, using the knowledge and training acquired to help the patient.

The tasks of removing drugs from a larger to smaller container and the typing of a label may be all there is to filling a prescription, as seen from the perspective of the ordinary citizen. For the professionally committed, there is no such thing as a simple prescription and the routine is symbolically transformed into a sacred trust.

The trouble is that *every* prescription, *every* situation, *every* question from a physician, nurse or patient, is potentially crucial. The pharmacist's response, his action, his answer can do the utmost good or cause the utmost harm or even death as a result. A major question for pharmacy and for pharmaceutical educators is how to orient the individual practitioner to view his practice in such a light (Italics are in the original) (6).

Clearly, this statement reflects a strong sense of responsibility. There are two dimensions to responsibility. First, there is the idea of careful work based on conscientiousness and avoiding unethical conduct, such as fee splitting with physicians who steer patients and illegal dispensing of desired medications. Second, there is the idea of sharing meaningful authority in providing health care, an authority now monopolized by the dominant profession of medicine. Some pharmacists seek increased responsibilities commensurate with their training, arguing that they be permitted to make generic drug substitutions for name brands, unless otherwise specified by the prescribing physician, to countersign the prescription after making sure that no medication error has been made, to advise all health care providers, including physicians, on the merits of new drugs, and to instruct and follow-up patients to insure medication compliance.

NEW DIRECTIONS

The two meanings of responsibility discussed above direct the field of pharmacy to enhancing the status of the field through self-improvement based on ethical behavior or to gaining power by being delegated meaningful responsibility. These two dimensions also represent two structural problems of all professionalization and reprofessionalization drives, namely, (1) how to gain recognition and approval for upgrading by demonstrating professional self-improvement (i.e. increased education and ethical conduct) and (2) how to gain control over resources so that members or adherents to the movement are sufficiently rewarded by participation to remain loyal (i.e. increased opportunity to receive higher pay and promotions for performing clinical roles). All modifications of pharmacy as a profession, it is hypothesized, will result from efforts to make the extraordinary behavior of pacemakers in pharmacy a part of the work of garden variety pharmacists and health care organizations.

The following predictions are made, based on the assumption that reprofessionalization in pharmacy will be in the direction of institutionalization, a social process which creates stabilized roles for the various leadership groups in efforts of professionals to gain power and status (7). It is not assumed that institutionalization through solving one problem (recognition or approval vs a stable reward system) will end all competition and conflict within the profession.

I.   A strong emphasis on inculcating professional values and techniques without acquiring opportunities to reward members through clinical practice will result in an inward looking effort to construct a more meaningful culture, similar to revitalization movements identified (8).

Wallace claims that these types of responses occur among dispossessed peoples and

. . . always originate in situations of social and cultural stress and are in fact, an effort on the part of the stress-laden to construct systems of dogma, myth, and ritual which are internally coherent as well as true descriptions of a world system and which thus will serve as guides to efficient action (9).

The specific form this direction will take in the field of pharmacy will be a strong emphasis on receiving deference and respect from patients, doctors and other significant role partners. Pharmacies both in the community and in hospitals will be so constructed to display the clinical concerns of practitioners, with consulting rooms and reference texts available. Public debate will focus on the ethical purity of the profession, manifested in discussions in professional journals and other forums of what is professional and unprofessional conduct.

II.   Alternatively, strong emphasis on sharing authority with physicians in health care organizations such as hospitals is likely to result in a process of segmentation within the field between the clinical pharmacists holding the rare Pharm. D. degree and the many licensed pharmacists with the bachelor's degree. Therefore, clinical pharmacy will be a special practice within the field, limited to clearly clinical settings.

To reach this outcome, there would have to be an opportunity for educated and trained clinical pharmacists to perform an expanded role in health care delivery, demonstrating effectiveness in terms of higher quality care than before and being able to save money in some other area of service.

Leadership from hospital pharmacy will focus on the organizational contribution that clinical pharmacy can make, particularly in the area of reducing the costs of care. Clinical pharmacists who improve patient compliance will reduce the likelihood of rehospitalization. Further, clinical competency will be based on holding the doctoral degree, a way of convincing the medical profession that pharmacy has a right to shared authority. Consequently, the Master's degree in clinical pharmacy, currently a popular advanced degree, will not be considered sufficient training for clinical responsibilities. Furthermore, the hospital-based leadership will seek to make their branch of pharmacy a doctoral-led profession, aided by pharmacy technicians and assistants. These efforts will further the process of segmentation in pharmacy.

It is also possible that the hospital-based segment will actively work within professional associations to upgrade the entire profession, creating in-service training programs for baccalaureate pharmacists, with the legal right to practice as a clinician dependent on the doctoral degree and internship: in addition, the current conventional role of the community pharmacist would produce great strain among those practitioners because they would be subject to some downgrading by the rise of the more credentialed (Pharm. D.) clinical pharmacist.

Clinical pharmacy cannot demonstrate this effectiveness in helping patients unless resources are allocated to support this practice. A number of studies which have appeared over the past 10 years justify the expanded role of pharmacists in increasing patient compliance, but there is little evidence suggesting that hospitals save money as a result of these activities. For example, a controlled study of compliance among hypertensive patients showed a significant improvement in the number of patients who complied with prescribed therapy and a significant increase in the number of study patients whose blood pressures were kept within normal range during the study period, when clinical services were provided by a pharmacist (10). Deviation from prescribed drug regimens among discharged hospital patients were found among a control group receiving no consultation prior to going home while two study groups showed 90% compliance (11). However, one study of efforts to teach a study group of patients about their medications and labeling their drug containers with the contents did not significantly decrease the number of medication errors made at home (12).

There is a great deal of evidence that medications are not always administered correctly, particularly by elderly people with chronic illnesses:

> Two studies of elderly patients receiving care in clinical settings revealed that 59 per cent of the patients had made one or more errors in taking medications and roughly one quarter had made errors that could be classified as potentially serious (13).

Currently, other clinical health care providers do not see the pharmacist's major role as involvement with patients on a direct or regular basis. The pharmacist was perceived in one survey as having very little patient involvement and was encouraged to become more involved. Reviewing drug utilization was considered by clinical providers as the major clinical activity for pharmacists and should remain as such (14). Despite this limited acceptance by other health care providers, as of 1978, at least one clinical service was offered by pharmacists in 23% of the nationally surveyed acute care hospitals (15).

Evaluations of new modes of clinical participation continue to be performed and reported by pharmacists; these efforts serve to document their capacity to perform useful clinical services. Specific studies have compared the readability of patient information materials in order to learn how to more effectively reduce patient medication errors (16–18). Direct clinical interventions were compared in a project which used patient counseling and special medication containers to see whether compliance among 100 hypertensive patients could be improved. Each intervention was measured in combination and separately in this controlled study. Rehder *et al.* (19) reported that combined interventions had an additive effect in increasing compliance.

Therapeutic pharmacy consultations with patients were also evaluated. Clinical pharmacists in a family practice office worked with physicians in providing information about a patient's drug therapy, and in some instances, making specific recommendations for immediate implementation. Sixteen physicians independently evaluated these consultations, concluding that the pharmacist's recommendations were appropriate and had favorable effects on patient care (20). In an unrelated study, patients in a family care practice were asked to evaluate the quality of health care received both with and without pharmacy consultations (21). Those patients who had encounters with pharmacists were significantly more satisfied with their health care than the control groups. Finally, McKenney *et al.* (22) compared drug therapy assessments for ambulatory patients made by pharmacists and primary physicians. Pharmacists were able to detect drug therapy problems and recommend appropriate actions for resolving them. The differences between the pharmacist's assessment and physician agreement were not significant.

Reprofessionalization in pharmacy faces considerable resistance because of three structural features of the carriers of this drive. First, the strongest advocates of the clinical role are among pharmacists who are most vulnerable to retaliation because they are young, are not well known to other health care providers at the workplace, and not protected by bureaucratic rules or seniority. Secondly, the strongest concentration of advocates for clinical roles are in academic posts and are not in direct practice. The Pharm. D. who educates does not face the day-to-day resistances found in hospitals. Finally, pharmacy students, by virtue of the location of their colleges on campus which often do not have medical colleges, have little opportunity to interact with physicians in training. Therefore, they only come into contact with physicians in superior-subordinate relationships, making it difficult for them to convince doctors that they can make a clinical contribution. Moreover, they cannot influence new generations of physicians when they are easily influenced and before they professionally close ranks as practicing physicians.

That the carriers of the ideas of clinical pharmacy may influence a new generation of graduates of colleges of pharmacies, there can be no doubt. Whether they will produce the results they intend may have more to do with their way of solving problems of adaptation in a stressful environment.

REFERENCES

1. Thompson EP. The Making of the English Working Class, Vintage, New York, 1963.
2. Larson MS. The Rise of Professionalism: A Sociological Analysis, University of California, Berkeley, 1977.
3. Larson MS. *ibid*, 67.
4. Millis J. Pharmacists for the Future: The Report of the Study Commission on Pharmacy, Health Administration Press, Ann Arbor, MI, 1975.
5. Editorial Effect of upgraded pharmacy education on pharmacy practice, Am J Hosp Pharm 1977;34:929.
6. Knapp DA, Knapp DE. An appraisal of the contemporary practice of pharmacy, Am J Hosp Pharm 1968;32:749.
7. Parson T. Professions, Int Encycl Soc Sci 1968;12:536-547.
8. Wallace AFC. Religion: An Antropologic View, p. 30, Random House, New York, 1966.
9. Wallace AFC. *ibid*.
10. McKenney JM, *et al*. The effect of clinical pharmacy services on patients with essential hypertension, Circulation 1973;48:1104.
11. Cole D, Emmanuel S. Drug consultation: Its significance to the discharged hospital patient and its relevance as a role for the pharmacist, Am J Hosp Pharm 1971;23:960.
12. Malahy B. The effect of instruction and labeling on the number of medication errors made by patients at home, Am J Hosp Pharm 1966;23:292.
13. Smith DB. A cooperative pharmacy project: An autopsy on a community health intervention, J Comm Hlth 1977;2:223.
14. Lambert EL, *et al*. The pharmacist's clinical role as seen by other health workers, Am J Publ Hlth 1977;67:253.
15. Stolar MM. National survey of hospital pharmaceutical services—1978, Am J Hosp Pharm 1979;36:316-325.
16. Spadaro DC, Robinson LA, Smith LT. Assessing readability of patient information materials, Am J Hosp Pharm 1980;37:215-221.
17. Eaton ML, Holloway RL. Patient comprehension of written drug information, Am J Hosp Pharm 1980;37:240-243.
18. Morris LA, Myers A, Thilmen DG. Application of the readability concept to patient-oriented drug information, Am J Hosp Pharm 1980;37:504-508.
19. Rehder T, *et al*. Improving medication compliance by counseling and special prescription container, Am J Hosp Pharm 1980;37:379-385.
20. Brown DJ, Helling DK, Jones ME. Evaluation of clinical pharmacist consultation in a family practice office, Am J Hosp Pharm 1974;36:912-915.
21. Helling DK, Hepler CD, Jones ME. Effect of direct clinical pharmaceutical services on patients' perceptions of health care quality, Am J Hosp Pharm 1979;36:325-329.
22. McKenney JM, *et al*. Drug therapy assessments by pharmacists, Am J Hosp Pharm 1980;37:824-828.

NEED FOR A THEORETICAL BASE FOR PHARMACY PRACTICE[e]

Donald C. Brodie

We have passed over the threshold into the 1980s. The only certainty of today is the uncertainty of tomorrow. Our nation probably has never entered a decade with more formidable

[e]Edited and reprinted with permission from Brodie DC: Need for a theoretical base for pharmacy practice. *Am J Hosp Pharm* 38:49-54, 1981. This paper was based on Dr. Brodie's 1980 Harvey A.K. Whitney Lecture.

issues to be solved than those which lie ahead in the 1980s. One of the issues of particular concern is the entire spectrum of problems involving health; changing roles of health professionals, the cost of health care and cost containment, health manpower and the use of support personnel, the role of government in health care delivery, the impact of computers and high technology, and the numerous problems in bio-ethics resulting from recombinant DNA research. For the profession of pharmacy as a whole, the central issue will continue to be the acceptance of the fact and reality of change and the determination to take an active role in shaping that change. The alternatives seem obvious: pharmacy either accepts what the future brings or works to shape the future in accordance with what pharmacists want that future to be. One of the difficult problems will be the identification of changes before and as they occur and the development of strategies to deal with them. One strategy that is available to us is the development of a theoretical base for pharmacy practice. To my knowledge, pharmacists have never been challenged by the idea that there might be a theory (or a family of theories) dealing with the practice of pharmacy and that such theory or theories could be useful in directing the course of our future.

A THEORETICAL BASE

I am defining "theoretical base" to mean an intellectual framework designed to serve the purpose and needs of future planning for pharmacy. The framework or structure is based on empirical information that is consistent with data available to support it either in the literature or elsewhere. You will sense from this definition that we are dealing with a structure composed of concepts and other sets of abstract ideas that, when brought together, form an ideal state. In fact, Dickoff and James (1), in their definition of "theory," emphasize the abstract nature of theory:

> . . . a conceptual system or framework invented to some purpose; and as the purpose varies so too must vary the structure and complexity of the system.

What a worthy objective for the profession were it to begin building a theoretical base for pharmacy practice during the decade of the 80s. Such an effort will not lead to a neatly bound compendium entitled, "A Theory of Pharmacy Practice." Rather, it will be in the form of a series of ideas, statements, hypotheses, and other forms of abstraction. When statements about pharmacists and pharmacy can be interrelated and describe a causal process (relationship), they can be studied, documented, and tested. If empirical data can be derived from causal processes and combined with existing data, they can be presented to members of the pharmacy profession for study, modification, and adoption. Where existing data are not adequate, research will be necessary to provide the documentation. What we are striving for is to develop a conceptual base in the form of ideas, constructs, and statements which describes, clarifies, and strengthens the societal position of pharmacy and its practitioners. It is part of the scientific body of knowledge about pharmacy developed by pharmacists in keeping with the purposes of pharmacy. In his introductory statement to his *Primer in Theory Construction,* Professor Paul Reynolds (2) states:

> A scientific body of knowledge consists of those concepts and statements that scientists consider useful for achieving the purposes of science.

As our statements and concepts lead to tangible evidence that documents the purpose and needs of pharmacy they begin to shape the framework which ultimately will encompass the theoretical base of pharmacy practice.

MODELS OF PROFESSIONAL BEHAVIOR

The construction of models of professional behavior is a useful step in the development of a theoretical base for pharmacy practice. Models, representations of reality or some hypothetical state of reality, are designed to provide clarity, understanding, and guidance. Models have been useful in studying social systems, such as systems of evaluation or patterns of human behavior. They can be constructed to represent new or modified roles for health professionals as a means of examining their proposed utility and general acceptance. A model for pharmacists, for example, would emphasize those contributions unique to pharmacists because of their education and training, such as monitoring drug therapy, applying pharmacokinetic principles to the design and adjustment of dose regimens, providing drug information to physicians and patients, and maintaining individual patient records of drug usage. It would include activities being developed by selected pharmacists in the care of certain classes of patients (oncology) in hospitals and ambulant patients in the out-of-hospital setting, and the reciprocal relationships between physicians and pharmacists designed to improve the level of patient care. The model would include those activities that are at variance with traditional pharmacist functions, such as the prescribing of drugs as currently being done legally on an experimental basis in California (3). In each instance, the uniqueness of the pharmacist's contribution to society would be emphasized as well as the desire and confidence pharmacists have in serving societal needs. Obviously, such a model would represent an alternative to pharmacists' traditional behavior, and if it were constructed, could be studied to determine its acceptability by present-day pharmacists, the public, and other health professionals. The degree of acceptability would provide justification and guidance to the profession for developing the modified role specified in the model. Similarly, it would guide the schools of pharmacy in adjusting the pharmacy curriculum in keeping with the new role.

PARADIGM FOR THE PROFESSIONS

If pharmacists were to begin construction of a theoretical base they would find a useful guideline in the generally accepted pattern of professional behavior usually referred to as the paradigm for the professions. The literary form in which the paradigm is presented will vary from scholar to scholar, but there is general agreement in terms of behavioral characteristics. I have chosen a model adapted from one presented by Argyris and Schön in their text, "Theory in Practice: Increasing Professional Effectiveness" (4).

1. An ideology—based on the original faith professed by a profession.
2. An ethic—that is binding on the practitioners of a profession.
3. A body of knowledge—unique to a given profession.
4. A set of skills—which, when combined, form the technique of a profession.
5. A guild—of those entitled to practice a profession—the brotherhood.
6. Authority—granted by society as a form of professional respect and licensure or certification.
7. An institutional setting—where a profession is practiced in a standardized environment such as hospital, courtroom, pharmacy, and church.
8. A theory—based on the societal benefits derived from the faith professed—the ideology.

Historically, the prototypical professional was the priest who practiced as a multiprofessional in an undifferentiated way, serving as minister, judge, healer, and teacher. In time, the professions of theology, law, medicine, and education were differentiated from the priesthood as secular institutions. The process of differentiation has been replicated many times in history with the growth of knowledge and skill where today we recognize some 200 professions, more than 50 of which are in the health field. Pharmacy was differentiated from medicine in the late Middle Ages and stands today as one of the autonomous health professions with a very specific mission in society (5). That mission, however, has suffered from the lack of definition over the past 50 years as the responsibility for making medicines has passed to the pharmaceutical industry. Some questions have been raised by social scientists and others regarding the professional status of pharmacy because of the passive attitudes and behavior of many pharmacists, the environment in which much pharmacy is practiced, and the apparent belief that the boundaries of the pharmacist's social responsibility are circumscribed by the act of pharmaceutical dispensing. These matters should be of concern to us as we begin to think of a theoretical base for pharmacy practice.

Because the professions have their roots in religion, Palmer (6) was prompted to say:

> A professional, as I understand it, is supposed to profess, to testify, to bear witness to some sort of faith or confidence or point of view. Traditionally, at least, it was only because he did so that he merited being called "professional."

Thus, medicine professed health, law professed justice, education professed truth, and the ministry professed salvation. And pharmacy—what did pharmacy profess? We have difficulty with this question in today's world. We do not have a clear picture of nor do we communicate with conviction that which we profess. As a result, the transformation of what we profess into a professional ideology seems distorted or in some way is incomplete. A question that has nagged me for years deals with the idea that at one time pharmacists did make a strong testimony of commitment to society that ultimately was transformed into an ideology for the profession. In the mid 60s I was searching for an answer by identifying a mainstream function for medicine, law, theology, and other professions; I could not identify one for pharmacy. In the report of the Commission on Pharmaceutical Services to Ambulant Patients by Hospitals and Related Facilities (7), I wrote:

> Does pharmacy practice have, in a historic sense, a mainstream component as have other professions? Has it had one only to lose it to time, science, technology, and social change? Has it had one only to lose it to professional neglect, such as over-indulgence in nonprofessional activities, or, perhaps, an attempt to serve the public on a part-time basis? Has it had one that in time has become so ill-defined in its outline that both practitioner and layman alike have difficulty in identifying the distinguishing marks?

I am forced to acknowledge that the faith pharmacists professed in my time has not led to a strong professional ideology that generates confidence in the values that are inherent in the services pharmacists provide. That ideology must be strengthened and restored for the 21st Century envisioned by Alvin Toffler (8) and other futurists. No doubt some of the historic ideology has eroded with the industrialization of pharmacy which stripped the practitioner of many creative functions unique to him.

Without a clear ideological component in the professional paradigm, the task of constructing a theoretical base for pharmacy practice is made difficult. The ideology, fully developed, envisions a better world because of the availability of drugs and drug-related services delivered by pharmacists who are educated and trained to fulfill these societal needs (9). Because of the availability of these services, society is the beneficiary; without them, the welfare of society is in jeopardy. As we think about our professional ideology and plan construction of a theoretical base for professional practice, there is yet another component that lacks clear definition in the minds of most people, including pharmacists. That component is an identified and articulated professional purpose. During my search for identity of a mainstream function for pharmacy, I proposed that drug-use control was that function:

> . . . the sum total of knowledge, understanding, judgments, procedures, skills, controls, and ethics that assures optimal safety in the distribution and use of medication.

This concept gave us light at the end of what seemed, at the time, to be a badly obscured tunnel. Penna (10) commented recently that this concept provided a ray of hope to "younger pharmacists" and "identified what pharmacists should be doing in serving the health needs of the American public." Is the concept of drug-use control our professional purpose? What is the object for which pharmacy exists? Is that object essential for the welfare of society or is it a convenience? I believe there is general agreement among pharmacists that their role in society is the delivery of the drug component of health care, but just what the limits of that role are is a question for which there is as yet no universal agreement. The answer, in my opinion, will direct the future course of pharmacy in our time. If that role expands as a result of progressive and responsible behavior, the slope of the curve of professionalism will be positive; if pharmacists choose to retain their traditional behavior, the slope almost surely will regress.

PHARMACISTS' BEHAVIOR

Pharmacists' behavior has changed perceptibly since World War II, undergoing the greatest change in the 1960s with the emergence of an expanded clinical role. If one lists the services pharmacists are providing today, he would find that they could be arranged in one of three categories:

1. Services mandated by law, rule, or regulation.
2. Discretionary services provided by a majority of pharmacists.
3. Discretionary services provided by a small minority of pharmacists.

He would find that there would not be a consensus among pharmacists that they should provide all the listed discretionary services. Even if the list were submitted to hospital pharmacists on the one hand and community practitioners on the other, still there would not be agreement among those in either group. But if the profession seeks guidance in the development of an expanded clinical role for its practitioners, it must rely particularly on its acceptability by pharmacists in addition to that by the public and other health professionals. This leads to a researchable question:

> What is the degree of consensus among pharmacists, consumers, and other health care providers on the acceptability of an expanded role for pharmacists, including the clinical services assumed in the current model?

The following,[f] or some such list of pharmacists' services, can be used to determine the degree of consensus. Whatever list is used, it should contain those clinical services already provided by pharmacists (to assess the minimal level of consensus) and a brief description of each service (to aid respondents). These services, incorporated into a scientifically designed and tested questionnaire, can be submitted to an agreed upon population of pharmacists,

---

[f]In compiling this list, I referred to Standards of Practice for the Profession of Pharmacy, *Am Pharm* 1979;NS19:22–35.

consumers, and physicians in order to answer two questions: Should the service be provided by any health professional? Should pharmacists provide the service?

1. Compounds and dispenses prescriptions.
2. Assumes custodial care and responsibility for the distribution of controlled substances.
3. Explains the directions for use of prescription medicines at the time of delivery of prescriptions to ambulant patients.
4. Delivers package inserts (PPIs) to patients at the time of delivery of estrogens and progestational agents.
5. Establishes and monitors a system to insure proper storage for perishable pharmacy items such as insulin and other biological products.
6. Selects the manufacturing source of drug products to be purchased under generic names.
7. Maintains prescription profile records for ambulant patients.
8. Refers to prescription profile records prior to dispensing refill prescriptions.
9. Obtains a drug history on selected inpatients and ambulant patients.
10. Conducts drug-use studies at periodic intervals using computer printouts and other sources of data.
11. Develops guidelines for the use of antibiotics.
12. Applies pharmacokinetic principles in determining or modifying the dose of selected drugs.
13. Provides patient counseling on an individual basis or through some form of mass media.
14. Provides formal and informal consultations with physicians regarding patient drug therapy problems.
15. Applies selected physical assessment techniques in evaluating patients responses to drug therapy.
16. Provides supplies and appropriate counseling services in the use of ostomy appliances and other surgical and sick room supplies.
17. Provides emergency services such as poison information, cardiovascular pulmonary resuscitation, and counseling regarding the appropriate use of drugs in emergent situations.
18. Reviews periodically the use of drugs in nursing homes, in accordance with professional and legal standards.
19. Participates in home health care programs with public health nurses.
20. Interprets drug levels for selected drugs in order to obtain optimal benefit in drug therapy.

Assuming that a scientifically valid study is conducted and the results showed a consensus ranging from 55 to 70% in support of pharmacists assuming an expanded role, what significance might these results have? They surely would lend support, confidence, and direction to the profession in its efforts to improve the utility of its practitioners. On the other hand, if one or both of the nonpharmacist groups believed that pharmacists should not provide the services, it would lead to an understanding of reality and simultaneously provide guidance in developing long-range strategy to shape that reality. But, in addition, such a study would contribute to the development of a theory for pharmacy practice. I have used this example because it illustrates how the profession of pharmacy can relate "theory development" to planning for the future. It places future planning in a broader frame of reference than we are accustomed to using.

The worth of pharmacy to society is judged by the actions and services of its practitioners. These actions justify or deny its recognition and acceptance as a profession. Pharmacists provide action; they are doers; they, as other professionals, define their scope of social concern through a more or less standardized pattern of professional behavior. They create, construct, and maintain reality. But the true professional does more than create, construct, and maintain the status quo. He shapes and changes reality and has before him those purposes that have been "invented" or "created" by and for his profession. Dickoff and James (1) summarize professional purpose as follows: ". . . a professional cannot just watch, cannot just do, and cannot just hope or dream. . . . A theory for a profession or practice discipline must provide for more than mere understanding or 'describing' or even predicting reality and must provide a conceptualization specially intended to guide the shaping of reality to that profession's professional purpose."

You in my audience tonight—pharmacists, scientists, and researchers—have the ability and the capacity to shape and change that reality; I challenge you to commit yourselves to such a goal because you have the vision and discipline to do so. But a theoretical base for pharmacy practice cannot be perceived according to traditional views of the world as we know it today. Our professional purpose and ideology must be perceived and articulated in view of that world we believe lies ahead. No one knows precisely the dimensions of that world but futurists are beginning to give us a glimpse of some of its characteristics. Alvin Toffler (8) says:

> Today, four clusters of related industries are poised for major growth and are likely to become the backbone industries of the Third Wave era, bringing with the, once more, major shifts in economic power and in social and political alignments.

Those industries—electronics and computers, space exploration, ocean exploration, and genetic engineering—all will have an impact on the future practice of pharmacy.

Futurist, Robert Theobald (11), said in 1978:

> We should recognize that we must move away from our industrial/mobile society toward a communication/community society. This shift will require modification in our social patterns which will be at least as great as those which occurred between the agricultural era and industrial era but they will take place far more rapidly. One of the most worrying aspects of the present period is the failure to understand the speed and scope of the microelectronic revolution which will change so much of our lives in the next decade.

Mr. Theobald's last sentence reminds us that the "future is now" (12). I am going into that future with hope and optimism notwithstanding the negative signs that surround us. I believe that you as hospital pharmacists and the Society which directs your professional destinies can share in my confidence. The experience, the successes, and the failures of the past justify our approach to the future, with the anticipation that the problems we find there will be solvable and that we can solve them. And that being so, justifies our hope and confidence for continued growth.

REFERENCES

1. Dickoff J, James P. A theory of theories: a position paper. In: Readings in nursing research I. Approaches to nursing research and theory development in nursing. New York: Nursing Research; 1969:31-7.

2. Reynolds PD. Primer in theory construction. Indianapolis: The Bobbs-Merrill Company, Inc.; 1971:3.
3. Assembly Bill 717, state of California health manpower projects. 1977 Sep 15.
4. Argyris C, Schön DA. Theory in practice: increasing professional effectiveness. San Francisco: Jossey-Bass Publishers; 1974:146-9.
5. Urdang G. Pharmacy's part in society. Madison, WI: American Institute of the History of Pharmacy; 1946:9.
6. Palmer P. Professions in the seventies. Church society for college work; 1973:2-6.
7. Report of the Commission on Pharmaceutical Services to Ambulant Patients by Hospitals and Related Facilities. The challenge to pharmacy in times of change. Washington, DC: the American Pharmaceutical Association and the American Society of Hospital Pharmacists; 1966.
8. Toffler A. The third wave. New York: William Morrow and Company, Inc.; 1980.
9. Brodie DC, Parish PA, Poston JW. Society needs for drugs and drug-related services. Am J Pharm Educ 1980;44:276-8.
10. Penna RP. Fifty years—has the profession come full circle? Address before the St. John's University College of Pharmacy and Allied Health Professions golden jubilee symposium. 1979 Oct 14.
11. Theobald R. Special study on economic change. Testimony before the joint economic committee, U.S. Congress; 1978, May 31. In: Sheppard CS, Carroll DC, eds. Working in the twenty-first century. New York: John Wiley and Sons; 1980:30-1.
12. The future is now. A conference of the Northeast Regional Assembly of constituent leagues for nursing. New York: National League for nursing; 1974.

4
Pharmacy

WILLIAM F. McGHAN

PHARMACY IN RETROSPECT

When reviewing the long history and evolution of the pharmacy profession, one has to consider that perhaps the longer the tail of a profession, the slower that profession is to respond to change in social need. Although a long history provides many interesting reflections, one might argue that history creates traditions and attitudes that may be difficult to modify. It may help protect the social domains of the pharmacy profession, but does history help the profession change as rapidly as a newer discipline, such as physician assistants and nurse practitioners? Perhaps every social group reminisces about the golden years or opportunities gone by, but many observers of pharmacy remark that we have given up too much control over drugs and drug therapy. Only by reviewing the history and assessing where the profession is now can we make better judgments for the future of the profession and its potential significance in society.

Each health profession, at least since the 1960s, seems to argue that it is expanding its functions to better meet the needs of society and, since medicine attempts to cover every professional function, so they always claim intrusion.

As a broad model, physicians may be viewed as the profession that interfaces between man and disease; priests intervene between man and spirit, and lawyers are the professional interface between man and man. Pharmacists then are the professionals that interface between man and medicines. There are different historical roles that relate to pharmacy, which have evolved from medicine man to the apothecary, pharmacist (compounder), and now clinical pharmacist. These titles reflect a stormy evolution for the profession that interfaces man with drugs, and the historical discussion below will elaborate on these descriptions.

The medicine man is a role that reaches back to prehistoric times of mankind and is a link between all health professions even today. These priestly healers or sorcerers, who among American Indians are still present as shamans, were familiar with spirit rituals and magic herbs. It is interesting to consider that this role existed back several millenia BC and then evolved into the three distinct professions of priest, physician, and pharmacist. Not until 1200 AD were physician and pharmacist professions officially first separated from one another by a German emperor. During the plague in England in the 1600s, many physicians died or immigrated out of the cities in fear of the disease, leaving apothecaries to provide a great deal of medical care to the citizens (1).

In the Colonial period of this country, the apothecary often performed the role of both physician and pharmacist for the community. It is interesting to consider that one thing that solidified the independence of pharmacy in the 1800s was when a medical school began encouraging pharmacists to enroll and raise their standards to that of physicians. The negative reaction of pharmacists toward medicine stimulated the founding of the first school of pharmacy, the Philadelphia College of Pharmacy, in 1821 (1).

From the Colonial days until the 1930s, pharmacists were the "compounders" in the "cottage pharmacy era." Pharmacists were experts in botanicals and various chemicals needed to compound the complicated medicines that, unfortunately, were often of questionable efficacy. Not until 1938 did the Federal Food and Drug Administration require that new drugs released on the market be proven safe, and not until 1962 did drugs have to be proven effective.

Just as concern for drug safety and efficacy was evolving between the 1930s and 1960s, also evolving was the role of the pharmacist. More medicines were being manufactured by a rapidly growing pharmaceutical industry, and there was far less compounding required by pharmacists. The dosage forms were thus already prepared and this led to a more mechanical pharmacy practice with terms like "count/pour" and "lick/stick." While this was occurring, pharmacy education also shifted from a 4- to a 5-year curriculum. These curricula were training the pharmacist to be more patient oriented, learning what drugs did in the human body, and how to use drug information to improve rational drug therapy.

It is disheartening that in 1952, two federal legislators who were also pharmacists, Durham and Humphrey, created a legal barrier to the expansion of pharmacist control over drugs on their own pharmacy shelves. They, and apparently the pharmacy associations at the time, were convinced that drugs were becoming more potent and needed to be limited to physician prescription. The legend of "Caution—Federal law prohibits dispensing without a prescription" has left the pharmacist in an indecisive, distributive role with drugs that they can only fill with a physician's order or over-the-counter (OTC) drugs that can be sold in supermarkets and vending machines with no pharmacist required (2).

CLINICAL PHARMACY

Since the 1960s, we have been entering the age of the clinical pharmacist in which we are dispensing knowledge as our product for patients and physicians. As new drugs were released on the market, pharmacy and pharmacy schools began to move to more pharmacology, clinical therapeutics, and pharmacokinetics. During the 1960s, some schools began 6-year curricula leading to the doctor of pharmacy degree. Hospital pharmacy seemed to take the lead in this clinical movement as several studies indicated that, with the many powerful drugs used in hospitals, adverse drug reactions were a serious problem that needed the involvement of pharmacy (3).

Although the Durham-Humphrey legislation has restricted the authority of the profession, most all states allow drug product selection by pharmacists and a few states have enacted limited pharmacist-prescribing legislation. These include California, Washington, Mississippi, and Florida. The laws in each state evolved differently. Washington slipped into their practice act a clause stating that the pharmacist could, under protocol, initiate and modify therapy. This terminology was later interpreted by the state government as allowing drug prescribing by pharmacists. After this happened, medical lobbyists in all states began previewing pharmacy acts more carefully. California pharmacy leaders negotiated directly with the medical society for a bill that allows pharmacists to prescribe drugs under protocol in institutional settings. Florida legislation now allows pharmacists to prescribe a limited number of drugs, such as antihistamines and several topical agents. The Mississippi law is similar to the California legislation and allows pharmacists to initiate and modify drug therapy under protocols approved by the board of pharmacy. Pharmacists have proposed expanding their state practice acts in numerous other states including Arizona, North Carolina, and Kentucky. Several pharmacy leaders have suggested that the prescribing role for the pharmacist is a natural progression of their expert knowledge about drugs. It may be that the attachment of pharmacy to traditional drug distribution roles has limited its control compared to the newer disciplines of physician assistants and nurse practitioners who can prescribe in 21 states compared to the four for pharmacy (4).

DEFINING PHARMACY TODAY

If a consumer checks on "pharmacy" in Webster's dictionary, he or she will find that lexicographers have not recognized the changing face of pharmacy and that they generally define the profession as the art or practice of preparing, preserving, compounding, and dispensing drugs.

The Millis Study Commission on Pharmacy defined pharmacy as both a service and a knowledge system, stating that pharmacy is "a system which renders a health service by concerning itself with knowledge about drugs and their effects on men and animals" (5).

The most assertive definition of the pharmacist role has been given through Dr. Donald C. Brodie's concept of *"drug use control* which involves the sum total of knowledge, judgment, procedures, skills, and ethics that assures optimal safety (and effectiveness) in the distribution and use of medication."

A national conference convened in February 1985 by the American Society of Hospital Pharmacists developed a high degree of consensus for the following statements (6):

- A fundamental purpose of the profession of pharmacy is to serve as a force in society for safe and appropriate use of drugs.
- Pharmacists should continue to have ultimate responsibility for drug-distribution and drug-control activities, but these functions should be carried out by technicians under pharmacists' general supervision, thus freeing the major portion of pharmacists' time for clinical services. Further, drug distribution should be mechanized and automated to as great an extent as possible (7).

Hepler, at the consensus conference, suggested that pharmacy, as any health profession, has a covenant, an agreement with society. Society asks a profession to abide by certain rules in providing very complex services and its profession is then given certain authority in the community (8). As pharmacy continues to document the cost-effectiveness of its services, society will grant pharmacists increased authority over drug use (9).

At this Hilton Head conference, Hepler argued that although pharmacy has often been defined in terms of informative and consultative functions, the discipline will best advance as a profession if it defines its service in terms of responsibility for the total drug-use control process, accepting responsibility for the appropriate use of drugs in patients, including providing medicines to the patients. These concepts are congruent with many leaders in the profession who have advocated that there should be a third class of drugs available only from a pharmacist and that more pharmacists should be able to prescribe drugs as they are able to do in just a few states now (10).

MANPOWER

There were an estimated 157,000 active registered pharmacists in the United States in 1984. Two-thirds of all active pharmacists worked in community pharmacies, of whom somewhat more than one-half were in chain store pharmacies with the remainder in independent pharmacies. The remaining one-third worked in hospitals, nursing homes, government, education, or manufacturing and were basically salaried employees (11).

The number of pharmacists working in independently owned pharmacies has decreased significantly in recent years. In 1966, 68.5% of the pharmacists either owned or worked in independent community pharmacies and in 1978, only 38% worked in independent settings. More than three in 10 active pharmacists worked in chain pharmacies in 1980, and the proportion in hospitals was more than two in 10. The number of pharmacists in hospitals nearly doubled between 1973 and 1980, from 17,000 to an estimated 30,000. In essence, in less than 20 years, pharmacy has changed from a profession characterized by practitioners who were pharmacy owners to one in which pharmacists are predominantly employees.

There has been a dramatic increase in the percentage of women joining the profession. In 1950, only 4% of active pharmacists were women; by 1980, the proportion had risen to 19% and they represent 57% of the pharmacy student enrollment. In 1985, there were 24,820 students enrolled in entry-level Pharm. D. or baccalaureate degree programs, and 2,852 of these students were in Pharm. D. programs for their first professional degree (11).

In a major national study of pharmacists, it was interesting to see what pharmacists do with their practice time. Based on an analysis of many activities, the results were aggregated into seven categories and percentage of time as depicted in Table 4.1 (12).

HOSPITAL PHARMACY PRACTICE CHARACTERISTICS

The American Society of Hospital Pharmacists has surveyed a random sample of hospitals 4 times between 1975 and 1985. As a measure of pharmacists' increasing interest and involvement in drug use control, the number of hospitals with complete unit dose distribution systems has increased from 17.6 to 62.4% over that 10-year period. The number of hospitals with computerized pharmacy systems continues to grow and by the spring of 1986, it is projected that 50% of all hospitals will have computerized pharmacy systems. In the last

Table 4.1   Time Spent by Pharmacists in Various Activities Based on a National Survey[a]

Activity	Overall Percentage of Time
Processing the prescription	48.1
Patient care functions	11.5
General management and administration	12.8
Inventory, record keeping, and control	8.0
Purchasing and receiving	7.2
Personnel administration	5.0
Education of public, etc.	7.4

[a]Adapted from American Pharmaceutical Association. A National Study of the Practice of Pharmacy. Washington DC, 1978.

several years, the surveys have shown significant increases in clinical services including written medication histories, counseling patients, monitoring of drug therapy, rounds with medical staff, and pharmacokinetic consultations (13).

COMMUNITY PHARMACY PRACTICE CHARACTERISTICS

Although there are nonrandom annual financial surveys, there is no periodic national random sample survey of services provided community and chain pharmacies that would provide longitudinal characteristics of pharmacy practice outside hospitals. There have been single state surveys of how pharmacists spend their time comparing hospitals to independent and chain pharmacies. Chain pharmacists report that they spend more time processing prescriptions than pharmacists in other settings, and hospital pharmacists spend more time in patient care functions, followed by independent, then chain pharmacists.

It is estimated that over 55% of all retail pharmacies, chain and independent, use a computer in their practice. By 1990, it is suggested that the computer will become as commonplace in pharmacies as the cash register. This is based on the projection that entrylevel systems are rapidly approaching the price of a cash register and, for pharmacists to remain competitive in the marketplace, they will need to have access to information that only a computer can provide. Computer programs can remind the pharmacist about refill times and check for drug interactions as the prescription is being processed. With a computer and telephone modem, pharmacists in even the most rural areas can access the huge clinical information sources available through the National Library of Medicine and other sources (14).

VIEWS FROM OUTSIDE PHARMACY: CONSUMERS

Although the pharmacy profession is undergoing internal turmoil concerning direction and definition, consumers still seem to have positive feelings about the pharmacist. For the last few years, pharmacists have been rated as the top health professional group in national surveys of the public on honesty and ethics. The only group to rate higher in the public mind is the clergy. The 1985 figures show that 65% of the American public rated "druggists, pharmacists" as "high, very high" in honesty and ethical standards, compared with a total of 67% for clergy. In the third position were physicians (58%), and some of the other categories evaluated included dentists (56%), college teachers (54%), policemen (47%), newspaper reporters (29%), and lawyers (27%) (15).

Further anecdotal discussions of how pharmacy is viewed come from classic works such as Koos' *The Health of Regionville* (16), and Studs Turkel's *Working* (17). In addition to the normal dispensing functions of the pharmacists in the rural community of Regionville, the pharmacist also helped families select over-the-counter drugs, advised on illnesses when a physician's care was not sought, and provided supplemental advice when physicians were being seen. In Turkel's portrayal of the fragmented workers in a technological society, the pharmacist he describes comes across as a personable figure who cares about his customers and enjoys his work.

On the more critical side, the Dichter Institute (1973) reported that consumers see the pharmacist more as a businessman than as a health professional. It recommended that pharmacists spend more time informing the public about the value of pharmaceutical services (18). With a sample of residents in Iowa, Yellin and Norwood (1974) studied the attitudes of consumers and factors related to those attitudes. They found that attitudes toward pharmacy were inversely associated with the educational level and family income of the consumers (19). Norwood followed up this cross-sectional survey with a prospective intervention in 1975, using two towns with families with one town serving as control and families in the other town serving as the treatment group that received expanded pharmacy services. Comparison of pre- and posttest data revealed no change in attitudes in the control group but, in the treatment group, there was significant improvement in the patients' attitudes toward pharmacy (20). Wertheimer et al. (1975), utilizing a consumer panel, found that consumers "want to converse directly with the pharmacist and want to know their pharmacist" (21).

A number of other studies have examined consumers' attitudes regarding pharmacy services. Knapp, Baird, and Winter (1976) found that two-thirds of consumers in a national survey obtained their information on OTC drugs from advertising or from friends. Only 20% mentioned the pharmacist as their source of information (22).

Gagnon (1977) found in a review of several studies that consumers wanted personalized, professional contact with their pharmacists, desired assurance of having the pharmacist available when they need him, and felt it important for the pharmacist to keep patient records (23). Patients in a family care practice were asked to evaluate the quality of health care received both with and without pharmacist consultation. Those patients who had pharmacist contact were significantly more satisfied with their health care than those who did not (24).

As an examination of the effects of national health insurance, Ricci, Enterline, and Henderson (1978) investigated the use of pharmacists before and after the introduction of national health insurance in the Province of Quebec. They found a dramatic reduction in advise seeking from the pharmacist once free medical care was introduced (25).

In 1978, Schering Laboratories undertook an ongoing series of survey studies designed to explore various attitudes about pharmacy. Their reports have covered such topics as consumers' perception of the pharmacists' role in OTC counseling, operational problems faced in pharmacies, and attitudes of physicians and pharmacists toward one another. The 1985 study revealed that the majority of consumers are very satisfied with the services they receive and, when selecting OTC drugs, the majority of consumers said they would buy the product the pharmacist recommends over the advice of friends or television. However, consumers said they would not dare take home a different product from the one specified by a spouse.

Going beyond attitudes, Schondelmeyer and Trinca (1983) (26) studied consumers' willingness to pay for pharmacist counseling by actually charging for the service separate from the price of the prescription. When counseling was offered for free, an average of 88.1% of patients used the service. When charged a fee, 25.9% participated. Various fee levels were charged, including $1, $2, and $3, and the mean rate of acceptance was 24.7%, 36.3%, and 16.7%, respectively. Greatest acceptance was demonstrated by patrons aged 36 to 45, and the larger amount they paid, the more they valued the service.

VIEWS FROM OUTSIDE PHARMACY: OTHER PROFESSIONALS

Knapp, Knapp, and Edwards (1969), concerned with the perceived occupational roles of pharmacists, conducted a study to assess attitudes toward pharmacists held by pharmacists, consumers, and physicians. They found that all groups, including pharmacists, placed the pharmacist closer to the concept of technician than that of professional. Most of the subject groups did not appear to hold the pharmacist in very high regard. The major exception to this finding was the strong, positive attitude toward the role held by pharmacy leaders. Knapp and coworkers suggested that pharmacists believed physicians to be more negative and critical than they actually were and that if pharmacists were aware of the willingness of some physicians to accept them on a more equal level, they might be less hesitant in offering more professional services (27).

Norwood et al. (1976) examined the attitudes of rural consumers and physicians and concluded that the enthusiasm of pharmacy for greatly enlarged roles (i.e., preliminary diagnosis, screening, and treatment) is not shared by rural consumers or physicians. Both groups, however, did support provision of health information and treatment in emergencies by the pharmacist (28).

Lambert and coworkers (1977) surveyed physicians, social workers, osteopaths, nurses, and other health professionals of the Minnesota Public Health Association and found that efforts to incorporate clinical pharmacy services into practice had not been entirely successful. These researchers suggested that pharmacists were not aware of their full range of possible activities and were not sufficiently aggressive in cultivating new areas (29).

Bernstein et al. (1978) categorized the type of physician most likely to use and have a positive attitude toward clinical pharmacy services and suggested that the optimal situation occurs when the physician is young, group-practice oriented, writes a large number of prescriptions, and has been exposed to the services of a clinical pharmacist (30).

McKay and Jackson (1978), in their study, found that physicians were more favorable toward the physician assistant, compared to the pharmacist, in performing the tasks of drug therapy monitoring and chronic disease maintenance (31).

Although generally physicians have been found to be somewhat negative toward most clinical pharmacy services, Ritchey and Raney (1981), in looking at factors associated with physicians' acceptance of pharmacy services, found that physicians were least supportive of tasks that allowed the pharmacist to make independent technical-therapy decisions, such as choice of drug, and most favorable toward traditional clerical tasks, such as maintaining patient drug profiles. Young physicians were found to be more favorable toward pharmacists becoming involved in direct patient care, but only in terms of adjunct tasks that facilitate the physician's role. They also found that physicians who spent a large part of their time in the hospital setting and those with past working experience with a clinical pharmacist were the most supportive (32).

Ritchey and Raney, in a second study, found that exposure to clinical pharmacists had a positive effect on physicians' attitudes toward clinical pharmacy (1981). The survey measured the extent to which physicians felt pharmacists in the hospital setting should maintain drug profiles, monitor prescribing patterns of physicians to prevent adverse reactions, counsel patients at the bedside, determine the frequency of use and dosage form of drugs prescribed by the physician, and independently select the drug to be prescribed based on the physician's diagnosis. Although physicians were generally unfavorable to pharmacists independently choosing drugs, those physicians exposed to a clinical pharmacist were significantly more positive toward pharmacists counseling patients and determining frequency of use and dosage form of prescribed drugs. Over 90% of physicians exposed to a clinical pharmacist ranked their quality of work as good or excellent (33, 34).

MICROEVALUATION OF THE IMPACT OF PHARMACY

Studies of pharmacists indicate inadequacies in their performance when it comes to such things as counseling or detecting drug interactions. At the same time, for the role of dispensing the orders as written by physicians, pharmacists are certainly highly trained for such a basic role. Although pharmacists are criticized as being underutilized, one could argue that being overtrained is safer than the alternative. Pharmacy is not the only health profession that has its problems. Nurses can certainly be linked to or at least partially responsible for many of the drug errors that occur in various institutional settings. Physicians have been found to have performance and quality of care problems as well. Their misprescribing has been an important reason for the evolution of clinical pharmacy. Studies have shown that they often prescribe antibiotics improperly. They even miss serious, yet one would think, recognizable problems such as myocardial infarction. Unnecessary surgery is another problem that has led many insurance companies to require second opinions (35-37).

MACROEVALUATION OF THE IMPACT OF PHARMACY

If we were to graph the amount spent on drugs as a percentage of the total health care expenditures in the United States, we would learn that the percentage for drugs and sundries peaked a few years ago. Does this mean that pharmacy is becoming less important in the health care system relative to other components? A positive way to examine this is to consider that, like nursing, clinical pharmacy costs are often built into the total hospital and nursing home costs. Drug costs, therefore, may no longer be a good index of all of the activities of pharmacy in the health care system.

So are we controlling more or less of the health care process? Borrowing an analogy from Victor Fuchs, suppose we put all of the medicines and pharmacists west of the Mississippi river and put all of the physicians east of the Mississippi without medicines. Where would patients want to go? This analogy can be made more complicated by playing the same scenario with different shades of "nurses with drugs in the west and no pharmacists." Would we still have a health care system? Probably. In reality, we must consider that improved health in any country is highly correlated with the appropriate use of drugs, and it may not matter to a significant degree which health professionals are prescribing or dispensing.

PHARMACY ORGANIZATIONS

Although the American Pharmaceutical Association claims to represent all aspects of pharmacy practice, there are several specialty organizations that are becoming increasingly strong. The American Society of Hospital Pharmacists (ASHP) has become a significant force in advancing and representing hospital pharmacists. The ASHP seems to be expanding its influence and is now claiming to represent pharmacists who work in organized health care settings. Because all health care is becoming interlinked and "organized," ASHP and American Pharmaceutical Association (APhA) are bound to overlap more in the future. The National Association of Retail Druggists, now officially called NARD, has been emphasizing management of community practice and is concerned with the survival of retail pharmacy.

Additional specialty groups include the American College of Apothecaries (ACA) and the American Society of Consultant Pharmacists (ASCP). The ACA upholds the highest standards for the maintenance of professional pharmacies and apothecaries. The ASCP had its roots in the development of consultant pharmacists for long-term care facilities, but now it seems to be expanding to pharmacists who consult in institutional and ambulatory settings. Another group that has formed over the last few years has been the American College of Clinical Pharmacy. It represents the more patient-oriented, clinical practitioners with a strong emphasis on clinical research.

Both the NARD and the ASHP were once part of the APhA structure before they broke away to form their own independent organizations. As a sign that the central role of the American Pharmaceutical Association has not yet stabilized, its own Academy of Pharmaceutical Sciences experienced a major upheaval in 1985 leading to the formation of the independent American Association of Pharmaceutical Scientists and leaving in APhA, a new Academy of Pharmaceutical Research and Science.

The profession is weak in the sociopolitical arena because these independent pharmacy groups make it difficult for outside players to get a solid, unified answer from the profession about what pharmacy wants and where pharmacy is headed.

CONCLUSIONS

The history and future of pharmacy are inseparable from drugs and medicines. It is expected that just as the power and usefulness of drugs improve, so should the potential impact of pharmacy.

Pharmacists seem well appreciated by the public, based on national polls regarding trustworthiness and ethics. Physicians seem to define their domain as encompassing all areas of health and disease, including drug dispensing, so it is expected that they will continue to resist attempts by pharmacists and other disciplines to encroach on the traditional medical roles of prescribing and diagnosis.

Although the pharmacy profession is beginning to define itself as a provider of information, the strength of a profession is often measured by the strength of its control over social objects (38, 39). With this social power model, it would be recommended that the pharmacy profession continue to increase its control over drug therapy as well as drug knowledge.

REFERENCES

1. Sonnedecker G. Evolution of Pharmacy. In: Remington's Pharmaceutical Sciences, 14th ed. Easton, PA: Mack Publishing Company, 1970, p 19.
2. Gagnon JP. Public health issues in medicine use control. In: Wertheimer AI, Bush PJ, eds., Perspectives on Medicines in Society. Hamilton, IL: Drug Intelligence Publications, 1977, pp 36–54.
3. Hepler CD. The third wave in pharmaceutical education: the clinical movement. Am J Pharm Educ 1987;51(4):369–385.
4. National Association of Boards of Pharmacy. Survey of Pharmacy Law 1986–1987. Park Ridge, IL.
5. Study Commission on Pharmacy. Pharmacists for the Future. Ann Arbor, MI: Health Administration Press, 1975.
6. Brodie DC. Need for a theoretical base for pharmacy practice. Am J Hosp Pharm 1981;38:49–54.
7. American Society of Hospital Pharmacists. Directions for clinical practice in pharmacy: proceedings of an invitational conference. Am J Hosp Pharm 1985;42:1287–1342.
8. Hepler DC. Pharmacy as a clinical profession. Am J Hosp Pharm 1985;42:1298–1306.
9. Schondelmeyer SW. Strategy to effect change in pharmacy practice. Am J Hosp Pharm 1982;39:2137–2142.
10. Penna RP. Don't call it prescribing. Am Pharm 1986;26:749–752.
11. US Department of Health and Human Services, Bureau of Health Professions. Fifth Report to the President and Congress on the Status of Health Professions Personnel in the United States. March, 1986;HRP No 0906767.
12. American Pharmaceutical Association. A National Study of the Practice of Pharmacy. Washington, DC:1978.

13. Stolar MA. National survey of hospital pharmaceutical services: 1985. Am J Hosp Pharm 1985;42:2667–2678.
14. Nelson AA. Computers in community pharmacy practice: will they affect your practice? In: Derner CH, ed., Lilly Digest. Eli Lilly and Company, 1986, pp 5–10.
15. Anon. Pharmacists at top in honesty/ethics poll. Pharm Weekly 1985;24(40):170.
16. Koos El. The Health of Regionville. New York, NY: Hafner Publishing Company, 1987.
17. Turkel S. Working. New York, NY: Pantheon Books, 1972.
18. Dichter Institute for Motivational Research, Inc. Communicating the Value of Comprehensive Pharmaceutical Services to the Consumer, Final Report. Washington, DC: American Pharmaceutical Association, 1973.
19. Yellin AK, Norwood GJ. The public's attitude toward pharmacy. J Am Pharm Assoc 1974;NS14:61–65.
20. Norwood GJ. Impact of a clinical pharmacists emphasis on patient communications on patients' attitude toward pharmacy. Drug Intell Clin Pharm 1975;9:601–604.
21. Wertheimer AI, Manasse HK, Smith MC. The quality of pharmaceutical services: an examination of myths and facts. Drugs in Health Care 1975;2:49.
22. Knapp DE, Baird JT, Winter WJ. How consumers view drugs. The Apothecary 1976;88:8–38.
23. Gagnon JP. Factors affecting pharmacy patronage motives: a literature review. J Am Pharm Assoc 1977;NS17:9.
24. Helling DK, Hepler CD, Jones ME. Effect of direct clinical pharmaceutical services on patients' perceptions of health care quality. Am J Hosp Pharm 1979;36:325–329.
25. Ricci EM, Enterline P, Henderson V. Contacts with pharmacists before and after "free" medical care: the Quebec experience. Med Care 1978;16:256–262.
26. Schondelmeyer SW, Trinca CE. Consumer demand for a pharmacist-conducted prescription counseling service. Am Pharm 1983;NS23:321–324.
27. Knapp DA, Knapp DE, Edwards JD. The pharmacist as perceived by physicians, patrons and other pharmacists. J Am Pharm Assoc 1969;NS9(2):80–84.
28. Norwood GJ, Seibert JJ, Gagnon JP. Attitudes of rural consumers and physicians toward expanded roles for pharmacists. J Am Pharm Assoc 1976;NS16:551–554.
29. Lambert RL, Wertheimer AI, Dobbert DJ, Church TR. The pharmacists' clinical role as seen by other health workers. Am J Public Health 1977; 67:252–253.
30. Bernstein LR, Klett EA, Jacoby KE. Physicians attitudes toward the use of clinical pharmaceutical services in private medical practice. Am J Hosp Pharm 1978;35:715–717.
31. McKay AB, Jackson RA. Attitudes of primary care physicians toward utilization of the pharmacist versus the physician assistant in patient care. Am J Pharm 1976;148:157–167.
32. Ritchey FJ, Raney MR. Medical role-task boundary maintenance: physician's opinions on clinical pharmacy. Med Care 1981;19:90–103.
33. Ritchey FJ, Raney MR. Effect of exposure on physicians' attitudes toward clinical pharmacists. Am J Hosp Pharm 1981;38:1459–1463.
34. Ritchey FJ, Raney MR, Keith TD. Physicians' opinions of expanded clinical pharmacy services, AJPH 1983;73:96–101.
35. Avorn J, Soumerai SB. Improving drug therapy through educational outreach. N Engl J Med 1983;308:1457–1463.
36. Schaffner W, Ray WA, Federspiel CF, Miller WO. Improving antibiotic prescribing in office practice. JAMA 1983;250:1728–1732.
37. Last JM. Hazards of health care. In: Public Health and Preventive Medicine, 12th ed. Norwalk, CT: Appleton-Century-Croft, 1986, pp 1577–1589.
38. Mumford D. Medical Sociology: Patients, Providers and Policies. New York, NY: Random House, 1983, pp 67–69.
39. McGhan WF. A theoretical model for the pharmacy profession. Consultant Pharmacist 1988;3(2):145–148.

SUGGESTED READINGS

1. Angorn RA, Thomison JE. Is pharmacy a "learned" profession? Am Pharm 1985;NS25:739–742.

2. Anonymous. Directions for clinical practice in pharmacy: proceedings of an invitational conference. Am J Hosp Pharm 1985;42:1287–1342.
3. Anonymous. Pharmacy in the twenty-first century: results of a strategic-planning conference. Am J Hosp Pharm 1985;42:71–80.
4. Avorn J, Soumerai SB. Improving drug therapy through educational outreach. N Engl J Med 1983;308:1457–1463.
5. Biles JA. The doctor of pharmacy. JAMA 1983;249:1157–1160.
6. Brodie DC. Need for a theoretical base for pharmacy practice. In: Harvey AK Whitney Award Lectures, 1950–84. Bethesda, MD: American Society of Hospital Pharmacists, 1984, pp 251-9.
7. Brodie DC. Pharmacy's societal purpose. Am J Hosp Pharm 1981;38:1893-6.
8. Fisher DJ, Pathak DS. Influence of attitudes, normative beliefs, and situational variables on physicians' use of pharmacists as drug information consultants. Am J Hosp Pharm 1980;37:483–491.
9. Gagnon JP. Factors affecting pharmacy patronage motives—a literature review. J Am Pharm Assoc 1977;NS17:556–566.
10. Goldberg T, DeVito C. The impact of state generic drug substitution laws. Drug Ther 1981;11:75–80.
11. Hatoum HT, Catizone C, Hutchinson RA, et al. An eleven year review of the pharmacy literature: documentation of the value and acceptance of clinical pharmacy. Drug Intell Clin Pharm 1986;20:33–48.
12. Jackson RA, Smith MC. Relations between price and quality in community pharmacy. Med Care 1974;12:32–39.
13. Knapp DA, Wolf HH, Knapp DE, Rudy TA. The pharmacist as a drug advisor. J Am Pharm Assoc 1969;NS9(10):502–505,543.
14. McGhan WF, Smith WE, Adams D. A randomized trial comparing pharmacists and technicians as dispensers of prescriptions for ambulatory patients. Med Care 1983;21(4):445-53.
15. **McGhan WF, Draugalis J, Bootman JL, et al. Identification of factors associated with student satisfaction and commitment to pharmacy practice. Am J Pharm Educ 1985;49(2):124–129.**
16. Ritchey FJ, Raney MR, Keith TD. Physicians' opinions of expanded clinical pharmacy services. Am J Pharm 1983;73:96–101.
17. Schaffner W, Ray WA, Federspiel CF, Miller WO. Improving antibiotic prescribing in office practice. JAMA 1983;250:1728–1732.
18. Stolar MH. National Survey of Hospital Pharmaceutical Services—1982. Am J Hosp Pharm 1983;40:963-9.
19. Thompson JF, McGhan WF, Ruffalo R. A comparison of pharmacists and physicians drug prescribing for patients in skilled nursing facilities. J Am Geriatr Soc 1984;32(2):154–159.
20. Zellmer WA. Achieving pharmacy's full potential. Am J Hosp Pharm 1985;42:1285.

SELECTED READINGS

THE PHARMACIST AS A DRUG ADVISOR[a]

D. A. Knapp
H. H. Wolf
D. E. Knapp
T. A. Rudy

The recent emphasis on demonstrating the effectiveness of drug products lends increased relevance to similar evaluations of practicing pharmacists since the safe and effective functioning of pharmacists is necessary for the patient to be able to receive the full benefits of a prescribed drug. This article deals with an analysis of the performance of pharmacists, with special attention to their role as drug advisors.

Since the available literature dealing with the effectiveness of the pharmacist as a drug advisor is limited, a three-phase field experiment was conducted to evaluate the pharmacist's performance as a drug advisor to (1) physicians, (2) patients on self-medication products and (3) patients on prescription medication.

DRUG ADVISOR TO PHYSICIANS

A group of 36 pharmacies in a large metropolitan area made up the sample. Because of the attention often given place of practice as a variable relevant to the quality of pharmaceutical services, the pharmacies were selected randomly within three categories—professional, traditional and discount-oriented.

The definitions used were (1) professional—an outlet dealing primarily in pharmaceutical goods and services and that projects an overall image that is unmistakably professional, (2) discount—an outlet characterized by price competition and volume, regardless of how many prescriptions dispensed and (3) traditional—a middle group encompassing all outlets not classified in either extreme category. All pharmacies in the test city were classified by two judges; high interjudge reliability was demonstrated.

The pharmacist-subjects were tested on their ability to provide answers to six drug-information questions telephoned to them at their place of practice by an investigator posing as a physician. The questions were of two types—pharmaceutical and therapeutic, and three levels of difficulty—easy, medium and hard.

The six questions were telephoned to each pharmacy one at a time over an eight-month period. If the pharmacist was unable to answer the question at once, he was asked to try to find the answer and told that he would be called back within two hours. The time required by the pharmacist to find the answer to the question was not considered a variable because of the many confounding factors that could affect. it. Instead, the two-hour time limit was set as a maximum period in which the information could reasonably be obtained.

---

[a]Edited with permission from Knapp DA, Wolff HH, Knapp DE, Rudy TA. The pharmacist as a drug advisor. J Am Pharm Assoc 1969;9:502–505,543.

Following, in condensed form, are the six questions. All were, of course, asked in a more realistic context.

Pharmaceutical easy—*Question:* Why does Asmolin epinephrine suspension contain phenol and sodium ascorbate?

Answer: Phenol is an antibacterial or preservative and sodium ascorbate is an antioxidant or preservative.

Pharmaceutical medium—*Question:* What are the chemical and therapeutic differences among Erythrocin, Ilosone and Ilotycin?

Answer: An acceptable answer consisted of the correct chemical names and a correct statement of absorption differences.

Pharmaceutical hard—*Question:* Is Orinase made up of the sodium salt of tolbutamide or is it the free base? If it is the base, why is this, since everyone knows that the sodium salt is more soluble?

Answer: The sodium salt is not used since slow absorption is desirable in this case. If the pharmacist volunteered that Orinase is actually a free *acid*, rather than a free base, he was given bonus points for the correction.

Therapeutic easy—*Question:* I am unfamiliar with a product named "Tridal." Can you tell me something about it?

Answer: A good answer required the correct generic names, amounts and pharmacologic classification of ingredients. Other factual information increased the score.

Therapeutic medium—*Question:* I have a patient taking Darvon-65 and Norgesic for back pain. Lately, he has developed traumas and dizziness. Is this common?

Answer: Simultaneous use of the compounds is contraindicated as stated in the Norgesic package insert.

Therapeutic hard—*Question:* I have tried several patients on Biphetamine-20 for appetite control and it seems to work well. However, some of these patients complain of excess nervousness. Do they make this product in combination with a sedative? If the pharmacist responded correctly by naming Biphetamine-T, he was then asked—Is the sedative a barbiturate? Some of my patients are extremely sensitive to barbiturates.

Answer: Besides identifying the product as Biphetamine-T, the pharmacist was required to identify the sedative ingredient as a nonbarbiturate which was not obvious from the product labeling alone.

Answers to easy questions could be found in the product labeling or in a standard reference such as the *PDR*. Medium questions required a greater effort, but answers could still be found in these sources. The hard questions could not be answered by referring to one source but required synthesis of information to arrive at an appropriate answer. Thus, only the hard questions actually required high-level professional activity on the part of the pharmacist.

The answers provided by the pharmacist were recorded verbatim, immediately after the conversation. They were graded independently by two judges on a ten-point scale. High interjudge agreement was demonstrated.

RESULTS

There were no statistically significant ($p > .25$) differences in performance among the three types of pharmacies (professional-, traditional- and discount-oriented). Therefore, the results from all 36 pharmacies were grouped. Pharmacists did best on the easy pharmaceutical question. However, if 60 percent were considered a liberal passing grade, the pharmacists in our sample would have failed five of the six questions. Responses were significantly lower ($p < .05$) on the therapeutic questions than on the pharmaceutical ones.

SELF-MEDICATION ADVICE

The same 36 pharmacies sampled in phase one were recontacted. A research assistant posing as a patient visited each pharmacy. He entered, picked up a bottle of Dristan tablets and proceeded to the prescription counter. When the pharmacist appeared, the patient explained that he was a college student majoring in archeology and that his class was about to depart for a two-week field trip in the wilds of the mexican jungle. Since he was a severe diabetic, he was concerned over whether his insulin would keep properly in such a hot climate with no means of refrigeration. After discussing this with the pharmacist and thanking him for the advice offered the patient then referred to the bottle of Dristan he had been holding and said to the pharmacist, "I've been bothered by a summer cold and the sniffles lately and wondered whether this Dristan would do me any good? The advice was received, a purchase was made if so advised and the patient left.

The first part of the incident served only to establish the patient as a severe diabetic. We were not interested in the advice given about insulin storage. We were, of course, interested in the pharmacist's response to the Dristan question, since this drug is contraindicated for this patient. It is a presumably well-known fact that the decongestant ingredients (sympathomimetic amines) of Dristan and several other popular cold and allergy remedies are contraindicated in diabetes. Since these drugs cause a rise in the blood sugar level, they might possible upset the control of the disease in certain diabetics. For this reason, products containing sympathomimetic amines are required to carry a prominent warning against their use in the presence of this disease.

Our patient had been instructed to respond favorably to whatever the pharmacist suggested. Thus, if the advice were to purchase another product, for any reason, he was to do so. If the pharmacist warned against Dristan, he was to inquire why, but in any case to follow the advice. If no components were offered, he was to purchase the Dristan. After leaving the pharmacy, the interviewer immediately recorded the conversation verbatim.

RESULTS

Of the 36 pharmacies contacted, only six knew of or noted the warning and refused to sell the Dristan. In these cases the patient was either sold an antihistamine with no indicated warning against use with diabetes or referred to his physician. The remaining 30 pharmacists—83 percent of the sample—either sold Dristan with their endorsement or switched the patient to a more expensive or private-brand product which was similarly contraindicated.

PRESCRIPTION MEDICATION ADVICE

A different sample of 12 pharmacies was used in this phase—five with a patient-record system and seven without. An investigator took a prescription calling for 24 Parnate tablets, *q.i.d.*, written by an Ohio State University physician to each pharmacy for dispensing. One week later the same investigator took a Tofránil prescription written by a different OSU physician to each of the same pharmacies for dispensing. On each occasion the comments and activities of each pharmacist were recorded verbatim.

Parnate (tranylcypromine) is a highly active monoamine oxidase inhibitor used for the symptomatic treatment of severe depression. Quoting from the package insert for the product— *"WARNING . . .: Parnate . . . is a potent agent with the capacity of producing serious side effects . . . .* Patients should be instructed to report promptly the occurrence of headache or other unusual symptoms. Patient should be warned against eating cheese . . . [or drinking] alcoholic beverages [while on Parnate]. Patients should be warned against self medication with proprietary . . . drugs such as cold, hay fever or weight-reducing preparations that contain pressor agents."

Of the 12 pharmacists dispensing this drug, only one gave any warning whatsoever regarding the medication.

Tofránil (imipramine hydrochloride) is a psychotherapeutic drug also recommended for the treatment of depression. The package insert of this product states— *"CONTRAINDICATIONS:* The concomitant use of monoamine oxidase inhibiting compounds is contraindicated. Hyperpyretic crises or severe convulsive seizures may occur in patients receiving such combinations. The potentiation of adverse effects can be serious or even fatal." The Parnate package insert states much the same thing and specifically lists Tofránil by brand name as contraindicated.

Goldberg[1] has stated in *JAMA* that

> The reactions observed with the combined therapy of MAO inhibitors and imipramine . . . have been particularly severe. Hypertension, seizures and hyperpyrexia frequently associated with death have often been reported . . . . Even though all patients do not experience adverse reactions when these drugs are administered together, concomitant administration is absolutely contraindicated because of the severity of the syndrome.

Eleven of the 12 pharmacists dispensed Tofránil to the same patient to whom they, or another pharmacist in the same pharmacy, had dispensed Parnate a week earlier. Only one man, using a patient-record system properly, detected the contraindication and called the physician. He then retained the prescription to insure that the patient did not have the drug dispensed elsewhere.

It is painfully and deadly obvious that the pharmacists in our sample utterly failed the tasks presented them—failed to the point of exposing their patients to the unnecessary risk of possible death in the third phase. Statistics are of little use in cases such as this, both because of the overwhelming nature of the incorrect responses and the severity of the consequences of the pharmacists' actions.

It would be easy to blame others and to make excuses at this point but such will not be done. It is irrelevant that the physician should have warned the patient, that educators should have done a better job of teaching, that the patient did not ask the right questions. All these things are irrelevant when you are faced with a patient in your practice. Suddenly it is up to you to see that this patient gets the proper drug therapy, to see that this patient knows how and when to take her medication, to see that this patient is warned and safeguarded against contraindications like the one we have just discussed.

You will note that we have been referring to a patient. Not a customer. Not someone buying a product. A patient! A human being who is going to be profoundly affected by what you are going to do for her (or to her). It is patient orientation that differentiates a truly professional health practitioner from his product-oriented colleague. It is patient orientation that is at the heart of drug-use control.

Patient orientation is an attitude and a way of practice which can only be actively implemented by complete personal commitment to the concept. It can not be forced upon you by a speaker at a professional meeting, a journal article or any other external force. Patient orientation means accepting a true professional's responsibility to place his patient's interest above his own, even if this is uneconomical or causes a confrontation with an angry, arrogant physician or a distressed, dissatisfied patient.

Certain tools also are required in order to be patient oriented. A complete up-to-date drug information library is necessary. A self-imposed regimen of continuing professional education is called for. A properly maintained and utilized patient-record system is vital. The Parnate-Tofránil problem could not be prevented any other way. As you have seen from the results, the record system alone is not a guarantee as such. It must be more than a public relations gimmick or a sales come-on. It must be used conscientiously and thoroughly every time it is called for, despite the time and despite the expense. No pharmacist can practice modern pharmacy without such a system.

Fortunately, today's pharmacists have access to these tools if they obtain and use them. Articles in recent journals have provided material about patient-record systems[2] drug information sources[3] and retrieval technics.[4,5] Continuing education meetings are becoming evermore frequent in all sections of the country.

More and more colleges of pharmacy throughout the United States are implementing professional curricula which include clinical pharmacy exposure.[6,7] Students at these institutions are gaining patient orientation through direct patient contact in medical center complexes. As these students graduate, they will be better prepared than any previous graduates in pharmacy's long history. In spite of their better educational background, however, contemporary pharmacy graduates must have the support and assistance of current pharmacy practitioners. Pharmacists practicing today must demonstrate that patient orientation is vital and must help the graduate carry over into every day practice the knowledge and attitudes learned in college.

We feel that the pharmacist must be patient-oriented if he is to survive the rigors of a constantly changing future. We are equally convinced that a prime reason why the pharmacists in our sample failed was because they were *not* patient oriented. This attitude of patient orientation must come primarily from within but it can be fostered in others with the help of practicing pharmacists. We ask for your personal self-examination on this point. We seek your support for the programs—in colleges, in local, state and national organizations and in the community—which are striving to better prepare pharmacists and prospective pharmacists for an expanded professional role in our health care system. We believe that the pharmacist is a professional person for whom the ultimate goal is successful treatment of the patient. But we also believe that pharmacists will be judged by their accomplishments and not by their potential.

REFERENCES

1. Goldberg, L.I., *JAMA,* **190,** 456-462 (Nov. 2, 1964).
2. Cain, R., Patient Record Systems," *JAPhA,* **NS4,** No. **4,** 164-168 (April 1964).
3. Burkholder, D.F., "Developing a Drug Information Service," *Hospitals,* **39,** 68-78 (Aug. 1, 1965).
4. Sewell, Winifred, "Medlars in Medicine," *JAPhA,* **NS4,** No. 6, 291-293 (June 1964).
5. Wicks, L.A., "Microfilm Service," *JAPhA,* **NS5,** No. 2, 84-85 (Feb. 1965).
6. Sister Emmanuel, "New Dimension for Pharmaceutical Education," *JAPhA,* **NS8,** No. 6, 284-287 (June 1968).
7. Parks, L.M., "Changing Concepts and Attitudes in Educating Pharmacists," *Am. J. Hosp. Pharm.,* **25,** 160-167 (April 1968).

ACHIEVING PHARMACY'S FULL POTENTIAL[b]

William A. Zellmer

The recent consensus-development conference on Directions for Clinical Practice in Pharmacy, the proceedings of which are featured in this issue of the *Journal,* turned out to be an important assessment of pharmacy itself, not just of clinical practice. The 150 conferees at the Hilton Head Island meeting concluded, in essence, that the value system fostered by the clinical movement should be assimilated by all practitioners so that pharmacy may become more fully professionalized.

The conferees agreed strongly on the following points:

- Pharmacy is *the* health-care profession most concerned with drugs and their clinical application.
- A fundamental purpose of the profession of pharmacy is to serve as a force in society for safe and appropriate use of drugs.
- A fundamental goal of the profession is to promote health, and pharmacists can best pursue that goal by working to promote optimal use of drugs (including prevention of improper or uncontrolled use of drugs).
- In pursuing the above goal, pharmacy should be expected to provide leadership to other health-care professions; this implies that pharmacists should be involved in a very positive way in advocating rational drug therapy, rather than just reacting to treatment decisions made by others.

The conferees were not ivory-tower types who found it convenient to overlook hard realities. As evidence of this, the group also strongly agreed that

- Pharmacists should continue to have ultimate responsibility for drug-distribution and drug-control activities, but these functions should be carried out by technicians under pharmacists' general supervision, thus freeing the major portion of pharmacists' time for clinical services. Further, drug distribution should be mechanized and automated to as great an extent as possible.

In several respects, the conference reflected an important notion that has begun to gel within pharmacy; namely, that clinical pharmacy should be thought of less in terms of discrete functions by discrete pharmacists and more in terms of responsibilities of a pharmaceutical services department. The management of the department is responsible for orchestrating comprehensive services that integrate drug dispensing and distribution with informative services. As the leader of a group of professionals, the department director seeks consensus among pharmacists on what level of service the department will provide, how pharmacists will spend their time, and what functions will be delegated to well-trained, well-supervised technical personnel. (Of little import within this construct is whether the pharmacy department is in a hospital, a medical clinic, or a drugstore. With respect to a drugstore, it is helpful not to think of the whole establishment as a pharmacy, but rather that there is a pharmacy department within the store.)

---

[b]Reprinted with permission from Zellmer WA. Achieving pharmacy's full potential. Am J Hosp Pharm 1985;42:1285.

One of the gems of the Hilton Head conference was Hepler's[1] discussion of the sociological and philosophical basis for the concept of a profession, coupled with an analysis of how pharmacy stacks up. Of particular interest to hospital pharmacists is his review of research on professionals employed by large organizations. one of the findings of this research, according to Hepler, is that

> . . . professionalization can occur in a bureacratic organization if the professionals are organized in a separate professional department headed by a person who is able and willing to insulate the professionals from the bureaucracy. This suggests a seldom-recognized dimension of hospital pharmacy management that could have great strategic importance in the future.

This idea makes a lot of sense given the continuing pressure that pharmacy faces from corporate management to standardize and mass-produce its services.[2]

Translating the philosophy of the Hilton head conference into changes in the way pharmacy is practiced will be a big challenge. As a first step, every pharmacy department should devote some time to reviewing and discussing the proceedings. Consider setting aside some time for a departmental meeting for this purpose within the next month or two. State and local pharmacy organizations may want to conduct programs patterned after the Hilton Head conference or review the conference findings in small group discussions.

ASHP will be building on the conference through its practice Spotlight Program for 1985–86 under the theme "Patient-Oriented Pharmacy Services." In September, the ASHP councils and SIG Cabinet will consider whether any policy recommendations should be issued as a result of the meeting. Further, the Society will be bringing the proceedings to the attention of Congress, federal health officials, colleges of pharmacy, and professional societies and trade associations in the health-care field.

The greatest force for change in pharmacy lies within pharmacists themselves. if they truly see themselves as practitioners of a clinical profession, they will behave accordingly, others will perceive them as such, and the pace of professionalization will accelerate. Widespread reading and thinking about the ideas of the Hilton Head conference could be an important catalyst in this process of enhancing the self-concept of pharmacists.

REFERENCES

1. Hepler CD. Pharmacy as a clinical profession. *Am J Hosp Pharm.* 1985; 42:1298–306.
2. Zellmer WA. Can pharmacy control its destiny? *Am J Hosp Pharm.* 1985; 42:69. Editorial.

LET'S SEPARATE PHARMACIES AND DRUGSTORES [c]

Don E. Francke

One characteristic of man is that he is eternally hopeful. Hopes, plans, thoughts, aspirations, dreams, and effort often go unfulfilled for years or even centuries but sometimes— when circumstances are right—they are brought into reality. Conditions are ripening rapidly for a separation of the American pharmacy from the drugstore, and by the beginning of the third millennium we may see the pharmacist much more fully accepted by society as a

---

[c]Reprinted from American Journal of Pharmacy, 1976;141(5):161–169 (September–October).

professional man serving the health needs of the public. But only if we plan now and make a concerted effort, can we change the image of pharmacy in America by the year 2000. . . .

Time, said St. Augustine, is a threefold present: the present as we experience it; the past as a present memory; and the future as a present expectation. By that criterion, the year 2000 has already arrived. By the decisions we make now we commit the future, for the future begins in the present though it is rooted in the past.

A man defines himself in part by the web of his relations with the past, the things for which he strives in the present and his expectations for the future. My credentials to speak on the American drugstore rest principally on a boyhood spent in my father's one-man drugstore in Pennsylvania during the depression years—an experience which some of you will recognize as qualifying me to at least speak my piece. While I have been associated with pharmacy practice in hospitals for many years, the memories of the lessons taught me by my father and by the experience in his pharmacy have never left me.

THE PAST AS A PRESENT MEMORY

Drugstores are the products of many complex interactions, and today I am going to discuss some of these under the headings of a) some developments in pharmaceutical education which helped to bring us where we are today, b) where we are as a profession, c) awakening concepts which show great promise for a richer professional future, d) reasons why we should separate pharmacies and drugstores, e) brief mention of some of the professional opportunities at hand, and f) suggested steps which colleges of pharmacy and pharmacists should take to accelerate the separation and prepare for the future.

In his famous distinction between fortune and courageous decision, Machiavelli (*The Prince*, 25) argues that half of man's actions are governed by chance, and the other half are ruled by men themselves. So it is with American pharmacy. And while I may say things today which may be offensive to the ears of some, I do not wish to be unkind or uncharitable to anyone, for I understand fully that the bell tolls for each of us and that we all must share collective responsibility for our profession.

The drugstore today is to a great extent a mirror of pharmaceutical education of past decades. It did not arise upon the scene yesterday—rather, it slowly evolved out of patterns of the past. It is a product of our educational system, a reflection of our scale of values and of our urge to make money at any cost. To shape it, American pharmacists have sold their professional heritage, or rather, they have failed to develop one because they have been held down, enmeshed, and drowned by the overwhelming number of drugstores that engulf all pharmacists.

For historical reasons, pharmacy in English-speaking countries has traditionally commanded little or no respect, but rather, as stated by Kremers (1) "became the butt of ridicule . . . as is clearly shown in English fiction. With English traditions as a guide, it was but natural, therefore, that Harvard and Yale, Columbia, and Pennsylvania, although they made provisions, not only for the traditional college course, but also for theology, law and medicine, paid no attention to the needs of the pharmacy."

This lack of respect for American pharmacy remains as true today as it was in the early 1900s when professor Kremers discussed it. In discussing "The Druggists' Dilemma" in 1956, McCormack (2) points out that:

> The young pharmacist today is trained as a professional, his interests and ability for scientific research are carefully developed, preparing him for the laboratory work required by hospitals, schools, and

pharmaceutical companies. Yet few pharmacists see themselves in this position. Most expect to become proprietors, with the status of independent professionals thus fusing the two systems and avoiding a final choice. . . . The professional drive is blunted by subordinating a service goal to individual achievement for its own sake.

At best this adjustment is not capable of providing the satisfaction of either pole.

Developments in Pharmaceutical Education

I want to mention only two developments in pharmaceutical education that have helped to mold American pharmacy to its form today. The first is its failure to follow the educational patterns of other health professions as laid down by Abraham Flexner (3) in his critical study of medical education published in 1910. When Flexner made his study, only a small percentage of physicians had graduated from medical school, not many had attended formal classes, laboratories for instruction were nonexistent, and most medical education was provided by proprietary schools. Medicine in America was neither taught nor practiced in keeping with the scientific knowledge already attained, particularly in Europe. At that time, both the Doctor of Medicine and the Doctor of Pharmacy were cheap degrees. Flexner believed that the way to change the practice of medicine was to change medical education, and I believe that pharmacy practice can be changed by the same method.

Although pharmaceutical education has made remarkable progress during recent years, it has never fully corrected the errors made several decades ago when it abandoned the professional degree of Doctor of Pharmacy to emulate the chemists by adopting the Bachelor of Science degree. At the same time, it did something else—it cast pharmacy into the role of a profession more firmly based on the physical sciences than on the biological sciences and thus deprived the profession of the required flexibility to adapt readily to change. Since the early 1930s, the center of science has passed from mathematical physics to biology, and our colleges of pharmacy have been extremely slow in adapting to this reality, and some even today have not begun the process.

Essentially all health professions except pharmacy retained the professional doctorate degree, as shown in Table 1.

Whereas medicine kept its professional degree of doctor of medicine and upgraded its educational program, pharmacy discarded its doctor of pharmacy degree. Had it retained the doctor's degree, as Tice points out, pharmacy may have been cast in a different mold than the one it settled for and the profession might have developed a sound professionally oriented program of education similar to the other health professions (4).

In 1948, the Report of the Pharmaceutical Survey again recommended that the curriculum in pharmacy consist of two years of general education followed by four years of professional studies leading to a Doctor of Pharmacy degree (5). Pharmaceutical education, however, continued to support the baccalaureate degree and thus turned down a second opportunity to restructure itself more in line with the other health professions. The five-year program that was adopted was a compromise which has held back the development of the profession. This was a tragic loss of opportunity.

A second error made by pharmaceutical education was the elimination of professional practitioners as teachers for professional courses in pharmacy, as we pointed out in our study published as *Mirror to Hospital Pharmacy* (6). In medical schools it is the Ph.D. who teaches the basic science courses such as anatomy, physiology, microbiology, and pharmacology. When these are completed, the education of the student is turned over to professional practitioners with the M.D. degree. It is these professional practitioners who instruct the student in the professional subjects such as medicine, pediatrics, and neurology. There is no substitute for well-educated practitioners for the teaching of clinical subjects.

With few exceptions, pharmaceutical education failed to do this. Rather, it has chosen Ph.D.s with little professional experience and motivation to teach professional subjects to pharmacy students. Advancement and other rewards for the Ph.D. are based on research, not on teaching. As a result, professional courses have been taught in a sterile atmosphere with little relationship to life, with no relationship to the patient, none to physicians nor to other members of the health team.

In most cases teachers of the terminal course in pharmacy have for years been those with strong orientation in the physical sciences. As a result, the major emphasis of the instruction was the physical and mechanical attributes of the drug product. The pharmacist was so poorly grounded in the biological sciences that he was unable to communicate with the physician. These two errors have tended to interact and reinforce each other to the detriment of the student and the profession. The needs of the professional practitioner of pharmacy were sacrificed to those of the pharmaceutical scientists.

In addition, as Brodie states, colleges of pharmacy showed little professional responsibility during the 1930s when the education and training offered were very similar in level to that of a technician (7). In 1942 Dean Rising raised his voice in protest when he commented about efforts of colleges to build up enrollment and to educate pharmacists when most drugstores were then filling only a few prescriptions a day (8). He asked, "Is it right, when there is so little pharmaceutical service for our graduates to perform, to be so concerned about increasing our enrollment and so thoughtless about the professional future of those we welcome within our halls?"

Where the Drugstore Is Today

With few exceptions, the American drugstore today can only be described as a commercialized jungle which dulls and tarnishes and blunts the professional drive of pharmacists as they seek to practice their profession within its walls. The participation of pharmacists in an environment of diverse nonprofessional activities such as the selling of lunches, hardware, women's clothing, garden tools, and other general-store items confuses the public as it does the pharmacist who practices in such a setting.

The drugstore, redefined and restructured, could be a respectable and acceptable institution. I bear no ill will against the drugstore per se. I protest strongly, however, its identification with pharmacy. It is this identification which is destroying pharmacy as a profession in America.

The public can associate neither the drugstore nor the pharmacist in it as serving the health needs of society. It cannot esteem a man who works in such an environment; he may sell a health-related product—but he is not accepted as a member of a health profession. Rather, such pharmacists stand outside the boundary of the profession—theirs indeed is a marginal profession—made marginal by the environment in which they practice. It is the drugstore which debases the profession of pharmacy in America.

Today's young pharmacists—both students and practitioners—are rebelling against the pattern of practice developed in this country, and are forcing a change in the pattern of pharmaceutical education. When they practice in the average drugstore, they count, pour, and label and, only in exceptional circumstances, do they have the opportunity to use the five years of specialized education acquired at some of the nation's most prestigious universities. Pharmacists represent a tremendous reservoir of health manpower and, as stated by

Dean Tom Rowe (9), he is "overeducated for his nonprofessional role and underutilized as a health profession." Eugene White (10), a community pharmacist, speaking at a conference at the University of Michigan in 1967, put it this way:

> It is evident today the pharmacist's abilities are not being utilized; a vast source of wasted professional talent is readily available. There must be a redirection of effort and a redefinition of his role in the total patient care concept.

This is the past as a present memory. Must the past always be the prologue for the future? Or can we take advantage of Machiavelli's teaching and not let things happen again by chance but rather mold the future by our own decision?

THE PRESENT AS WE EXPERIENCE IT

During the past 30-some years—which is my present—there have been many interacting forces and developments which now give us the opportunity to make a change, to separate the pharmacy from the drugstore, for the pharmacist to recapture some of his lost prestige, for pharmacy to enter the mainstream of health care and to become one of the recognized professions serving the health needs of the people.

I will mention briefly some of the more important of these changes and postulate that similar changes will continue to occur for the next 30 years so that by the year 2000 pharmacy will be completely different than we know it today in America.

Physical and Biological Knowledge

Within the past three decades the mixture of knowledge brewed by thousands of physical scientists has brought true the dreams of ancient alchemists and enabled man to achieve the age-old dream of the transmutation of the elements. But it was not gold that was produced but rather atomic energy with sufficient power either to destroy the world or, by converting the energy to peaceful uses, to make the deserts of the world bloom and to release man from burdensome toil for all time to come. The physical scientists have made it possible for man to circumnavigate the moon, and soon he will be exploring the outer reaches of the universe.

Within the same period of time the biological scientists have been doing all sorts of wonderful things such as the transplantation of hearts and other organs, and predictions are that artificial hearts made of silicone or natural rubber with a synthetic valve system will be developed before the turn of the century. More than a thousand types of birth defects are known and cause damage to a quarter million babies each year. Medicine for the unborn baby as well as the geriatric patient is a rapidly expanding field. The enzyme ribonuclease has been synthesized, and this will eventually unfold a new generation of therapeutic agents and may open new fields of research into the most intimate chemical processes of life. The cure rate for cancer is expected to rise to about 60% by the end of the century. About 50,000 people are now using blood vessels made of nylon and Dacron. There is growing confidence that new drugs can be tailor-made to fit specific biochemical pathways. Genetic research may make it possible—for better or worse—to alter the heredity factors of our children. The golden age of virus research is just beginning (11).

One could go on reciting developments of these kinds, but they would all only show the tremendous advances in the field of biochemical pharmacology, genetics, and related fields affecting the development of new drugs, and each new development increases by exponential proportions the new advances that then become possible.

Development of New Drugs

During the past 30-some years, great impetus was given to the development of new therapeutic agents when the French workers Trefouel and colleagues discovered that the inactive complex azo dye, Prontosil, was metabolized to the active sulfanilamide. This discovery opened the floodgates of research for other synthetic antibacterial agents and led to the discovery and synthesis of hundreds of other potent drugs such as penicillin and other antibiotics, cortisone and other steroids, the tranquilizers, remarkably effective diuretic agents, and a host of other therapeutic agents. Today, more than 90% of the drugs used were unknown 10 years ago, so rapid are the developments. These significant developments in the history of medicine have occurred during the recent past, since it is only a few years ago I heard Dr. Domagk—who first reported the antibacterial effects of Prontosil and thus set the stage for many of these developments—speak at the meeting of the Congress of Pharmaceutical Sciences in Germany.

Information Explosion

So rapidly have drugs been developed and progress in research made that there is indeed an information explosion. Ninety percent of the scientists of all time are living and publishing today. Most of the scientific literature of the world has been published during the past 10 years, generated by increased research.

The pharmacist traditionally has served as a consultant on drugs to the medical profession, and this was not a very difficult task 30 years ago. There were not too many potent drugs, not much was known about drug metabolism, there were not too many adverse drug reactions, few drug interactions were recognized, and bipharmaceutics, or the effect of formulation on therapeutic activity, had not been explored. Today the pharmacist finds himself in an entirely different ballpark, and he needs a far better education than ever before if he is going to be of value to society and to participate with the physician and nurse in the care of the patient.

Medication Error Study

One of the pioneering studies which first gave pharmacists an inkling that they may be of value working in closer association with physicians and nurses was that done on the incidence of medication errors by McConnell and Barker (12) at the University of Florida in 1961. These men showed that mistakes in administering drugs to hospitalized patients occur much oftener than anyone had realized.

The high incidence of adverse drug reactions has also been a factor in bringing the pharmacist closer to the patient, the physician and the nurse. Several studies showed that the patient receives from 10 to 25 different drugs during his stay in the hospital, and there is a direct proportional increase in adverse reactions with an increase in the number of drugs prescribed. The incidence of adverse reactions suffered by patients has been reported to be from 15 to 25%—which is significant enough to produce great concern and even alarm.

The relatively recent recognition of the complex interaction of many drugs which may antagonize, potentiate, modify, inhibit, or destroy the action of another drug has opened up a whole new area of knowledge for the pharmacist. Here he can serve a most useful function by becoming knowledgeable about drug interactions.

Adverse drug reactions and drug interactions both emphasize the importance of relatively new professional function of the pharmacist—that of maintaining a patient profile of the drugs being taken. This has a great social significance because it is an important professional service to both the patient and the physician—and it can lead to detection of the causes of malaise suffered by patients and can sometimes even be lifesaving.

Clinical Pharmacy

One of the most dramatic events of recent years is the emergence of the concept of clinical pharmacy and its belated adoption by colleges of pharmacy as an educational tool. Dean Martin Barr has been a leader in this, and Sister Emmanuel has been a pioneer in teaching pharmacy students this concept.

It is sad to have to say, however, that it was the narrow provincialism of pharmaceutical educators themselves which held back the development of the concept of clinical pharmacy for more than a quarter of a century. Clinical pharmacy as an educational tool was begun by Professor L. Wait Rising (13-15) of the University of Washington in 1944 but was disapproved by resolution by both the American Association of Colleges of Pharmacy and the American Council on Pharmaceutical Education in 1946 (16). This action abruptly terminated an imaginative research program in teaching methods without even giving the professor who originated it, the students taking the course, or the pharmacists participating in it an opportunity to be heard. The value of the clinical pharmacy experiment at the University of Washington was again brought to the attention of pharmaceutical educators in 1953 by Professor H. W. Youngken, Jr. (17) then at the University of Washington, but the idea lay dormant for many years until recently resurrected.

Educationally, clinical pharmacy may be defined as a concept which considers the treatment and care of patients by members of the health team in the presence of pharmacy students, with particular emphasis on the safe and appropriate use of drugs. Clinical pharmacy can best be taught using the hospital as a laboratory for the education of pharmacy students in a manner similar to its use for the education of medical and nursing students. This provides a new and rich educational experience for pharmacy students. It centers attention on the patient and his needs and on all knowledge concerned with the use of drugs in patients. It teaches the pharmacist the language of the patient-centered biologist and helps him in developing his skills to communicate with the physician and nurse. Wherever they practice throughout their life, pharmacists trained in clinical pharmacy will always be able to use the knowledge obtained. It adds relevance to their entire educational program.

Social Legislation

Although serious debate relative to compulsory health insurance started in this country around 1912, it was the passage of the Medicare amendments to the Social Security Act in 1965 that ushered in the beginnings of a new way of life for millions of Americans over 65 years of age. During its second year of operation, from July 1967 to June 1968, about $3.7 billion were paid for health care for about 19,700,000 people. Of these, there were 5,600,000 hospital admissions, 450,000 admissions to extended care facilities, and 260,000 home health services.

Traditionally, when societies become wealthy and knowledgeable about disease, they devote more time and money and effort to its prevention and control for the benefit of members. I remember well the lectures in public health presented by Dr. Nathan Sinai at Michigan many years ago and how he lamented the fact that the nation was doing very little toward the prevention of disease, except pestilential ones such as smallpox and a few others. It is also a paradox that a wealthy and sophisticated country as the United States only now recognizes the principles laid down by the World Health Organization as early as 1948. The preamble (18) to the constitution of WHO states:

> The enjoyment of the highest attainable standard of health is one of the fundamental rights of every human being without distinction of race, religion, political belief, economic or social conditions. . . . Governments have a responsibility for the health of their peoples.

Passage of Medicare is only the first step toward providing adequate health care in the United States. As enabling legislation continues to be passed by the several states, the impact of Medicaid upon the health of the nation is expected to far exceed that of Medicare. It will provide matching federal-state funds for the care of children and youth of medically indigent families, for dental care, for mental health services, for health services for the disabled, the crippled and the afflicted, and, in effect, for anyone who needs it. Acceptance of this new, broad concept of health as the right of every citizen provides great opportunities for pharmacy as a profession.

Although Medicare and Medicaid remain the main focus of health care legislation, there is additional legislation, much of which preceded these acts, which has generated and continues to generate great ferment and activity, all of which produce great opportunities for pharmacy as a health profession. Included among these are the extensive grant programs of the Public Health Service, the National Institutes of Health, and other agencies for vast research activity; the Hill-Burton hospital construction act; the Health Professions Educational Assistance Act; scholarships and loans for students of the health professions; construction and equipment grants for health schools; the Regional Heart Disease, Cancer and Stroke Act; and a host of others that have poured hundreds of millions of dollars in the support of health care.

Public's Concern About Drugs

From time immemorial people have been concerned about drugs and have always attributed certain magic properties to them and to those who handle them.

Society's attitude toward drugs and their use is a complex subject. As a whole, society believes that drugs are essential to health and well-being. Individuals and groups are concerned about any factor which tends to deprive anyone of needed drugs, whether these factors are related to poverty, cost of drugs, or the failure of the system which cares for the indigent.

Drug addiction is one of the most highly publicized and morally condemned social problems in America today. On the other hand, drug addiction and dependence are so widespread that they may be a part of some larger social problem, those of poverty and the presence of such a large number of disadvantaged, deprived, and unassimilated members of minority groups in our great urban areas. In fact, 10 cities account for 75% of all active narcotic addicts in the United States according to federal figures (19). Between half and two-thirds of the male prisoners and 95% of women prisoners at the city of Washington's Lorton reformatory are narcotic addicts (20). Consolidation of the old Bureau of Narcotics and Bureau of Drug Abuse Control into a new Bureau of Narcotics and Dangerous Drugs in the Department of Justice is evidence of the seriousness of this problem.

Paul Parker (21) in his article "Drugs and the People" discusses how pharmacy, which has always had the basic elements of a monopoly on drugs, became more obsessed with the business aspects than with the principle of protecting the public, and as a result, advertised drugs directly to the public, mass-merchandised them in drugstores, and placed itself in direct competition with the people who had a business advantage to gain from loosening its monopoly. Pharmacy can only regain its monopoly on drugs if it exercises control of them in the interest of public health. This could be done if pharmacies and drugstores were separated. "We must provide," as parker has said, "a drug emphasis that is consistent with the importance of drugs in the total concept of health care" (21).

THE FUTURE AS A PRESENT EXPECTATION

In view of the past and considering the present, what can we expect of pharmacy in the future? One does not have to be an angel to be a saint. Nor does one have to be able to divine precisely the future as a present expectation. This will evolve with commitment to professional practice, with changes in educational patterns and with research related to the ability of pharmacists to perform beyond the present demands placed upon them.

According to a physician, Ward Darley, ". . . the future of the pharmacist—if imaginatively approached—could be exciting indeed" (22). Dr. Darley makes several other comments about the pharmacist and pharmacy which I believe reflect quite accurately the attitude of the health professions and of society toward us.

> As a rule, the pharmacist has not been considered a professional in the mainstream of person-to-person patient care. His principal task has been to count or measure a prescribed brand of precompounded pills, capsules, liquids or powders, to prepare the proper labels, and to keep appropriate records. . . .
>
> With prescription drugs increasing in their effectiveness and, unless properly used, becoming increasingly dangerous, it is time for the pharmacist to become a more important member of the medical-care team. He should be used for what he knows as much as, if not more, than for what he does—indeed, under his supervision, many of the things the pharmacist does now could be done by other, less skilled assistants.
>
> This would free the trained pharmacist to play a truly significant part in patient care. He should be prepared to participate in the evaluation and distribution of drugs in the clinical setting. He should be active on the clinical floors of the hospital interpreting chart orders for medication; when necessary, preparing medications for the nursing staff; and providing consultative services to both physicians and nurses. . . .
>
> The pharmacist diluting his talents running the nonmedical aspects of a drugstore, would rapidly lose status as a professional. . . . The need for more pharmacists is clearly related to an upgraded and more professionalized role of the type suggested above. The pharmacist's future—quantitatively as well as qualitatively—may depend on his willingness and initiative in assuming these larger challenges and responsibilities and on his willingness and ability to become a meaningful member of the comprehensive medical-care team.

Once again in history, American pharmacy is faced with an opportunity and a challenge to change its path. We cannot continue to grasp simultaneously at the best of the professional world and at the best of the business world. In attempting to grasp both we lose both. We must decide either to follow the paths of the other health professions and concentrate our efforts on the health needs of the people, or to follow the paths of the entrepreneur.

The stimulating events of the recent past—particularly the social legislation—give us new hope for a rich professional future.

Pharmacy in America has not yet been united by a strong professional organization and has suffered as a result. There is a big question in my mind as to whether unification can take place with the great dichotomy we have today in pharmacy—and by that I mean the great number of drugstores in relationship to the number of pharmacies. In the absence of this, the continuing professionalization of pharmacy must depend more heavily on the influence of a small group of highly inspired and aspiring members. There is some evidence that a significant number of colleges of pharmacy are beginning to attract clusters of highly motivated practitioners with advanced professional degrees to their faculties to teach clinical pharmacy courses. Although these practitioners rarely possess the authority of power, they do possess the authority of ideas, which may have even greater influence with students. These practitioner-teachers may provide the spark needed to set pharmacy's course toward full professionalism. In due time, I anticipate that the professional degree of Doctor of Pharmacy will be as acceptable for a dean of a college of pharmacy as a degree of Doctor of Medicine is appropriate for a dean of a college of medicine today.

We must look to colleges of pharmacy for leadership to guide pharmacy's future. We can no longer afford to leave the future development of pharmacy to chance. We must take advantage of the new opportunities, of the aggressive social legislation and of the great interest in professional practice shown by today's pharmacy students. Several projects must be started simultaneously—efforts to separate legally the pharmacy and the drugstore, changes in pharmaceutical education and research in the community practice of pharmacy.

Separation of Pharmacies from Drugstores

The United States has more than 50,000 retail establishments known as drugstores with which are included a few thousand pharmacies. This great heterogeneous mass makes it impossible for the public and the allied professions to discern clearly, to distinguish carefully, or to recognize in any way the pharmacist practicing in one of them as a professional person. Drugstores in America so greatly outnumber the pharmacies that when pharmacies are called drugstores and drugstores are called pharmacies the terms pharmacist and pharmacy become meaningless to the public because they are equated with druggist and drugstores.

America is a land of many peoples of European heritage, and part of this heritage is the concept of the pharmacy and drugstore. In Europe, the pharmacy is a dignified setting in which a professional man serves the health needs of the people. The drugstore is an establishment that sells a variety of goods including certain herbs and household remedies and is operated by a person with principally vocational training. When these two establishments are put together, as they are in America, the dignity of pharmacy and the pharmacist is lost completely, especially since they are so greatly outnumbered. The relatively few pharmacies are engulfed, enmeshed, submerged, and choked by the many drugstores.

Brodie has said that one of the first things pharmacy must do is to get the pharmacist out of the drugstore and into a professional setting so that he can be readily identified as a pharmaceutical specialist by the public and by the practitioners of other health professions (23). To do this effectively, we must legally separate pharmacies from drugstores. This is indeed an arduous and complicated undertaking in a country with 50 sets of state laws, but it must be done. This is not the time nor am I the person to discuss legal questions, but essentially I would like to see the pharmacies licensed to sell prescription drugs with the privilege of handling nonprescription drugs and other health-related services. The drugstore could sell anything except prescription drugs and would not be required nor permitted to employ a pharmacist. Whether drugstores would employ a person with a special training as is done in Europe must be decided. For example, the general pattern of training for the druggist in Europe is three years of practical training in a drugstore, during which time the druggist goes to school one full day a week, he is allowed to manage a drugstore and to handle crude drugs, chemicals, herbs, certain poisons, and other miscellaneous goods.

Community Pharmacies for Education, Training, and Research

Each qualified college of pharmacy in the nation should establish a community prescription pharmacy for the education and training of professional practitioners under controlled conditions, and for the conduct of research. I am not talking about a college-operated student-health-service pharmacy, but rather, one that serves the population of a town or city and thus would be a pharmacy servicing a representative population. There must be a concerted, nationwide effort on the part of the colleges to train pharmacists in clinical practice under ideal conditions in an establishment operated, controlled, and supervised by the college. The pharmacy should be designated and constructed for teaching and research purposes and should be operated by professional practitioners holding appointments on the faculty.

Such a pharmacy would reflect the best in pharmaceutical practice for students to emulate. It would establish patterns, explore new possibilities, conduct research, investigate unmet health needs, and test new potential roles for pharmacists. It would be a living, viable, dynamic part of the college's instructional program with which the prospective community pharmacist could identify, in a manner similar to the way in which hospital pharmacists identify with the hospital in which they serve their residency. The pharmaceutical center could provide a model for all undergraduate students and would be an essential tool for the training of Doctor of Pharmacy candidates. I know the arguments against colleges engaging in activities of this type, but those in favor of it are so overwhelming that it could gain strong support from community pharmacists if properly explained.

Research in Community Practice

There is great need for research in pharmacy practice. Colleges must begin to pay appropriate attention to the needs of pharmacy practitioners for research as they have heretofore to the pharmaceutical sciences. Research will be possible if the colleges operate pharmacies under controlled conditions.

A very important question is the expanded role the pharmacist can play in the handling of drugs for the benefit of society. What other health services can be appropriately rendered by a pharmacist? Is there a place for clinical laboratory services in a pharmacy? What can he do to help relieve the health manpower shortage? What can he do to help the physician, nurse, or other health personnel function more effectively? What is his relationship to the medical center of his community? What is his role in the broad aspects of public health? How could he serve the public more effectively in the use of nonprescription drugs? What relationships can be developed with extended-care facilities, nursing homes, and small hospitals? What influence can he have on the abuse of drugs by the public? What type of education will he need for these new roles? How will he be compensated? Brodie has said that "the classical professional purpose for pharmacy as we have known it will not sustain us in the future" (23).

The need for research in pharmacy was recognized by the Task Force on Prescription Drugs, which stated that the public sees the role of the pharmacist as simply transferring pills from a large bottle to a small one, typing labels, and calculating the price (24). The real question for pharmacy, says Hubbard, is whether the pharmacist will function at a high technical level or whether he will serve a professional role (25). In this connection it is interesting that the United States is one of the last of the developed countries which does not have a trained pharmacy technician. In many countries, technicians do the work of pharmacists here. What can be done to raise the level of the pharmacist's contributions to public health to take advantage of his level of education?

The major problem which prevents pharmacy from stepping across the line of marginality is its failure to gain control over the social object which justified the existence of its professional qualities in the first place, according to the social scientists Denzin and Mettlin (26). Pharmacists view the drugs as a product to be sold rather than an object of service for a patient. Can pharmacists perform a socially useful function for society by accepting the responsibility for the control of drugs for the benefit of the public health? I believe that society would give this function to pharmacists if it could readily identify them. Here is a subject worthy of the greatest research effort.

The role of the hospital pharmacist has been expanding, evolving, developing, and maturing until now it represents a base from which we may think about the evolution of pharmacy as a profession. What roles of the hospital pharmacist can be transferred, with or without adaptation, to community practice? Brodie has called attention to some of the advantages in rendering a professional service a pharmacist in a pharmaceutical center has over the hospital pharmacist—particularly the highly personalized service possible from a community pharmacist (27). What use can be taken of these?

The Future as a Present Expectation

Pharmacy can become a meaningful profession only if it is separated from the drugstore. For years pharmacists have tried to serve two masters and failed. Pharmaceutical educators have encouraged the merging of these two paths—business and professional. In turn, students recruited to colleges of pharmacy have the same mixed interest ranging from a purely business to a professional, highly humanitarian orientation. According to the sociologists Denzin and Mettlin (26):

> It is not surprising then that pharmacy has failed to send practitioners out into the field who could correct the deficient aspects of its professional image. 'True' professions demand greater commitment from their students than does pharmacy—and similarly, 'true' professions—like medicine, organize the activities of their members around consenually held supra-individual humanitarian goals and values. On both of these counts pharmacy has failed to achieve a stance which would accord it the status of a profession.

To a great extent we have failed because we have sought to serve two masters. Pharmacy must recognize that its future lies with the professional world. The world of commerce unrelated to health should be left to the drugstore. Pharmacists must commit themselves to take the road toward full professionalization. "You may hold yourselves fit for the palaces of princes," Oliver Wendell Holmes told a group of young doctors in 1858, "or you may creep back to the Hall of the Barber Surgeons, just as you like. It depends on how the profession bears itself whether its members are peers of the highest, or barely tolerated operatives of society."

We now have great opportunities to change our past patterns, a chance to make our profession meaningful and rich in dignity and inspiration and service to the health needs of society. Merely changing the locus of practice of pharmacists from a drugstore to a pharmacy will have great psychological impact on physicians and patients and upon society in general. We will either rise to new heights or sink to a new low. Society will not permit the expensive luxury of a five- and six-year educational program if our practitioners do essentially nothing more than count, pour, and label. It will demand much more of us, and we must determine our destiny through a program of intensive research. Our objective should be to answer the question: What role can the pharmacist play in fostering the safe and appropriate use of drugs by patients and by the public? Can we develop answers to this question by the beginning of the third millennium? Two out of three of us here will see the dawn of that day.

REFERENCES

1. Kremers E, cited by Blauch, LE and Webster GL., The pharmaceutical curriculum. p. 12, American Council on Education, Washington, D.C. (1942).
2. McCormack T. H., "The Druggists' Dilemma: Problems of a Marginal Ocupation," *Am. J. Sociol.* 61:308–315 (1956).
3. Flexner, Abraham, *Medical Education in the United States and Canada,* The Carnegie Foundation for the Advance of Teaching, New York (1910).
4. Tice, L. F., cited by Brodie, Donald C., *The Challenge to Pharmacy in Times of Change,* p. 45, American Pharmaceutical Association and American Society of Hospital Pharmacists, Washington, D.C. (1966).
5. Elliott, Edward C., *The General Report of the Pharmaceutical Survey 1946-49,* p. 230, American Council on Education, Washington, D.C. (1950).
6. Francke, Don E., et al., *Mirror to Hospital Pharmacy,* p. 17, American Society of Hospital Pharmacists, Washington, D.C. (1964).
7. Brodie, Donald C., *The Challenge to Pharmacy in Times of Change,* p. 45, American Pharmaceutical Association and American Society of Hospital Pharmacists, Washington, D.C. (1966).
8. Rising, L. Wait, "A Situation and a Plea," *Am. J. Pharm. Educ.* 6:253–254 (1942).
9. Rowe, Tom D., Introduction, p. 2, Proceedings Pharmacy-Medicine-Nursing Conference on Health Education, University of Michigan (1967).
10. White, Eugene V., "Conceptual Design of Pharmaceutical Practice in the Community," pp. 69–77, *Proceedings-Medicine-Nursing Conference on Health Education,* University of Michigan (1967).
11. Kahn, Herman and Wiener, Anthony J., *The Year 2000: A Framework for Speculation on the Next Thirty-Three Years,* pp.105–117, The Macmillan Co., New York (1967).
12. Barker, Kenneth N. and McConnell, Warren E., "The Problems of Detecting Medication Errors in Hospitals," *Am. J. Hosp. Pharm.* 19:360–369 (1962).
13. Rising, L. Wait, "Theory and Practice Can Be Combined," *Am. J. Pharm. Educ.* 9:557–559 (1945).
14. Rising L. Wait, Editor's Mail, *Am. J. Pharm. Educ.* 9:579 (1945).
15. Rising L. Wait, "The Washington Experiment," *Am. J. Pharm. Educ.* 1:257–264 (1947).
16. Anon., "Report of the Committee on Educational and Membership Standards, *Am. J. Pharm. Educ.* 10:80–89 (1946).
17. Youngken, H. W., Jr., "The Washington Experiment—Clinical Pharmacy," *Am. J. Pharm. Educ.* 17:64–70 (1953).
18. World Health Organization, *The International Governmental Organizations,* 2nd ed., vol. II, p. 1881.
19. Barber, Bernard, *Drugs and Society,* p. 117, Russell Sage Foundation, New York. (1967).
20. Weil, Martin, "D.C. Health Chief Says Majority of Lorton Inmates Are Addicts," *Washington Post,* Feb. 2 (1969).

21. Parker, Paul F., "Drugs and the People," *Am. J. Hosp. Pharm.* 24:350–355 (1967).
22. Darley, Ward and Somers, Anne R., "Medicine, Money and Manpower—The Challenge to Professional Education. III. Increasing Personnel," *New Engl. J. Med.* 276:1414–1423 (1967).
23. Brodie, Donald C., "Emerging Patterns of Education and Practice in the Helth Professions—Pharmacy," pp. 23–35, *Proceedings Pharmacy-Medicine-Nursing Conference on Health Education,* University of Michigan (1967).
24. Task Force on Prescription Drugs, *Second Interim Report and Recommendations,* p. 54. U.S. Department of Health, Education, and Welfare, Washington, D.C. (1968).
25. Hubbard, W. N., Jr., "Emerging Patterns of Education and Practice in the Health Profesions—Medicine," pp. 5–9, *Proceedings Pharmacy-Medicine-Nursing Conference on Health Education,* University of Michigan (1967).
26. Denzin, Norman K. and Mettlin, Curtis, J., "Incomplete Professionalization: The Case of Pharmacy," *Social Forces* 46:375–381 (1968).
27. Brodie, Donald C., *The Challenge to Pharmacy in Times of Change,* p. 20, American Pharmaceutical Association and American Society of Hospital Pharmacists, Washington, D.C. (1966).

IS PHARMACY A "LEARNED" PROFESSION[d]?

Richard A. Angorn
James E. Thomison

Is pharmacy a "learned" profession? One might wonder what difference it makes whether pharmacy is considered a "learned" profession, or any other kind of profession, as long as pharmacy continues to be a respected calling. In fact, the question is more than rhetorical.

It must be answered with certainty and decisiveness, and the answer must be able to withstand the test of legal challenge, because the ramifications are important. An affirmative answer places pharmacy in the advantageous position of being able to chart its own future with minimum interference from either the courts or from state legislatures. A negative answer serves, at best, to maintain the status quo, and, at worst, reduces pharmacy to the status of a nonprofession.

STATUS QUESTIONED

From time to time, the professional status of pharmacy has been called into question. Pharmacy has generally been regarded as a profession, but questions have arisen as to whether it is a "statutory" or a "learned" profession. A bill was recently introduced in the Alabama legislature declaring pharmacy to be a "learned" profession. Until the bill passes and is signed into law, pharmacy, in Alabama, will continue to be a "statutory" profession and thus more susceptible to legislative caprice.

Classification of the practice of pharmacy into an occupational category depends on the definitions given to it by the courts, state legislatures, and Federal administrative agencies. An examination of the pertinent occupational categories is in order at this point.

---

[d]Reprinted with permission from Angorn RA, Thomison JE. Is pharmacy a "learned" profession? Am Pharm 1985;25:27–30.

OCCUPATIONAL CATEGORIES

Traditionally, both courts and legislatures have categorized certain occupations as trades, professions, statutory professions, or learned professions. These distinctions assume greater importance than ordinary societal classifications, because they affect the way the courts and legislatures view the appropriateness of both self-regulation and governmental regulation.

Trade: The dictionary defines trade as "an occupation requiring manual or mechanical skill."[1] The courts have held that a trade is an "occupation or employment, particularly mechanical employment," that can be "distinguished from the liberal arts and learned professions and from agriculture.[2]

The U.S. Supreme Court has continued to recognize its early definition of trade: "Wherever any occupation, employment, or business is carried on for the purpose of profit, or gain, or a livelihood, not in the liberal arts or in the learned professions, it is constantly called a trade."[3]

Carpentry, shipbuilding, tailoring, blacksmithing, and shoemaking are cited as examples of trades, although "some of these may be, and sometimes are, carried on without buying or selling goods."[4] The definition is broad; it can encompass both manual and mechanical skills as well as commercial activities.

Profession: A profession has been defined as a "calling requiring specialized knowledge and often long and intensive academic preparation."[5] According to one court, a profession is "A vocation, calling, occupation or employment involving labor, skill, education, special knowledge and compensation or profit, but the labor and skill involved in predominantly mental or intellectual, rather than physical or manual.[6]

"The term originally contemplated only theology, law, and medicine, but as applications of science and learning are extended. . . , other vocations also receive the name which implies professed attainments in special knowledge as distinguished from mere skill."[7]

Pharmacy practice, most people would agree, is not a trade, despite the commercial activity that is usually involved. Pharmacists have long been recognized as professionals, and pharmacy has been recognized as a profession, by both courts and state legislatures. Nevertheless, the courts have found it necessary to distinguish between "statutory" professions and "learned" professions.

Statutory Profession: A "statutory" profession is an occupation or vocation that has been accorded professional status by legislative action. Courts have defined "statutory" professions as any occupation other than law, medicine, or theology, for which entry restrictions are reasonable because of the skill or knowledge required for their competent practice.[8] The Supreme Court of Alabama views pharmacy as a "statutory" profession.[9]

Learned Profession: Originally, only law, medicine, and theology were recognized as "learned" professions. The modifier "learned" came into use to distinguish them from the other vocations, callings, or employments that were generally recognized as professions, but which did not require a high degree of literacy and long years of academic preparation as prerequisites for admission.

The Supreme Judicial Court of Massachusetts, in a 1939 antitrust decision, cited an 1896 U.S. Supreme Court case which noted that "Traditionally, the learned professions were theology, law and medicine; but some other occupations have climbed, and still others may climb to the professional plane."[10]

It went on to say that "learned professions are characterized by the need of unusual learning, the existence of confidential relations" and "the adherence to a standard of ethics higher than that of the market place . . ."[11]

The court also noted that the learned professions create a personal relationship of trust and confidence between the practitioner and the client, and this relationship promotes a degree of intimacy not normally required of other occupations.[12]

Whether pharmacy attains uniform status as a "learned" profession in the United States ultimately depends on the public's perception of the practice of pharmacy and the extent to which the courts and legislatures are willing to reflect the public's views. A look at the traditional as compared with the modern legal views of pharmacy shows that the public's perception of pharmacy has undergone a significant change.

TRADITIONAL VIEW

Traditionally, courts have viewed a pharmacist as a "compounder" of drugs. For example, in 1886 the Kentucky Court of Appeals stated that a pharmacist is a person who possesses the knowledge and skills necessary to compound and dispense medicines.[13] This view of pharmacy has left a legacy of problems.

In the past, the practice of pharmacy required special knowledge about the preparation of medications, but today many of these medications are available in prepared dosage forms. Some people believe that the availability of these prepared dosage forms diminishes the need for pharmacists. This view is reflected in U.S. Supreme Court Chief Justice Berger's comment that pharmacists primarily perform a packaging function.[14]

In applying the traditional test for determining whether an occupation is a "learned profession" to pharmacy, three conditions must be satisfied.

The test will be met and pharmacy will have "climbed to that professional plane" if: (1) pharmacists require "unusual learning" in order to practice; (2) pharmacists "adhere to a standard of ethics higher than that of the marketplace;" and (3) a "confidential relationship" of trust and confidence arises between pharmacists and patients through the disclosure of "intimate information."

In the case of pharmacy all three conditions have been satisfied: (1) both the U.S. Supreme Court and the Federal government have recognized the pharmacy curriculum as a prolonged course of specialized study;[15] (2) the U.S. Supreme Court has recognized the codes of professional ethics of the American Pharmaceutical Association and the state pharmacy associations;[16] and (3) intimate information is frequently revealed to pharmacists when a physician or patient seeks drug counseling.

Finally, although no jurisdiction has any specific pharmacist-patient confidentiality privilege, either by common law or by statute, some courts have recognized the intimate nature of a pharmacist's role by extending the physician-patient confidentiality privilege to include a pharmacist's records of a patient's medical history.[17]

MODERN VIEW

In 1975, the U.S. Supreme Court noted that the states have a particular interest in preserving the professionalism of licensed pharmacists.[18] The court recognized that today's pharmacist has been clinically trained in basic pharmacology, clinical pharmacology, drug toxicity, drug monitoring, and patient education. Extensive academic and practical exposure in these areas has produced pharmacists capable of educating physicians and patients on the selection of rational, cost-effective, and therapeutic drug regimens.

Table 1.   Professional degrees of some health professions

Professional degree	Preprofessional study (years)	Professional study (years)
M.D. (Medicine)	3	4
D.D.S. (Dentistry)	2	4
D.V.M. (Veterinary medicine)	2	4
O.D. (Optometry)	2	4
Pharm. D. (Pharmacy)	2	4
B.Sc. (Pharmacy)	2	3

As more drug patents expire, the number of generic alternatives on the market will increase. Trained pharmacists, who can assess the consequences of complex bioavailability data on these products, are well qualified to distinguish the clinically important from the clinically insignificant differences in drug products.

Awareness of drug interactions that have potential clinical importance is growing rapidly; pharmacists' drug expertise allows them to recognize and help prevent the additive or antagonistic actions that can happen when the patient is taking several drugs.

Another new area in pharmacy practice is the preparation of parenteral solutions and the monitoring of their use. Pharmacists are also in the forefront in clinical applications of plasma drug levels and formulation of dosing regimens for individual patients. Most important, pharmacists are the best source—for both physicians and patients—for general information on the relative benefits, adverse effects, and costs of various therapeutic compounds.

EMERGING MODERN VIEW

Just as the profession of pharmacy has evolved, so has the legal system's view of what constitutes a "learned" profession. The scope of the "learned" professions has continued to expand, as modern courts have come to appreciate burgeoning educational requirements and evolution of more specialized occupations. For example, optometry[19] and dentistry,[20] two callings of relatively recent origin, were not included among the original three "learned" professions, but are now recognized as "learned" professions in various jurisdictions.

The Federal government has specifically defined "learned" professions as "those requiring knowledge of an advanced type in a field of science or learning customarily acquired by a prolonged course of specialized intellectual instruction and study as distinguished from a general academic education and from an apprenticeship and from training in the performance of routine mental, manual, or physical processes."[21]

The U.S. Supreme Court has adopted this definition: it expressly recognizes engineering as a "learned" profession.[22] The *Code of Federal Regulations* specifically lists pharmacy as a "learned" profession.[23]

PHARMACY A "LEARNED" PROFESSION

Given the modern legal view of the "learned" profession, is pharmacy really a "learned" profession?

Pharmacy is obviously a dynamic profession that has changed immensely over the past century. That the U.S. Supreme Court has chosen to recognize the state's strong interest in the preservation of pharmacy's professionalism greatly enhances the stature of pharmacy. For example, recognition of the pharmacist's expertise on drugs prompted the Florida legislature to enact a statute that gives Florida pharmacists the right to prescribe certain drugs from a specified formulary.[24]

As the practice of pharmacy has become more complex, educational and licensing requirements have correspondingly become more exacting. In fact, the Federal government expressly recognizes pharmacy as meeting "the requirement for prolonged course of specialized intellectual instruction" in its definition of the "learned" professions.[25]

Therefore, as the "learned" professions have expanded beyond medicine, law, and theology, to encompass dentistry, optometry, and engineering, it seems reasonable that the states should concur with the Federal government in recognizing pharmacy as a "learned" profession.

STATE LEGISLATION

The pharmacy practice act of Florida alludes to the "practice of the *profession* of pharmacy."[26] Other states' pharmacy practice acts declare outright that pharmacy is a profession,[27] while many states' pharmacy practice acts are completely silent on the issue. So far, no states have enacted a legislation which says that pharmacy is a "learned" profession.

In its battle to attain "learned" profession status in statutes, optometry, a profession of recent origin, has so far succeeded in getting a toehold in a handful of states. Pharmacy, however, an ancient profession that quite possibly predates medicine, is not so recognized in any state's statutes and is only now beginning to assert itself.

HISTORICAL COMPARISON

Sometime between 1231 and 1240, Frederick II, Emperor of the Holy Roman Empire, issued an edict to establish pharmacy as a distinct and separate profession, wholly independent from medicine.[28]

Although the edict applied only to a portion of the Empire, the Kingdom of the Two Sicilies (Sicily and lower Italy), in the ensuing years the concept spread and became firmly entrenched throughout continental Europe.

From the beginnings of history, pharmacy and medicine had been intertwined. They were, in all practicality, one and the same "learned" profession. However, as scientific knowledge continued to increase, the tasks allotted to each began to diverge so it became logical to separate medicine and pharmacy into two independent "learned professions." In continental Europe, pharmacy continues to be a "learned" profession.

Modern pharmacy, in England, has other roots:[29] it developed from an alliance of the spicers and chemists, the purveyors of crude drugs and chemicals.

The United States, to a great extent, was influenced by its British heritage. However, until the twentieth century, it was predominantly a frontier country. The rules that had worked so well in continental Europe did not seem to make much sense on the frontier. A laissez-faire attitude dominated the marketplace. There were no well-established or long-entrenched pharmaceutical and medical professions; licensing was practically unknown.

Physician dispensing paralleled the practice of the British apothecaries and competed directly with that of pharmacists.

Pharmacists, in turn, responded to the competition from dispensing physicians and the vendors of patent medicines by engaging in general merchandising.

It wasn't until after the 1820s, and the establishment of the first colleges of pharmacy, that the practice of pharmacy began to emerge as a distinct profession. The United States, settled for slightly more than 200 years, was beginning to show its first stirrings toward professional status for pharmacy.

The advances in medicine and pharmacy in the twentieth century were truly phenomenal; the post-World War II explosion in pharmaceutical scientific knowledge drastically changed the complexion of pharmacy and gave it a new, highly professional image.

VITAL MEMBER

Under all modern legal tests, pharmacy is indeed a "learned" profession. Pharmacy has long been acknowledged as a profession. It requires long years of academic training as a prerequisite for entry and a commitment to continuing education in order to keep up with the continuum of its scientific knowledge base.

The pharmacist is a vital member of the health care team, and pharmacy must make its role known by educating both the public and the legal system. If pharmacy is ever to attain its proper recognition as a "learned" profession in all fifty states, individual pharmacists, professional associations, and colleges of pharmacy must take concerted action to propose enlightened legislation in order to advance pharmacy to its proper status.

REFERENCES

1. *"Webster's Seventh New Collegiate Dictionary,"* G&C Merriam Co., Springfield, MA, 1967.
2. *Woodfield v. Colzey,* 47 Ga. 112.
3. *U.S. v. National Association of Real Estate Boards,* 339 U.S. 485 (1950).
4. *Id.,* at 491.
5. *Supra,* note 1.
6. *Maryland Casualty Co. v Crazy Water Co.,* Tex. Civ. App., 160 S.W. 2d 102.
7. *U.S. v. Laws,* 163 U.S. 258 (1896).
8. *Lee Optical Company of Alabama, Inc. v. State Board of Optometry,* 261 So. 2d 17 (Ala. Sup. Ct. 1972).
9. *ID.* at 24.
10. *Commonwealth v. Brown,* 20 N.E. 2d 478 (Mass. Sup. Ct. 1939).
11. *Id.*
12. *Id.*
13. *State Board of Pharmacy v. White,* 84 Ky. 626.
14. *Virginia State Board of Pharmacy v. Virginia Citizens Consumer Council, Inc.* 425 U.S. 748 (1975).
15. *Id.* at 751; 29 C.F.R. Sec. 541.302 (1984).
16. *Id.* at 751.
17. *Rudnik v. Superior Court of Kern County,* 114 Cal. Rptr. 603 (Cal. 1974).
18. *Supra,* note 14 at 766.
19. Arkansas Stats, Anno., Chapter 8, Sec. 72-801; Colorado Rev. Stats., Chapter 102, Sec. 102-1-1; Georgia Code Anno., Title 84, Sec. 1101; Nevada Rev. Stats., Title 54, Sec. 636.010.
20. *Graves v. Minnesota,* 272 U.S. 425; *Commonwealth v. Brown, supra,* note 10; *State v. Kindy Optical Co.,* 248 N.W. 332.
21. 29 C.F.R. Sec. 541.302 (1984).
22. *National Society of Professional Engineers v. U.S.,* 435 U.S. 679 (1978).

23. *Supra,* note 21.
24. Florida statute Sec. 465.186 (1985).
25. *Supra,* note 21.
26. Florida Statute Sec. 465.003(12) (1983).
27. See, e.g., pharmacy practice acts of AK, AZ, CO, GA, ID, IA, KS, ME, MS, NH, NY, ND, TN, TX, and VA.
28. G. Sonnedecker, *"Kremers and Urdang's History of Pharmacy,"* 4th ed., J. B. Lippincott, Philadelphia (1976), pp. 34–35.
29. G. E. Trease, *"Pharmacy in History,"* Bailiére, Tindall and Cox, London (1964), p. 181.

5
Psychosocial Aspects of the Illness Experience

DONNA DOLINSKY, Ph.D.

Patients understand their illness within their own conceptual framework, which includes their own beliefs, thoughts, and feelings. They process that information using their own algorithms, which may not correspond to those of Baysian statistics (1), and then make their own decision and act.

The purpose of this chapter is to describe these experiences, these psychosocial aspects of the illness experience that influence patient decisions, and also to describe and analyze the decision making process.

People experience symptoms that they may label as portending illness and then decide whether they will become a patient or will treat themselves. Those who become patients make further decisions about how faithfully they will follow their prescribed treatment. The series of events that patients experience and take part in on their path from sickness to wellness is not necessarily direct, simple, or even logical. It is influenced by multiple factors, external and internal to the patient. Internal factors, the psychosocial factors, are the patients' thoughts, beliefs, and feelings about their sickness and drug therapy, and the process of making decisions about their medications and health behaviors. The external factors or systems factors that have an impact on a patient's health include quality of health care services, appropriateness of drug therapy, and quality of interaction with various health professionals.

The systems factors influencing health outcomes, such as quality of health care services and quality of interaction with health professionals, are addressed in other chapters in this volume. This chapter addresses patients' experiences, perceptions, feelings, decisions, and behaviors that are related to the maximizing of their own health outcomes.

The following personal accounts of illness and medication taking (Refs. 2 and 3, respectively) will illustrate what is meant by the psychosocial aspects of the illness experience, i.e., the illness experience from the patient's perspective.

PATIENT 1

"Yes, I am a pharmacy student. But yes, I have been diagnosed as schizophrenic. . . . In lectures on antipsychotic drugs, I want to tell faculty and fellow students what it feels like to take medicines and have to depend on them to function "outside" and what it is like to be titrated as an individual to the proper to the proper medication and dosage and the problems involved. I want to talk about schizophrenia and let them know it is not so far removed from them and correct some of the common misconceptions held about people who have schizophrenia. . . . During my first semester of pharmacy school I was on 2 mg of Haldol and 2 mg of Cogentin h.s. . . . .I found I could neither read the board nor my notes; everything was blurred no matter where I sat. . . . I also had problems with what a friend of mine called "the Stelazine stroll"—akathisia. In an effort to be self-destructive, and perhaps as part of the uncontrolled disease process, I stopped my psychotherapy and medication for 3 months. I was a pharmacy student with probably one of the worst compliance problems possible. . . . I didn't take the medicine at times because I didn't want the disease, its problems, and its stigma. I wanted to be normal. . . it would probably shock many people to know a schizophrenic was in their class. . . . I have been on the dean's list, and have friends, and expect to receive my pharmacy degree from a major university."

PATIENT 2

"From the age of 8 months to 26 years I was an intractable asthmatic. . . . . . . the burden of never really feeling good, of being frail, and a "sickly runt" began to affect my personality. . . . I began to lose [sic] confidence in any future. . . . I could distinguish those doctors who were interested in a creative solution and those who relied on routine procedures and could not conceal their attitude toward a kid who knew *a lot* about what worked *for him* and what did not."

A pharmacist might describe the above cases in terms of accurate medical diagnosis, rational drug therapy, appropriate drug product selection, technically correct dispensing, accurate and understandable presentation of medication information, and effective drug therapy monitoring. The patients above perceive and describe their situations quite differently. They talk about feelings, e.g., fear, anger, and low self-esteem. They express their own thoughts and beliefs about their illness: "I would like to talk about schizophrenia and let them know it is not so far removed from them. . . ," (2), and "I could distinguish those doctors who. . . could not conceal their attitude toward a kid who knew *a lot*." (3) Behavior is also described: "I was a pharmacy student with probably one of the worst compliance problems possible." (2).

As with all human actions, the decisions regarding health behaviors are influenced in part by external stimuli, e.g., a pharmacist advises a patient to "take your medicine as indicated," and also by internal states, such as those thoughts and feelings and beliefs described above. When confronted with a health problem and a rational drug therapy solution designed by an expert health professional, it is not uncommon for patients to choose to not accept the advice exactly as dispensed. Patients often choose to modify their treatment plan to meet their needs as they perceive them, within their own conceptual framework based upon their own experiences.

Thus, the patient's health outcomes may ultimately be more dependent upon what the patient feels, thinks, believes, decides, and does than on accurate medical diagnosis, rational drug therapy, appropriate drug product selection, technically correct dispensing, and accurate and understandable presentation of medication information.

Humans experience symptoms, label them, do something about the symptoms, or do not, consider themselves either to be or not to be ill, do or do not seek out and accept treatment, have thoughts, feelings, and beliefs about their illness, treatment, health professionals, and environments, make decisions, act, and then interpret the outcome of their actions within their own frame of reference. All of these experiences have a tremendous influence on patients' future decisions regarding their medication taking and health related behaviors.

Why do pharmacists need to know this? As pharmacy is evolving toward a strong clinical orientation, many pharmacists are talking to patients about the drugs they dispense. The dialogue that occurs between patient and practitioner often is one of pharmacist telling and patient listening. The purpose of this "telling" has been to ensure that patients will know how to take their medications and take them properly. Unfortunately, there is not a one-to-one correspondence between telling and knowing, or knowing and doing. Patients take information and process it within their own cognitive framework, which is based upon their interpretation of their own experiences. The meaning that the patient attaches to the information may be quite different from the meaning that the pharmacist attaches to the information. An understanding of the patient's feelings and thinking process will enable the pharmacist to move beyond information and product dispensing to taking on the additional role of "helping professional." Understanding the drug-taking process from the patient's point of view can help the pharmacist help the patients make better decisions about their medication taking and related health behaviors. To practice as a "helping professional," the pharmacist needs to know what kinds of communications to be sensitive to, that is, the kinds of messages that patients send about their illness experience that may influence how they decide to carry out their medication regimen. Pharmacists who choose to practice as "helping professionals" need to better understand the psychosocial aspects of their patients illness experience, and through appropriate counseling, can increase the likelihood that their patients will make better decisions about their medication-taking behavior.

The psychosocial aspects of the illness experience that have been investigated within disciplines of social psychology, medical sociology, health psychology, behavioral pharmacy and that will be addressed in this chapter follow. They roughly parallel stages that a patient may go through, from experiencing symptoms and seeking (or not seeking) treatment to deciding on the degree to which a treatment plan will be followed. The sequence does not imply linearity, but exists as a means of grouping concepts. Decisions, for example, are occurring constantly, not just after a patient has been treated and given a medication.

The psychosocial aspects of the illness experience that will be discussed are:

1. the difference between disease and illness
2. illness behavior—how people interpret and respond to symptoms
3. sick role—how people behave and are expected to behave when ill
4. group differences in interpretation of illness
5. affective and cognitive reactions to illness
6. health beliefs
7. models of health-related behaviors
8. how patients decide

DISEASE AND ILLNESS

Illness happens to humans. Disease happens to organs. Most health professionals, including pharmacists, seldom come into direct contact with a disease, diseased tissue, or a diseased organ to the degree that a pathologist does. But they do come in contact with humans who are taking medicines to alleviate symptoms of disease. Thus in dispensing medications, counseling patients, and monitoring drug therapy, the pharmacist needs to understand not only the disease, but also the illness, i.e., patients' perception and interpretation of their disease. To efficiently perform in the role of the helping professional, one must deal with, communicate with, that intermediary between the health professional and the disease, i.e., the human, and that human's developing feelings, thoughts, beliefs, decisions, and behaviors related to his or her interpretation of the disease. This somewhat nebulous idea of illness can be operationalized by the concept of illness behavior.

ILLNESS BEHAVIOR

Muscle soreness, tiredness, and a moderately altered sense of reality will be interpreted differently by persons in different contexts. A person who has just completed running a 6½-mile race attributes the symptoms to having succeeded in reaching a "personal goal" in completing a race, wears the "pain" proudly, and does nothing more perhaps than take a hot bath. A person awakening on a winter morning with those symptoms interprets the symptoms as flu, predicts that this may mean at least 1 day's loss of work and several days of discomfort, and then takes some antibiotics that were not completed from an earlier prescription. A person who has just begun a new chemotherapy regimen attributes the symptoms to the drug, reacts with a feeling of loss of control over his or her own health, which, in turn, leads to feelings of depression. The person continues the regimen and does not mention the symptoms to his physician because he is aware that many chemotherapy agents have side effects and he or she does not want to be a bother.

These three different interpretations of the same symptoms appear to make sense in each of the above cases to each individual. The definition of the illness, the decisions made, and subsequent behavior were primarily influenced by the patient's perceptions of and interpretation of symptoms, within the patient's experience, cognitive processing, and organization of those experiences. The behavior was not automatically triggered by the pain and discomfort. "Generally it is agreed that objective pathology of disease is neither a necessary nor a sufficient condition to prompt the seeking of medical care (4). The inclusion of the patient's framework in identifying symptoms, decision making, and behavior is encompassed in the concept of illness behavior.

> "The term *illness behavior* describes the way persons respond to bodily indications which they experience as abnormal. Illness behavior thus involves the manner in which persons monitor their bodies, define and interpret their symptoms, take remedial actions, and use the health-care system. People differentially perceive, evaluate, and respond to bodily changes, and such behaviors have enormous influence on the extent of the interference of symptoms with usual life routines, the chronicity of the condition, the attainment of appropriate care, and the cooperation of the patient in the treatment situation." (5)

In the example presented above, the athlete's evaluation of the muscle soreness, tiredness, and moderately altered sense of reality was that the pain and symptoms were not serious. She defined them as a normal response to running a race and then decided that she did not need to utilize the health care system.

The second person's interpretation and evaluation of the symptoms resulted in the belief that he had "flu" and that the disorder needed to be treated. He treated himself with a leftover antibiotic.

The last person, the patient on chemotherapy, attributed the symptoms to his medication, evaluated the symptoms as moderately serious, and chose to not take remedial actions or to communicate his symptoms to a health care professional. The symptoms were interpreted and evaluated differently by each person, different decisions were made, and different actions were taken as a function of the differential interpretation and evaluation of the patient.

Differences in illness behavior occur as a function of the immediate experience, past experiences, and patients' information processing and resultant cognitive structures, i.e., how information is organized and recalled by the patient. *The subjective and psychosocial aspects of the incident were more important in determining decision and action than the symptoms themselves.*

There are differences among patients in how they focus their attention on symptoms and also differences between patients and health professionals. Patients and health professionals may focus upon and stress the response to different types of symptoms, with the health professional's stress on symptoms that may occur after long periods of time, such as long-term symptoms from smoking. The patient may focus upon symptoms that have short-term consequences, such as a cough.

Health professionals may be more likely to focus on long-term gains at the expense of a short-term loss for the patient, such as discomfort, whereas patients may be more likely to focus on short-term gains at the expense of long-term losses. Health professionals have more experience with a greater number of illnesses and ill patients and have seen patients' health worsen as a function of taking risks. Patients decisions are more often based upon their own illness experience. They have not seen many progressions along the health-wellness continuum change as a function of risky behavior, as the health professional has, and make decisions to take short- or long-term gains based upon their own experience.

Thus, adolescent smokers may not be influenced by arguments related to long-term consequences of smoking, such as lung cancer, but may be influenced by discussion of short-term consequences of smoking, such as performing less well athletically or being less socially desirable.

An understanding of illness behavior can help the pharmacist appreciate and accept why patients respond differently to what appear to be similar stimuli, e.g., pain or discomfort. The knowledge can also help a pharmacist understand why patients sometimes behave in ways that appear, to the pharmacist, to be illogical.

SICK ROLE

Once patients decide they are ill, they decide how they are going to act. As students' behaviors change as they switch from the student role to the role of worker, athlete, or spouse at the end of a day of classes, people's behaviors also change as they move from the healthy role to the sick role (6). Parsons found specific types of behaviors that occurred when people perceived themselves to be sick. These were:

1. The patient is not blamed for the sickness since they did not choose to become ill.
2. The patient is exempted from work and social and personal responsibilities.
3. As long as the patient accepts the undesirability of the illness, it is recognized that the illness is legitimate.
4. The patient and the family of the patient are expected to seek competent help and work to get well.

These behaviors are psychological, not logical, and are quite normal and relatively common in the general population. Subsequent studies on specific populations found that all people did not follow Parsons' patterns of sick role.

Cockerham (7) concluded that "although Parsons' concept of the sick role has provided a useful framework for understanding illness behavior, it has not been generally useful, or in all cases sufficient because of its failure to (a) explain the variation within illness behavior; (b) apply to chronic illness; (c) account for the variety of settings and situations affecting the patient-physician relationship; and (d) explain the behavior of lower class patients. Meile (8) found that the sick role also was not applicable to mentally ill patients who are reluctant to ask for help and try to get well. Although exceptions occur, the sick role does exist and many but not all patients do take on the role.

Pharmacists and pharmacy students should be cautious in using group data from research to make decisions about individuals, e.g., believing that a specific mentally ill patient will not ask for help. As indicated above (8), groups of mentally ill patients were less likely to ask for help than were groups of physically ill patients yet as seen in the article written by the schizophrenic pharmacy student at the beginning of this chapter (2), a pharmacist using those group data to make a decision about that patient would have been in error, as that patient did seek help and did try to get well. The stereotyping that can occur by overgeneralizing group data to individual patients can interfere with the patient-health professional relationship required in the "helping" professions. Evidence of stereotyping by health professionals has been documented in textbooks and in practice, with health professionals having negative attitudes toward certain patient groups (9). When given more in-depth information on individual patients, (individuating information), health professionals' stereotyping decreased.

Understanding the reality of these patterns of behavior may keep a pharmacist from labeling a patient as "lazy" or "irresponsible" when, in fact, the patient is behaving quite normally.

Armed with knowledge of the dangers of stereotyping, one can approach the following studies with the understanding that a profile of a group represents an average of that group. It does not apply to every individual in that group.

GROUP DIFFERENCES IN INTERPRETATIONS OF ILLNESS

Although the concepts of illness behavior and sick role are useful in understanding broad patterns of the illness experience, medical sociologists have found that people's perceptions of and reactions to symptoms and illness are also influenced by ethnic and cultural backgrounds, class, and gender. For example, cultural and social influences appear to influence the type of helping professional selected by students experiencing psychological distress. Variables of gender, religious background, affiliation, education, and area of the country could be used to predict psychologically distressed students' choice of counselor, psychiatrist, clergyman, or physician (10). Studies on cultural, socioeconomic, and gender influences follow.

Cultural Influences

A classic study conducted by Zborowski (11) indicated that Jewish and Italian hospitalized patients were more likely to respond emotionally to pain than Irish and Yankee (Old American) patients. The Jewish and Italian patients were considered to have had a more expressive response to pain whereas the Irish and Yankee patients were labeled as stoical and denying of pain. Italian and Jewish patients emphasized the perception of pain, whereas the Old American and Irish tended to deemphasize it. Irish and Old American patients said that they preferred to hide their pain, while Jewish and Italian patients admitted freely that they showed their pain by crying, complaining about it, being more demanding, and by stating that they could not tolerate pain. Withdrawal from others when in pain was most characteristic of the Old American. Those patients who are easily given to emotional expressiveness for cultural, social, or psychological reasons may, in the view of the pharmacist who is not from that culture, overstate their distress and distort the description of their physical experience when speaking to or communicating with a health professional.

Thirty years later, Lipton and Marback (12) also found cultural and ethnic differences in response to symptoms. They obtained verbal descriptions of patients' pain sensations, related behaviors, attitudes, and meaning attached to pain by different ethnic groups and found the following:

- Black patients were more likely to seek care from lay (nonmedical) individuals when ill. There was also greater dependency during sickness on members of one's social and ethnic group. Emotional and expressive responses to pain were accepted, and it was acceptable to have daily functioning disrupted by pain.
- Irish patients found it was acceptable that pain caused disruption in daily functioning. Their response to pain was generally nonemotional.
- To Italian patients, chronic pain was reacted to strongly with both emotional and expressive responses and with disruption in performing usual activities.
- Jewish patients explained pain experience in terms of level of psychological distress, e.g., the pain caused the patient to become upset. Patients responded expressively and emotionally to the pain and allowed pain to interfere with daily functioning.
- Puerto Rican patients expressed high levels of distress when in pain. They were highly likely to depend on strong friendship and group solidarity as supports when in pain. Emotional expressiveness to pain was common, and great disruption in daily activities was attributable to the pain.

The behavior of the groups of Italian, Jewish, and Irish patients was not unlike that found earlier by Zborowski.

Swedish patients were found to have stronger beliefs in personal responsibility for health than Australian patients, which was likely to be due to the emphasis by the Swedish Health Care System on preventive health through exercise and good nutrition (13). It also was hypothesized that with the greater emphasis on psychosocial aspects of health care in the Australian system, patients may be more likely to demonstrate emotional distress because of expectations that it would be addressed.

Spector (14) reviewed and summarized several additional studies describing cultural and ethnic beliefs and behaviors in illness for the following groups: American Indian, Asian American, Greek American, Mexican American, and Filipino Americans.

WHAT THIS MEANS FOR THE PHARMACIST.   Different patients may react differently to what appears to be a similar degree of discomfort from a drug, e.g., frequent urination after taking a diuretic. As indicated above, those differences in reaction may be influenced by ethnic and cultural differences. However, when one uses group data from these studies to predict how an individual patient may behave, one is likely to make an error because one would be attributing the mean of the group to any member, including those three standard deviations above and below the mean.

The value of the studies discussed in this chapter lies in their potential to sensitize the pharmacist to the fact that we are all influenced by our ethnic and cultural backgrounds, and that we often consider our own attitudes and behaviors to be the "correct" attitudes and behavior, and those from other ethnic and cultural backgrounds to be different, strange, or wrong. The second point to remember is that not all people from a group behave in the same way, and by generalizing from a group to an individual, we are likely to make an error.

Socioeconomic Differences

Koos (15) found that people in lower socioeconomic groups, as defined by their educational level and income, were less likely to visit a physician when experiencing physical symptoms such as loss of appetite, coughing, and fainting. DiMatteo and Friedman (16) suggest that this behavior is probably not due to differences in attitude toward health care among different classes, but probably due to their ability to pay. Although third party payment plans exist for low income people, payments to physicians through these plans are usually less than what would be paid by a private insurance company, and some physicians will not accept these patients. Physician utilization by the poor has increased since Medicaid and Medicare, however, the poor are more likely to be seen in emergency rooms or in outpatient clinics, whereas higher income groups are more likely to receive medical services in private doctors' offices and in group practice.

There also is lower utilization of health prevention services among the poor (7). Curbow (17) found that health care presented within the context of not having a choice was devalued and influenced intentions to seek care. Welfare services were considered to be of inferior quality and to be avoided. Intended utilization of health care services was lowered for all women in a no-choice condition. "Health care that is forced upon clients is potentially stigmatizing and likely to be avoided" (17). Thus, decisions to avoid using the health care system by the poor, appear to be related to their perception of the inferior nature of health care available to the poor.

Gender Differences

Mechanic (5) reviewed the literature on gender differences in utilization of health care services and found that women were more likely to report symptoms than men. Several interpretations have been hypothesized to account for this occurrence, i.e., women are more likely to become ill than men, women have lower thresholds of pain and discomfort, women are more likely to seek care because it is more acceptable for them to ask for help, or women cope differently than men. Mechanic indicated that few studies have been conducted that actually compare and validate these reasons.

Women are also more likely to receive a prescription for common ailments than are men (18), are more likely to be prescribed tranquilizers than men (19), and also less likely than men to receive answers to direct questions from male physicians (20). At this point, it is known that women are more likely than men to report symptoms, but it is not known why.

Meininger (21) found that illness behavior interacted with sex and social class. The relationships between social class and illness behaviors were very different for men and women. Other things being equal, women who sought lay consultation as opposed to doing nothing or using medical care and those who treated themselves instead of having a physician treat them were of higher social class. A very different pattern was observed for men. Those who used medical care were of significantly higher social class than those who did not, and those who sought lay consultation instead of medical advice had significantly lower social class scores. Some men may have equated going to the doctor for symptoms with taking on the sick role, which was not compatible with their definition of the appropriate male role and thus avoided if possible. This effect may have been more pronounced among men in the lower social class groups due to the fact that the degree of sex role differentiation is inversely related to social class (22).

Other things being equal, those women in higher social class groups may be more selective about seeking medical care for their symptoms. In this instance, social class could be serving as a proxy variable for greater knowledge about health matters or availability of lay consultants with such knowledge.

As seen in the previous studies, patterns exist that describe, but do not explain, average behavior of groups on psychosocial aspects of the illness experience. It has been shown that groups of women when compared with groups of men behave differently in certain health-related situations, however, that difference cannot be explained with the information available, nor should those group data be used to make a prediction or decision about an individual woman or man.

AFFECTIVE AND COGNITIVE REACTIONS TO ILLNESS

In the studies and examples above, we have seen patients experiencing symptoms, demonstrating illness behavior, i.e., labeling symptoms and signs, making decisions regarding whether or not to seek help, and selecting the type of help to seek. The patients may have taken on the sick role, to some greater or lesser degree, and choices may have been influenced by cultural, class, and social variables. The experience of illness involves affective and cognitive reactions to the illness, in which the patient will undergo emotional changes and also attempt to understand the illness. Family members also experience some of these emotional reactions. Bernstein and Bernstein (23) described the following common emotional reactions to illness and treatment:

1. emotional reactions directly related to illness or treatment
   a. fear and anxiety
   b. feelings of damage
   c. frustration caused by loss of habitual gratification and pleasure
2. Reactions determined primarily by life experience before or during illness
   a. anger
   b. dependency
   c. guilt
3. Complications
   a. depression
   b. loss of self-esteem

Mechanic (5) found that psychological distress, i.e., anxiety and depression, were correlated with symptom reporting.

Many of these emotions are expressed by the two patients in their statements at the introduction to this chapter. They are common reactions to illness and influence patients' behavior. Zoller (3) expressed guilt about his illness, "As I got older, I began to be aware of the fact that hospital costs exceeded medical insurance and felt that I was a financial drain on the family." He also expressed frustration ". . . the burden of never really feeling good, of being frail, and a "sickly runt" began to affect my personality." In an anonymous account, another individual (2) expressed feelings of depression: "The schizophrenia worsened and I became depressed in addition, due to my inability to cope."

An example of patient fear was illustrated by Tagliacozzo and Mauksch (24) who interviewed 86 hospitalized patients and found that they were apprehensive about the reliability of the health professionals responsible for their care and often feared for their safety. Yet, because of the expectations of the patient to "trust and have confidence" in their health professional, the patients did not permit themselves to express their fears.

Lederer (25) identified three main periods of illness and described the psychological responses patients experienced as they moved through those stages. During the first period, *transition from health to illness,* along with physical responses, patients experienced anxiety, denied that they were ill, were aggressive and irritable or passive. During the second period, *acceptance of illness,* patients demonstrated behavior that could have been described as "sick role," e.g., temporary withdrawal from adult responsibility. Other behaviors also were demonstrated. Patients became **egocentric** in that they became concerned with their own needs such as eating, drinking, resting, and the need for physical comfort. Their personal needs took precedence over their social needs. Some patients believed that people around them were focused primarily upon their (the patients') needs and would become hurt if they found this to not be true. There was a **constriction of interests** in that patients became apathetic about work, business, friends, and social events. Patients became **dependent** and were willing to let others make decisions for them, which created both a sense of comfort for the patient and also a contradictory feeling of resentment at having to be dependent. Patients also demonstrated **hypochondriacal behavior** as indicated in the following statement (26) of the wife of an AIDS patient.

> Hypochondriasis, meanwhile, has become our favorite pastime. AIDS is unlike cancer, leukemia, and tuberculosis in that one never knows what ailment may ultimately lead to death. Every hangnail, pimple, rash, cough, or pain becomes a matter of serious discussion. My husband, who abhorred calling a doctor if he was sick, now must immediately report any temperature over 100°.

The third period of illness described was *convalescence.* During this period, physical strength along with personality integration returned. The dependent and egocentric behavior ended. The period was likened to adolescence in that adolescents are ambivalent about growing up and taking responsibility even though they want the freedom that comes with adulthood. Some patients also expressed repressed hostility toward health professionals at this time, in much the same way that adolescents react toward authority.

As stated earlier, members of the patient's family also experience emotional reactions to the patient's illness. The following quote (26) is from the wife and mother whose husband has AIDS.

> Then there is the anger, rational and irrational. Some days I am consumed with anger at just about everyone and everything—anger at my husband for dying and, however unwillingly, exiting the center stage of my life; anger at society for not doing more to fight this disease; anger at the insurance companies for approaching AIDS as a drain on their profits; anger at religious ostriches who fail to realize that AIDS is a medical, not moral, problem.

While patients are experiencing emotional reactions to illness, they are forming hypotheses in an attempt to understand their disorders. Myer, Leventhal, and Gutmann (27) found that 88% of people in continuing treatment for high blood pressure believed they knew when their blood pressure was elevated if they experienced headaches, face flushing, or heart pounding, even though they agreed with the statement that "people cannot tell when their blood pressure is elevated." The authors' explanation for this apparent contradiction was that patients build their own schemas or representations of what they believe to be occurring, and that these beliefs are based upon their interpretation of their own experiences within the framework of their past experiences. Patients' models were designed upon their interpretation of their own personal experience and not "facts" or "scientific principles."

HEALTH BELIEFS

While experiencing the psychological and sociological aspects of illness and generating hypotheses to explain their illnesses, patients eventually accept some of their own hypotheses and form beliefs, that are judgments they hold to be true concerning their illnesses. Those beliefs, which have been found to correlate with preventive health behaviors and sick-role behaviors (behaviors whose intent is to restore health or prevent further disease progress), are listed below (28):

1. perceived susceptibility of contracting a disease
2. perceived severity of medical and social consequences of the disease
3. perceived benefits of related behaviors
4. perceived barriers

The concept of "perception" is an important concept in the Health Belief Model. It is the patient's perception that drives decisions and behaviors, not the pharmacist's perceptions. The responsibility of the pharmacist who chooses to act in the role of a "helping professional" is to go beyond giving information about his or her own perceptions of the drug and disorder and to enter into the patient's world and address that patient's perceptions from within. These components of the Health Belief Model are discussed elsewhere in this volume (see Kimberlin, "Communications," pp. 00–00).

MODELS OF HEALTH-RELATED BEHAVIORS

Although common sense might tell us that patients' decisions to seek health care, accept a diagnosis, and engage in health-related behaviors would be related to the severity of a disease, the studies described above indicate that this is generally not true. Patients' health behaviors are a function of many psychosocial variables, as indicated in the research reviewed above. Most of these studies focused upon individual variables such as gender, social class, and hypothesis generation concerning the illness. There is another means of analyzing the psychosocial aspects of the illness experience, and that is through models of health-related behaviors.

An analysis of systems-related variables that influence health behaviors is beyond the scope of this chapter, however, models of health-related variables have addressed psychosocial variables along with systems variables. Efforts to systematically study predictors of health behaviors have been undertaken by numerous investigators.

Models have been generated to explain correlates of health-related behaviors, and extensive research has been conducted to test the effect of elements of these models. Becker and Maiman (29) discussed those models that were most effective in predicting health-related behaviors (health behaviors, illness and sick role) and were cited most often. Cummings et al. (30) asked eight living authors of the models discussed to group the 109 variables extracted from the models. These variables were then clustered into the following six major groupings:

1. accessibility of health services
2. attitudes toward health care
3. perception of threat of illness
4. knowledge about disease
5. social interactions, norms, and structure
6. demographics, i.e., social status, income, and education

Although attitudes toward health care and perception of threat of illness are represented in these models, the other psychosocial aspects of illness are missing. Health behaviors are explained primarily in terms of systems variables and other variables external to the patient.

Thus, the patient is not seen to be the decision maker in charge of his or her own health behaviors, but rather is seen as influenced by forces outside him- or herself. While patients' health behaviors are influenced by variables external to them, the patient alone makes the final decision about medication taking and health behaviors.

HOW PATIENTS DECIDE

All of the previous information on psychosocial aspects of the illness experience is valuable in helping the pharmacist to understand what leads up to the process patients go through when making decisions about taking their medication. At this point, the pharmacist can choose to dispense medications and give information on the medication to the patient, ending the interaction with the patient at that point, or the pharmacist can choose to become involved in helping the patient to make a "better" decision about taking medication.

Once a patient accepts symptoms and is diagnosed, treatment is prescribed, medication is dispensed, and the patient is counseled regarding the medication, the hand of the health care system is removed and the patient is expected to comply with the medication regimen. First, the patient decides.

There is increased evidence that patients want to become involved in decisions regarding their own medical treatment and that this increased role in decision making may lead to greater rates of patient compliance, greater satisfaction with their health care, and better health outcomes.

Leventhal (31) hypothesized that the reason that early compliance research was not successful in identifying the "noncompliant personality" was that an inappropriate model of human behavior was posited to explain the behavior. The model presented humans as passive organisms that respond to stimuli (instructions to take medication in a certain way) and then are reinforced (getting well) for behaving appropriately. Leventhal believes that patients choose and uses control theory to explain patient medication-taking behavior. The major principle in control (self-regulation) theory is that the individual forms a representation or schema of his or her illness and uses that schema to evaluate information and choice of coping behaviors. This is the patient's private illness model. Representations or understandings of the patient's illness are generated by comparing and fitting current symptoms to past representations of illness. These representations are our own theories of how and why we are ill, not automatically ingested chunks of information presented to us by our health professionals. They include "at least four features: (31)

1. an identity, consisting of a symptom pattern and an illness label
2. a perceived cause
3. expectations about the severity or consequences of the illness
4. time lines or expectations about the duration of the illness (acute, cyclic, or chronic) and the other features, such as how long it takes the cause to operate and consequences to develop."

These representations were illustrated by Meyer, Leventhal, and Gutmann (27), who found that 88% of patients in treatment for high blood pressure believed that they could monitor their pressure by attending to symptoms such as headache, face flushing, and heart pounding. Eighty percent of this group of patients agreed that "people cannot tell when their blood pressure is elevated." Bauman and Leventhal (32) further investigated the relationship between patient representations of their illnesses and medication taking and pathology and found that even though patients believed that they could tell when their blood pressure was increasing, the majority could not, as was indicated by blood pressure readings being taken as patients predicted a rise in pressure. When patients were told that their blood pressure had not increased, their beliefs in their ability to monitor their own pressure were influenced little. They continued to hold their representations of their illnesses despite factual information to the contrary.

Wolfe (33) reported studies in which patients' anxiety about their illnesses was reduced and they were more likely to be careful about following specific recommendations for medications when given copies of their medical records. Once the paternalism that has traditionally existed in patient-health practitioner relationships has been reduced and patients openly participate in decision making regarding treatment, desirable health outcomes increase as patients take greater responsibility for their health care.

The reality of patient decision making regarding health outcomes is illustrated by the *Health Decision Model* (34), which combines the Health Belief Model discussed earlier, decision analysis, and behavioral decision theory.

Decision analysis is a systematic means of studying the process of decision making. It is a means for patients, pharmacists, and physicians to assign numbers to their perceived value of therapeutic outcomes and also to the probability that that outcome would occur. One can compute the utility (value and probability of occurrence) of each outcome. Theoretically the decision maker will choose the outcome with the highest utility (35). A problem with decision analysis occurs because humans do not always make decisions logically or treat information objectively or value free (1).

Behavioral decision theory (36–38) may be shown to be more effective in understanding how patients make decisions about their medication and health-related behaviors because it is a body of research and theory on how people actually make decisions. Behaviors that have been studied include acquisition of information, information processing (including thinking about probabilities), responses to situations requiring making decisions under uncertainty, and finally, interpreting outcomes of that decision. Common biases in decision making also have been investigated and described. Examples of patterns of bias in decision making are presented below (3).

1. Risks involving gains and losses. Patients are more likely to take a health risk to avoid an aversive situation rather than to gain a positive health outcome. An example of this principle would be a patient who would take a medication when faced with a life-threatening disease (a possible loss) even though the medication is highly likely (the risk) to have a very bad side effect. The same patient, however, would not take the risk of suffering from the same side effect of a medication if no life-threatening disease were involved (no loss) and if the purpose of taking the medication was to gain a benefit, such as increased well-being.

2. Certainty effect. Patients are more likely to choose a certain outcome rather than an outcome with a high probability of occurrence, even if the certain outcome is less valued then that one with a high probability of occurrence. This directly contradicts the expected utility theory, which is the basis of decision analysis, explained above.

3. Sunk costs. When a person has already invested time and money into a product or activity, he is likely to continue it, even if it does not appear to be effective. A person who continues to wear a disliked article of clothing because he paid a considerable sum of money for it is behaving according to the principle of sunk costs. A cancer patient may continue to take Laetril because she paid a considerable

amount of money for the product, even though there are no observable benefits from the product.

Why do humans behave so illogically? Hogarth (36) explained that humans are biased when making decisions under uncertainty because we fail to "appreciate randomness." We believe that there are known causes and effects for all phenomena, and we have a need to be able to explain outcomes. It is more comfortable to attempt to explain, even though incorrectly, than to have to deal with an ambiguous situation. Humans also tend to be inconsistent in judgment, often because it is not always possible to remember how a judgment was made in the past. Logical rules, which are designed by humans to help other humans make better decisions, seldom explain how human decision making actually occurs. Machines that humans design are often logical, but humans themselves are psychological.

Another reason that humans tend to be biased in their decision making is that we seldom have feedback from negative decisions. That is, if we decide not to elect to follow a treatment regimen, we do not know how effective it would have been if we had followed the regimen. Yet, there is a propensity to prefer the outcome chosen.

Additional biases are described by Hogarth (36) that could be useful in understanding patients' choices about their health behaviors. Some of these follow:

1. Availability. Well-publicized events tend to be believed more than less-publicized. A patient may choose to buy a highly advertised over the counter (OTC) product rather than a house brand.
2. Selective perception. We tend to believe what matches our existing beliefs.
3. Concrete versus abstract information. A real incident will be believed more than abstract statistics. A patient may be more likely to change a dietary habit if it helped a family member than if given outcomes of a research study supported following the diet.
4. Two incidents occurring close in time and place tend to be seen as causal, even though they may have nothing to do with each other.
5. We tend to be reluctant to revise our beliefs, even given new data, and would rather discount the new information rather than discount our belief. If a patient believes that aspirin helps "nerves" and is told otherwise, a patient may believe that it does not help most people with "nerves," but it works for him. The hypertensive patients discussed earlier (27) continued to believe that they could monitor their own blood pressure by responding to symptoms, even when their blood pressure was taken and they were shown that they were not successful in their monitoring.
6. Very few instances of an occurrence are needed for us to form a new belief if it has a strong impact upon us.
7. We believe something is more likely to happen if we want it to happen.
8. A decision resulting in success is more likely to be considered to be due to the knowledge and wisdom of the decision maker. A decision resulting in loss is likely to be blamed upon another.

These are a few examples of principles of human decision making that influence how patients may make decisions about their medication-taking behaviors and health outcomes. Human decision making under uncertainty, with its many common biases, is very different from the logical process used by computers, or from the way in which we feel we should make decisions.

Human decision making is influenced by a myriad of psychological and sociological factors that interact in many nonlogical ways. Pharmacists who want to better understand patient medication taking and health-related behaviors need to sensitize themselves to this process of decision making, in order to help their patients make better decisions.

SUMMARY

The goal of this chapter was to sensitize pharmacists to the many psychological and socio-logical factors involved in patients' interpretations of their illnesses, emotional reactions to illness, decision making, and subsequent medication taking and health-related behaviors. As more pharmacists choose to practice as members of the health care team and develop into "helping professionals," they need to understand patient behavior in order to help their patients make better decisions about their own health care.

Common patterns of human reactions to illness were described and explained in this chapter. Patients were found to differ in how they labeled symptoms (illness behavior) and how they reacted to illness once they had accepted the fact that they were ill (sick role). These behaviors were found to be linked to cultural, class, and gender differences. The studies presented average behaviors for groups, and readers were cautioned against over-generalizing the mean of that group to every member of that group (stereotyping). Common affective or feeling responses to illness, e.g., depression, anxiety, and frustration, were de-scribed and illustrated with examples. The role of patients' health beliefs in health behav-iors was presented. Finally, common biases in human decision making were described, with examples of applications to medication-taking behaviors.

As pharmacists become sensitized to the psychological needs of the patient, they can move from the dispensing role, beyond the information-giving role, to the role of health professional and helping professional, i.e., with primary interest is in the well-being of the patient.

REFERENCES

1. Viscusi WK. Are individuals Bayesian decision makers? Am Econ Assoc Papers Proc 1985;75:381–385.
2. Anonymous. First person account: schizophrenia—a pharmacy student's view. Schizophrenia Bull 1983;9(1):152–155.
3. Zoller JE. Ill and well, with or without doctors. Asthma 1984;21(1):53–57.
4. Alonzo AA. Everyday illness behavior: a situational approach to health status deviations. Soc Sci 1979;13A:397–404.
5. Mechanic D. The experience and expression of distress: the study of illness behavior and medi-cal utilization. In: Mechanic D, ed. Handbook of health, health care, and the health profes-sions. New York: The Free Press, 1983, p 591.
6. Parsons T. Definitions of health and illness in the light of American values and social structure. In: Jaco EG, eds. Patients, physicians and illness. New York: The Free Press, 1958, pp 165–187.
7. Cocherham WC. Medical sociology. Englewood Cliffs, New Jersey: Prentice-Hall, Inc., 1986, pp 95–98.
8. Meile RL. Pathways to patienthood: sick role and labeling perspectives. Soc Sci Med 1986;22:35–40.
9. Blalock SJ, Devellis B. Stereotyping: the link between theory and practice. Patient Educ Coun-seling 1986;8:17–25.
10. Greenley JR, Mechanic D. Social selection in seeking help for psychological problems. Health Soc Behav 1976;17:249–262.
11. Zborowski M. Cultural components in response to pain. J Soc Issues 1952;8:16–30.
12. Lipton JA, Marback JJ. Ethnicity and the pain experience. Soc Sci Med 1984;19:1279–1295.

13. Westbrookm MT, Nordholm LA, McGee, JE. Cultural differences in reactions to patient behavior: a comparison of Swedish and Australian health professionals. Soc Sci Med 1984;9:939-947.
14. Spector R. Cultural diversity in health and illness. New York: Appleton-Century Crofts, 1985.
15. Koos E. The health of regionville. New York: Columbia University Press, 1954.
16. DiMatteo MR, Friedman HS. Social psychology and medicine. Cambridge, MA: Oelgeschlager, Gunn, & Hain, 1982, p 123.
17. Curbow B. Health care and the poor: psychological implications of restrictive policies. Health Psych 1986;5(4):375-391.
18. Verbrugge LM, Steiner RP. Prescribing drugs to men and women. Health Psych 1985; 4(1):79-98.
19. Anderson JE. Prescribing of tranquillizers to women and men. Can Med Assoc J 1981;125:1229-1232.
20. Wallen J., Waitzkin H, Stoeckle JD. Physician stereotypes about female health and illness: a study of patient's sex and the informative process during medical interviews. Women Health 1979;4:135-146.
21. Meininger JC. Sex differences in factors associated with use of medical care and alternate illness behaviors. Soc Sci Med 1986;22:285-292.
22. Troll LE. Early and middle adulthood. Monterey CA: Brooks/Cole, 1975, p 290.
23. Bernstein L, Bernstein RS. Interviewing: A guide for health professionals. 1980, pp 128-144.
24. Tagliacozzo DL, Mauksch HO. The patient's view of the patient's role. In: Jaco EG, ed, Patients, physicians and illness. New York: The Free Press, 1972, pp 162-175.
25. Lederer HD. How the sick view their world—social interaction and patient care. Philadelphia: Lippincott, 1965.
26. Day, S. My husband has AIDS. The New York Times, 1987, March 29, p 25.
27. Meyer D, Leventhal H, Gutmann M. Common-Sense Models of Illness: The Example of Hypertension, Health Psych 1985;4(2):115-135.
28. Janz NK, Becker MH. The health belief model: a decade later. Health Educ Q 1984;11(1):1-47.
29. Becker MH, Maiman LA. Models of health-related behaviors. In D. Mechanic ed, Handbook of health, health care, and the health professions. New York: The Free Press, 1983, p 591.
30. Cummings KM, Becker MH, Maile MC. Bringing the models together: an empirical approach to combining variables used to explain health actions. Behav Med 1980;3(2):123-145.
31. Leventhal HL. Behavioral medicine: psychology in health care. In: Mechanic D, ed, Handbook of health, health care, and the health professions. New York: The Free Press, 1983, pp 714-717.
32. Baumann LJ, Leventhal H. "I can tell when my blood pressure is up, can't I?" Health Psych 1985;4(3):203-218.
33. Wolfe SM. Why you need a copy of your medical records. Health Let 1986;2(4):5.
34. Eraker SA, Kirscht JP, Becker MH. Understanding and improving patient compliance. Ann Intern Med 1984;100:258-268.
35. Einarson TR, McGhan WR, Bootman JL. Decision analysis applied to pharmacy practice. Am J Hosp Pharm 1984;42:364-371.
36. Hogarth R. Judgment and Choice. New York: John Wiley & Sons, 1983.
37. Wright G, eds. Behavioral decision making. New York: Plenum Press, 1985.
38. Eraker SA, Politser P. How decisions are reached: physician and patient. Ann Intern Med 1982;97:262-268.

SELECTED READING

THE PATIENT'S VIEW OF THE PATIENT'S ROLE [a]

Daisy L. Tagliacozzo
Hans O. Mauksch

Every society grants to the sick person special privileges and every society also imposes on the sick person certain obligations.[1] An understanding of such general norms can provide an effective guide to the study of the behavior and attitudes of the sick in our society. However, general norms gain meaning in a specific social setting, or may be modified by intra-institutional expectations. The extent to which a sick person may feel free to seek satisfaction for his emotional needs and to assume the "rights and privileges of the sick role" may thus depend on the social context within which behavior unfolds. Even if general rules for behavior remain the same, the patient may be influenced by considerations which involve efforts to accommodate to real or imagined expectations of significant others.

The experience of being hospitalized adds another dimension to the experience of being ill. This dimension consists of the rights and obligations which are legitimated by organizational forces and which are based on the fact that admission to the hospital is tantamount to assuming an organizational position with all the implications for normative compliance and sanctions. This discussion is based on a study which sought to ascertain to what extent the attitudes and needs which are organized around these two experiences, being ill and being hospitalized, may differ or even come into conflict with each other. The attitudes and reactions of patients were viewed within the context of a system of roles and as a consequence of the patient's efforts to conform to perceived systems of expectations. The study concentrated on the implications of hospitalization, with less concern for the illness role *per se*. It explored to what extent the role of the hospitilized patient may be lacking clear definitions of rights and easily definable criteria for legitimate claims. The question was raised whether the position and the attitudes of patients deprive them of genuine means to control others in the system and thus limit their readiness to express their claims and desires without fear of sanction.

Throughout the study the patient is shown to be aware of the degree to which he is dependent on those who care for him. This dependency is based largely on the power to heal and to cure. It is also based on the power ascribed to hospital functionaries to give or to withhold those daily services which, for the hospitalized patient, can embrace some basic survival needs. The single or double rooms and the rapid patient turnover in the modern hospital do not foster an effective patient community which could serve as interpreter and modifier of hospital rules. The patient, therefore, is much more dependent on his previous

[a]Reprinted with permission from Jaco EG, ed. Patients, Physicians and Illness. 2nd ed. New York: The Free Press, 1972.

Based on a study conducted by the authors through the Department of Patient Care Research, Presbyterian-St. Luke's Hospital, Chicago, Ill. This study was supported by a grant from the Commonwealth Fund.

[1]Parsons, T., "Definitions of Health and Illness in the Light of American Values and Social Structure," in E. G. Jaco (ed.), *Patients, Physicians and Illness,* New York: Free Press, 1958, pp. 165–187 (chap. 8 in this volume).

learning, be it from direct or indirect experiences with the patient role. More importantly, the absence of adequate interpretations by the patient community makes the patient more dependent on hospital functionaries for clues about the appropriateness of his behavior, demands and expectations.

The fact that patients frequently remain strangers in the hospital community tends to add to the power of those who, as functionaries, are intimately familiar with the rules and expectations of the organization. The power which is vested in them can inhibit the patient to seek clarification and guidance. Also, those who are informed tend to become oblivious to the needs of their clients to be initiated into the "rules of the game."

The study was conducted in a metropolitan voluntary hospital with a capacity of 850 beds. The hospital is part of a large Midwest medical center. It is a teaching hospital for nurses and physicians. Patients occupy predominantly two-bed or private rooms.[2] This discussion rests on the analysis of 132 interviews which were administered to 86 patients. The sample was limited to patients who were admitted with cardio-vascular or gastro-intestinal diagnoses. All patients in the sample were Caucasian, American-born males or females between 40 and 60 years of age. All patients had been previously hospitalized and all were married. They paid for their hospitalization in part with private or industrial insurance. During the semi-structured interview, the patient was asked to express himself freely on present and previous hospital experiences. The interviews averaged one hour and were recorded and transcribed. The average day of interviewing was the fifth day of hospitalization. When possible, second interviews were conducted.

PHYSICIANS AND NURSES: THEIR SIGNIFICANCE

Physicians and nurses are among the significant others in the network of role relationships in which the hospitalized patient becomes involved. Their significance is derived from different sources. The physician represents authority and prestige. His orders legitimize the patient's demands on others and justify otherwise deviant aspects of illness behavior. The physician is not only the "court of appeal" for exemption from normal role responsibilities,[3] he also functions as the major legitimizing agent for the patient's demands during hospitalization. Yet his orders generally do not constitute guides to behavior in specific situations and they do not consider or modify the patient's understanding of the formal and informal expectations of nurses. Although the physician's authority ranks supreme in the eyes of most patients, they are also aware that he is only intermittently present and thus not in a position to evaluate the behavior of both patients and nurses and to sanction this behavior during the everyday procedures of hospital care.

The significance of the nurse stems not only from her authority in interpreting, applying and enforcing the orders of the physician but, in addition, from the fact that she can judge and react to the patient's behavior more continuously than the physician. From the patient's point of view, he also depends upon the nurse as an intermediary in the provision of many other institutional services.

For most patients it is of greatest importance to feel that they adjust to the expectations of the nurse and of the physician. To accommodate themselves to what they feel is expected of them, patients must be able to perceive these expectations as congruent or they must cope

---

[2]Thirty-two per cent of the patients in this sample occupied a private room; 61 per cent occupied a two-bed room and 7 percent shared a room with two other patients.

[3]Parsons, T., *The Social System,* New York: Free Press, 1951, pp. 433–477.

with the strains involved in efforts to adjust to what may appear to them as conflicting demands. Conflict is thus likely to rise if the nurse executes a plan of care which, from the point of view of the patient, deviates in detail or emphasis from the patient's interpretation of the physician's orders.

Close adherence to the orders of the physician was not equally important for all patients and not all patients appear to be equally intense in their sensitivity to congruence in the plan of care and cure. Those patients who expressed concern for complete adherence to the physician's word and expected strictest observance and literal interpretation of medical orders typically expressed distrust in the reliability and efficiency of anyone except the physician. These patients frequently feared that even minor deviations may result in further physical harm. For some patients, close adherence to medical orders appeared congruent with their conceptions of themselves; as did some patients, who resisted following certain medical orders, they used this area of conformity to convey something essential about themselves.

Demands for rigid adherence to medical orders were associated with the desire for "reliable" nursing care and "efficiency." The eagerly co-operative patient not only emphasized that he followed all orders willingly, he also expected the nurse to "co-operate" with him in his efforts to carry out the orders of the physician as he understood them. The patient's concern typically expressed itself in close observations of hospital personnel, in emphasis on observance of punctuality and in worry whether "orders have been written" and "charts double-checked." Such efforts to "co-operate with the physician" by seeing that "things get done" may become a source of stress. The patient who is ready to act on behalf of medical orders may have to call for services from the nurse and impose demands on her time or ask her to alter behavior. Thus, if the patient hears from the physician that the "specimen should be warm," he may feel obligated to insist that a "cooling-off" delay be avoided. If the physician has told him that he may "stay in bed another day," the patient's interpretation may lead him to actively resist a nurse's urging that he do some things for himself: "My doctor said that I can stay in bed another day." Patients' insistence on rigid adherence to the orders of the physician were frequently defended in the light of one implication of the sick role—the obligation to make efforts towards the restoration of health. Thus, patients who were critical of deviations from medical orders justified their criticism by pointing out that they did not want to be "complainers" or "troublemakers"—but that they, after all, "want to get well."

When a patient's efforts to co-operate fully and to observe the details of medical orders expressed themselves in more frequent demands, he also reacted to the risks involved in violating his obligation not to be demanding of nurses. Those patients who reported that they had expressed their desire for compliance with medical orders in active demands or complaints also tended to be very observant of the reactions of members of the nursing staff. Praise and criticism of "good" and "bad" nurses revealed that these patients rejected the nurse who "grumbled" and that they praised enthusiastically the nurse who responded "willingly" and who "smiled" when she was asked to do things for the patient. Patients also praised the nurse who "helped the patient to co-operate" and who "did not mind" when she was reminded of an order.

Those patients for whom co-operation with a physician's order became the guiding principle during hospitalization tended to be very sensitized to the reactions of others. They appeared to be "on the alert" and reacted quickly to facial expression, a tone of voice and the general manner in which a request was received. If they felt that their demands were not well received, they frequently became angered and, when given an opportunity, expressed their antagonism in attacks on those members of the nursing staff who "do not treat you like a person," who "make you feel that you are at their mercy" and "who consider you just a case."

The conflict between the felt obligation to insist on precise implementation of medical orders and efforts not to appear demanding or inconsiderate *vis à vis* the nursing staff was often resolved in favor of striving for approval by nurses. The data indicate that many patients prefer not to risk appearing too demanding or too dependent. They accept what appears to them to be deviations from the physician's orders, and even violate what they believe is expected of them by the physician. They anxiously watch a medication being late, rather than object to the delay, and they watch the specimen get cold rather than pointing this out to a nurse. Frequently this endeavor to "please" the nurse may backfire. Patients who disobey the physician's orders and get up to do "small things" for themselves rather than call the nurse may find themselves reprimanded by her because she may view this as lack of co-operation or even protest. She also may consider such behavior an incident which could incur the anger of the physician.

Thus, patients may pay for the security of "being liked" by nurses and of having them "know that I am not demanding" with concerns over arousing the physician's criticism or harming their own recovery. But even where the obligation to be cooperative with the physician is not immediately at stake, patients may somewhat reluctantly forego the privileges which they could claim as a result of being sick. As one patient expressed it:

> If it is a hotel you won't hesitate to pick up a phone or to complain; in a hospital you think twice about it—you figure maybe they are busy or shorthanded. . . .It's a much more human thing, the hospital. . . .it's more personal.

EXPECTATIONS AND CONSTRAINTS

When patients were asked what was expected of them by their physicians and by nurses, they responded with considerable consistency, indicating that several rules for "proper" conduct of patients were well defined and widely shared. The physician was seen as expecting "co-operation" and "trust and confidence." A large group of patients felt that the nurse, too, expected "co-operation." On the other hand, many patients were convinced that nurses expected them "not to be demanding" to be "respectful" and to be "considerate." Only very few patients listed these latter three categories for physicians.

Self-descriptions which patients introjected into the interviews followed a similar pattern. It was most important to patients that the interviewer saw them as having "trust and confidence" in those who took care of them. This was particularly true of those patients who also admitted to some negative reactions toward nurses or physicians. Many patients were eager to mention that they were not demanding, co-operative, not dependent and considerate. In spontaneous discussions of the obligations of the hospitalized patient, the pattern did not change significantly.

One of the factors underlying the patient's hesitation to impose demands on hospital personnel is his awareness of the presence of other, often sicker patients. Observation of other patients introduces restraints. Comparisons of "my illness" with the illness of the roommate appeared to intensify the moral obligation to "leave them free to take care of the seriously ill" and comparisons of one's own claims or criticisms with the behavior of a very ill person seemed to intensify restrained behavior: "After I observed him I felt kind of bad. I felt that I should be grateful and not ask for anything." It is well nigh impossible and a latent source of difficulty for the patient to judge his comparative status relative to patients in other rooms. The nurse summoned to give him a glass of water may have been called away from "a critical case." The isolation of the patient and the ensuing inability to establish relatives claims serve as restraining forces on the expression of needs,[4] even though this concern is counterbalanced with an occasionally voiced concern about "getting one's share."

The patient's perceived entitlement for service is also linked to his definition of the severity of his illness. Patients apparently feel more secure in ascertaining their rights if their understanding of their condition permits them to rank themselves in the upper strata of a "hierarchy of illness." However, a secure assessment of "my case" may be difficult. Communications from the physician are general and understanding of the relative severity of the illness does not appear to be facilitated by his explanations. In many cases, a statement such as "I want you to stay in bed" does not legitimize the demand for a glass of water—the patient gets up to avoid being considered "too demanding."

Patients thereforefore seem to link the extent of their claims on service to readily perceived and objectively visible indices. Thus, being in traction, having tubes attached or being restrained by dressings are highly ranked legitimators for patients' demands. Fever also serves as a criterion for claims; the patient who asks the nurse what his temperature might be not only may inquire about the severity of his illness but indirectly may also ask: "To what services am I entitled today?" Hospital rules which prevent the nurse from giving such information may deny the patient guidelines for the rules applicable to his behavior.

Two-thirds of all patients in the sample indicated that they had refrained from expressing their needs and criticisms at least once. The observation that nurses are too busy, rushed and overworked was given as the most frequent reason for this reluctance. Beliefs about the conditions under which hospital personnel work serve thus as another limiting factor in the patient's expression of demands. One has to keep in mind the admiration for nurses and for "all those who do such difficult work" to understand why some patients may spend a night helping another patient when being told "that there is a shortage on the nightshift." Some patients did not engage in these activities without some conflict. They admitted that they were concerned with the physician's reactions "if he finds out," and that they were fearful of the consequences of such activity for their health. Even though they never admitted it directly, many responses revealed indirectly their desire to take more advantage of the privileges of the sick.

Constraint in voicing demands was also reinforced by the patient's assessment of the power of hospital personnel and physicians relative to his own. Over one-fourth of those patients who admitted to restraint of their demands also expressed their often resentful assessment of their own helplessness. Efforts to be "considerate" of the conditions which limit services may thus be convenient rationalizations of the patient's fears of offending others and of endangering his good relationship with them. "Being on good terms" was seen by these patients not only as a convenient but as an essential factor for their welfare. They directly expressed their awareness of their inability to control those who are in charge of their care. Patients felt that they were subject to rewards and punishment and that essential services can be withheld unless they make themselves acceptable. Some of these patients were dependent upon intimate forms of physical assistance, and their points of view reflected their awareness of this dependence upon others.

---

[4]This phenomenon suggests a parallel to the concept of "relative deprivation" described by R. K. Merton and P. Lazarsfeld (eds.), *Continuities in Social Research*, New York: Free Press, 1950. Just as deprivation is experienced in relation to relative norms, legitimacy of claims rests on a relative basis. If this basis is not ascertainable, uncertainty functions as restraining force.

Feelings of helplessness were directly expressed in observations that "one is at their mercy," that "trying to change things is futile" and "won't get you anywhere" and that patients feel "helpless." The recognition of the power of others to withhold services also found expression in fears that one does not want to be considered a "complainer," or "trouble-maker" or a "demanding patient," and in such apprehensions as "they can refuse to answer your bell, you know," or "they can refuse to make your bed." The same fears were expressed in efforts "to save that button so they come when I really need them" or in enthusiastic reactions to nurses who "come in to inquire why you never call for them" or who "do not mind if you ring once too often."

Patients very rarely expressed openly a concern that their physician may impose sanctions on inappropriate behavior. They tried to be intensely considerate toward him, since he, too, is considered "very busy" and "on his way" to other sick patients. Attempts to accommodate demands to these pressures on the physician serve as a considerable restraint on the patient's willingness to ask questions.

The admiration for the physician was in most cases tied to a very personal and emotionally charged attachment to the man who is "so kind and understanding." Gratitude intensified efforts to "make things easy" for him. Although hostility or annoyances toward nurses was often directly expressed, patients actively resisted direct verbalization of any negative feelings toward "the physician." Typically, complaints were expressed reluctantly and in terms of "I wish he could" coupled with quick modifications such as "I know he can't—he is too busy."

Patients may also be concretely limited by the observation that the physician is "on the go." Thus, a patient may want to ask questions and feel that "taking his time" is legitimate, but may feel that the time is simply not made available:

> He'll say well, we'll talk about it next time. And next time he'll talk fast, he out-talks you—and rushes out of the room and then when he's out of the room you think, well, I was supposed to ask him what he's going to do about my medicine . . . you run in the hall and he has disappeared that fast.

A patient who was impressed with the fact that his physician was "overburdened and rushed" tried to describe how the resulting pressure of his own tensions and anxiety prevented him from fully comprehending what he was told:

> All I know is that your mind sort of runs ahead. You sort of anticipate what they are going to say, and you finish what they are going to say in your mind. I guess it's because perhaps sometimes you have trouble following them or maybe you would want them to say certain things, and you are listening— well, I don't know . . . you try to think what they are going to say, because otherwise, you have difficulty understanding them, but then, when they are out of the room, you don't remember a thing about what they have said.

In view of the above, it is not surprising that patients who were asked directly what they "considered their rights" had some difficulties responding. One-fourth of the respondents admitted that they did not know what their rights were; some patients stated outright that they had no rights. The majority of respondents limited themselves to general answers such as "good care," followed by the modification that specific claims depended upon the "seriousness of the illness." The belief that claims for service had to be justified in terms of immediate physical needs over-shadowed any inclination to voice the rights of paying consumers. Few patients justified their demands in relation to their monetary payment and many of those who introduced the criteria of a paying consumer quickly added to their demands other legitimizing factors, such as the nature of their illness or the fact that they had been considerate in other respects. Conceptions of rights and obligations provide guidelines for alternative actions. They are used and "fitted" in accordance with the exigencies of situations and the developing meanings which individuals and groups bring to bear upon them. The general patterns which have been discussed should not conceal that differences in the characteristics of patients may contribute to significant variations in the more general theme. The following observations will illustrate the importance of further research in this area.

Patients who do not experience active and well-defined symptoms and whose activities are not visibly impaired may hesitate to present themselves to others as seriously ill and may find "co-operation" at times more difficult. Patients with cardio–vascular illness tended to focus more frequently on behavior involving co-operation with physicians and nurses; particularly in relation to the physician, this obligation appeared to preoccupy these patients. They were also more intent on presenting themselves as co-operative to the interviewer. Some of these patients were severely ill from the medical point of view, requiring complete bed rest and its concomitant extensive services. However, they seemed to have a difficult time accepting this state without concern that they may be considered "too dependent" or overly "demanding." At times, these difficulties appeared enhanced by social and economic pressures to leave the hospital, and by psychological needs for denial which also seemed to find expression in the insistence that they "really did not need any special attention" and that they were "not worried about their illness."

Some of the subtle difficulties of these patients are not easily verbalized. Only rarely can a patient formulate as forcefully the aftermath of a heart attack as did the patient quoted below. His statement sums up the allusions and hints dropped by other patients with a cardiac problem:

> Well, you know, a heart patient is a peculiar animal. That heart attack has done something to him, not only physically but mentally. I can tell you this because I have been through it. It brings up something which you don't want to let go of. If he tells you you must stay in bed, well, how come this sudden change? I don't want to stay in bed, and if he tells you that you cannot walk upstairs, he is telling you that you are weak, that you are no longer strong. He has taken something away from you—ah, your pride. You suddenly want to do what you are not supposed to do, what you have been doing all your life and that you have every right to do. Besides, a heart patient has an excitability built up in him.

Patients with cardio–vascular conditions verbalized criticisms less frequently than other patients. On the other hand, they stressed the importance of "dedication and interest" when discussing their ideal expectations of nurses and physicians.

One explanation for these tendencies may be found in some common fears which occur among patients who suffer from a type of illness in which the onset of a crisis can be sudden and unpredictable. For a patient with a cardio–vascular illness, as probably for all patients who fear a sudden turn for the worse, it is of utmost importance to know that someone will be there when the patient really needs help. The need for this type of security is revealed in the following responses of cardio–vascular patients:

> I think that there should be somebody out in front there all the time. I think the hospital would back me up on that. . . . If the patient was really ill, rang the buzzer and nobody was there to get it—no telling what would happen.
>
> Well, as I said, some patients may need more care because they have a more serious illness and when you have a heart disease then you need to be watched much more, also you are more frightened and it is important that somebody is around to watch your pulse.

Patients with non-specific gastro–intestinal conditions were more likely to be preoccupied with cancer. At times this was accompanied by the suspicion that the physician "really knows but will not tell me." Such apprehensions seemed to make it more difficult for the patient to sustain trust and confidence in personnel, particularly the physician.

Openly anxious and critical patients were found more frequently within the gastro-intestinal category. While patients with cardio-vascular conditions appeared to focus attention on concrete services which assured their safety, gastro-intestinal patients seemed more inclined to focus on the qualitative nature of their interactions with nurses and physicians. They were more easily threatened by the attitudes of others, more responsive to "personalized care" and more openly critical when these areas of expectations were not satisfied.

In each culture there is the recognition that it is legitimate to deviate from normal behavior under certain extreme conditions. For these conditions most societies develop differential standards for men and women. In our society men and women are generally not expected to respond in an identical fashion to pain nor are they expected to react identically to illness. We expect that expressive behavior (complaining or moaning) should be more controlled by men, and we frown less when women appear to exploit the illness role through passive and dependent behavior. All patients generally agreed that it was more difficult for men to be patients.

The data indicate that the sex of a patient may substantially affect orientations, needs and reactions to physicians and nurses. Evidence for such differences can be found in many areas. Women were considerably more critical of nursing care than were men, and more frequently expressed fear of negative sanctions from nurses. Women, more than men, emphasized personalized relationships when they discussed the needs of patients. Women were less concerned with problems of co-operation. On the other hand, they tended to focus on nurses' expectations for consideration and respect. When describing their expectations of nurses or when evaluating them, women focused more on personality attributes than men and also gave more emphasis to efficient and prompt care. Women were more critical when a quick response was not forthcoming and they were generally more concerned with efficiency. It is compatible with the male role to receive care and to have someone else maintain the physical surroundings. Women, however, are typically the managers of the home and the performers of major house-keeping tasks. They "know" from experience the standards of personal care and house-keeping, and thus tend to apply them to their judgment of the nursing team. The female patient's concern that the nurse may be critical of her may be indirectly an expression of her awareness that she tends to be demanding.

The more intense emphasis of women on "personality" and "personalized care" may also stem from a relationship which tends to be less personal and less informal than the relationship between nurses and male patients. Unlike his female counterpart, the male patient is probably not too critical of the technical aspect of those functions of the nurse which are reminiscent of the homemaker and mother. He may also derive satisfaction from his relationship to a member of the opposite sex. All this may not only contribute to tolerance of nursing care in general but may give the appearance of more "personalized" relationships. These conjectures may also help to explain the well-known preference nurses have for male patients.

FEARS AND APPREHENSIONS

Apprehensions and fears are the frequent companions of illness. The nature of the patient's concern springs, on the one hand, from his intense preoccupations with himself, with *his* body and with *his* state of mind. His dependence on others, on the other hand, prompts simultaneous concern with the meaning and consequences of their activities. Once the patient enters the hospital his attention may shift back and forth from himself to others. He is sensitive to any physical changes and watchful of any new and unexplained symptoms. He wonders about the outcome of an examination and about the effectiveness of his treatment. He ponders the reliability of those who are responsible for the many procedures and activities which to the patient remain unknown or unknowable, albeit essential.

Patients are preoccupied with safety in the hospital. This is revealed in the preoccupation with protection from mistakes and neglect which prevails when patients talk about their own needs or the needs of other patients. It is expressed in the nature of their recall of past experiences. Not only do patients concentrate on negative experiences, but they select those occurrences which signify the dangers of neglect and lack of attention. Although patients generally deny that they, themselves, are fearful, they have a tendency to ascribe such feelings to other patients.

These apprehensions cannot be entirely alleviated by admiration for the professional groups who are responsible for his treatment, or by a very favorable relationship to the personal physician. Realistic awareness of the complexity of large organizations or simply the fact that among many competent and interested doctors and nurses there may always be a "few who are not competent" may at least put the patient on the alert. In the words of a male patient with gastrointestinal illness this fear is expressed as follows:

When you are really sick, you are at the mercy of the hospital staff. In my opinion, you've got to have luck on your side. You've got to be lucky enough to get key people in the hospital who are really alert and who wish to do a job; and have someone on the shift at the time you need them who want to give the service or you are just out of luck. I think you could die in one of these hospitals of a heart attack before anybody came in to help you.

Perceptions of the patient role make it unlikely that such fears will be openly expressed by many patients. It is one of the obligations of a patient to have "trust and confidence" in those who care for him. The expression of these concerns could thus be interpreted as a failure to conform to these obligations. Also a free expression of concerns is inhibited by the belief that the courageous, sick persons rather than "sissies" are valued and rewarded.

Apprehensions of certain "dangers" may be directly derived from previous experiences which were, to the patient, indicative of lack of competence, neglect, or lack of interest. They also may be derived indirectly from certain widely held conceptions about the nature of "some" doctors and nurses and the conditions under which they work. Thus, the belief that some nurses do not like "demanding patients" leads to the concern of many patients that asking for too much may result in a slow response to a call or in reduced attention to their needs. The belief that some nurses and some physicians may be prone to oversights because they are inevitably overworked and rushed may further contribute to insecurity. Some patients observed with concern that physicians occasionally are "too busy" to spend enough time to listen to the patients or that a nurse "under the pressure of work" may overlook a physician's order or fail to carry it out in time.

There is evidence in the data that both physicians and nurses, in effect, continuously have to prove themselves. Beliefs such as "some doctors are only interested in money," "some doctors are not interested in their patients," "some doctors are hard-hearted," appear as conceptions about "possibilities" which the patient is ready to have dispelled or confirmed upon first contact with a nurse or a physician in the hospital. Negative conceptions about physicians and nurses, therefore, are typically limited to specific individuals. Without this "specificity" in orientation, patients would find it difficult to sustain the trust and confidence which they consider so important.

The patient's search for safety and security in the hospital may also be indirectly expressed in expectations of good physicians and good nurses. Their behavior or attitudes are seen by the patient as being instrumental in recovery and recuperation. The attitudes of others in the hospital function as clues which are symbolic of good care. From the patient's point of view, the "dedicated nurse" or the nurse who gives "spontaneous and willing services" is a reliable nurse; the "kind" physician who visits the patient regularly is "trustworthy" and "thorough." Mistakes and neglect are more obviously avoided if the nurse responds promptly, if the physician "knows what is going on" and if the nurse is informed about the doctor's intent. A "prompt response" from a nurse appears as one of the most significant indices for establishing trust and confidence in nursing care.

Patient's perspectives are also shaped by the nature of the social process into which they have entered and by the nature of the interactions to which they are exposed. Those patients who were very responsive to the more impersonal phases of patient care also tended to be among the more apprehensive. Such patients often felt that they were functioning in a situation in which they could not establish effective and meaningful relationships with others. Feelings of "unrelatedness" were expressed directly in the observation that other patients are often "lonely" and "fearful" or that one sometimes feels like "just a case":

> You're no more . . . no more a patient but just a number . . . you dare not ask a question; you know, they're too busy. And they come around, fine, that's it, "we'll see you next time" and that's it. . . .

The very isolation he fears may be aggravated by the patient himself. In his efforts to be "considerate" and "not demanding" he may intensify the consequences of the anonymity and segmentalization he observes in the modern hospital. Efforts to be a "good patient" may, therefore, trigger disappointments and criticisms of those who do not provide services "spontaneously." The demand for "spontaneous services" appears also to stem from the desire to obtain all necessary services and attentions without having to initiate action. Spontaneous services curtail those interactions in which the patient may be viewed as "too demanding" or "difficult."

The interviews suggest that conformity to the patient role may lead to discrepancies between the behavior and the emotional condition of a patient. The calm appearance of the "good patient" may often hide anxieties and tensions which may not come to the attention of physicians or nurses unless relationships develop which do not trigger fear of criticism or sanction. When patients fail to exercise the restraints on behavior which they think appropriate, guilt or fear may be the consequence. Deviation from the good patient model can be threatening to a patient, unless he is convinced that his behavior was, in the eyes of others, legitimate and/or justified by the condition of his illness:

> I know myself that I talked very rudely to my doctor on one occasion. Afterwards I was ashamed of myself. I was sick or I would never act that way. He is kind and understanding. When I apologized, he acted as if nothing happened. He didn't walk out of the room or tell me off or any of the things that I might do after someone talked to me that way. But I know they have to have a lot of patience with us.

Patients practice an economy of demands, based on their own "principles of exchange." They will indeed curtail their less urgent demands to assure for themselves a prompt response during times when they "really need it." Some patients appear to consider themselves entitled to a certain finite quantity of services which they use sparingly to draw upon during periods of crisis, and many patients seem to feel that their entitlement to service is more severely cut by a demand which does not meet the approval of doctors and nurses:

I says, "I'm saving that button," I says, "When I push that thing you'll know I need help." She smiled . . . they kind of appreciate that. And from that day, all the times I've been in the hospital I have never pushed the button unless it was something that I actually needed . . . not like some people that drive these nurses crazy; pushing it to raise the bed up; five minutes later push it again. "Oh, that's a little too high." To me it paid dividends, because every time I pushed that button I got service, every dog-gone time.

DISCUSSION

The hospitalized patient is a "captive" who cannot leave the hospital without serious consequence to himself. These consequences do not only apply to the patient's physical condition. Our society expects efforts of the sick to do everything in their power to get well as soon as possible. Open rebellion against the care by competent professional personnel is, therefore, subject to severe criticism. The obligation to be a "co-operative patient" is learned early in life and, as has been indicated, apparently taken very seriously by most patients. More aggressive interpretations of the patient role are not easily verbalized and, apparently, not often realistic alternatives for the patient. Prevalent images of the hospital as a crisis institution, the conception that rights and demands should be governed by the seriousness of the illness and consideration for other, possibly sicker patients, makes it extremely difficult to play the "consumer role" openly and without fear of criticism. Thus, self-assertion as a "client" is controlled by moral commitments to the hospital community as well as by considerations of practical and necessary self-interest.

The norms of our society permit the sick person conditionally passive withdrawal and dependence but, at the same time, emphasize the sick person's responsibility to co-operate in efforts to regain his health.[5] The prevaling image of the hospital increases the pressure to get well fast by enhancing the patient's awareness of the relative degree of the seriousness of his case. Many patients do not have to look far to find and hear about patients who seem more seriously ill. This pressure to get well also is intensified by the observation of "overworked" and "rushed" nurses and physicians. The pattern of hospital relationships which, for the most part, prevents the development of those relationships which would reduce fears of being rejected or criticized, further discourage patients from exploiting the leniency to which illness *per se* may entitle them. A moral commitment to physicians and nurses is also strengthened by the gratitude and admiration of the sick for those who are "trying to help."

Patterns of interaction are also affected by the controls which the participants can exert over each other and the understanding which they can have of the function of others. For a variety of reasons, the patient sees few areas in which he has control.

A prerequisite for controlling the actions of others is the capacity to feel competent to judge their achievements. Most patients feel quite helpless in evaluating the knowledge, skill and competence of nurses and physicians. This may be one reason for their intense emphasis on "personality." "Personality" is felt to be associated with, and an indicator of, those more technical qualities which patients do not feel qualified to judge.

Control does not only depend on the capacity to judge the competence or efficiency of others. It also involves the freedom to convey and impose judgments. Even if patients feel quite certain about their judgments, they may feel reluctant to express them if such action may portend a reduction in good patient care.

[5]Parsons, T., and R. Fox, "Illness, Therapy and the Modern Urban American Family," in E. G. Jaco (ed.), *Patients, Physicians and Illness,* New York: Free Press, 1st ed., 1958, p. 236.

The institutional context affects the way the patients balance their perceived claims and obligations. They manage to communicate the conditional nature of their claims, the undesirability of their state and, therefore, the importance of their obligations. Their persistent verbal assertions that they should co-operate, that they must not be demanding, underscore their motivation to get well. The problem of patients does not stem from a rejection of major social values but rather from the dissonance created between the desire to broaden the boundaries of what seems a legitimate sphere of control and the tendency to adhere compulsively to behavior which reflects conformity to obligations.[6] The data confirm Parsons' contention that dependence is, in our society, a primary threat to the valued achievement capacity and that the sick, to this extent, are called upon to work for their own recovery.[7]

Efforts to adhere to obligations are accompanied by the complementary hope that others will meet their obligations in turn and thus will satisfy the patient's expectations. Recognition of the limitations under which hospital functionaries work does not prevent patients from forming "ideal" expectations which call for a model of care which the on-going work processes of the hospital do not readily approximate.[8] The restraint which is exercised by the hospitalized patient is partly an expression of his fears that he may be deprived of important service if he should deviate from acceptable behavior. However, while patients have some notions of the sanctions which can be applied should they violate standards for appropriate behavior, they appear much less certain what they could do if nurses or physicians do not meet their obligations. The feeling of helplessness of patients is partly derived from an incapacity to judge adequately the competence of those who take care of them—in part, from the fact that their experiences do not provide easily defendable criteria for asserting their rights; and partly from their reluctance to use the controls which are available to them.

The interviews showed that patients always knew what they should not be like or what qualities or behavior would make them acceptable to others. Even much more difficult for them was to define what specific tasks they had a right to expect and what expectations could be transformed into active demands without deviating from general norms for behavior. A lack of familiarity with what constitutes proper care and cure procedures as well as the fact that a slight change in their condition could alter the legitimacy of demands appears to contribute to this difficulty. Rigid adherence to general rules of conduct appeared to be one way out of this dilemma.

Patients were also limited in the expression of their feelings by the fact that personalized and supportive care was not considered to lie within the sphere of the essential. They clearly felt that they had to subordinate such demands to their own or other patients' needs for physical care. The point of view of patients parallels the common distinction between the legitimacy of somatic and mental illness—a distinction which is accompanied by the notion that somatic illness legitimately entitles the ill to accept dependence as a result of manifestly impaired *physical* capacity for task performance. This dependence is narrowly defined in terms of permitting hospital functionaries to do things for the patient only as long as it is

---

[6]At times the patient and his significant others among hospital functionaries may be less in disagreement over proper role relationships than significant others involved in their social network. Thus, in some cases patients were found to define their obligations in terms of all the previously discussed considerations. Their relatives, however, emphasized the rights of the paying consumer and expressed their opinion that the patient was "not asking for enough." For a discussion of the role of the third party see W. J. Goode, "A Theory of Role Strain," *American Sociological Review,* 25:483–496, August, 1960.

[7]Parsons, "Definitions of Health and Illness. . . .," *op. cit.,* p. 185.

[8]Reactions to experiences in the hospital assume, therefore, meaning not only in relation to "realistic" anticipations but also in relation to more subtly held "ideal" expectations. The relative discrepancy between "realistic" and "ideal" experiences is a significant variable in the patients' responses to actual experiences.

really *physically* necessary. Emotional dependence or other deviations from adult role performance are considered legitimate by most patients only in cases of extreme illness.[9]

The opportunities to obtain personalized care are limited and they are further restricted by patients who as "good patients" withdraw from those on whom they depend and with whom they wish to communicate but whom they do not wish "to bother." The control of the desire to obtain and demand more personal care tends to intensify alienation.[10] The expression of such emotional needs is checked not only by the various pressures to conform to the patient role, but also by the fact that those patient-care activities which direct themselves to the emotional needs of the patient are not institutionalized as role obligations of personnel in the general hospital. Personal concern, support or other emotionally therapeutic efforts tend to be from the patient's point of view pleasant (often unexpected) attributes of otherwise task-oriented personnel. Such activities are quickly praised and even "ideally" seen as the major attributes of the "good" nurse and of the "good" physician. But, since these do not really belong to the manifestly legitimate obligations, they are only reluctantly criticized when missing and rarely directly demanded.

Efforts to adhere to rules of conduct involve also the desire to project a specific image of self.[11] Being accepted is of more than passing importance to the hospitalized patient.[12] Self-consciousness about the norms to which one tries to conform may also suggest that the role is in certain respects alien to the performers and that they are not secure in essential social relationships. Efforts to reiterate conformity to general rules of conduct may thus, at least in part, stem from the patient's limited knowledge of the reality of the institutional setting and from fears that he may not be able to measure up to institutionalized expectations. Thus, uncertain about how far he can go before violating prescribed rules for behavior, patients may find their security in efforts to live up to the "letter of the law."[13]

The frequently expressed obligation to co-operate and the persistent attempt to seek approval is, within this frame of reference, not only a diplomatic effort to manipulate relationships to one's own advantage, but also an expression of the patient's perception of the degree of dependency associated with his status. The associated attitudes are thus not

[9]Patients were not interviewed during the critical phases of their illness when, indeed, their claims may have been different. However, only a few patients in the sample considered themselves recovered. The majority of patients in the cardio-vascular category were recuperating from severe illness and were under orders for bedrest. The majority of the patients in the gastro-intestinal category were under treatment for ulcers or hospitalized for other chronic or acute gastro-intestinal conditions. In all of these cases the conditional nature of rights was bound to create some difficulties—either because of the absence of visible symptoms of illness or because the illness was not considered very serious. Case studies of the more seriously ill patients indicate that anxiety may cause them to "break through" the limits set by their role but that such a breakthrough often demands added efforts since claims, demands or irritations have to be justified. To reestablish an acceptable view of themselves seems to often constitute a major effort for these patients.

[10]Parsons, "Definitions of Health and Illness . . . ," *op. cit.*, p. 186. The author points out that the supportive treatment of the sick person "undercuts the alienative component of the motivational structure of his illness."

[11]Goffman, E., "The Nature of Deference and Demeanor," *Amer. Anthropologist*, 58:473-502, June, 1956; E. Goffman, *Encounters: Two Studies in the Sociology of Interaction*, Indianapolis, Ind.: Bobbs-Merrill, 1961, pp. 99-105.

[12]Efforts to give verbal evidence of conformity may aim at protection from criticism. Deviations tend to be viewed as forgiveable as long as a person gives evidence of "good will." Goode emphasized that failure in role behavior tends to arouse less criticism than failure in emotional commitment to general norms. This principle may be particularly applicable to situations where it is also an obligation of alters to tolerate failures in role behavior. See W. J. Goode, "Norm Commitment and Conformity to Role Status Obligations," *Amer. J. Soc.*, 66:246-258, November, 1960.

[13]See Merton's discussion of ritualism. Anxiety over the ability to live up to institutional expectations may contribute to compulsive adherence to institutional norms. R. K. Merton, *Social Theory and Social Structure*, New York: Free Press, Rev. Ed., 1957, pp. 184-187.

merely psychological consequences of the sick role but also reflect the patient's common sense assessments of the abrogation of independence and decision-making associated with his status in the hospital.[14] These deprivations are communicated to the patient beginning with the possessive gesture of the identification bracelet affixed during admission to the hospital, and they are continuously reinforced in daily experiences. The hospital preempts control and jurisdiction, ranging from the assumption of accountability of body functions to the withholding of information about medical procedures.[15]

The interviews reflect a degree of uncertainty whether physicians and nurses operate as effective teams in close communication or whether the patient ought to function as interpreter and intermediary between these two all important functionaries. Sometimes patients wonder whether they are sources of conflict and competition between medicine and nursing. The physician is seen as supreme authority and patients repeatedly stress that "if something is really seriously wrong," they would turn to the physician. The physician, however, is for the most part not present to observe, respond or intervene. The nurse is continually present, or at least within reach of the call system. She is the physician's representative and interpreter, but she also is the one who has to bear the brunt of work resulting from the physician's orders. She represents hospital rules, and yet she is not infrequently seen by the patient as a potential spokesman for his needs and interests. These perceptions reflect remarkably well the organization of the hospital and the ambiguous position of the nurse at the crossroads of the care and cure structures.[16]

This study suggests that the patient role, like other comparable behavior syndromes organized around a status, are not adequately described by isolating attitudinal and normative responses to the role theme itself, i.e., illness. The full repertory of role behavior must be placed into the context of organizational processes if it is to encompass realistic orientations and behavior display.

The patient role described in this paper is specific to the hospital. The data support and amplify the implication of Merton's use of the role-set as an analytic concept.[17] The patient gropes for appropriate criteria and distinctions in defining his role with reference to a variety of significant relationships. The concept points to the importance of the difference in the power of the members of the role-set *vis-à-vis* the status occupant who has to manipulate between correspondents and to the significance of the support which the status occupant receives from others in like circumstances. However, the relatively isolated patient in the modern single or double hospital room is frequently left to his own devices in coping with differences in real or perceived expectations. This adds to the conditions favoring manifestations of withdrawal or dependence on the approval of others as realistic responses to institutionalized impotence.

The data also suggest a further elaboration of certain aspects of the theoretical model of role behavior. The concept of the role-set refines the differential system of expectations attached to a status from the point of view of the range of counter roles. The data reported in

[14]Parsons and Fox stressed the need for a "well-timed, well-chosen, well-balanced exercise of supportive and the disciplinary components of the therapeutic process." Institutional factors as well as widely held social values may tend to shift the emphasis too much to the disciplinary components particularly in the setting of the general hospital which incorporate structurally as well as in terms of explicitly or implicitly held attitudes the distinction between the emotionally sick and the physically sick (Parsons and Fox, *op. cit.*, p. 244).

[15]Mauksch, H. O., "Patients View Their Roles," *Hospital Progress,* 43:136–138, October, 1962.

[16]Mauksch, H. O., "The Organizational Context of Nursing Practice," in F. Davis (ed.), *The Nursing Profession,* New York: Wiley, 1966, pp. 109–137.

[17]Merton, R. K., "The Role Set," *British J. Sociology,* 8:106–120, June, 1957.

this paper suggest that an additional dimension of role expectation would be a useful addition to theory. Expectations which define a role are normally attributed to the social system surrounding a status.[18] It is suggested that a distinguishable difference exists between the pattern of expectations arising from the structural aspects of the status and those expectations which are attached to the function ascribed to the role. Thus, the role concomitants of being ill can be defined as the functional role segment of the patient role while the consequences of hospitalization, be they perceived or real, could be termed positional role segments.

Concern with the functional segment of the patient role has been evidenced in most previous treatments of the sick role in the literature.[19] The positional role segment in this study is specific to the hospital. Yet in other settings for patient behavior—be it the home, the clinic or the physician's office—these structural components of the patient role would also bear fruitful sociological investigation. This conceptual scheme aids in structuring the observations of potential strain and conflict between different aspects of the patient role.

This study suggests that a prevailing theme of successful role behavior is the ability of the status occupant to integrate into his own behavior and responses different components from the system of expectations surrounding him. In the case of the patient his efforts to be "a good patient," to meet the obligations as he perceives them and to strive to co-operate in recovery are handicapped by the inadequacy of the communications system within which he functions.[20] Were it more effective, it may permit the patient to cope with his role with greater certainty about rights and obligations, the controls at his disposal and the risks inherent in behavioral experimentation.

[18]*Ibid*, p. 113f.

[19]Parsons, *The Social System, loc. cit.* Other writers, notably R. Coser, *Life in the Ward*, Lansing, Mich.: Michigan State Univ. Press, 1962, include positional considerations to a greater extent.

[20]Skipper, Jr., J. K., D. L. Tagliacozzo and H. O. Mauksch, "Some Possible Consequences of Limited Communication Between Patients and Hospital Functionaries," *J. Health and Human Behavior*, 5:34–39, Spring, 1964; J. K. Skipper, Jr., "Communication and the Hospitalized Patient", in J. K. Skipper and R. C. Leonard (eds.), *Social Interaction and Patient Care*, Philadelphia: Lippincott, 1965, pp. 61–82.

6
Communications

CAROLE L. KIMBERLIN

BACKGROUND

Health professionals, including pharmacists, have become increasingly concerned with how well they communicate with patients—and with good reason. Evidence is overwhelming that patients frequently do not follow health advice or comply with therapeutic regimens (1–3) and, in fact, frequently do not understand what is required of them in order to comply with treatment (4). For years researchers asked the question, "What distinguishes noncompliant from compliant patients" (What is wrong with *them*)? The results were disappointing and often conflicting. The general conclusion has been that characteristics of the patient such as education level, socioeconomic status, and personality characteristics (5) do *not* reliably discriminate compliant from noncompliant patients. Patient knowledge of the medication regimen demands is considered to be a necessary condition for compliance but is certainly not always sufficient to ensure appropriate behavior (6).

A more promising (and practical) line of inquiry evolved when researchers began asking, "What do health professionals *do* in their interactions with patients that enhances patient knowledge and compliance?" These findings at least pointed out ways for health professionals to improve patient care.

Along with concern on the part of health professionals about patient nonadherence with recommendations, patients themselves became more demanding of information from health professionals. The era of "consumerism" affected the health care industry. Demands for more information from patients (7) and concerns about liability for "failure to warn" among health professionals (8, 9) likely contributed to increased concern about the quality and effectiveness of patient education activities. Recent court decisions reinforcing the pharmacist's duty to warn patients (10) about potential side effects will further emphasize the professional and legal responsibilities they have to communicate effectively with patients. The notion that health professionals can tell patients "Do what I say because I say so" without explanation or question seems to have been abandoned by all health professionals as inadequate, ineffective, and unethical patient care.

College courses and other educational programs are now offered to teach pharmacists and other health professionals better patient communication techniques (11–15). This chapter will begin by outlining some of the theoretical underpinnings of communications skills training and will then examine the specific skills and techniques that are necessary in enhancing the communication skills of health professionals.

CONCEPTUAL FRAMEWORKS

Communication Process

Miller (16) developed a simple model to represent communication that is similar to that used or adapted by various authors in the pharmacy literature (17, 18). The model, diagramed below, shows the speaker and listener in a communication, each with a set of attitudes that affects communication. They also have a set of skills that affects their abilities to adequately encode or send and decode or receive messages. As part of the total process, both speaker and listener are constantly providing each other feedback, both positive and negative, on the effects of the messages. This feedback serves to modify and clarify the communication messages. Although the model leaves undefined the attitudinal components of speaker and listener and the specific nature of the encoding and decoding skills, it does highlight the importance of feedback. The fact that constantly transmitted feedback alters the communication both sent and received and is a crucial part of the process is depicted in the model.

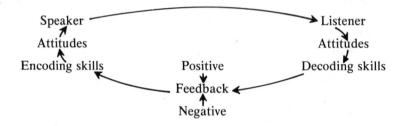

Therapeutic Communication

Many of the skills taught in communication skills classes, particularly those of empathy, warmth, and acceptance, are founded in the person-centered psychotherapy advocated by Carl Rogers (19, 20). Person-centered therapy is itself part of a humanistic tradition in psychology. Central to this tradition is the belief that human beings will naturally grow in healthy, self-actualizing directions unless thwarted by their environments. The way to help is to provide a psychologically safe environment in which a person feels genuinely cared for and nonjudgmentally understood. In such an atmosphere, people can activate their potentials to solve their own problems and find meaning in their lives.

The core skills of person-centered therapy such as attending, listening, conveying respect, clarifying, and reflecting feelings are easy to understand and helpful in the work done by a variety of health professionals. Even other schools of psychotherapy acknowledge these skills as crucial in establishing a therapeutic or helping relationship with a patient (21).

One caution to the person-centered approach is that it involves more than skills and techniques. The techniques are based on a set of attitudes that the therapist must bring to the relationship. Genuineness is required so that the therapist must actually *feel* warmth and concern for patients. Also required is trust in patients' abilities to cope with their own feelings and, to a large extent, solve their own emotional problems.

Nonverbal Communication

A number of disciplines, including anthropology, psychology, and sociology, have examined the role nonverbal behavior plays in human communication. Researchers have estimated that the majority of meaning in a communication, particularly that involving feelings or attitudes, is conveyed nonverbally (22). The study of nonverbal communication has focused on a number of distinct areas, each of which has communicative meaning. Some of these areas are:

1. Vocal characteristics. It is generally recognized that the *way* we say something sometimes conveys more than the words we use. This area studies how characteristics such as the tone, rate, pitch, hesitations, etc. of speech convey meaning.
2. Facial cues. The amount of eye contact and type of facial expression also convey meaning. To a considerable degree, we think people are interested in us to the extent that they maintain eye contact during conversation.
3. Interpersonal space. The distance between people and the presence or absence of physical barriers affect communication. A distance of $1^{1}/_{2}$ to $2^{1}/_{2}$ feet is probably most appropriate when conducting patient interviewing or education (23).
4. Body motions. This area examines the meaning that gestures, body posture, touch, etc. have in communication.

Behavior Change

Behaviorism

Many of the specific techniques taught in communications skills training are grounded in behavior therapy. Central to this approach is the belief that the way we communicate (including nonverbal communication) is learned behavior. As such, if a particular type of communicative response is not appropriate or effective, we can learn a better type of response.

Behaviorism has been a dominant, driving force in psychology in the United States since the 1950s. B. F. Skinner, whose influence has been overwhelming, contends that behavior is established and maintained by its consequences (24). In essence, behaviors that are reinforced are repeated. While antecedent conditions or cues may serve as reminders for a particular behavior to occur, it is the consequence of the behavior that is the controlling influence.

Communications training in pharmacy and other health professions utilizes analysis of behavior, modeling, tailoring, cuing, assertion training, relaxation training, systematic desensitization, positive reinforcement, and behavior rehearsal, as well as various self-management techniques such as self-monitoring (25–30), which are adapted from the behaviorist tradition.

Cognitive Components

Behavior therapy has begun to broaden beyond the operant conditioning models of Skinner to include cognition as a focus of intervention. Thoughts are now viewed as part of learned behavior and, as such, modifiable. Cognitive-behavioral therapy is based on the assumption that a change in one's self-statements or thoughts will result in a corresponding change in one's behavior (31, 32). Therapeutic interventions attempt to help people examine events and their responses more rationally and change some of the basic, but irrational, values and beliefs that serve to keep them disturbed. In the pharmacy literature, cognitive-behavioral intervention techniques are used most extensively in the area of assertiveness training.

Assertiveness Training

Assertive behavior has been defined as "the outward expression of practically all feelings other than anxiety" toward others (33). Certain specific skill areas have been identified as central, and frequently problematic, in nonassertive individuals. These include: (*a*) responding appropriately to criticism, (*b*) giving negative feedback, (*c*) expressing appreciation or pleasure, (*d*) refusing requests, (*e*) making requests, (*f*) conveying confidence, (*g*) initiating and maintaining conversations, and (*h*) expressing opinions.

The techniques used in assertiveness training center around goal setting, which forces the individual to identify personal problem areas and define more appropriate, assertive responses to these situations. The individual is then guided through behavioral rehearsals by the therapist or trainer. These might involve the trainer role playing with the student situations in which the student must practice the appropriate behavior defined in the goal statements. These rehearsals serve to reinforce the assertive behavior and decondition the anxiety in response to the situations.

When the level of anxiety or communication apprehension is so high that individuals are incapable of emitting appropriate behaviors, relaxation training or systematic desensitization (34) may be initiated to counteract the anxiety. In these procedures, nonassertive persons are taught deep muscle relaxation and then mentally imagine themselves in the particular situations that create anxiety. While imagining these situations, the individuals practice relaxation as a way of counterconditioning the anxiety response.

In addition to these more traditional behaviorist techniques, assertiveness training usually includes cognitive restructuring as a treatment strategy. This stems from the theoretical position that nonassertiveness is the result of an inhibition of appropriate behavior by self-defeating thoughts that produce counterproductive anxiety.

Support for this theoretical assumption exists in research, which has shown that low-assertive people differ from those who are appropriately assertive in certain key beliefs or cognitive themes. These include:

1. Fear of rejection and need for approval (35–37)
2. Overconcern for the feelings and needs of others (35)
3. Negative thoughts of one's self (38) and high, perfectionistic expectations of performance of both oneself and others (36, 39)

Cognitive restructuring teaches people to identify their self-defeating thoughts that produce anxiety in assertive situations and replace them with more reasonable thoughts. With practice, these thoughts become incorporated into the person's belief system. For example, a pharmacist who feels "used" by the boss who always counts on him or her for emergency coverage might currently say to him- or herself, "I don't want to come in to work on my day off, but if I say no the boss will get angry and that would be awful." This causes anxiety at the imagined catastrophic consequences of saying "no" so he or she inhibits this response. A more rational thought process when faced with such a request would be, "I don't want to work on my day off this week. It is my right to say no. I am not responsible for solving the problems my manager has in finding back-up coverage." A combination of cognitive restructuring and behavioral rehearsal is often used in training and has been shown to improve assertiveness more than either technique used independently (40).

Health Beliefs

Probably the crucial function of the health provider's communication with a patient involves information exchange. However, other elements of the communication are intended to persuade patients in certain ways. Health providers seek to persuade patients to accept a certain set of beliefs and to adopt a certain way of behaving in following therapeutic recommendations. One conceptual model that attempts to explain a patient's adoption of particular health behaviors is the Health Belief Model (41, 42). Although not a communication model as such, some of the elements of the model are viewed as being modifiable by health professionals (43) and thus become a focus for intervention in the provider-patient relationship. Changing those patient beliefs that interfere with appropriate self-care, such as their compliance with medication regimens, could have a significant impact on patient care.

The major elements in the Health Belief Model that are potentially modifiable are reviewed below. An example of how these elements might affect compliance with antihypertensive medications is also provided. The critical elements necessary for appropriate self-care are:

1. Patients must perceive themselves as susceptible to negative health outcomes if they do not behave in a certain way. For example, hypertensive patients must perceive themselves as susceptible to stroke and heart disease if their blood pressure readings are not brought within the normal range.
2. Patients must perceive these health outcomes as serious.
3. Patients must perceive treatment as being effective. Hypertensive patients must believe that they can avoid or significantly reduce the possibility of strokes or heart disease by taking medication.
4. Patients must perceive the benefits of treatment as outweighing the costs. These costs may be monetary, they may be enduring side effects of medication, they may be psychosocial costs, and so on. In order for hypertensive patients to be compliant, they must perceive the costs of side effects as *not* being too great to tolerate. In addition, they must be willing to pay the psychological "cost" of labeling themselves as hypertensive and thus dependent on medications for the rest of their lives (even when they do not feel "sick"). Finally, they must perceive the monetary costs as being within their means.
5. Patients must have cues to action. This may take many forms, such as reminder postcards from pharmacists that their prescriptions are due to be refilled.

COMMUNICATION WITH PATIENTS

This section will first review some of the research on the nature and quality of the communication that takes place between health providers and patients. Then, research on the specific communication factors affecting the quality of patient care will be reviewed. Finally, these research findings will be translated into specific recommendations to the pharmacist on ways to improve communication with patients.

Quality of Patient Communication

Considerable research has been conducted examining the physician-patient relationship. Many of these findings would probably apply as well to the pharmacist-patient relationship. Research has indicated a relationship between patient satisfaction with physician care and compliance with medical advice (44–46). Research findings suggest that the quality of the communication and information given by physicians is related to patient satisfaction (47–50). Relationships also have been found between measures of the quality or thoroughness of physician communication with patients and patient compliance with advice (51, 52). Svarstad (52), in her analysis of physician instructions to patients about medication taking, found evidence that physicians frequently failed to explain or discuss even critical information such as how regularly medications should be taken or the duration of therapy.

A number of studies also have examined the relationships of pharmacists and patients and the communication that takes place between them. Much of this literature has been critical of pharmacists in terms of the small percentage of patients who receive any consultation from pharmacists, the brevity of the consultations that do take place, and the inadequacy or inappropriateness of the pharmacists' decisions in regard to patient care.

The shopper technique in which trained observers are sent into pharmacies and present themselves as patients has been widely used in examining the quality of pharmacists' consultations. Such a technique has been used to evaluate the quality of consultation given by pharmacists when "patients" have requested assistance in purchasing nonprescription products. Results have indicated that a large proportion of pharmacists do not adequately assess problems before recommending nonprescription products, or they sell products that are clearly contraindicated (53–56).

The shopper technique also has been used to evaluate the consulting skills of pharmacists when they are dispensing prescription medications. Again, conclusions drawn by researchers have often been critical of pharmacists' performance (55–60) even when pharmacists were functioning under state regulations mandating that they counsel patients on the proper use of medications (59, 60). Reports on the incidence of verbal counseling when dispensing new prescriptions varies, with the reviewed research indicating a range from approximately 30% (58) to 70% (61). The mean length of interaction per patient when consultation is initiated in the routine provision of pharmacy services has been found to be approximately 20–30 seconds (61).

Some researchers have used independent observers to examine pharmacists' behavior. One pioneering observational study of pharmacists indicated that pharmacists devote little of their work time to patient communication and half of the time they do spend talking with patients is in nonprofessional communication (63). An observational study of pharmacists in a Veterans Administration hospital (Svarstad BL, Mason HL, Schuna A. Factors affecting the pharmacists' consultation behavior: an observational study. Unpublished manuscript.) found that pharmacists provided no oral instructions with $1/2$ of the prescriptions and asked no questions of the patient when delivering 78% of the prescriptions. This finding of very little attempt on the part of pharmacists to ask questions of patients in order to assess understanding of regimen demands, allergies, other medications being taken, etc. has been found in other studies as well (61).

In addition to describing the incidence of consultation, research has attempted to identify what variables might be related to the amount of consultation performed by pharmacists. Pharmacists' attitudes toward patient consultation have been found to predict the amount of counseling done (64). The amount of privacy available to the pharmacist also has been found to relate to the amount of time spent with patients and the amount of information discussed (65–67).

The evidence on the effect of the pharmacists' age and the type of practice setting is mixed. Some studies have suggested that younger pharmacists are more competent as patient educators (53, 57) while others have noted no differences based on the pharmacist's age (55, 59, 68). Some researchers have found that chain pharmacists or those practicing in discount outlets do not perform as well as those practicing in independent or service-oriented pharmacies (57, 59, 68), while others have found no differences in different types of settings (53, 69).

When researchers have surveyed patients regarding the information they receive from pharmacists about their medications, the majority (greater than 70%) reported receiving no information from their pharmacists (70-72). This report of receiving no information has been found to be more frequently the case for older than younger patients (71). Although patients seem to feel that pharmacists are available to answer questions, they perceive them as not voluntarily offering counseling (73).

In apparent contradiction to the findings that actual communication with patients is minimal, research has found that pharmacists consider patient communication to be an important part of practice (74). They also perceive themselves as willing to provide and competent in providing patient consultation services (75). In addition, they believe the patient counseling services they already provide are effective and oppose regulations to mandate counseling (76). They estimate that they orally counsel about 40-50% of patients with new prescriptions (77, 78) and that these counseling sessions last 1-2 minutes (77). These estimates, with the exception of the incidence of counseling reported by Mason and Svarstad (61) among rural pharmacists, are inflated when compared with data on observed counseling behavior.

When pharmacists have been taught skills of patient counseling, they have been found to improve their counseling (79). Finally, when intervention studies have been conducted that have increased the level of patient education conducted by pharmacists, researchers have found significant effects on patient knowledge of medication regimens and compliance with those regimens (67-84) and patient satisfaction with pharmacy care (85) and with health care in general (86).

Factors Affecting Patient Care

The research on the relationships between practitioner-patient communication characteristics and patient care outcomes will be divided into two areas—those factors related to the establishment of an amicable, satisfying relationship and those related to specific techniques used in interviewing and presenting medication information to patients.

Establishing Positive Patient-Practitioner Relationships

The importance of empathy in establishing a trusting relationship between pharmacist and patient has been frequently emphasized (87-89). In addition, the ability of the pharmacist and patient to communicate effectively is dependent on the physical setting in which the communication takes place. Several studies in pharmacy have shown that the degree of privacy in communication affects the quality of the communication (65-67). Patients are more willing to ask questions, are able to remember more information, and are more compliant with treatment if they have more privacy in conversations with the pharmacist. One study also found telephone consultation with patients after they had returned home superior to face-to-face consultation without privacy (67).

Other research on the practitioner-patient relationship has found that a friendly rather than a businesslike attitude on the part of physicians (52, 45) and an ongoing relationship between patient and physician (90) are associated with better patient outcome. Willingness to listen and respond to patient complaints or concerns about treatment also has been associated with higher levels of adherence (52), as has physician expression of sincere concern or sympathy (5). Finally, encouraging patients to take greater responsibility in their own care and establishing a more "collaborative" relationship have been found to be related to increased compliance (91), more patient-initiated questioning of practitioners (92), and increased involvement in follow-up care (93).

Educational Techniques Used

Ley has conducted numerous studies examining how aspects of communication with a physician affect patient understanding and compliance with instructions. Many of the techniques used, such as advanced organizers or categorization, are supported by basic research in learning. The findings of his research and related research by others are summarized in the reading by Garrity found later in this chapter. In one study, Svarstad (52) found that patient understanding and compliance were related to the direct, comprehensible, and explicit communication of directions and expectations from physician to patient. Careful monitoring of medication taking on follow-up visits and assessment of problems with compliance also were found to relate to adherence. Her research also provided evidence that justification or provision of reasons for advice assists in compliance.

Tailoring or establishing a cuing system for medication taking has been found to help with establishing compliance (94, 95) as has implementation of self-monitoring procedures (96, 97) and the use of a reinforcement schedule in a contingency contract (98, 99). Finally, some evidence exists that a combination of explicit written information along with oral consultation is best (100, 101), although other research has disputed this claim of the superiority of using a combination of both types of communication (102).

Recommendations for Pharmacist-Patient Communication

The research findings have obvious application in pharmacist-patient communication. First, those aspects of the communication that set a positive tone for the relationship will be discussed. Then specific techniques to improve the interviewing and educational skills of pharmacists will be briefly described.

Establishing Rapport

Providing a sense of privacy when communicating with patients is essential. A completely private room is impractical for most pharmacist consultations, but a feeling of privacy can be established if the conversation is held away from other patients waiting in a prescription area or by drawing curtains between beds in a hospital room.

There are a number of ways in which we nonverbally convey our interest and concern. Establishing eye contact, leaning toward the patient with no physical barriers between you, having a relaxed, open posture all help to put the patient at ease.

Sensitivity to the nonverbal cues of patients is also necessary. Ask yourself "How is this person feeling?" during the course of a conversation. Does the patient seem upset? . . . anxious? . . . depressed? Your awareness of this "silent" communication can help you reach a deeper understanding of the patient and can point out circumstances that require further investigation, such as indications of depression.

The ability to convey understanding of patients and their concerns is the basis of helping relationships. Although so important it is also rare. Rather than conveying understanding, we do or say various things to try to change or stop patients' feelings. We try to reassure them that things are not so bad or that things will get better, we try to give advice that will "solve" their problems, or we change the subject to something we feel comfortable with, such as the medication regimen. These responses tend to convey to the patient that we are not really listening. An empathic response, on the other hand, makes patients feel that we are listening, that we care about them and, to a large extent, that we understand their concerns.

A technique for communicating empathy is to capsulize in fresh words the essence of what you understand the patient's feelings to be. For example, a patient tells you, "My husband is having bypass surgery tomorrow. I've been so nervous about it I haven't slept for days." You respond, "You sound really frightened about the surgery." Such a response conveys that you understand her concern and take it seriously. You do not downplay it ("Don't worry. Lots of people have bypass surgery nowadays and do fine") nor subtly criticize or give glib advice ("You're going to have to be more positive. You don't want to concern your husband with your fears")—both of which would convey that she should *not* feel as she does and would probably stop her from further confiding in you.

It is also important in day-to-day contact with patients to attempt to establish an ongoing relationship with them. This can be facilitated by introducing yourself, calling patients by name, and updating your profile records on return visits. When engaged in a particular activity, such as establishing patient profiles, tell the patient the purpose of the interview, convey how long it will take, and elicit their consent to proceed. When patients are treated as having some control in the relationship, it establishes the perception of a more positive, equal relationship.

Interviewing

The varied tasks that pharmacists perform frequently require interviewing of patients. Often interviewing is thought of in terms of thorough medication histories taken in hospitalized patients. However, if interviewing is thought of as a process of gathering information from patients regarding their health and medication use, there are numerous pharmacist activities that require interviewing skills. In addition to obtaining medication histories for patient charts, the community pharmacist interviews a patient before recommending a nonprescription product. Gathering information on the nature of the symptoms, their severity and duration, what has already been done to treat the condition, other medications being taken, as well as allergies or conditions the patient might have is routine before recommending self-care products.

In addition, there are various assessments that pharmacists must make relative to a patient's care. As part of their efforts to assure that patients understand the requirements of their treatment, pharmacists should assess patients' knowledge of their medication regimens. Usually patients will have obtained some information from their physicians or other sources before they come into contact with the pharmacist. Assessing current levels of knowledge as well as assessing understanding of information provided during a pharmacist consultation are important activities. Such assessments require that patients tell the pharmacist what they know about their medications. Open-ended questions that require such descriptions are necessary—a "yes" response to "Do you understand how to take this?" is not adequate. Instead, an open-ended probe would be more effective, such as: "I would like to take just a few minutes to discuss the medication with you. Rather than repeating a lot of things you already know, could you tell me what your physician has told you about this medication?" Pharmacists, by such questions, let patients take the lead in communication and at the same time gather information on the understanding (or misunderstandings) of patients. With such information, they can focus their own communication on gaps that need to be filled or areas in which misunderstandings might exist.

On follow-up visits, the pharmacist should assess how the patient has actually been taking the medication. Because self-reported problems with compliance can be touchy, prefacing questions with accepting phrases can help. Such a line of questioning might go something like this: "It's difficult for most people to take medication exactly on schedule. We forget or have other problems with the medication. How many doses would you estimate you missed in the last week?" It is also important to have patients report on any problems they have experienced that may point to adverse effects of the medication. Finally, assessing patients' beliefs about treatment, such as their perceptions of the effectiveness of the medication or perceptions of barriers to taking the medication, may point out problems that require the pharmacist's attention. When problems are reported, it is important for pharmacists to treat these reports with concern and to try to address the problems. Such an effort might involve urging the patient to tolerate side effects for several more weeks to see if they disappear, suggesting ways to alleviate the side effects, or consulting with the physician on alternative treatment if the adverse effects are serious or are leading to noncompliance.

Providing Information

There are various techniques that can be used when conducting patient education that will help patients recall and comply with instructions.

1. Categorize information for the patient as it is being provided. For example, say, "First I'd like to go over directions for use. . . . Next I'll list a few possible side effects to be aware of." Giving patients these organizers in advance of information aids in learning and memory (103).
2. Make information as concrete as possible. Any information that we can form a "picture" of mentally is more easily remembered (104). This may require the use of visual aids or demonstrations in teaching. For example, showing a patient how to pull the lower eyelid down to form a pocket for eye drops will be more easily learned and remembered than a verbal description. Encourage patients to try to form pictures in their minds of key points as a way of helping them remember. In addition, making instructions specific rather than general (e.g., "Drink at least 8 large glasses of liquid a day" versus "Drink a lot of liquid") aids in recall (105).
3. Help patients identify events that occur consistently in their daily routines that they can use as cues or reminders to take their medication. For example, if the instructions are to "Take 3 times a day with meals" but the patient does not eat lunch, the dose to be taken at midday will likely be difficult to remember. The patient may, however, always watch the news on television at noon, which could serve as a reminder to take the medication. If no event can be identified, suggesting an alarm or other reminder system, perhaps with the help of family members, can assist in patient adherence.
4. Use simple words and short sentences. Short words and sentences that are easy to understand have been shown to facilitate learning (105). Avoid complex words and medical terminology or jargon. One investigator concluded that 35 to 87% of patients do not understand instructions for taking prescription medications (106). What may happen in a consultation is, rather than asking clinicians to clarify unclear instructions, patients will feel a personal inadequacy and will be reluctant to show their "ignorance" by asking questions. In any case, information that is understandable, and therefore meaningful, to the patient is going to be

more easily learned and remembered than information only vaguely understood (107).

5.   Give reasons for important advice. Rather than saying only, "Take 1 hour before or 2 hours after meals," give the patient some simple understanding of why it is desirable to take the drug on an empty stomach. When explaining duration of therapy, tell why it is important to take an antibiotic for the full duration even when symptoms disappear. Again, information that is clearly understood is more easily remembered. The technique of explaining reasons for advice also has been shown to assist not only in improving patient knowledge of medications but also in improving compliance.

6.   Do not overload with information. Pare verbal consultations down to the essential elements and make sure written information is concise with important points highlighted.

7.   Emphasize when a specific point is particularly important to remember (108). Saying to a person *before* giving information, "Now, this is very important" assists in recall of the information that follows.

8.   Do not use scare tactics. Too high a level of anxiety is thought to interfere with learning (109). Give information on why it is important to take medication in a certain way, but do not scold patients if they have not taken medication as directed in the past. On the other hand, some anxiety may be beneficial to patients if it is based on realistic concern and if patients know they can control the problem through compliance with therapeutic regimens. Emphasizing both the patient's susceptibility to problems if medications are not taken appropriately and the effectiveness of treatment have been shown to be a positive force in motivating adherence (110, 111). The important thing once problems are identified is to correct the misconceptions or other barriers to taking medications appropriately. This should be done without having the patient view you as a source of criticism, which may simply serve to create anxiety when the patient is in your presence.

9.   Try to put patients at ease. Be friendly and concerned rather than brisk and businesslike. This attitude on the part of health professionals has been found to promote better learning and better compliance. If patients seem anxious, try to assess the cause and alleviate worry or concern before trying to provide education.

10. With chronic care medications, conduct ongoing monitoring of patient medication-taking behaviors, perceptions of effectiveness, and problems encountered. Even when patients have shown no problems with compliance when beginning a regimen, we cannot assume they will continue to comply over the long term. Research has indicated that patients who were compliant while receiving ongoing attention and counseling from a pharmacist became noncompliant when the pharmacist intervention was not continued (81). In addition, reinforcement from you for positive behaviors, for the ability to manage therapy, may be a more potent force than giving attention only when problems exist.

INTERPROFESSIONAL COMMUNICATION

Although most of the writings and research in pharmacy communications focus on communication with patients, a crucial aspect of professional practice is the ability to communicate effectively with other health professionals. This section will first examine some of the barriers to effective interprofessional communication, some research related to pharmacists' relationships with other health professionals, and finally some techniques to assure more effective interprofessional communication.

Barriers to Communication

Although there are a number of barriers that might exist in communication with other health professionals, three will be discussed here: (*a*) environmental barriers, (*b*) pharmacist hesitancy in initiating communication, and (*c*) interprofessional struggles for power and autonomy.

Environmental Barriers

Pharmacists often find themselves communicating with other health professionals primarily over the telephone. The community pharmacist who notes a problem with a patient's medication regimen calls the physician. The nurse in the hospital who is inquiring about a drug order phones the pharmacy. This type of communication maintains and may exacerbate the distance that already exists among health professionals. In addition, the physical distance from the primary provider in community pharmacy results in a pharmacist who may remain ignorant of patient information that may help evaluate the appropriateness and effectiveness of the medication therapy.

Pharmacist Hesitancy to Communicate

Pharmacists have been accused of hiding behind prescription counters, avoiding communication with patients and health professionals. There is some evidence that many pharmacists are apprehensive in situations requiring interpersonal communication (25). Although there is certainly great individual variation, the practice of pharmacy behind the counter in the community or in the basement of the hospital may have, at least in the past, allowed pharmacists to avoid interpersonal contact.

Struggles for Power and Autonomy

Of all of the health professionals, physicians have been, without question, the dominant and most autonomous of health professionals. Some of this may be due to the educational process wherein physicians are taught to perceive themselves as autonomous (112, 113). In addition, the hierarchical structure of health care delivery has physicians at the top of the pyramid with the bulk of health care personnel at the base. Finally, physicians are the only ones who meet all of the following criteria that assure power and autonomy among health professionals (113).

1. They have broad permissible scopes of practice, legitimized by state licensing laws.
2. They have access to necessary health facilities, such as practice privileges in hospitals.
3. They are able to obtain reimbursement from governmental and private third party payers.

Some writers have noted that other health professionals have themselves contributed to the power of the physician by being deferent and unassertive in communication with physicians (114). The discrepancy in power and autonomy can lead to tension among professionals as well as a tendency for health professionals to interact primarily with members of their own group, with only limited interchange across professions (113). This in turn can lead to numerous misunderstandings as well as an "us versus them" mindset.

Research on Interprofessional Relationships

Very little research has been done examining the communication between pharmacists and other health professionals. Research that relates somewhat indirectly has examined the degree to which pharmacists are used by other professionals as sources of information and research on the attitudes toward pharmacists held by other health professionals.

Results of studies examining physicians' sources of information about medications have found among other things that pharmaceutical company sales representatives are frequently used as sources of information (115) as opposed to sources such as pharmacists. However, a survey of physician assistants' ratings of different potential sources of information gave pharmacists higher ratings than detail persons and, in general, pharmacists were given high marks as sources of information (116).

In hospital pharmacy practice, pharmacists have been found to be primary information sources for physicians (117) and nurses (118). Older physicians have been found to be less favorable toward expanded roles (119), something that also has been found in attitudes of private practice physicians (120). However, even younger physicians were favorable only toward those tasks that facilitated the physician role and did not involve independent therapeutic decision making on the part of pharmacists (119). Those physicians with more exposure to clinical pharmacists seem to be more positive about the contributions of pharmacists (121). Physicians have been found to change their attitudes in a more positive direction after implementation of clinical services in hospitals, with the exception of their attitudes related to pharmacist decision making on choice of drugs (122). Surveys of private practice physicians have revealed similar negative attitudes toward screening and therapeutic decision-making roles of community pharmacists (123).

Physicians in practice in hospitals or nursing homes have been found in numerous studies to accept pharmacist recommendations on drug therapy changes (124-128). One community-based study found that face-to-face meetings of clinical pharmacists and physicians were effective in improving the prescribing practices of physicians who were identified as having problems through review of Medicaid records (129).

Studies that have examined interprofessional attitudes have had mixed results, perhaps due to the diversity of techniques used and attitudinal dimensions examined. Some reports have claimed that generally positive attitudes toward pharmacists exist among physicians and other health professionals (130) although some problems have been highlighted. Physicians have been reported to be critical about pharmacists advising patients about drugs or recommending certain drugs (131, 132). A study in Florida after passage of legislation allowing pharmacists a limited independent prescribing privilege indicated that physicians were more negative about this law than were either pharmacist or consumer groups (133).

Although the research was conducted many years ago, Knapp et al. (134) found that physicians viewed the ideal pharmacist role in a more favorable light than certain pharmacist groups expected them to. A more recent report indicated that although physicians often believed pharmacists should be performing many clinical activities (except prescribing), they do not perceive them as *actually* functioning in those capacities (135). It seems from the research that pharmacists are probably viewed in a positive or at least acceptant light as long as their activities are not seen to encroach on areas physicians view as their exclusive purview. Interestingly, however, even activities such as patient counseling, which pharmacists see as part of their professional responsibilities, seem to be viewed by some physicians as encroaching on their territory (131, 132).

Improving Interprofessional Communication

Because the research on pharmacists' communication with other health professionals has not examined specific techniques for improving communication, recommendations will be based on a logical analysis of the interprofessional communication process. Because conflicts involving struggles for power and autonomy have already been noted as a key concern in interprofessional relationships, techniques to ameliorate such conflicts will be addressed.

Empathy is as important in relationships among equals as in communication with patients. The ability to understand other people without personally judging them, even when you disagree on issues, is part of effective communication. The ability to step outside your own frame of reference, to set aside stereotypes you hold, to listen to people, understand them, and convey that understanding back to them will assist any communication.

However, when conflicts arise, it is also necessary to be assertive in communication. The ability to express opinions in a straightforward manner, to give recommendations on therapy, and to persist in attempts to get the best therapy for patients is part of effective interprofessional communication. An apologetic, defensive tone, a defeatist attitude, or an "us versus them" point of view when conflict arises is not conducive to problem solving. Even though your best efforts to influence physicians may fail, it is necessary to persist in trying simply for your own sense of professional self-esteem.

CONCLUSION

The need for better provision of patient education services and more careful monitoring of medication use by health professionals is obvious. Pharmacists are in a position to have positive effects on the quality of care. To do so, however, would require that they be able to effectively communicate with patients and other health care providers. Although this chapter has primarily considered communication with patients, the problems and shortcomings revealed apply to communicating with health professionals as well. Pharmacists have generally not been found to be as involved as they could or should be in communication with patients or other health professionals. However, when they *are* involved, they have been found to significantly improve patient care.

Efforts have been made in colleges to improve the communication skills of pharmacy students. Hopefully, these efforts will lead to a more active and effective role for pharmacists in counseling patients, monitoring their drug use, and advising other health professionals on drug therapy.

REFERENCES

1. Haynes RB, Taylor DW, Sackett DL, eds. Compliance in health care. Baltimore: Johns Hopkins University Press, 1979.
2. Christensen DB. Drug-taking compliance: a review and synthesis. Health Serv Res 1978;13:171–187.
3. Blackwell B. The drug defaulter. Clin Pharm Ther 1972;13:841–848.
4. Ley P, Spelman MS. Communicating with the patient. London: Staples Press, 1967.

5. Becker MH, Maiman LA. Sociobehavioral determinants of compliance with health and medical care recommendations, Med Care 1975;13(1):10–24.
6. Kirscht JP, Rosenstock IM. Patients' problems in following recommendations of health experts. In Stone GC, Cohen F, Adler NE, eds. Health psychology—a handbook. San Francisco: Jossey-Bass, 1979.
7. Lander L. Defective medicine: risks, anger, and the malpractice crisis. New York: Farrar, Straus and Giroux, 1978.
8. Angorn RA. Does the pharmacist have a legal duty to consult with prescription patients about potential drug risks? Florida Pharm J 1981;53:6–8, 13.
9. Brushwood DB. The pharmacist's duty to warn the patient. U.S. Pharmacist 1984;9:21–29.
10. Brushwood DB. The pharmacist's duty to counsel patients: recent legal developments. Patient Counseling Commun Pharm 1985;4:13–14.
11. Fedo DA, Lezberg AK. Using communication skills. Apothecary 1978;90:12–15, 50–53.
12. Kauss DR, Robbins AS, Abrass I, Bakaitis RF, Anderson LA. The long-term effectiveness of interpersonal skills training in medical schools. J Med Educ 1980;55:595–601.
13. McKenzie MW. Competency-based, self-instructional modules on medication history interviewing, patient counseling, and drug therapy monitoring for pharmacy students. Am J Pharm Educ 1985;49:66–73.
14. Giannetti VJ. The effect of empathy training upon pharmacy student response styles. Am J Pharm Educ 1986;50:261–264.
15. Kahn GS, Cohen B, Jason H. The teaching of interpersonal skills in U.S. medical schools. J Med Educ 1979;54:29–35.
16. Miller GR. An introduction to speech communication. 2nd ed. New York: The Bobbs-Merrill Co, Inc, 1972.
17. Tindall WN. Principles and elements of interpersonal communication. In Tindall WN, Beardsley RS, Curtiss FR, eds. Communication in Pharmacy Practice: A Practical Guide for Students and Practitioners. Philadelphia: Lea & Febiger, 1984.
18. Barnard D, Barr JT, Schumacher GE. Person to person: empathy. Bethesda, Maryland: American Association of Colleges of Pharmacy, 1982.
19. Rogers CB. Client-centered therapy. Boston: Houghton-Mifflin, 1951.
20. Rogers CB. The necessary and sufficient conditions of therapeutic personality change. J Consulting Psych 1957;21:95.
21. Corey G. Theory and practice of counseling and psychotherapy, 3rd ed. Monterey, CA: Brooks/Cole Publishing, 1986.
22. McCroskey JC, Larson CE, Knapp ML. Introduction to interpersonal communication. Englewood Cliffs, NJ: Prentice-Hall, Inc, 1971.
23. Hall ET. The silent language. Garden City, NY: Doubleday, 1959.
24. Skinner BF. Science and human behavior. New York: Free Press, 1953.
25. Berger BA, Baldwin HJ, McCroskey JC, Richmond VP. Implementation of a systematic desensitization program and classroom instruction to reduce communication apprehension in pharmacy students. Am J Pharm Educ 1982;46:227–234.
26. Penwarden JR, Rowland CR, Shaffer W. Results of comprehensive communications training for pharmacy students. Am J Pharm Educ 1982;46:142–145.
27. Berger BA, Baldwin HJ, Richmond VP, McCroskey JC. Reducing communication apprehension: is there a better way? Am J Pharm Educ 1984;48:46–50.
28. Kimberlin CL. Assertiveness training for pharmacy students. Am J Pharm Educ 1982;46:137–141.
29. Zifferblatt SM. Increasing patient compliance through the applied analysis of behavior. Prev Med 1975;4:173–182.
30. Mastria MA, Drabman RS. The development of behavioral competence in medical settings. In McNamara JR, ed. Behavioral approaches to medicine: application and analysis. New York: Plenum, 1979.
31. Ellis A. Reason and emotion in psychotherapy. New York: Lyle Stuart, 1962.
32. Meichenbaum D. Cognitive behavior modification: an integrative approach. New York: Plenum, 1977.
33. Wolpe, J. The practice of behavior therapy. New York: Pergamon Press, 1969.
34. Lazarus AA. Behavior therapy and beyond. New York: McGraw-Hill, 1971.

35. Schwartz RM, Gottman JM. A task analysis approach to clinical problems: a study of assertive behavior. J Consulting Clin Psych 1976;44:910-920.
36. Alden L, Safran J. Irrational beliefs and nonassertive behavior. Cognit Ther Res 1978;2:257-264.
37. Heisler G, Shipley RH. The ABC model of assertive behavior. Behav Ther 1977;8:509-512.
38. Mongomery D, Heimberg RC. Prof Psych 1978;9:220.
39. Ludwig LD, Lazarus AA. A cognitive and behavioral approach to the treatment of social inhibition. Psychother Theory Res Pract 1972;9:204-206.
40. Bruch MA. A task analysis of assertive behavior revisited: replication and extension. Behav Ther 1981;12:217-230.
41. Maiman LA, Becker MH. The health belief model: origins and correlates in psychological theory. Health Educ Monogr 1974;2:336-353.
42. Rosenstock IM. The health belief model and preventive health behavior. Health Educ Monogr 1974;2:354-386.
43. Becker MH, Maiman LA. Strategies for enhancing patient compliance. J Commun Health 1980;6:113-135.
44. Ley, P. Improving communications: effects of altering doctor behavior. In Osborne DJ, Gruneberg MM, Eiser JR, eds. Research in psychology and medicine. London: Academic Press, 1979.
45. Francis V, Korsch BM, Morris MJ. Gaps in doctor-patient communication: patients' response to medical advice. N Engl J Med 1969;280:535-540.
46. Freemon B, Negrete VF, Davis M, Korsch BM. Gaps in doctor-patient communication: doctor-patient interaction analysis. Pediatr Res 1971;5:298-311.
47. Boreham P, Gibson D. The informative process in private medical consultations: a preliminary investigation. Soc Sci Med 1978;12:409-416.
48. Smith C, Polis E, Hadac R. Characteristics of the initial medical interview associated with patient satisfaction and understanding. J Fam Pract 1981;12:283-288.
49. Stiles W, Putnam S, Jacobs M. Verbal exchange structure of initial medical interviews. Health Psych 1982;1:315-336.
50. DiMatteo MR, Hays RD, Prince LM. Relationship of physicians' nonverbal communication skill to patient satisfaction, appointment noncompliance and physician workload. Health Psych 1986;5:581-594.
51. Hulka B. Patient-clinician interactions and compliance. In Haynes RB, Taylor DW, Sackett DL, eds. Compliance in Health Care. Baltimore: Johns Hopkins University Press, 1979.
52. Svarstad B. Physician-patient communication and patient conformity with medical advice. In Mechanic D, ed. The growth of bureaucratic medicine. New York: Wiley, 1976.
53. Wertheimer AI, Shefter E, Cooper RM. More on the pharmacist as a drug consultant: three case studies. Drug Intell Clin Pharm 1973;7:58-61.
54. Vanderveen RL, Adams C, Sanborn M. The pharmacist as drug consultant—five years later. Drug Intell Clin Pharm 1978;12:718-719.
55. Knapp DA, Wolf HH, Knapp DE, Rudy TA. The pharmacist as drug advisor. J Am Pharm Assoc 1969;NS9:502.
56. Jang R, Knapp DA, Knapp DE. An evaluation of the quality of drug-related services in neighborhood pharmacies. Drugs Health Care 1975;2:21-38.
57. Rowles B, Keller SM, Gavin PW. The pharmacist as compounder and consultant. Drug Intell Clin Pharm 1974;8:242-244.
58. Puckett FJ, White SJ, Mossberg HE, Matchett JA. Pharmacist/patient counseling practices. Contemp Pharm Pract 1978;1:67-71.
59. Campbell RK, Grisafe JA. Compliance with the Washington State Patient Information Regulation. J Am Pharm Assoc 1975;NS15:494.
60. Ross SR, White SJ, Hogan LC, Godwin HN. The effect of a mandatory patient counseling regulation on the counseling practices of pharmacy practitioners. Contemp Pharm Pract 1981:64-68.
61. Mason HL, Svarstad BL. Medication counseling behaviors and attitudes of rural community pharmacists. Drug Intell Clin Pharm 1984;18:409-414.
62. Deleted in proof.

63. Dickson WM, Rodowskas C. Verbal communications of community pharmacists. Med Care 1975;13:486–498.

64. Mason HL. Using attitudes and subjective norms to predict pharmacist counseling behaviors. Patient Counseling Health Educ 1985;1:190–196.

65. Ludy JA, Gagnon JP, Caiola SM. The patient–pharmacist interaction in two ambulatory settings—its relationship to patient satisfaction and drug misuse. Drug Intell Clin Pharm 1977;11:81–89.

66. Beardsley RS, Johnson CA, Wise G. Privacy as a factor in patient counseling. J Am Pharm Assoc 1977;NS17:366–368.

67. McBean BJ, Blackburn JL. An evaluation of four methods of pharmacist-conducted patient education. Can Pharm J 1982;115:167–172.

68. Watkins RL, Norwood GJ. Impact of environment and age on quality of consultant behavior among pharmacists. Am J Pharm Educ 1977;41:19–22.

69. Linn LS, Davis MS. Occupational orientation and overt behavior—the pharmacist as drug advisor to patients. Am J Pub Health 1973;63:502–508.

70. Smith MC, Sharpe TR. A study of pharmacists' involvement in drug use by the elderly. Drug Intell Clin Pharm 1984;18:525–529.

71. Morris LA. A survey of patients' receipt of prescription drug information. Med Care 1982;20:596–605.

72. Moore SR, Kalu M, Yavaprabba S. Receipt of prescription drug information by the elderly, 1983;17:920–923.

73. Carroll NV, Gagnon JP. The relationship between patient variables and frequency of pharmacist counseling. Drug Intell Clin Pharm 1983;17:648–652.

74. Oliver CH, Barnes BA. Communication attitudes, practices and training needs of working pharmacists. Am J Pharm Educ 1983;47:119–122.

75. Zelnio RN, Nelson AA, Beno CE. Clinical pharmaceutical services in retail practice. I. Pharmacists' willingness and abilities to provide services. Drug Intell Clin Pharm 1984;18:917–922.

76. Robinson JD, McKenzie MW. Pharmacists' views on mandatory patient counseling. Drug Intell Clin Pharm 1984;18:913–917.

77. Kirking DM. Pharmacists perceptions of their patient counseling activities. Contemp Pharm Pract 1982;5:230–238.

78. Ascione FJ, Kirking DM, Duzey OM, Wenzloff NJ. A survey of patient education activities of community pharmacists. Patient Educ Counsel 1985;7:359–366.

79. Watkins RL, Norwood GJ, Meister FL. Improving the quality of the pharmacist as a drug advisor to patients and physicians through continuing education. Am J Pharm Educ 1976;40:34–39.

80. Rantucci MJ, Segal HJ. Over-the-counter medication: outcome and effectiveness of patient counseling. J Soc Admin Pharm 1986;3:81–91.

81. McKenney JM, Slining JM, Henderson HR, Divins D, Bass M. The effects of clinical pharmacy services on patients with essential hypertension. Circulation 1973;XLVII:1104–1111.

82. McKenney JM, Brown ED, Necsary R, Reavis HL. Effect of pharmacist drug monitoring and patient education on hypertensive patients. Contemp Pharm Pract 1978;1:50–56.

83. Sharpe TR, Mikeal KL. Patient compliance with antibiotic regimens. Am J Hosp Pharm 1974;31:479–484.

84. Hammarlund ER, Ostrom JA, Kethley AJ. The effects of drug counseling and other educational strategies on drug utilization of the elderly. Med Care 1985;23:165–170.

85. Norwood GJ. Impact of a clinical pharmacist's emphasis on patient communication on the patient's attitude toward pharmacy. Drug Intell Clin Pharm 1975;9:601–604.

86. Helling DK, Hepler CD, Jones ME. Effect of direct clinical pharmacy services on patient's perceptions of health care quality. Paper presented at the American Society of Hospital Pharmacists Annual Midyear Clinical Meeting, San Antonio, TX, December 6, 1978.

87. Kimberlin CL. Empathy. In Tindall WN, Beardsley RS, Curtiss FR, eds. Communication in pharmacy practice: a practical guide for students and practitioners. Philadelphia: Lea and Febiger, 1984.

88. Lawrence GD. If I were in his shoes, how would I feel? J Am Pharm Assoc 1976;16:453–454.

89. Barnard D, Barr JT, Schumacher GE. Empathy: person to person. Bethesda, Maryland: American Association of Colleges of Pharmacy, 1982.

90. Becker MH, Drachman RH, Kirscht JP. A field experiment to evaluate various outcomes of continuity of physician care. Am J Pub Health 1974;64:1062–1070.

91. Schulman B. Active patient orientation and outcomes in hypertensive treatment. Med Care 1979;17:267.

92. Roter DL. Patient question asking in physician–patient interaction. Health Psych 1984;3:395–409.

93. Tracy J. Impact of intake procedures upon client attrition in a community mental health center. J Consult Clin Psych 1977;45:192–95.

94. Azrin NH, Powell J. Behavioral engineering: the use of response priming to improve prescribed self-medication. J Appl Behav Anal 1969;2:39–42.

95. Fink DL. Tailoring the consensual regimen. In Sackett DL, Haynes RB, eds. Compliance with therapeutic regimens. Baltimore: Johns Hopkins University Press, 1976.

96. Epstein LH, Masek BJ. Behavioral control of medicine compliance. J Appl Behav Anal 1978;II:1–9.

97. Schafer LC, Glasgow RE, McCaul KD. Increasing the adherence of diabetic adolescents. J Behav Med 1982;5:353–362.

98. Haynes RB, Sackett DL, Gibson ES, et al. Improvement of medication compliance in uncontrolled hypertension. Lancet 1976;1:1265–1268.

99. Steckel SB, Swain MA. Contracting with patients to improve compliance. J Am Hosp Assoc 1977;51:81–84.

100. Clinite JC, Kabat HF. Improving patient compliance. J Am Pharm Assoc 1976;16:74–76, 85.

101. Kimberlin CL, Berardo DH. A comparison of patient education methods used in community pharmacies. J Pharm Market Management, in press.

102. Ascione FJ, Shimp LA. The effectiveness of four education strategies in the elderly. Drug Intell Clin Pharm 1984;18:926–931.

103. Ley P, Bradshaw PW, Eaves D, Walker CM. A method for increasing patient recall of information presented by doctors. Psych Med 1973;3:217–220.

104. Paivio A. Mental imagery in associative learning and memory. Psych Rev 1969;76:241–263.

105. Bradshaw PW, Ley P, Kincey JA, Bradshaw J. Recall of medical advice: comprehensibility and specificity. Br J Soc Clin Psych 1975;14:55–62.

106. Ley P. Patients' understanding and recall in clinical communication failure. In Pendleton D, Hasler J, eds. Doctor–patient communication. London: Academic Press, 1983.

107. Ley P. Giving information to patients. In Eiser JK, ed. Social psychology and behavioral medicine. New York: John Wiley and Sons, 1982.

108. Ley P. What the patient forgets. Med Opinion Rev 1966;1:71–73.

109. Eisdorfer C, Nowlin J, Wilkie F. Improvement of learning in the aged by modification of autonomic nervous system activity. Science (Wash DC) 1970;170:1327–1329.

110. Innui TS, Yourtee EL, Williamson JW. Improved outcomes in hypertension after physician outcomes in hypertension after physician tutorials: a controlled trial. Ann Intern Med 1976;84:646–651.

111. Becker MH, Drachman RH, Kirscht JP. A new approach to explaining sick-role behavior in low-income populations. Am J Pub Health 1974;64:205–216.

112. Weiss S. Role differentiation between nurse and physician: implications for nursing, Nurs Res 1983;32:133–139.

113. Northouse PG, Northouse LL. Health Communication: A handbook for health related professionals. Englewood Cliffs, NJ: Prentice-Hall, 1985.

114. Mauksch, I. Nurse-physician collaboration: a changing relationship. J Nurs Admin 1981;11:35–38.

115. Avorn J, Chen M, Hartley R. Scientific versus commercial sources of influence on the prescribing behavior of physicians. Am J Med 1982;73:4–8.

116. Fincham JE. How pharmacists are rated as a source of drug information by physician assistants. Drug Intell Clin Pharm 1986;20:379–383.

117. Shearer SW, Gagnon JP, Eckel FM. Community, hospital and clinical pharmacists and drug information centers as physician drug information sources. Am J Hosp Pharm 1978;35:909–914.

118. Roth CP. Nurses and pharmacists: a study of consultation patterns on patient units. Nurs Health Care 1982;34:438–442.

119. Ritchey FJ, Raney MR. Medical role—task boundary maintenance: physicians' opinions on clinical pharmacy. Med Care 1981;19:90-103.
120. Bernstein LR, Klett EA, Jacoby KE. Physicians' attitudes toward the use of clinical pharmaceutical services in private medical practice. Am J Hosp Pharm 1978;35:715-717.
121. Ritchey FJ, Raney MR. Effect of exposure on physicians' attitudes toward clinical pharmacists. Am J Hosp Pharm 38:1459-1463.
122. Nelson AA, Meinhold JM, Hutchinson RA. Changes in physicians' attitudes toward pharmacists as drug information consultants following implementation of clinical pharmaceutical services. Am J Hosp Pharm 1978;35:1201-1206.
123. Norwood GJ, Seibert JJ, Gagnon JP. Attitudes of rural consumers and physicians toward expanded roles for pharmacists. J Am Pharm Assoc 1976;16:551-554.
124. Hull JH, Eckel FM. Evaluation of the pharmacists as a drug therapy advisor on ward rounds. Am J Hosp Pharm 1973;30:687-694.
125. Schweigert BF, Oppenheimer PR, Smith WE. Hospital pharmacists as a source of drug information for physicians and nurses. Am J Hosp Pharm 1982;39:74-77.
126. Briggs GG, Smith WE. Pharmacist-physician drug consultations in a community hospital. Am J Hosp Pharm 1974;31:247-253.
127. Taylor AT, Martell PH. Physician acceptance of clinical pharmacy service in a skilled nursing home. J Am Geriatri Soc 1980;18:227-229.
128. Miller DA, Lucarotti RL, Vlasses PH, Krigstein DJ, McKercher PL. Perceived clinical significance of consultant pharmacist recommendations in the skilled nursing facility. Drug Intell Clin Pharm 1980;14:182-186.
129. Avorn J, Soumerai SB. Improving drug therapy decisions through education outreach: a randomized controlled trial of academically based "detailing." N Engl J Med 1983;308:1457-1463.
130. Dickinson JG. How pharmacists relate to other health professionals. Drug Topics 1981;11:28-30, 35.
131. R.Ph-MD relations are good, but some frictions exist. Am Druggist 1983;188:49.
132. Schering Report Explores Pharmacist-Physician Relationships. Am Pharm 1984;NS24:13-14.
133. Pharmacist Prescribing Law: An attitude survey of Florida consumers, physicians and pharmacists. Unpublished report of survey done by C/IR research firm, commissioned by Upjohn, 1985.
134. Knapp DE, Knapp DA, Edwards JD. The pharmacist as perceived by physicians, patrons and other pharmacists. J Am Pharm Assoc 1969;9:80-82, 84.
135. Lambert RL, Wertheimer AI, Dobbert DJ, Church TR. The pharmacist clinical role as seen by other health workers. Am J Pub Health 1977;67:252-253.

SELECTED READINGS

ATTENDING TO THE UNSPOKEN [a]

David Barnard

To judge by some accounts, pharmacists ought to be psychoanalysts. As people have begun to question the emotionally distant, interpersonally passive, task-oriented role they traditionally adopt, there is increasing emphasis on forming a bond of understanding and empathy with patients and consumers, and reverence for the inner world of individuals experiencing illness. While I would not advocate a psychoanalytic model for pharmacy practice, I do believe that some deep and sophisticated understanding of patients' *unspoken agenda* in health care interactions is the basis for effective communication. I would claim that such understanding is not only a specific indicator of some communications skills competencies, but the condition for all of them. Without this understanding, communications skills may simply degenerate into rote behaviors or manipulative strategies little different from the mechanistic technologies of health care they are intended to enrich. I intend to sketch briefly patients' unspoken agenda, and then to suggest some of the specific competencies that seem to be implied by the analysis.

Notwithstanding the undeniable (and quite pertinent) diversity in personal and cultural responses to illness, three crucial issues can reliably be expected to engage at least part of the attention of the person standing or lying before a practicing pharmacist. These are:

- the problem of uncertainty;
- the fear of helplessness and dependency;
- the need for meaning and order.

Does illness entail uncertainty? We need only consider the expression of the patient contemplating an experimental protocol for treatment of his or her cancer; or the convalescent coronary patient gingerly seeking tolerable levels of physical exertion.

Does illness entail the fear of helplessness and dependency? We need only consider the look in the eyes of the recently bereaved child; or the countenance of the erstwhile household provider coming to grips with chronic disability.

Does illness entail the need for meaning and order? We need only consider the person in intractable, incurable pain; or recall our own experiences of "hanging fire" until unusual sensations reveal their ominous or (more commonly) harmless message. Eric Cassell, in *The Healer's Art*, has captured this core of anxious preoccupation:

> "You may be able, if you so decide, not to think about, say, the Pittsburgh Symphony, but it is virtually impossible not to think about your own unresolved symptoms."

It has become a commonplace to observe that the importance *patients* attach to these issues is rarely matched by a corresponding concern on the part of health care personnel, who more frequently define their role in terms of technical and scientific, rather than inter-

---

[a]This paper was presented to the AACP-Lilly Invitational Conference on Communications Skills Competencies, Kansas City, November, 1980. Printed with permission of the author.

personal, expertise. Emphasis on the superficial, task-specific interpersonal transactions in pharmacy practice may be readily explained by pharmacists' busy schedules, personal reticence, technical and quantitative biases, or comparative lack of training for anything else. Patients contribute to this pattern, too, however. They are quickly taught to be scrupulously respectful of busy professionals, and are often desperately fearful of "taking too much time." They may even carefully rehearse their visit to the pharmacy or clinic in order to be able to complete their transaction as quickly and inconspicuously as possible. More significant, perhaps, is the fact that many of the deeper issues and feelings associated with illness are only dimly sensed by patients themselves, who, on one level, may be only too happy to dilute them with the trivial busy-work of therapeutic regimens. Those issues and feelings persist, however, in steady counterpoint to the public transactions of patienthood, and they constitute an internal frame of reference for experiencing and evaluating health care. Unattended, they frequently account for patients' ultimate feelings of isolation, manipulation, or dehumanization in the health care system.

A paradox of health care is the patient who feels lonely and confused, while surrounded by scores of health professionals, relentlessly providing information. In my view, emphasis on communications skills can go astray if it considers only the optimum strategies and techniques for teaching people about complex medications, or giving technical advice on treatment, referrals, and product selection. As critical as these skills are, they can suggest the *appearance* of excellent communication even as they smother the patient's deeper, silent agenda beneath the weight of the pharmacist's technical one. Yet for patients, the burdens of private wrestling with problems of uncertainty, dependency, and meaning are increased by the conviction that they must be borne silently and alone, that no one else cares much or understands. And, depending on a patient's personality, these feelings can actually nullify the pharmacist's otherwise excellent communicative efforts. This can occur through the listlessness of hopelessness and depression, or through a heightened anxiety that distorts, resists, or mistrusts the information that is transmitted.

In this context, the pharmacist represents to the patient—before he or she represents anything else—*human contact:* a voice, a presence, a potential ally in the face of suffering. To realize this potential requires that professionals suspend their technical agendas to enable patients to apprehend the possibility—and *permissibility*—of expressing *their* deeper doubts and concerns. Even if patients do not respond to this offering immediately, it exists to remind them that they are *not* fundamentally alone. And, I want to repeat, it is *the conviction of enduring relationship and companionship during illness* that underlies any serious professional intervention, be it of a therapeutic, educational, or consultative nature. The professional commitments and interpersonal behaviors that nourish this conviction in patients are not luxuries, to be rationed or employed when the "essential" technical tasks are finished. They are the prerequisites for the effective and thorough performance of every aspect of patient care.

Let me now conclude, equally dogmatically, with a set of attitudinal and behavioral implications that I draw from this brief account, related to pharmacists' skill development in communications. I hope they will provoke some lively discussion.

1) Pharmacists ought to cultivate basic knowledge of the psychosocial aspects of illness and treatment, with special emphasis on the issues of uncertainty, dependency, and meaning for patients within the health system.

2) Pharmacists' ought to develop *an expectation of psychosocial relevance* to the patient's experience of health care, rather than assuming this dimension will always be attended to by others.

3) Pharmacists ought to move from a *task-orientation* to a *person-orientation* in professional practice.
4) Pharmacists ought routinely to communicate *emotional availability* and *expectant attention* to their patients and consumers.
5) Pharmacists ought to become familiar and comfortable with their own anxieties and associations with illness and with the various personality types encountered in clinical practice.
6) Pharmacists ought to identify a network of continuing support from peers, allied professionals, or personal relationships who can provide consultation, supervision, and personal renewal amid the rigors and demands of competent, thorough, and *emotionally present* professional work.

PHARMACY PRACTICE—THE IMPORTANCE OF EFFECTIVE COMMUNICATIONS[b]

Daniel A. Hussar

WITH OTHER PHARMACISTS

The subject of "communication" has received considerable attention within the profession of pharmacy and well it should. Major emphasis has been placed on the need for pharmacists to communicate effectively with patients in an effort to assure the optimal use of drugs. Likewise, communication between the pharmacist and other health professionals has been stressed. These efforts are extremely important and the success of our professional endeavors will depend to a large extent on the effectiveness of our communication with patients and other health professionals.

There is another type of communication that is often overlooked in our enthusiasm to pursue some of the opportunities that are available to us—a type of communication that also is very important to the profession of pharmacy and to each of us as individual pharmacists. I refer to the communication that occurs or does *not* occur *between pharmacists*.

In many respects, pharmacy is a divided or fragmented profession. There is too little communication and cooperation between pharmacists who practice in different settings and/or have differing primary responsibilities. In spite of the fact that we share a common background and have many similar responsibilities and goals, we, within the profession, seem to concentrate on the differences. It is reasonable to expect that the public, our legislators, and others outside the profession do not identify or differentiate the various roles and responsibilities that pharmacists assume or the practice settings in which they function. Yet *we* tend to magnify these differences with the result that we lose the benefit of achieving certain goals that are seemingly without our grasp were we to pursue them in a united fashion.

Independent pharmacists, chain pharmacists, hospital pharmacists, industrial pharmacists, pharmacy educators, employer pharmacists, employee pharmacists—the list goes

[b]Reprinted with permission from Hussar DA. Pharmacy practice—the importance of effective communications. Am J Pharm 1976;148:136–147.

on and on. Too often, we place ourselves in one of these groups and feel that our activities and existence is independent and exclusive of the others. Even within a single one of these groups we sometimes view each other as competitors rather than colleagues.

Certainly it is understandable that some grouping of pharmacists based on type and location of practice will exist. We must also recognize that change and progress will not occur uniformly in all practice settings and with regard to all types of responsibilities. Yet, this should not be used as a reason for one group to set itself apart from the others, but rather viewed as a reason to encourage others to pursue progressive change.

We need not look any further than the division, and even conflict, that exists between pharmacy associations for an example of how we are slowed in our progress toward accomplishments for the *profession* of which we are all a part and with which we are identified regardless of our specific responsibilities. It is sobering to consider that this is the situation that exists which involves those pharmacists who at least have the interest and take the responsibility of belonging to their professional associations and thereby have the benefit of a certain level of communication.

Have the associations caused the problem? Certainly not! However, the lack of support of a large number of pharmacists has limited the extent to which the associations can be effective. We see now, and can anticipate more, issues that will be controversial and difficult to resolve and the associations often are unable to work from a position of strength. Progress has been slow, but it is occurring, and we can be encouraged by the types of activities and the success of efforts in which our associations are now involved.

It is not pleasant to imagine what would happen if we did not have our associations to deal with the issues, and it is my feeling that every pharmacist has a responsibility to belong to his local, state, and national professional associations.

We have been talking about those pharmacists who are members of professional associations and who continuously receive information and become aware of the issues facing the profession even though some of them may be difficult to understand and resolve. But what about those pharmacists who are not members, who may not even know what the issues *are*, let alone understand them?

More and more frequently it is necessary for us to go to our patients, the general public, and our legislators to describe what we are prepared to offer in the way of professional services and to describe some of the problems that we are encountering and need to have addressed. Yet is it any wonder that our effectiveness in communicating with and achieving consumer and legislative support is limited when we have not identified an effective way to communicate with and bring the issues to the attention of many within our own profession? There are many pharmacists who do not know what PSRO's and MAC are, let alone have an appreciation for the impact they can have on their individual practices.

In our view, the need to increase communications and cooperation among pharmacists represents *the* major challenge before the profession. It is tempting to take an attitude that we should forget about those pharmacists who have not done anything for their profession, who have not joined the professional associations, since actually they have benefited from our efforts without paying their own way. However, we cannot afford to take this attitude but must accept the challenge to do even more than we have done in the past.

WITH PHYSICIANS AND OTHER HEALTH PROFESSIONALS

Many health professionals become involved directly or indirectly with various aspects of drug therapy.

The pharmacist has had the most extensive training in this area and by maintaining this expertise he can develop and strengthen communications and a working relationship with other health professionals.

There will be many situations in which the pharmacist will have occasion to discuss a patient's drug therapy with the physician. Indeed in an increasng number of circumstances the pharmacist is involved in the development of treatment plans.

This communication should be viewed as a cooperative effort in the patient's behalf. Too often when a pharmacist contacts a physician about a patient's drug therapy it is viewed as a challenge rather than an overture of wishing to cooperate in providing the best therapy for the patient.

In addition to the situations regarding therapy for patients, numerous other opportunities exist for strengthening communications with physicians and include: (1) inviting physicians into the pharmacy and explaining services and policies; (2) developing newsletters for physicians with pertinent information on medications and services; (3) holding joint meetings of local medical and pharmaceutical societies; and (4) exploring the possibility of having input into local and state medical journals, newsletters, etc.

It is essential for pharmacy associations to have effective communications with the medical associations. At a time when we are encouraging individual pharmacists to assume additional responsibilities that necessitate a close working relationship with the physicians, it is important that our professional associations have effective channels of communication.

Similar opportunities are available for the development of cooperative efforts with other professions.

WITH PHARMACEUTICAL MANUFACTURERS

During the last several years there has been considerable attention directed towards some of the differences of opinion between the manufacturers and practicing pharmacists, particularly pertaining to the issues of drug product selection and pricing policies. It is unfortunate that these differences have led to a significant breakdown in communications. The apparent inability of the manufacturers and practicing pharmacists to resolve these differences among themselves has contributed to a situation where someone else, namely the government, will be making important decisions regarding the provision of and reimbursement for pharmaceutical services. At this point the specific implications of this for the profession are uncertain.

Differences on certain issues should not be permitted to obscure the numerous areas of mutual interest and concern shared by the manufacturers and practicing pharmacists. The development and dissemination of information on drugs via drug information services (at the manufacturer's level and at the practitioner level), and continuing education programs, many of which are sponsored by manufacturers are examples of such efforts.

These remarks should not be interpreted to mean that we should only be discussing issues on which we agree. It is important that differences of opinion be expressed and problems resolved. However, to achieve this it is essential that open channels of communication be maintained.

WITH LEGISLATORS AND GOVERNMENT AGENCIES

It is important for pharmacists to be politically aware and active. We must take the initiative in meeting legislators and in influencing the development of legislation.

Pharmacy often finds itself reacting after the fact. We cannot afford to *wait* to have someone tell us when legislation is developing that will affect pharmacy practice or to have legislators ask us our opinion on various issues—usually they won't.

Most of us are politically naive and we have learned some hard lessons as a result. It is essential that the profession be aware of proposed legislation and involved in the development of legislation not only at the national level but also at the state and local levels.

WITH ADMINISTRATORS OF THIRD-PARTY PRESCRIPTION PROGRAMS

It is recognized that the number of prescriptions for which the pharmacist receives reimbursement from a third party has sharply increased.

The type and value of pharmaceutical services must be communicated to those responsible for financing and administering these programs and we should be able to effectively demonstrate how these services contribute to patient care.

We need also to anticipate what type of information and data will be requested by those evaluating the scope and value of pharmaceutical services.

Pharmacists often complain that the fee in many of the programs is too low and there is no doubt that they are correct. Yet when pharmacists are asked how much it costs them to dispense a prescription and provide pharmaceutical services, most do not really know. There is relatively little in the way of individual or collective data regarding these costs. Therefore, it is imperative that efforts be pursued to obtain such information as it will certainly become more important for us to be able to provide it. It certainly will be advantageous to have hard data that pharmacists have developed than to have someone else estimate the cost of dispensing a prescription because of the lack of such data.

WITH PATIENTS

First of all the terminology is important as it relates to the attitude towards the individuals we serve.

To be considered a true professional the pharmacist must regard those who come to him for pharmaceutical services as patients, not customers.

One observer has identified several of the most important criteria for establishing whether an individual is deserving of the designation "health professional." One criterion is whether in all instances the health and welfare of the patient are held paramount. It must be kept in mind that the pharmacist, as other licensed health practitioners, is granted a license by the state conferring on him a special privilege to practice his profession. It is therefore to the public, and more specifically to his own patients, that he owes his primary allegiance.

Another characteristic of a professional practice is the existence of a one-to-one relationship between the patient and practitioner. It is disturbing to note how often pharmacists jealously guard what they feel to be their professional prerogatives of counting, pouring, and labeling and then find no time left for patient counseling or for telephone calls to the physician when there might be questions about the therapy.

Reference will be made several times to the Dichter study (1) of consumer attitudes toward pharmacists and pharmacy practice that was commissioned several years ago by the American Pharmaceutical Association. One finding of this study was "that the pharmacist has lost contact with his patients." However, it was also identified that "patients expect— and indeed want—contact, personal attention and professional services from the pharmacist."

Studies indicate that the public is generally unaware of what the pharmacist really does. Patients also often have the impression that there are secrets regarding their illness and drug therapy that they are not privy to. Therefore, in addition to counseling the patient regarding his drug therapy, the pharmacist should explain the nature of the services he provides. Too often, pharmacists who maintain good patient medication records never make the patient aware of this service or how the records are used for the patient's benefit. We talk a lot among ourselves about pharmaceutical services, but to what extent do we discuss these services with patients?

Consideration should also be given to the removal of certain other barriers that may detract from the pharmacist–patient relationship. The "secrecy" concerning the prescription may be increased in the eyes of the patient when the pharmacist disappears behind a high counter to work on the prescription. The Dichter study notes that one of the public's most prevalent perceptions is that the pharmacist hides behind a specialized counter in a corner of the establishment, makes a little bit of noise, and comes up with a small bottle and a large bill.

These recognitions led those conducting the Dichter study to state: "the single most important recommendation of our study is that communication has to be reestablished between the public and the pharmacist. It is necessary to explain to the public in considerable detail exactly what the pharmacist does. To achieve this, all modern available channels of communication should be utilized."

The communication between the pharmacist and the patient must be of the type that a personal interest on the part of the pharmacist is evident. There is ample evidence that the patient desires this type of interest and attention. In many instances the patient's visit to the pharmacy, whether at the community level or in a hospital as an outpatient, is the last step in what may have been a lengthy, tiring, and sometimes unpleasant series of consultations, tests, and diagnostic procedures used to identify the nature of the disease. If then in the last step of this process to restore or maintain health the relationship is one which is not on a high professional plane and in a professional atmosphere with an interest in the patient being evident, the patient's progress may be harmed and the image of the pharmacist as a health professional will suffer.

A number of situations could be identified to demonstrate the need for effective pharmacist–patient communications. However, the problems of patient noncompliance very clearly and meaningfully illustrate not only some of our shortcomings in addressing our professional responsibilities, but also the opportunities to enhance our contribution to patient care.

Patient Noncompliance

With the considerable advances that have been made in the development of new therapeutic agents that are more efficacious and potent than previously available drugs, it is ironic to note that in many circumstances drugs are not being used in a manner that is conducive to optimal benefit and safety. Increasing attention has been directed to the problems of adverse drug reactions and drug interactions and there have been many reports and commentaries in the recent literature regarding these occurrences.

However, more and more frequently even more basic questions regarding drug usage are being asked. Does the patient understand how to take his medication and if so, is he taking it according to the directions provided? Although problems concerning patient compliance with instructions have been recognized for years, these problems continue to be prevalent and it has only been relatively recently that this issue has begun to receive the attention it deserves.

When the complexity of the patient's illnesses and the action of modern therapeutic agents is taken into account, it seems understandable that the physician and other health professionals can easily become preoccupied with the diagnosis of the disease state as well as the selection and implications of drug therapy and assume that the patient will follow instructions provided him. After all, the medication is being provided to improve and/or maintain the patient's health so why would the patient not cooperate by following instructions? Yet studies continue to show that a large percentage of patients, for a variety of reasons, do not take their medication according to instructions. Although the studies reported to date have indicated a wide variation in the degree of noncompliance, in most studies at least a third of the patients failed to comply with instructions and in some studies the rate of noncompliance exceeded 50%.

Several studies involving the use of digoxin present some interesting implications. In one study (2), the mean serum digoxin concentrations were determined to be significantly lower in the group of noncompliant patients leading the investigators to conclude that "patient compliance is a major (if not the major) determinant of outpatient serum digoxin concentration." The therapeutic equivalence and bioavailability of digoxin preparations have received considerable study and publicity during the last several years. Although attention to these matters should continue to receive high priority, it would appear that the factor of noncompliance is much more likely to be responsible for unexpected or altered therapeutic responses.

CONSEQUENCES OF NONCOMPLIANCE

The consequences of noncompliance, although seemingly apparent, are often not fully appreciated. In many cases noncompliance will result in the underutilization of a drug, thereby depriving the patient of the anticipated therapeutic benefits and possibly resulting in a progressive worsening of the condition being treated. Several examples of problems can be cited. A patient may discontinue taking an antibiotic for the treatment of an infection when the symptoms subside and, therefore, not use all the prescribed medication. This could result in a reoccurrence of the infection since the shorter course of therapy was not sufficient to eradicate it.

Hypertensive patients have frequently been found to be noncompliant. If the physician is unaware that the patient is not taking the medication according to directions and sees that the elevated blood pressure is not well controlled, he may prescribe larger doses of the same agent(s) or prescribe more potent antihypertensive medications. This will expose the patient to a greater risk of adverse effects. Therefore, before a patient is judged to be unresponsive or not optimally controlled with the initial therapy prescribed, it should be ascertained that the medication is being taken according to instructions.

Noncompliance may also result in the overutilization of a drug. When excessive doses are employed or when the medication is given more frequently than intended, there is an increased risk of adverse reactions. These problems may develop rather innocently as in the case where a patient recognizes that he has forgotten a dose of medication and doubles the next dose to make up for it. Some other patients apparently subscribe to a philosophy that if the one-tablet dose that has been prescribed provides some relief of symptoms, two or three tablets will be even more effective.

THE NONCOMPLIANT PATIENT

Efforts have been made to demonstrate the relationship of noncompliance to a number of variables such as age, sex, religion, race, marital status, education, occupation, socioeconomic status, personality factors, physiologic variables, and the number, types, and severity of illnesses. Although certain patterns have been noted in some studies, the results, in general, have been inconsistent and it continues to be difficult to identify which patients are most likely to be noncompliant. In several studies in which physicians were asked to predict whether patients would be compliant, the predictions were little better than could be obtained by chance and the complexity of the problem has led one investigator to observe (3), "It has not proved possible to identify an uncooperative type. Every patient is a potential defaulter; compliance can never be assumed."

FACTORS CONTRIBUTING TO NONCOMPLIANCE

A number of factors pertaining to patient noncompliance have been identified and these are considered in the following discussion:

Failure to Comprehend Importance of Therapy—It would appear that a major reason for noncompliance is that the importance of the drug therapy and the potential consequences if the medication was not used according to instructions have not been impressed upon the patient. Patients usually know relatively little about their diseases let alone the therapeutic benefits and problems that could result from drug therapy. Therefore, they establish their own ideas regarding their condition and their own objectives that they expect from the drug therapy. If the therapy does not meet these expectations they are more inclined to become noncompliant. Greater attention to educating the patient regarding his condition as well as the benefits and limitations of drug therapy will contribute to a more cooperative attitude on the part of the patient.

Poor Understanding of Instructions—Numerous investigations have described problems of this type. In one study (4) of approximately 6000 prescriptions, 4% were written with the designation for patient instructions being "as directed." In following up on 151 of these prescriptions it was found that in 36 cases the patients had received auxiliary written instructions from the prescriber. Of the other 115 prescriptions the patient gave the same instructions that the physician intended (as determined by contacting the physician) in 71 cases but in 44 cases the understanding of the directions on the part of the patient was different than that intended by the prescriber.

Even when directions to the patient are more specific than "as directed," confusion can still occur. In a study (5) of interpretation of prescription instructions it was shown that there were frequent errors of interpretation even when the instructions were not ambiguous. For example, in interpreting a prescription that read "tetracycline, 250 mg every 6 hours," only 36% of the 67 patients in the study indicated they would take the drug every 6 hours around the clock for a total of four doses each day. About 25% of the patients would not take a night-time dose since they divided the time that they were awake into three 6-hour periods.

These and other studies point out the confusion that may exist on the part of the patient even when instructions are seemingly clear. However, many prescriptions are written and labeled to indicate how many doses are to be taken each day with no additional clarification as to how the doses are to be scheduled. For example, how should instructions to take one tablet three times daily be interpreted? Does this mean every 8 hours, or with meals, or possibly some other schedule? If the drug is to be given with meals or at a specified time before or after meals, it is usually assumed that the patient eats three meals a day. Yet this is not always the case. Some drugs that are given several times a day include a bedtime dose. However, there can be a wide variation among patients in the time that this dose would be administered.

Multiple Drug Therapy—It is generally agreed that the greater the number of drugs the patient is taking the higher the risk of noncompliance. Even when rather specific dosage instructions for the medications are provided, problems can still occur. For example, many geriatric patients are taking five or six or more medications several times a day at different times. When one considers how often healthy young women have difficulty in taking oral contraceptives according to a simple dosage schedule using specially designed packages, it is easy to understand how the geriatric patient can become confused regarding his therapeutic regimen. In addition some geriatric patients may experience lapses of memory which make noncompliance even more likely.

Although combination drug products have a number of disadvantages and have received quite a bit of negative publicity in recent years, their use may help improve compliance with therapy since only one tablet need be administered rather than several. The issue of compliance provides one of the strongest arguments for the continued availability of combination products. However, in most cases, therapy should not be initiated with such products but rather with the individual agents so that optimal dosage levels can be determined.

Frequency of Administration—Just as the use of multiple drugs contributes to noncompliance so does the use of an individual drug at frequent intervals. This situation makes it more likely that the patient's normal routine or work schedule will have to be interrupted to take a dose of medication and in many cases the patient will forget, not want to be inconvenienced, or even be embarrassed to do so.

Many drugs must be given at frequent intervals to maintain the desired blood and tissue levels. However, some drugs which have traditionally been administered three or four times daily such as the tricyclic antidepressants and isoniazid have been found to produce just as good a respponse when administered once daily.

Duration of Therapy—Several studies have shown that the rate of noncompliance becomes greater when the treatment period is long. This is most likely to be true in the management of chronic conditions such as hypertension which are often not associated with significant symptomatology. Patients understandably tend to become discouraged with extended therapeutic programs that do not produce "cures" of the conditions.

Adverse Effects—The development of unpleasant effects of a drug is an obvious deterrent to patient compliance. In some situations it may be possible to change the dosage or use alternative drugs to minimize these problems. However, in other cases these alternatives may not exist and the benefits expected from therapy must be weighed against the risks. Particularly disconcerting are those situations in which the development of side effects makes the patient feel worse than he did before therapy was initiated. This is often the case in hypertensive patients.

Patients May Be Asymptomatic or Symptoms Subside—It is understandably difficult to convince a patient of the value of drug therapy when the patient had not experienced symptoms prior to the initiation of therapy. Such is the case in the treatment of hypertension and the lack of previous symptoms coupled with the lack of appearance of symptoms if therapy is discontinued contributes to the high rate of noncompliance in these patients.

Other situations in which the benefits of drug therapy are not directly apparent include those circumstances in which a drug is used on a prophylactic basis. Noncompliance is often seen in children for whom penicillin has been prescribed prophylactically to prevent the reoccurrence of rheumatic fever. Since the cooperation of the mother in giving penicillin to the child is often difficult to achieve, many physicians prefer to give monthly injections of penicillin G benzathine (*Bicillin*).

Fear of Becoming Drug Dependent—The increasing problems of drug abuse and addiction have increased the awareness and concern about becoming dependent on agents that are prescribed for legitimate medical reasons. Although drugs that carry a potential for abuse and the development of dependence are often prescribed and utilized too casually, patients often develop a fear of dependence regarding the use of *any* drug that is to be employed for a prolonged period. To avoid such a possibility or to prove to themselves that they are not dependent, they may stop the therapy or use it in smaller amounts.

Unpleasant Taste of Medication—Taste problems of medications are most commonly encountered with the use of oral liquids by children. Getting a child to take a dose of medication may be such a difficult task for a parent that noncompliance may result or the administration of the drug is discontinued as soon as the parent sees any sign of improvement. However, compliance problems relating to the taste of medication are not limited to children. Objections to the taste of liquid potassium chloride preparations have often been raised and a number of patients discontinue taking this medication because of this factor.

Illness—The nature of the patient's illness may also contribute to noncompliance. For example, the incidence of these problems may be expected to be higher in patients with psychiatric disorders who are often less cooperative than patients with other disorders.

Cost of Medication—Although noncompliance does frequently exist with the use of drugs that are relatively inexpensive, it might be anticipated that patients will be even more reluctant to comply with instructions for the use of more expensive agents.

The expense involved has been cited by some patients as the reason for not having the prescriptions filled at all whereas in other cases the medication is taken less frequently than intended or prematurely discontinued because of the cost. Antibiotics are among the higher priced drugs and it is understandable that some patients will discontinue taking the drug as soon as the symptoms subside so that they can save the balance of the medication for similar problems they may encounter in the future.

Measurement of Medication—Although a patient may fully intend to comply with instructions, he may inadvertently receive the wrong quantity of medication due to the incorrect measurement of medication or the use of inappropriate measuring devices. In one study (6) of the use of medications in pediatric patients it was found that in only one-third of 74 "teaspoons" measured was the capacity found to be within the 4.5–5.4-ml range. The importance of providing the patient with calibrated teaspoons or measuring cups for the use of oral liquids is evident.

Another situation in which the measurement of medication has presented problems is seen with the use of insulin. The confusion or misunderstanding that has resulted in the administration of incorrect doses of insulin is well recognized, although it is anticipated that the use of the U-100 insulins will minimize these problems.

Although not a complete listing of all the factors that result in noncompliance, those discussed give an indication of the complexity of trying to assure optimal drug therapy. Inherent in many of the factors considered is the matter of communication of the physician and pharmacist with the patient. This communication is in many cases not only incomplete and ineffective but the patient is often left with the impression that physicians and pharmacists are too busy or not interested in talking with him. Improving communications must be considered the key to increasing compliance and several approaches and recommendations are offered.

IMPROVING COMPLIANCE

In most situations both the physician and the pharmacist have the opportunity to talk with the patient about the drugs that have been prescribed and the effectiveness of this communication will be a major determinant of patient compliance. Not to be overlooked is the desirability of also having effective communication between the physician and the pharmacist so that their efforts in the patient's behalf are consistent and harmonious.

Although the physician's role in minimizing noncompliance should not be underestimated, the pharmacist has a particularly valuable opportunity to encourage compliance since his advice accompanies the actual dispensing of the medication and he is the last health professional to see the patient prior to the time the medication is to be used.

All patients should be viewed as potential noncompliers. However, a first step in efforts to improve compliance should be to recognize those individuals who are most likely to be noncompliant as judged by a consideration of the risk factors noted earlier.

These risk factors should also be taken into account in planning the patient's therapy so that the simplest regimen that is, to the extent possible, compatible with the patient's normal activities can be developed. Although developing the treatment plan has traditionally been the responsibility of physicians, pharmacists have become increasingly involved in this aspect of patient care.

When prescriptions are written the instructions should be as specific as possible. Instructions such as "as directed" or other directions that can easily be misinterpreted should be avoided. Even such seemingly specific instructions as "one tablet three times daily" are often misinterpreted as discussed previously. Where possible and with a recognition of the patient's normal routine, the specific times of day at which the patient is to take the medication should be indicated. In all cases the pharmacist should ascertain that the patient understands how to use the medication.

In discussing an illness or drug therapy with a patient, a distinction should be made between "information" and "education." Patients may receive information but not understand it and utilize it correctly whereas education implies understanding and behavioral change. Patients should be encouraged to participate in the discussion and where possible they should be brought in on the decision-making process. They should also be encouraged to ask questions and it would seem desirable for the pharmacist, after he has explained the directions for using a drug, to ask the patient if he has any questions as to how the drug is to be used.

The goal of communications with the patient is to provide information that the patient is able to understand and utilize. The approach should be one that will be reassuring to the patient and will not unnecessarily alarm him. With regard to the latter possibility, it is easy to anticipate that an over-enthusiastic discussion of adverse effects may make the patient afraid to use the drug. Thus, the provision of too much information or an inappropriate approach in presenting it could actually contribute to noncompliance rather than minimize it.

Communication between the pharmacist and patient regarding the use of medication can be both verbal and written. Although it may be supplemented and reinforced by written instructions, verbal communication is a very important aspect of patient education since it directly involves both the patient and the pharmacist in a two-way exchange and provides the opportunity for the patient to raise questions. For such communication to be most effective it should be conducted in a setting that provides privacy and is free of distractions. Although most pharmacies do not presently have a separate patient consultation area, this would seem to be a desirable goal. Not only will this reinforce to the patient the importance the pharmacist attaches to the information being discussed but it will also further strengthen the recognition of the pharmacist as one who is contributing to the patient's health care. Even in the absence of such a separate area, however, there must be an awareness of the need for a setting that is conducive to effective communication.

Medication is often obtained in a manner that does not lend itself to verbal communication. For example, the pharmacist may receive a telephoned prescription from a physician that is to be delivered to the patient's home or picked up at the pharmacy by a relative or friend. In these circumstances, when appropriate, the pharmacist might call the patient to discuss the use of the medication.

The emphasis on verbal communication should not be interpreted to indicate that written communication is not important. Although the patient may understand how the medication is to be used he may not remember the details relating to administration considered in the discussion with the pharmacist. Therefore, specific instructions for use should be placed on the prescription label. In addition it is often desirable to provide supplementary written instructions or other information pertaining to the patient's illness or drug therapy.

Verbal and written communication should be used to complement each other and both should be viewed as important components of the effort to educate the patient regarding his drug therapy.

The pharmacist's role in minimizing noncompliance does not end when the prescription is dispensed. If he becomes aware that the patient is not using the drug as intended he should endeavor to determine the reason and resolve any problem that may exist. The pharmacist is in an excellent position to detect noncompliance pertaining to the use of drugs used in the management of chronic conditions such as hypertension and diabetes by paying close attention to the frequency with which a patient gets his medication renewed.

If a pharmacist becomes aware that a patient has not had his medication renewed by the time that his supply should have been exhausted, he might contact the patient regarding it. Indeed it would seem desirable for pharmacists to develop systems whereby the renewal frequency for chronic medications could be quickly checked so that potential problems could be identified at an early point. When inconsistencies are noted and the matter pursued with the patient, it may be found that there is a valid reasson for the patient not renewing the prescription at the expected time. Nevertheless, the awareness of the patient that the pharmacist is paying attention to his therapy and has taken a personal interest in contacting him should not only contribute to compliance but also increase the respect of the patient for the pharmacist.

Situations in which drug usage would seem to be excessive, as evidenced by the patient desiring to renew his prescription more frequently than the directions would suggest, represent equally important problems that are easier to detect. Again the pharmacist should attempt to identify the reason for the inconsistency and any problem that may exist.

The manner in which medication is packaged may also have an influence on patient compliance. Specially designed packaging for oral contraceptives has been valuable in increasing patient understanding of how these agents are to be taken. Special packages of certain steroids to be used for a treatment period of 6 days (*Medrol Dosepak*) or in an alternate-day regimen (*Medrol ADT Pak, Aristo-Pak*) have been designed to facilitate the use of steroids in dosage regimens that may be difficult to understand or remember.

A possible negative effect of drug packaging on patient compliance is seen with the use of the child-resistant containers. Some patients, particularly the elderly and those with conditions like arthritis and parkinsonism, have difficulty in opening some of these containers and may not persist in their efforts to do so. Pharmacists should be alert to problems of this type and where appropriate, suggest the use of standard containers.

New dosage forms of certain drugs have also been developed in large part as a recognition of problems of noncompliance. The increasingly accepted practice of using tricyclic antidepressants in larger single evening doses to increase compliance and minimize certain adverse effects has led to the introduction of *Tofranil-PM*, a dosage form containing larger quantities of imipramine.

CONCLUSION

Considerable time, energy, and expense have often gone into the diagnosis of a patient's illnesses and the development of his treatment program. Yet the goals of therapy will not be reached unless the patient understands and follows the instructions for use of the drugs prescribed. One cannot also help but wonder how often patients have been categorized as treatment failures and have had their therapy changed, possibly to more potent and toxic agents, when the reason for the lack of response or an unanticipated altered response has been noncompliance.

Despite the increasing attention directed to the matter of noncompliance the problem is still not accorded the attention it deserves and it continues to be prevalent. Although the approaches taken and suggestions advanced in an effort to decrease noncompliance have met with varying success, they have significantly contributed to a recognition of the problem and provide a valuable base on which to develop modified or new approaches to the problem. Certain approaches that involve a significantly increased commitment of time on the part of physicians and pharmacists, may be viewed by some as impractical. Yet can this compare with the commitment of time and expense that is presently wasted as a result of noncompliance?

The pharmacist is the logical health professional to assume the major responsibility in minimizing noncompliance. Of priority importance is the need to strengthen communications with patients and physicians.

Many pharmacists are reluctant to accept and sometimes even resist opportunities to become more involved in advising patients or contributing to decisions regarding drug therapy because they do not feel adequately prepared. The desirability of pharmacists increasing their knowledge about disease states and the properties of drugs cannot be too strongly emphasized. However, there is no reason why every pharmacist cannot have at least some initial involvement in decreasing the problem of noncompliance even if it is limited to reviewing the directions with the patient or determining the frequency of renewal of chronic medications. The satisfaction that this contribution to patient care can bring will serve as a challenge to further increase one's knowledge and professional involvement.

The problem has been identified and is receiving increasing attention. Patients for too long have been deprived of a close attention to and monitoring of their drug therapy. This observer cannot accept the excuse that pharmacists are too busy to advise patients regarding their drug therapy. If pharmacists do not assume the responsibility for decreasing noncompliance, someone else will. The profession cannot afford to default on this valuable opportunity to enhance its contribution to patient care.

REFERENCES

1. The Dichter Institute for Motivational Research, Inc.: Communicating the Value of Comprehensive Pharmaceutical Services to the Consumer, American Pharmaceutical Association, Washington, D.C., 1973.
2. Weintraub M, Au WYW, Lasagna L. Compliance as a determinant of serum digoxin concentration. J Am Med Assoc 1973;224:481.
3. Porter AMW. Drug defaulting in a general practice. Brit Med J 1969;1:218.
4. Powell JR, Cali TJ, Linkewich JA. Inadequately written prescriptions. J Am Med Assoc 1973;226:999.
5. Mazzullo JM III, Lasagna L, Griner PF. Variations in interpretation of prescription instructions. J Am Med Assoc 1974;227:929.
6. Arnhold RG, Adebonjo FO, Callas ER, Callas J, Carte E, Stein RC. Patients and prescriptions. Clin Pediatr 1970;9:648.

MEDICAL COMPLIANCE AND THE CLINICIAN-PATIENT RELATIONSHIP: A REVIEW[c]

Thomas F. Garrity

INTRODUCTION

Reviews of the literature on medical compliance (1, 2) suggest that correlates of compliance fall into categories such as patient characteristics (e.g. demographic, cognitive), regimen characteristics (e.g. duration, complexity, intrusiveness), characteristics of the clinical setting (e.g. waiting time, continuity of care) and characteristics of the clinician-patient interaction (e.g. emphasis on teaching, interpersonal warmth). Studies of clinician-patient interaction, the focus of this review, are not very numerous in the literature. One reason for this may be the persistent assumption that nonadherence is a problem rooted in the *patient's failure* to carry out physician recommendations. From this perspective, the task of the investigator is to uncover reasons for this failure, usually sought in the patient's knowledge, attitudes and behavior and their mesh with his social and material environments. The clinician-patient interaction, on the other hand, is simply the context within which the recommendations are conferred, a process infrequently viewed as problematic in itself.

A second reason for neglect of studies of clinician-patient interaction is no doubt the difficulty in monitoring what happens during this encounter. First, the encounter is traditionally surrounded by the ethical veil of privacy and confidentiality not lightly breached by researchers. Second, as physicians tend to be gatekeepers of research in the clinical setting, study of physician performance risks the loss of their sponsorship for this and less threatening sorts of clinical-behavioral research. Finally, *in vivo* measurement of characteristics of the interaction process has always presented a supreme challenge to behavioral science because of its complexity and dynamism.

---

[c]Edited and reprinted with permission from Garrity TF. Medical compliance and the clinician-patient relationship: a review. Soc Sci Med 1981;15E:215-222.

In spite of these difficulties, there is now a modest number of studies of compliance and clinician–patient interaction. They are predominantly descriptive and correlational in design, though a few recent intervention studies can be identified. In the following pages the literature extending back to the early 1960's has been brought together and discussed under 4 headings. First are studies that deal with the clinician–patient interaction as a pedagogical encounter in which the clinician employs various approaches aimed at conveying clearly the specifics of the recommended regimen. This cluster of studies views the very act of conveying information as a process fraught with impediments to the patient's learning what is expected of him. Second, studies dealing with the sorts of expectations brought to the medical encounter by patient and provider are presented. This literature views compatibility of clinician and patient expectations as crucial for patient follow-through on medical advice. Third, we discuss studies that measure the balance and sharing of responsibility between clinician and patient, and attempt to examine associations between greater patient activeness and adherence. Fourth, research dealing with the affective tone of the clinician–patient interaction is summarized. While such a classification model is inevitably somewhat arbitrary, it is hoped that it will help to bring some greater order to the compliance literature on clinician–patient interaction.

A CLASSIFICATION MODEL

Pedagogical Technique

A great part of compliance research makes the assumption that patients receive medical recommendations clearly and unequivocally from their health care agents, usually the physicians. From this perspective failure to act in the recommended fashion is primarily a problem in the patient or his environment. Recently a few authors have begun to question the assumption that recommendations are clearly communicated to and grasped by patients. In general, these authors have examined the physician's communicative behavior as well as the patient's characteristics and attempts to follow through with perceived medical advice.

Ley and coworkers have been active since the mid-1960's studying the links between the comprehensibility of the physician's medical recommendations and the compliance of patients. These researchers have argued that appropriate patient follow-through is not logically possible in the absence of clear and understandable advice.

In a second study, of different design, Ley and coworkers (3) also found a comprehensibility–compliance association. The 4 physicians of a British family practice studied the recommendations of the researcher on ways to increase the clarify of communication. This written material advised the physicians to (1) give medical advice early in the interview, (2) emphasize its importance, (3) employ simple sentences, (4) arrange advice in categories, (5) use repetition and (6) give specific advice. Evidence emerged that this intervention did improve patient recall of physician advice although it did not improve comprehension or compliance. On the other hand, patient comprehension was correlated both before and after the intervention with level of compliance.

Just as patient *understanding* of medical recommendations is often limited and limiting of compliance, the same appears true of *recall* of advice. Ley listed several determinants of poor recall; they include large numbers of statements presented to the patient, high anxiety of the patient, low medical knowledge of the patient, but not age or 'intellectual level' of the patient (4, 5).

Caution, however, needs to be exercised in inferring from the data *causal* links between explicit instruction and good compliance. Most studies that demonstrate associations between these two factors fail to control simultaneously for possibly correlated factors such as the increased interest shown by practitioner, increased satisfaction with and liking of the clinician and the like. Such variables as these may not only operate to produce spurious correlations between practitioner instruction and adherence, but also to mediate between the two. So, although the precise causal order linking instruction and adherence cannot now be deduced from the literature, it seems clear that attempts to develop causal models of these relationships must include practitioner instructional effectiveness.

Mutuality of Expectations

Symbolic interactionism, a sociologically-oriented school of thought within social psychology, provides a framework for understanding interpersonal behavior (26). This perspective suggests that people bringing noncomplementary expectations to the interpersonal encounter are likely to experience conflict. For example, if the patient expects the clinician to spend time answering questions but the clinician neither expects nor does this, then some discord, even if unexpressed, is likely. This discord may result in open quarreling, feelings of dissatisfaction and failure to follow through on the practitioner's advice.

An early example of this research perspective is given by Overall and Aronson (6) in the context of the university outpatient psychiatry clinic. Questions tapping patient expectations of the therapist's activeness (e.g. therapist will instruct patient), medical orientation (e.g. therapist will be interested in physical–organic problems), supportiveness (therapist will avoid discomforting or 'charged' issues), and others were asked before the first doctor–patient encounter. Afterward, the patients were asked corresponding questions about the extent to which expectation had been fulfilled. (Therapist reports generally supported the accuracy of patient reports.) It was found that patients with unfulfilled expectations were significantly less likely to return for the next scheduled appointment. Others have reported similar associations between expectations regarding conduct or results of psychotherapy and dropping out of therapy (7, 8).

Strategies for increasing compliance derived specifically from the expectation literature just described have not yet been tested. Although this aspect of the clinician–patient interaction literature is not extensive in numbers of studies, the findings are consistent complementary expectations regularly yield patient satisfaction and following of advice. Intervention trials now seem warranted. The specifics of such strategies might vary widely though all variations would attempt to bring therapist and patient expectation into closer agreement. The process might attempt to prepare new patients for the relatively rigid expectations of the medical institution through use of media or direct communication with the therapist. In more flexible medical care settings, therapist behavior might be able to be tailored more closely to reasonable patient expectations.

Raising Patient Responsibility

In their classic paper on the doctor–patient relationship, Szasz and Hollender (9) described the types of relationship that varied in the relative responsibility of each person in this dyad. The 'activity–passivity' model is characterized by physician taking complete responsibility for care of the patient. In this type there is an extreme imbalance of power between doctor and patient, with the initiative and control totally in the doctor's hands. Although this model is seen in doctor–patient encounters in a variety of settings and with various types of presenting problems, it is most clearly appropriate when the patient is incapable of response, as in trauma, coma and the like. The 'guidance–cooperation' model is characterized by physician giving advice that the patient is expected to obey. This configuration of responsibility is the traditional one in our society and the one that comes closest to Parsons' description of the normative 'sick role' (10). It is also the notion of doctor–patient relating to which the word 'compliance', with all of its connotations of patient subservience, seems traceable. Szasz and Hollender see this model most appropriately implemented in situations such as presentation of acute infection in which the physician diagnoses and prescribes short-term therapy making only modest demands on patient responsibility. In the 'mutual participation' model the parties share equally in the responsibility of patient care. Implementation of this approach is most clearly appropriate in chronic disease problems such as diabetes in which the physician must depend on the patient for information needed to adjust therapy and for long-term follow-through for health maintenance.

Affective Tone of the Interaction

A fourth and final aspect of interpersonal relating to be taken up in this review concerns the affective tone of the clinician–patient encounter. In this category we will be dealing with an aspect of clinician–patient relating similar, perhaps identical, to what others call social support (11–14). In its broad sense, social support refers to material, intellectual and emotional resources people find through the agency of others. Other people may offer goods and services useful in dealing with challenge. They may also offer information for meeting the challenge. Finally, they may offer a measure of sympathy, understanding and encouragement. All of them have been discussed in the literature as aspects of social support (15). For the purpose of the present discussion, 'emotional support' between therapist and patient comes closest to capturing the essence of this correlate of compliance.

Once again the work of Svarstad (16) makes an important contribution. She developed an index of physician approachability. The physician's index is raised if he solicits patient questions, does not 'clockwatch' and does not mumble or cut patients off in response to their questions. Further, the physician who greets the patient, responds to his first question, smiles or laughs with the patient and bids farewell to the patient on closing the interaction is given points that raise the approachability index. Finally, when the physician makes an unexpected departure from the interaction, what Svarstad terms a 'quick getaway', a deduction from the approachability index is made. These characteristics of the doctor's interpersonal behavior, it will be recalled, were measured by direct observation of the interaction. The investigator found that there was considerable variation in the approachability of the 8 physicians in the study.

This measure of approachability, an amalgamation of signs of friendliness, interest and respect for the patient, was found directly associated with level of patient compliance. Approachability, in turn, was associated with amount of patient questioning of the physician. Svarstad's analysis led her to suggest that the physician's cues signal the patient about the doctor's willingness to deal with questions. It may be that the increased give-and-take facilitates patient learning of doctor's advice and rationale for mode of treatment, thus helping to account for improved compliance. Evidence was also presented that approachability responds to situational pressures on the doctor, such that doctors under pressure are less approachable.

CONCLUSION

As future work is contemplated on compliance and clinician–patient relationships at least two cautionary comments are needed. First, the 'clinician' to whom we have most often referred was the physician, though occasionally nurses and health educators were the subjects of study. The foregoing discussions did not emphasize that differences may exist as clinicians of differing professional status and responsibility interact with patients. On the contrary, we have generally made statements that imply generalizability across professions. Nonetheless such an assumption will need examination in future research. Second, the research reports presented in this review described patients with a variety of illnesses. Again, we have not emphasized the variations that may exist as clinicians try to induce maximum compliance in patients with different diseases. Instead, we have made statements that imply similarity of compliance issues across diseases. But here too the need for empirical testing of this position is needed. It seems clear, for example, that illnesses requiring more complex and enduring therapeutic regimens present greater adherence challenges (1, 2). Is it not also possible that techniques based in clinician–patient relation may have sundry results depending on illness type and regimen characteristics?

This review has presented evidence that several sorts of interventions in the context of clinician–patient interaction bring benefits for both behavioral compliance and clinical outcomes. The evidence seems to justify continued, carefully evaluated interventions in the clinician–patient relationship aimed at improving compliance. At the same time there is still the need to learn more about the specific elements that make these strategies work. This 2-fold approach to future work permits immediate dissemination and application of apparently useful compliance-boosting strategies as well as studies of basic mechanisms and the conditions that influence their operation.

REFERENCES

1. Dunbar J, Stunkard A. Adherence to diet and drug regimen. In Nutrition, Lipids and Coronary Heart Disease (Edited by Levy R, et al.). Raven, New York, 1979.
2. Becker M, Maiman L. Sociobehavioral determinants of compliance with health and medical care recommendations. Med Care 1975;13:10.
3. Ley P, et al. Improving doctor–patient communication in general practice. Jl R Coll Gen Pract 1976;26:720.
4. Ley P. Psychological studies of doctor–patient communication. In Contributions to Medical Psychology (Edited by Rachman S). Pergamon, Oxford, 1977.
5. Ley P, Spelman M. Communicating with Patient. Staples, London, 1967.
6. Overall B, Aronson H. Expectations of psychotherapy in patients of lower socioeconomic class. Am J Orthopsychiat 1963;33:421.
7. Caine T, Wijesinghe B. Personality, expectancies and group psychotherapy. Br J Psychiat 1976;129:384.
8. Farley O, Peterson K, Spanos G. Self-termination from a child guidance center. Commun Ment Hlth J 1975;11:325.
9. Szasz T, Hollender M. A contribution to the philosophy of medicine: the basic models of the doctor–patient relationship. Archs Intern Med 1956;97:585.
10. Parson T. The Social System, Chap. 10, Free Press, Glencoe, IL, 1951.
11. Kaplan B, Cassel J, Gore S. Social support and health. Med Care 1977;15:47.
12. Pattison E, Llamas R, Hurd G. Social network mediation of anxiety. Psychiat. Ann 1979;9:474.
13. Dimsdale J, et al. The role of social supports in medical care, Soc Psychiat 1979;14:75.
14. Andrews G, et al. Life event stress, social support coping style, and risk of psychological impairment. Nerv Ment Dis 1978;166:307.
15. Caplan R, et al. Adhering to Medical Regimens. Institute for Social Research, Ann Arbor, 1976.
16. Svarstad B. The doctor–patient encounter: an observational study of communication and outcome. Doctoral dissertation, University of Wisconsin, 1974.

7
Sociology of Drugs in Health Care

BONNIE L. SVARSTAD

Although social scientists have done a considerable amount of research on the nonmedical use and abuse of psychoactive drugs (1-4), it is only recently that they have begun to seriously study the full range of social and behavioral issues surrounding the development and utilization of drug technology in the health care context. Thus, our understanding of and ability to resolve drug-related problems is still very limited, as implied in chapter 1. The purposes of this chapter then are to discuss the need for theory and research in this area, to outline some of the differences in the orientation of social scientists and researchers in other pharmaceutical fields, and to provide an overview of some of the sociological and social psychological frameworks that can be used to broaden and improve our understanding of drug processes. The theme is that many drugs are prescribed and taken in a less than optimal manner and that previous attempts to prevent and reduce these problems have been only partially successful. Therefore we need to develop a better understanding of how practitioners and patients view drugs and their roles in the drug use process, why practitioners and patients do not always use drugs in an appropriate manner, and what specific steps can be taken to stimulate and maintain optimal drug practices.

NEED FOR SOCIAL SCIENTIFIC THEORY AND RESEARCH

Why do we need more social scientific theory and research when we could rely on "common sense" and/or other practical approaches to the prevention or resolution of drug use problems? This is a reasonable question. After all, social scientific research requires considerable training, financial support, cooperation, and time. And we know that many health professionals lack time and are under considerable pressure to generate quick, simple, and inexpensive solutions to drug use problems.

Given these considerations, it is not surprising that health professionals have traditionally ignored social scientific approaches and simply relied on their common sense and a trial and error approach. For example, many health professionals have conducted patient compliance studies in the past 5-10 years. Instead of studying *why* patients behave as they do, they simply tested or tried a given technique or set of techniques in which they were interested. Sometimes the technique was based on sound behavioral science principles and in other cases it was not.

If the first technique failed, then a second technique was tried. This trial and error process continued until the researchers found an acceptable solution or reached the bottom of their list of techniques. Although this approach has yielded some useful and interesting results, health professionals have shown increased interest in the social sciences in the past few years. There are three major reasons for this increased interest.

1. The need for a systems approach. Early efforts to improve the quality of drug use were focused almost entirely on patients and their presumed "failure" to comply with medical advice. But it now appears that patient compliance is associated with the ways in which physicians and pharmacists relate to their patients. How should physicians and pharmacists be trained for these roles and what are the factors that will facilitate or inhibit the building of better relationships and communication among physicians, pharmacists, and patients?

   We need a better understanding of the processes that are required to stimulate and maintain adherence to long-term drug regimens as well as the processes that precede and follow drug use. Indeed it appears that there are unresolved problems from the time a drug is developed and tested to the time that it is consumed and evaluated. Studies still show that about 50% of all patients do not follow their drug regimen and that this noncompliance is linked to poorer treatment outcomes, a larger number of physician visits, and a higher rate of hospitalization or admission to a nursing home (5–7). Recent surveys have demonstrated that elderly patients still do not receive basic information from their physician and pharmacist and, as a result, experience a wide variety of other medication-related problems that are preventable (8, 9).

   Other problems include: the extensive use of vitamins and other dietary supplements that may not be necessary (10); the less than optimal prescribing of non-narcotic analgesics, antibiotics, and vasodilators (11, 12); the prescribing of heavily promoted and costly drugs instead of less expensive but equally effective drugs (12, 13); the underprescribing of narcotic analgesics for severe cancer pain (14, 15); the potentially excessive use of psychotropic medications in nursing homes (16); and numerous other problems related to the prescribing and administration of drugs in geriatric long-term care facilities (17). Analyses of the pharmaceutical industry have also revealed questionable marketing practices and instances of bribery and fraud in the testing of drugs (18–22).

2. The failure of previous efforts to change behavior. Perhaps the main reason for the increased interest in social science theory is that previous efforts to change patient and professional behavior have been only partially successful, perhaps because the trial and error approach ignores the complex steps that are involved in stimulating and maintaining behavioral change (23, 24).

   This is not to say that previous work has not yielded any effective methods, because it has. On the other hand, we need a better understanding of many things. The use of written information sheets leads to higher patient compliance with short-term drug regimens but has no effect on compliance with long-term drug regimens (25). We also know that compliance can be improved through the use of medication containers and compliance aids, blood pressure monitoring techniques, and other compliance-gaining strategies, but sometimes these efforts fail (26). Why is that?

   Recent efforts to influence the behavior of health professionals also have yielded somewhat mixed results. Controlled studies have shown that an educational visit by a clinical pharmacist or another physician can significantly improve physician prescribing of antibiotics, nonnarcotic analgesics, vasodilators, and diazepam (12, 27). But this method failed to improve the prescribing of antipsychotic medications in nursing homes (28). Why is that? Does the physician really determine the level and quality of psychotropic drug use in the nursing home? Or does the nurse play a more important role than previously assumed?

Other investigators have been disappointed to learn that physicians and nurses do not always respond to pharmacists' recommendations, governmental warnings and regulations, computerized feedback, and other cost-containment and quality assurance methods (13, 29–31). But why is that? And why is it that generic substitution laws and other regulatory and educational efforts aimed at pharmacists have also failed to produce the desired results, even though there is impressive evidence that pharmacists can have a substantial impact if they decide to assume new responsibilities (32–37)?

3. Unexplained variations in drug use. We also need a blueprint for understanding or interpreting cultural or historic variations in drug use, variations from one health care setting to another, and differences among practitioners and consumers. It is known that there are wide variations in the use of psychotropics from one hospital to another (38), that the level of psychotropic prescribing varies widely from one nursing home to another (16), and that medication administration errors also vary from one long-term care facility to another (39). But we do not know why. It should be possible to sort out and systematically test alternative hypotheses based on sociological and social psychological theories about behavior under different environmental conditions.

SOCIAL SCIENTIFIC AND BIOPHARMACEUTICAL ORIENTATIONS: A COMPARISON

Like research in the other pharmaceutical fields, social scientific work on drugs can encompass at least four general subjects: (a) the definition and classification of drugs; (b) the dynamics of various drug processes; (c) the factors affecting drug response; and (d) the evaluation of drugs and their effects. When analyzing and classifying drugs, the specialists in the biopharmaceutical sciences emphasize the chemical structure, solubility, stability, potency, pharmacologic action, and other physical or pharmacologic features of a drug (see Table 7.1). In contrast, social scientists emphasize the importance of the social and cultural meanings and functions served by drug giving and taking. Their assumption is that prescribers, patients, and others are influenced by scientific facts and the inherent features of a drug as well as the social and cultural meanings and labels that have been assigned to the drug. Thus it is very important to determine how patients, professionals, and others perceive and evaluate the drug.

Basic pharmaceutical scientists focus their attention on the drug and the animal or human ingesting the drug, whereas social scientists take a broader approach, which explicitly considers the larger systems in which drugs are developed and used. In particular, social scientists have been interested in the social issues surrounding the development and testing of drugs, issues regarding drug marketing and promotion, the diffusion of drug innovations, the impact of drug policies and regulation, the dynamics of clinical decision making (including physician, pharmacist, and nurse decision making), the dynamics of prescription and nonprescription drug use, and drug information and communication processes.

Unlike physical or biologically oriented scientists who focus on the physical, chemical, or biopharmaceutic factors affecting drug response, social scientists focus on the social,

Table 7.1.   Study of Drugs: An Overview of the Biopharmaceutical and Social Scientific Orientations

Subject	Biopharmaceutical Orientation	Social Scientific Orientation
Definition/classification of drugs	Physical, chemical, and/or pharmacologic properties (e.g., chemical structure, pharmacologic action, solubility, stability, potency)	Social and cultural meanings and functions (e.g., how individuals and society view the drug and its use, the social and psychological functions of prescribing and use)
Drug research, development, commercialization, regulation, and use	How drugs are isolated, purified, synthesized, absorbed, metabolized, excreted, etc.	Social issues regarding drug marketing, control, prescribing, dispensing, drug-taking monitoring, etc.
Factors affecting drug response	Physical, chemical, or biopharmaceutic factors (e.g., product variability, age, size, and metabolic status of user)	Social, cultural, and social psychological factors (e.g., what consumer expects, the social context in which drugs are given and taken)
Evaluation of drugs and their effects	Physiological effects (e.g., therapeutic effects, adverse drug reactions)	Social, cultural, and social psychological effect (e.g., how drug use affects self-concept, motivation, stigma, quality of life, satisfaction with care)

cultural, and social psychological factors that might influence the response to drug therapy. These factors can include the physician's and patient's expectations regarding drug efficacy and toxicity, the social context in which the drug is given or taken, and other factors.

Social scientists also take a somewhat broader view of drug effects. In contrast to basic pharmaceutical scientists who focus on the physiological effects of drugs, social scientists emphasize the importance of including the social, cultural, and psychological consequences of drug use. They have suggested, for example, that drug use can influence the person's self-concept, feelings of control and competence, motivation, stigma, quality of life, and satisfaction with care.

OVERVIEW OF SOCIAL SCIENTIFIC PERSPECTIVES USED TO EXPLAIN DRUG PROCESSES

There are many potentially relevant perspectives within the social sciences. As a result, I will only briefly describe and illustrate some of the general theoretical perspectives that have been used to explain drug processes and that seem relevant at this stage. These perspectives, along with specific examples from the literature, are listed in Table 7.2. Because each of the perspectives has been critically reviewed elsewhere, the review will not be a critical one. Rather, I will briefly introduce each perspective and illustrate how it can be used to gain

Table 7.2. Studies Using Social Scientific Theories to Explain Drug Process

Type of Theory	Level of Decision Making and Behavior [a]			
	Patients/ Consumers	Health Workers	Drug Industry	Government/ Others
Cultural/subcultural	40–49	50, 51		
Functional	54, 55	56–58		
Symbolic interaction	64, 65	64, 65		
Social learning	66, 67			
Cognitive	72–79	80–83		
Social influence, exchange, and power	75, 76, 87, 88	58, 89, 90		
Stress, social support, and coping	10, 48, 92–95			
Diffusion of innovation		96		
Roles and social organization		16, 99–104		
Theories of deviance and crime	2–4	51	21, 51	21, 51

[a]Numbers refer to references listed at the end of the chapter.

insights into various drug processes. Each perspective provides a slightly different perspective on drug use, thereby making a unique contribution. How adequate a theory is depends on the question that is being addressed, among other things.

Cultural/Subcultural Perspective

This perspective can provide insight into various cultural, subcultural, or historic variations. It has been used to understand the ways in which popular medical and pharmaceutical concepts impact on the use of Western drugs in developing and developed countries (40–46), ethnic and gender differences in the use of pain relievers and tranquilizers (47, 48), how psychiatric patients view their medications and the stigma that occurs as a result of using these medications (49), the ways in which physicians view drugs (50, 51), and other social and cultural consequences of drug use (52, 53). According to this perspective, drugs and drug behaviors have cultural and symbolic meanings that are learned or passed on as part of social and cultural traditions, values, roles, and belief systems. These conceptions can then influence both professionals and patients during any stage of the drug use process, including the perceived need for a drug, how the person presents his/her complaints or requests for medication to the practitioner, drug preferences, what regimen is preferred, patterns of use, perceptions of drug efficacy and safety, and the social consequences of drug use.

Functionalist Perspective

Sociologists, anthropologists, and psychologists have advanced a variety of theories that basically suggest that certain behaviors (including deviant behaviors) serve important, *la-*

tent functions for society and individuals in society. According to this perspective, drug giving and taking can serve diverse medical and nonmedical functions, some of which are latent or unrecognized (54). The functions that are actually served by drugs may or may not be consistent with the "intended" or "approved" functions and may vary over time. In other words, drug taking can serve diverse therapeutic functions as well as a means of coping with personal failure or stress, gaining pleasure and relaxation, improving work performance, and other functions listed in Table 7.3. Likewise, drug prescribing can serve therapeutic functions as well as a means of gaining status or income (status-conferring function), satisfying the patient (placebo function), managing clinical uncertainty (diagnostic-research function), and controlling or avoiding difficult patients (social control function).

These concepts can be useful in understanding how some patients may view drug compliance and noncompliance. As illustrated in the reading by Conrad (55), patient *noncompliance* may serve an important function for epileptic patients who view noncompliance as a means of exercising some control over their disorder or life. In other words, noncompliance serves a "self-regulatory function." Other interesting examples have been suggested by researchers who have studied physician prescribing. They suggest that writing a prescription may be considered a means of managing clinical uncertainties or ambiguities and satisfying the patient (56–59). In fact, several British authorities have suggested that certain vitamin preparations are prescribed so frequently that they can be considered the "modern placebo" (59).

Although there has not yet been a systematic study of the different functions that might be served by the prescribing of psychotropic drugs in nursing homes, there is anecdotal evidence suggesting that overworked and undertrained nursing staff administer these drugs

Table 7.3. Human Motives and the Functions of Drugs

Motive	Function
Prevent, treat, and cure disease; relieve pain and discomfort	Therapeutic function
Relieve feelings of personal failure, grief, stress, fear, loneliness, sadness, or inferiority	Coping function
Relax and enjoy the company of others; experience pleasurable sensations, satisfy curiosity	Recreational function
Improve academic, athletic, or work performance	Instrumental function
Beautify the skin, hair, or body image	Cosmetic function
Seek religious meaning or experience	Religious function
Allay hunger or control the desire for food	Appetitive function
Control fertility	Fertility function
Exercise control over disorder or life	Self-regulatory function
Gain social status, prestige, income	Status-conferring function
Satisfy the patient or show concern	Placebo function
Help make diagnosis; manage uncertainty; gain knowledge	Diagnostic research function
Control the behavior of disruptive or problem patients; avoid contact with problem patients; terminate visit	Social control function

for the purposes of controlling noisy or disruptive residents (60). This would be consistent with survey data, which show that nurses are more likely to administer tranquilizers to residents whom they consider to be "unfriendly" (61). Others have indicated that prescriptions serve as objects of negotiation between doctors and patients (62, 63).

Symbolic Interaction Perspective

The symbolic interaction framework emphasizes the importance of analyzing objects and events from the *actor's perspective*. Proponents of this approach suggest that people actively search for and assign meaning to things and that these meanings develop through social interaction and have important implications for a person's self-concept and behavior (64). People make an active effort to manipulate these meanings in an effort to present themselves in a manner that allows them to retain their self-esteem. In other words, people actively engage in "impression management."

According to this perspective, drug use can be considered a "symbolic action" that has implications for the patient's self-concept and behavior. This perspective is perhaps most useful in helping us to better understand why patients *underreport* or *overreport* certain symptoms and why they *underestimate* or *overestimate* their compliance with the drug regimen. According to this perspective, patients will make an active effort to present themselves as "good patients" who are not "complainers" or people who take too much or too little medication. Given the difficulties associated with evaluating pain and the pain relievers, it is perhaps understandable that the researchers using this perspective both examined staff–patient interaction surrounding chronic pain and its management (62, 65). One of the patients in these studies described a bad experience with his physician. After explaining why he felt it was necessary to "con" the doctor, the patient told the interviewer:

> First of all, you never tell a doctor that it hurts only some of the time. If you do, he'll think that your problem is not all that bad. . . . Always tell the doctor that you are using less drugs than you actually do, just to make sure he doesn't think you're just a "popper" looking for a prescription. Act real cheerful in the office. Let them know that you're handling the pain OK. . . . It really seems like they look for any little excuse to send you to a shrink (Ref. 64, p. 77).

Social Learning Perspective

This perspective encompasses a variety of theories that focus on the rewards, punishments, and environmental stimuli or cues that are presumably required in order for learning and behavioral change to occur (66, 67). According to this approach, drug use is more likely to occur if there are strong cues to use the drug and if taking the drug brings only obvious and immediate rewards (relief, praise, etc.). Medication that is associated with few obvious rewards and many bothersome side effects would yield the opposite result. Recent reviews of this approach suggest that it is not as predictive as other theories of patient compliance, thereby limiting its potential usefulness to practitioners. However, we present it here for the sake of completeness and because it provides at least one key insight that has been successfully applied in a variety of patient education programs. The key point is that patients will be better able to remember their medications if they develop a system for "cuing" or reminding them to take the medicine at specific times throughout the day (26).

Cognitive Perspective

This perspective also encompasses a wide variety of theories that deal with different aspects of information processing, decision making, risk taking, and other processes of relevance to our understanding of various drug processes (68–83). According to this perspective, professionals and patients are both viewed as rational decision makers. The important concepts include information processing, internal representations (schema) of illness and treatment, rational decision making through an assessment of benefits and risks, beliefs, intentions, and attitudes. Because there are so many theoretical frameworks that fit under this rubric, it might be helpful to identify what I believe are the unique contributions of this perspective.

1. Communication is a process involving multiple steps. One of the most important insights provided by this perspective is that effective communication requires multiple steps, including exposure to a message, attention to the message, comprehension of the message, agreement with the recommendation (attitude change), recall of the recommendation, and behavioral action (70, 71). Unfortunately, many practitioners and policy makers fail to address one or more of these necessary steps when designing their educational or drug information materials. The result is that some programs are successful in achieving the cognitive outcomes (attention, comprehension, and recall) but fail to achieve the necessary affective and behavioral outcomes (attitude change and behavior). Other programs succeed in changing the patient's attitude but neglect the cognitive side of the equation.

2. Patients (and providers) have multiple sources of information. Another point that is often overlooked is that patients (and providers) have multiple sources of information that they utilize when making their decisions about illness and treatment (72). The main sources of information are threefold: communication with health professionals and others, personal experience with the illness and treatment (drug), and other information obtained through the larger culture and health care system. Although most people now agree that communication with health professionals is perhaps the most important of the three sources of information, the work by Leventhal and his colleagues (72) indicates that health professionals must begin to devote more attention to patients' personal experiences with their illnesses and treatment because patients develop their own common sense theories and become actively involved in monitoring their bodily sensations.

3. Health professionals will be more successful in achieving the specified cognitive outcomes if they adhere to several basic principles derived from cognitive theory and subsequently confirmed in compliance studies (70, 71, 73–76). The key principles for maximizing the various cognitive outcomes include 10 practical techniques that can and have been used by pharmacists and other health professionals. They are listed below:

Principles for Gaining Attention/Comprehension/Recall

- Provide explicit oral directions about how to take the drug.
- Orally explain the purpose and importance of the drug.
- Provide written or visual reinforcement of directions/purpose.
- Provide special compliance aids (if appropriate).
- Repeat key points.
- Simplify the regimen as much as possible.
- Make sure that consistent advice is given.
- Solicit and respond positively to patient feedback.

- Use a credible/trustworthy source of information.
- Use multiple techniques and channels.

4. Another set of principles relates to the effects of certain beliefs, expectancies about treatment, and normative influences. These concepts can be found in three theories: the Health Belief Model, Fishbein's theory of reasoned action, and Vroom's expectancy–value theory (77, 80–83). These theories suggest that drug giving and taking are rational actions that are influenced by one's beliefs, values, and normative influences. If the patient or prescriber has positive beliefs, values, and normative influences that are positively disposed toward the drug, then we would expect a high intention to comply or use the drug.

   The Health Belief Model suggests patients will not take a recommended health action (such as a prescribed medication) unless they believe that they are susceptible to the disease being treated, the disease is a serious one, the benefits of the recommended action will outweigh the costs, and there is a cue to action (77). Fishbein's theory of reasoned action includes some of the same elements in the sense that it stresses the person's positive beliefs and attitudes about the treatment. However, it adds another important element—the extent to which the actor's normative influences are positive (e.g., the patient's physician, family, and friends are positively disposed toward the drug). Other models that have been used in explaining the drug use process include Vroom's valence and force propositions (81, 82).

   Although certain aspects of the Health Belief Model have been heavily criticized in recent years (7), its straightforward emphasis on the patient's assessment of treatment benefits and costs (including social and psychological costs) remains a unique and important contribution to our understanding of patient drug-taking behavior. It is doubtful that any practitioner can effectively communicate with patients *without* close attention to and discussion of these aspects of the treatment process.

   There have been several attempts to predict physician-prescribing behavior through the use of theories that emphasize expectancy, and they all have been quite successful, suggesting that the physicians' beliefs need to be examined further (80–83). Because there have not yet been any experimental studies to determine whether it is possible to improve the quality of prescribing using these theories of decision making, it is too early to determine the potential contribution of such theories to our understanding and improvement of prescribing.

5. The cognitive perspective can also provide insight into the patient's evaluation of bodily symptoms and drug effects, including the "placebo effect" (78, 79). This should become a more important area for work as researchers from various disciplines begin to explore new ways of evaluating the outcomes of drug therapy, including measurement of "quality of life."

   In summary, the cognitive perspective can offer a variety of insights into the ways in which patients and providers process information and make decisions. Specific patient principles have been identified and could be applied in practice. Finally, it is of interest to note that many of the principles found to be effective in improving patient compliance seem to be the same ones that appear to be useful in the improvement of physician prescribing. For example, controlled trials of prescribing have recently shown that better results are obtained when there is face-to-face communication with written reinforcement (12, 27) and when there is a second follow-up visit to reinforce earlier advice and resolve any problems (84).

Social Influence, Exchange, and Power

Theories in this group take a different approach in that they focus on the dynamics and outcome of the professional–patient relationship (75, 76, 85). They are interested in determining how physicians use their authority and power, whether they share their expertise and information, and the effects of different styles of decision making. A specific hypothesis is that health professionals will have a more positive influence on their patients if they adopt a "participatory approach" as opposed to an "authoritarian approach" when counseling their patients. This participatory approach involves the use of five interpersonal strategies that can be applied by health professionals in various settings:

Participatory Strategies for Influencing Patients

- Provide positive rationale and reinforcement.
- Provide positive expectations and direction.
- Show positive affect/interest in patient.
- Seek feedback and check compliance at next visit.
- Help patient resolve barriers to compliance.

There have been only a few studies examining the nature and outcome of professional–patient interactions, but they tend to support the notion that patient satisfaction and compliance will be higher if the physician or pharmacist establishes a warm and friendly relationship that includes the provision of clear instructions and explanation and regular monitoring and resolution of drug-taking problems (6, 7, 75, 76, 86–88). In addition, researchers have shown that these concepts are also useful in understanding physicians' prescribing and willingness to give information (89, 90).

Stress, Support, and Coping

The work in this area suggests that drug use can be viewed as a means of coping with stress and that use will be affected by the level of stress, the availability of social support (which minimizes the effects of stress), and the availability or attractiveness of other coping styles (91). The implication is that one can influence the level of drug use in three ways—by reducing the stressors, by increasing the availability of social support, or by making other coping methods or styles more available or attractive.

This type of approach (or parts of it) has been applied to the study of nonprescription drugs (10), the use of alcohol and other psychoactive drugs in the community (48), the use of antiasthmatic drugs (92), the use of analgesics and other medications after surgery (93, 94), and the use of tranquilizers (95). What is most interesting about this work is that health professionals can have a rather dramatic effect on the level of drug use in a hospital by providing more information and support before patients experience stressful events such as surgery.

Other Theoretical Perspectives

As shown in Table 7.2, there are a few other theoretical perspectives that have been used to study drug processes. However, the studies using these theories are scattered and few in number. Interestingly enough, there is only one published study that applies Roger's theory regarding the diffusion of innovation (96, 97). This is a particularly interesting theory because it can help us to understand why some doctors are quicker than other doctors to adopt new drugs as well as other issues regarding the adoption of new ideas or practices. For example, it might help us to understand why some pharmacists are eager to innovate, while others would prefer to keep things the way they are.

Although sociology offers a number of useful theories that pertain to roles and social organization (98), there are only a few studies using such approaches (16, 99-105). The results of these studies suggest that it would be fruitful to do further investigations along these lines, especially if we want to gain a better understanding about why professionals often appear reluctant to assume roles or why there are differences in the use of drugs from one organization to another.

Finally, there are many studies examining various theories of deviant behavior as these theories can be applied to the abuse of various drugs (2-4). In the past few years, there also have appeared several interesting studies that examine the sociological aspects of corruption in the pharmaceutical industry (21) and among health workers in a developing country (51).

NEED FOR INTEGRATION

Although most of the discussed theories have something to contribute to our understanding of drug processes, none takes a very comprehensive view. Thus, it is likely that we will need to integrate these perspectives so that we can obtain a fuller picture of certain processes. For example, it makes sense to integrate the cognitive and social influence perspectives as they tend to complement each other quite well (106). It also seems important to develop a more comprehensive and integrated view of the drug use system (107). A future goal would be to link the micro-level perspectives and the macro-level perspectives. But much remains to be done before that can take place.

CONCLUSION

It is clear that many drugs are prescribed and taken in a less than optimal manner and that previous attempts to resolve these problems have been only partially successful. Thus we need to begin doing research of various kinds, including studies of the social meaning and function of drugs, the dynamics of drug prescribing and use, the social factors affecting drug response, and the social consequences of drug taking. Given the diversity and complexity of the problems that confront us, it is unlikely that a single perspective or approach will suffice. Thus we need to consider a wide range of frameworks, each of which makes a contribution to our understanding of drug processes.

REFERENCES

1. Clinard M, Meier R. The sociology of deviant behavior. 5th ed. New York: Holt, Rinehart, and Winston, 1979.
2. Stephens R. Mind-altering drugs: use, abuse, and treatment. Newbury Park: Sage Publications, 1987.
3. Josephson E, Carroll EE, eds. Drug use: epidemiological and sociological approaches. New York: John Wiley & Sons, Inc., 1974.
4. Winick C. The deviance model of drug-taking behavior: a critique. In Segal B, ed. Drugs and society, No 1, Vol 1, 1986, pp 29-49.
5. Burrell C, Levy R. Therapeutic consequences of noncompliance. In Improving medication compliance—proceedings of a symposium. Washington, DC: National Pharmaceutical Council, 1985, pp 7-16.
6. Smith M. The cost of noncompliance and the capacity of improved compliance to reduce health

care expenditures. In Improving medication compliance—proceedings of a symposium. Washington, DC: National Pharmaceutical Council, 1985, pp 35–44.

7. Haynes RB, Taylor D, Sackett D, eds. Baltimore: Compliance in health care, Johns Hopkins Press, 1979.

8. Ostrom J, Hammarlund ER, Christensen D, Plein J, Kethley, A. Medication usage in an elderly population. Med Care 1985;23:157–164.

9. Ascione F. An assessment of different components of patient medication knowledge. Med Care 1986;24:1018–1028.

10. Svarstad B. Stress and the use of nonprescription drugs. In Greenley J, ed. Research in community mental health. Greenwich, CT: J.A.I. Press, 1983, pp 233–254.

11. Schaffner W, Ray W, Federspiel C. Antibiotic prescribing in office practice: modifying inappropriate use. In: Morgan J and Kagan D (eds.), Society and medication: conflicting signals for prescribers and patients. Lexington, MA: Lexington Books, 1983, pp 327–341.

12. Avorn J, Soumerai S. Improving drug-therapy decisions through educational outreach: a randomized trial of academically based "detailing." N Engl J Med 1983;308:1457–1463.

13. Hershey C, Porter D, Breslau D, Cohen D. Influence of simple computerized feedback on prescription charges in an ambulatory clinic: a randomized clinical trial. Med Care 1986;24:472–481.

14. Marks R, Sacher E. Undertreatment of medical inpatients with narcotic analgesics. Ann Intern Med 1973;78:173.

15. Morgan J, Pleet D. Opiophobia in the United States: the undertreatment of severe pain. In Morgan J, Kagan D, eds. Society and medication: conflicting signals for prescribers and patients. Lexington, MA: Lexington Books, 1983, pp 313–318.

16. Ray W, Federspiel C, Schaffner W. A study of antipsychotic drug use in nursing homes: epidemiologic evidence suggesting misuse. Am J Public Health 1980;70:485–491.

17. Cooper J. Drug-related problems in a geriatric long term care facility. J Geriatr Drug Ther 1986;1:47–68.

18. Silverman M, Lee PR. Pills, profits, and politics. Berkeley: University of California Press, 1974.

19. Silverman M. The drugging of the Americas. Berkeley: University of California Press, 1976.

20. Silverman M, Lee P, Lydecker M. Prescriptions for death. Berkeley: University of California Press, 1982.

21. Braithwaite J. Corporate crime in the pharmaceutical industry. London: Routledge and Kegan Paul, 1984.

22. Melrose D. Bitter pills: medicines and the third world poor. Oxford: Oxfam, 1982.

23. Svarstad B. Pharmaceutical sociology: issues in research, education, and service. Am J Pharm Educ 1979;43:252–256.

24. Leventhal H, Hirschman R. Social psychology and prevention. In Sanders G, Suls J, eds. Social psychology of health and illness. Hillsdale, NJ: L Erlbaum Associates, 1982, pp 183–226.

25. Morris L. Patient package inserts: a review and a perspective. In Moran J, Kagan D, eds. Society and medication: conflicting signals for prescribers and patients. Lexington, MA: Lexington Books, 1983, pp 205–219.

26. Svarstad B. Patient-practitioner relationships and compliance with prescribed medical regimens. In Aiken L, Mechanic D, eds. Applications of social science to clinical medicine and health policy. New Brunswick, NJ: Rutgers University Press, 1986, pp 438–459.

27. Schaffner W, Ray W, Federspiel C, Miller W. Improving antibiotic prescribing in office practice: a controlled trial of three educational methods JAMA 1983;250:1728.

28. Ray W, Blazer D, Schaffner W, Federspiel C. Reducing antipsychotic drug prescribing for nursing homes patients: a controlled trial of the effect of an educational visit. Am J Public Health 1987;77:1448–1450.

29. Swenson E, Gooch M, Higbee M, Walsh P. Compliance of neonatal nurse practitioners with gentamicin pharmacokinetic recommendations. Am J Hosp Pharm 1986;43:1472–1475.

30. Haaijer-Ruskamp F, Dukes G. Drugs and money: a preliminary survey and research proposal. Copenhagen: World Health Organization Regional Office for Europe, 1986.

31. Soumerai S, Avorn J, Gortmaker S, Hawley S. Effect of government and commercial warnings on reducing prescription misuse: the case of propoxyphene. Am J Pub Health 1987;77:1518–1523.

32. Morris L. A survey of patients' receipt of prescription drug information. Med Care 1982;20:596–604.
33. Morris L, Myers A, Gibbs P, Lao C. Estrogen PPIs: an FDA survey. Am Pharm 1980;NS20:318–26.
34. Bernardo D. Observations on the behavior of pharmacists—implications for better patient counseling. Patient Counseling Commun Pharm 1986;4:3–10.
35. Cooper J. Consulting to long-term care patients. In Brown T, Smith M, eds. Handbook of institutional pharmacy practice. 2nd ed. Baltimore: Williams & Wilkins, 1986, pp 17–25.
36. Shannon R, DeMuth J. Application of federal indicators in nursing home drug regimen review. Am J Hosp Pharm 1984;41:912–916.
37. Goldberg T, DeVito C. The impact of state generic drug substitution laws. In Morgan J, Kagan D, eds. Society and medication: conflicting signals for prescribers and patients. Lexington, MA: Lexington Books, 1983, pp 99–110.
38. Derogatis L, Feldstein M, Morrow G, et al. A survey of psychotropic drug prescriptions in an oncology population. Cancer (Phila) 1979;44:1919–1929.
39. Shannon R, DeMuth J. Comparison of medication-error detection methods in the long-term care facility. Consult Pharm 1987;2:148–151.
40. Logan M. Humoral medicine in Guatemala and peasant acceptance of modern medicine. Human Organ 1973;32:385–95.
41. Nichter M. The layperson's perception of medicine as perspective into the utilization of multiple therapy systems in the Indian context. Soc Sci Med 1980;14B:225–233.
42. Ferguson A. Commercial pharmaceutical medicine and medicalization: a case study from El Salvador. Culture, Med Psychiatry 1981;5:105–134.
43. Mitchell F. Popular medical concepts in Jamaica and their impact on drug use. W J Med 1983;139:841–847.
44. Welsch R. Traditional medicine and Western medical options among the Ningerum of Papua New Guinea. In Romanucci-Ross L, Moerman D, Tancredi L, eds. The anthropology of medicine. New York: Praeger, 1983.
45. Bledsoe C, Goubaud M. The reinterpretation of Western pharmaceuticals among the Mende of Sierra Leone. Soc Sci Med 1985;21:275–282.
46. Sachs L. Perceptions of pharmaceuticals: a theoretical framework for studies on the use of Western drugs in developing and developed countries. Stockholm, Sweden: Division of International Health Care Research, Karolinska Institute, Unpublished manuscript, 1987.
47. Zborowski M. Cultural components in response to pain. J Soc Issues 1952;8:16–30.
48. Parry H, Cisin I, Balter M, Mellinger G, Manheimer D. Increasing alcohol intake as a coping mechanism for psychic distress. In Cooperstock R, ed. Social aspects of the medical use of psychotropic drugs. Toronto: Addiction Research Foundation of Ontario, 1974, pp 119–144.
49. Estroff S. Making it crazy: an ethnography of psychiatric clients in an American community. Berkeley: University of California Press, 1981.
50. Linn L. Physician characteristics and attitudes toward legitimate use of psychotherapeutic drugs. J Health Soc Behav 1971;12:132–140.
51. Van Der Geest S. The efficiency of inefficiency: medicine distribution in South Cameroon. Soc Sci Med 1982;16:2145–2153.
52. Lennard HL, Bernstein A. Perspectives on the new psychoactive drug technology. In Cooperstock R, ed. Social aspects of the medical use of psychotropic drugs. Toronto: Addiction Research Foundation of Ontario, 1974, pp 149–165.
53. Whalen CK, Henker B. Psychostimulants and children: A review and analysis. Psych Bull 1976;83:1113–1130.
54. Barber B. Drugs and society. New York: Russell Sage Foundation, 1967.
55. Conrad P. The meaning of medications: another look at compliance. Soc Sci Med 1985;20:29–37.
56. Raynes N. What can I do for you? In Mapes R, ed. Prescribing practice and drug usage. London: Croom Helm, 1980, p 83.
57. Comaroff J. A bitter pill to swallow: placebo therapy in general practice. Soc Rev 1976;24:79–96.
58. Hall D. Prescribing as social exchange. In Mapes R, ed. Prescribing practice and drug usage. London: Croom Helm, 1980, pp 39–57.

59. Dunnell K, Cartwright A. Medicine takers, prescribers, and hoarders. London: Routledge and Kegan Paul, 1972.

60. US Senate, Special Committee on Aging, Subcommittee on Long-Term Care. Nursing home care in the United States: failure in public policy. Supporting Paper No. 2, Drugs in nursing homes: misuse, costs and kickbacks, Washington, DC: US Government Printing Office, 1975.

61. Milliren J. Some contingencies affecting the utilization of tranquilizers in long-term care of the elderly. J Health Soc Behav 1977;18:206-211.

62. Kotarba J. Chronic pain: its social dimensions. Beverly Hills: Sage Publications, 1983.

63. Haaijer-Ruskamp F, Stewart R, Wesselilng H. Does indirect consultation lead to overprescribing in general practice? Soc Sci Med 1987;25:43-46.

64. Stryker S, Statham A. Symbolic interaction and role theory. In Lindzey G, Aronson E, eds. Handbook of social psychology. Vol 1, 3rd ed. New York: Random House, 1985, pp 311-378.

65. Fagerhaugh S, Strauss A. Politics of pain management: staff-patient interaction. Menlo Park: Addison-Wesley, 1977.

66. Dunbar J, Marshall G, Hovell M. Behavioral strategies for improving compliance. In Haynes R, Taylor D, Sackett D, eds. Compliance in health care. Baltimore: Johns Hopkins University, 1979, pp 174-190.

67. Wallston B, Wallston K. Social psychological models of health behavior: an examination and integration. In Baum A, Taylor S, Singer J, eds. Handbook of psychology and health. Vol 4. Hillsdale, NJ: L Erlbaum Associates, 1984, pp 23-53.

68. DiNicola DD, DiMatteo MR. Practitioners, patients, and compliance with medical regimens: a social psychological perspective. In Baum A, Taylor S, Singer J, eds. Handbook of psychology and health. Vol 4. Hillsdale, NJ: L Erlbaum Associates, 1984, pp 55-84.

69. Rodin J. The application of social psychology. In Lindzey G, Aronson R, eds. Handbook of social psychology. Vol 2. Special fields and applications. 3rd ed. New York: Random House, 1985, pp 805-881.

70. McGuire W. The communication-persuasion model and health-risk labeling. In Morris L, Mazis M, Barofsky I, eds. Banbury Report No. 6: Product labeling and health risks. Cold Spring Harbor Laboratory, 1980, pp 99-122.

71. McGuire W. Attitudes and attitude change. In Lindzey G, Aronson R, eds. Handbook of social psychology. Vol 2. Special fields and applications. 3rd ed. New York: Random House, 1985, pp 233-246.

72. Leventhal H, Nerenz D, Steele D. Illness representations and coping with health threats. In Baum A, Taylor S, Singer J, eds. Handbook of psychology and health. Social psychological aspects of health. Vol 4. Hillsdale, NJ: L Erlbaum Associates, 1984, pp 219-252.

73. Ley P. Psychological studies of doctor-patient communication. In Rachman S, ed. Contributions to medical psychology. Oxford: Pergamon Press, 1977, pp 9-42.

74. Ley P. Satisfaction, compliance and communication. Br J Clin Psych 1982;21:241-254.

75. Svarstad B. Physician-patient communication and patient conformity with medical advice. In Mechanic D, ed. The growth of bureaucratic medicine. New York: J. Wiley and Sons, 1976, pp 220-238.

76. Svarstad B. Doctor-patient communication. In Currie B, ed. Patient education in the primary care setting. Madison, WI: Proceedings of the Second Conference 1978, pp 17-29.

77. Becker M, Maiman L, Kirscht J, Haefner D, Drachman R, Taylor D. Recent studies of the Health Belief Model. In Haynes R, Taylor D, Sackett D, eds. Compliance in health care. Baltimore: Johns Hopkins University Press, 1979.

78. Jospe M. The placebo effect in healing. Lexington, MA: Lexington Books, 1978.

79. Skelton J, Pennebaker J. The psychology of physical symptoms and sensations. In Sanders G, Suls J, eds. Social psychology of health and illness. L Erlbaum Associates, Hillsdale, NJ: 1982, pp 99-128.

80. Knapp DE, Oeltjen P. Benefits to risks ratio in physician drug selection. Am J Public Health 1972;62:1346-1347.

81. Segal R, Hepler C. Prescribers' beliefs and values as predictors of drug choices. Am J Hosp Pharm 1982;39:1891-1897.

82. Segal R, Hepler C. Drug choice as a problem-solving process. Med Care 1985;23:967-976.

83. Denig P, Zijsling D, Haaijer-Ruskamp F. Use of a prescribing behavior model to evaluate the effect of information for physicians. Paper presented at the annual meeting of Federation International Pharmaceutique. Amsterdam, Netherlands, September 1987.

84. Soumerai S, Avorn R. Predictors of physician prescribing change in an educational experiment to improve medication use. Med Care 1987;25:210–221.
85. Rodin J, Janis I. The social power of health-care practitioners as agents of change. J Soc Issues 1979;35:60–81.
86. Inui T, Carter W. Problems and prospects for health services research on provider-patient communication. Med Care 1985;23:521–538.
87. Davis M. Variations in patients' compliance with doctors' advice: an empirical analysis of patterns of communication. Am J Public Health 1968;50:274–288.
88. Inui T, Carter W, Kukall W, Haigh V. Outcome-based doctor-patient interaction analysis. Med Care 1982;20:535–549.
89. Heath C. On prescription writing in social interaction. In Mapes R, ed. Prescribing practice and drug usage. London: Croom Helm, 1980, pp 59–69.
90. Waitzkin H. Information giving in medical care. J Health Soc Behav 1985;26:81–101.
91. Svarstad B. The institutionalized patient. In Brown T, Smith M, eds. Handbook of institutional pharmacy practice. 2nd ed. Baltimore: Williams & Wilkins, 1986, pp 17–25.
92. Dahlem N, Kinsman R, Horton D. Panic-fear in asthma: requests for as-needed medications in relation to pulmonary function measurements. J Allergy Clin Immunol 1977;60:295–300.
93. Mumford E, Schlesinger H, Glass G. The effects of psychological intervention on recovery from surgery and heart attacks: an analysis of the literature. Am J Public Health 1982;72:141–151.
94. Egbert L, Battit G, Welch C, et al. Reduction of postoperative pain by encouragement and instruction of patients. N Engl J Med 1964;270:825–827.
95. Caplan R, Abbey A, Abramis D, Andrews F, Conway T, French J, Jr. Tranquilizer use and well being. Ann Arbor, MI: Institute for Social Research, 1984.
96. Rogers E. Diffusion of innovations. 3rd ed. New York: Free Press, 1983.
97. Coleman J, Katz E, Menzel H. Medical innovation: a diffusion study. Indianapolis: Bobbs-Merrill Company Inc, 1966.
98. Pfeffer J. Organizations and organization theory. In Lindzey G, Aronson E, eds. Handbook of social psychology. Vol 1. Theory and method. 3rd ed. New York: Random House, 1985, pp 379–440.
99. Mason H, Svarstad B. Medication counseling and attitudes of rural community pharmacists. Drug Intell Clin Pharm 1984;18:409–414.
100. Robers P. The use of sleep medications in skilled nursing facilities: a study of biomedical and psychosocial factors. Unpublished PhD dissertation, School of Pharmacy, University of Wisconsin-Madison, 1985.
101. Parker W. Effect of hospitalization on patient use of hypnotics. Am J Hosp Pharm 1983;40:446–447.
102. Wack J, Rodin J. Nursing homes for the aged: the human consequences of legislation-shaped environments. J Soc Issues 1978;34:6–21.
103. Rodin J, Langer E. Long term effects of a control-relevant intervention with the institutionalized aged. J Pers Soc Psych 1977;35:897–902.
104. Svarstad B, Bond C, Peterson R. The use of hypnotic drugs in proprietary and church-related nursing homes. Paper presented at the annual meeting of Academy of Pharmaceutical Sciences. Philadelphia, October 1984.
105. Van Der Geest S. Anthropology and pharmaceuticals in developing countries: Part I. Med Anthropol Q 1984;15:59–62.
106. Svarstad B. The relationship between patient communication and compliance. In Breimer D, Speiser P, eds. Topics in pharmaceutical sciences. Amsterdam: Elsevier Science Publishers, 1985.
107. Hemminki E. The role of prescriptions in therapy. Med Care 1979;13:151.

SELECTED READINGS

WHO'S USING NONPRESCRIBED MEDICINES? [a]

Patricia J. Bush
David L. Rabin

Little is known about health and illness behavior outside of the formal system of health care provided through physicians. In the informal system, self-medication is a frequent response to either illness or its prevention that may substitute for use of physicians or prescribed medicines. Most illnesses are treated in part with a nonprescribed medicine that is the first response in almost half of illness incidents (8). The use of nonprescribed drugs is not without risk. A three-year study of adverse drug reactions as a cause of hospitalization at the University of Florida Hospital medical service showed that 18 per cent were caused by nonprescribed drugs (2). Concomitant use of prescribed and nonprescribed drugs is common in the population (11) and in persons referred to doctors (12), suggesting the importance of physicians inquiring into the nonprescribed drug use of their patients. In view of the extent of nonprescribed medicine use and the likelihood of substitution of physician visits and prescribed drugs by nonprescribed drugs, more should be known about the characteristics of users and the relationships of nonprescribed medicines to physicians and prescribed medicines.

The two United States areas studied as part of the World Health Organization International Collaborative Study of Medical Care Utilization (WHO/ICS-MCU), were found to have the highest two-day rates of medicine use of the 12 areas in seven countries surveyed in 1968-69 (9). The age-sex standardized two-day rate of persons using medicines in one of these, the Baltimore SMSA, was 533 ± 9 per 1,000 population. Thirty-six per cent of the population reported they had used a nonprescribed medicine in the two days prior to interview as compared with 33 per cent reporting use of prescribed medicine. Nonprescribed medicine users averaged 1.4 different kinds per person (11). While healthy persons were less likely to use nonprescribed medicines than those with morbidity, use did not increase with increasing severity of acute and chronic illness.

In the few surveys where nonprescribed medicines have been a subject of inquiry, the primary correlate of use has been illness. In a panel of Ohio families, Knapp and Knapp (8) found that in 12 months, 70 per cent of illnesses were treated with nonprescribed medicine. In two English studies (4, 13), as the number of symptoms increased, the use of nonprescribed medicine increased. Age, sex, race, and social class have been related to nonprescribed medicine use as well; in general, women and the elderly having highest rates of use. However, rates are high in other groups. In a two-week period, one of the English surveys (4)

[a] Reprinted from *Medical Care,* 14(12):1014–1023 (December) 1976. Baltimore data were drawn from the World Health Organization/International Collaborative Study of Medical Care Utilization, supported in the Baltimore Study Area by Grants 8-R01-HS-00110 and 5-Y01-HS-00012 from the National Center for Health Services Research and Development. Analysis of the data was supported by Grant I-R01-HS-01408-01.

Part of this paper was presented at the 122nd Annual Meeting of the American Pharmaceutical Association, San Francisco, California, April 22, 1975.

found that 75 per cent of children less than two years old had been given a nonprescribed medicine. Upper-class persons were found by Knapp and Knapp (8) to use more kinds of nonprescribed medicines, while the NCHS (3) reported that upper-class persons spend more money on them. The NCHS also reported less use by nonwhites than by whites.

Information on the substitution of nonprescribed medicines for other care is mixed, one English survey finding that persons using prescribed medicines are more likely to use nonprescribed medicines as well (7), and another finding that persons with similar numbers of symptoms using prescribed medicines are less likely to use nonprescribed medicines than are those without prescribed medicine use (4).

In view of the lack of knowledge about the use of nonprescribed medicines in the United States, either about the rates of use, the characteristics of users or how nonprescribed medicines relate to prescribed medicines, physicians and insurance, an analysis of data from the WHO/ICS-MCU survey of the Baltimore area was undertaken. While Baltimore has, along with the Northeast, a higher ratio of physician and hospital services than the national averages which can be expected to affect prescribing patterns, there is little reason to believe that factors relating to nonprescribed medicine use should be atypical of the nation's SMSAs.

METHODS

Questionnaires were completed on the use of health services, morbidity, content of recent physician visit, fiscal resources, and social relationships and attitudes by 3,481 persons representing 90 percent of the noninstitutionalized nontransient residents of the Baltimore SMSA (14). Eligibility of households was determined by means of a multistage, area-probability cluster design. The sample was obtained from six subdivisions of the SMSA, Baltimore City, and the five counties, so that each was proportionately represented. Through sequential selection, clusters of three households were drawn from census tracts and enumeration districts that made up the primary sampling units within the six subdivisions. The questions were asked of each adult respondent during the survey of 1,239 households in four quarterly probability samples between June 1, 1968 and May 31, 1969. A separate questionnaire was used for proxy administration to children (defined as < 15 years). Of 3,951 persons contacted, 79 individuals were excluded because they did not meet definitional requirements. Eight per cent of eligible respondents refused to be interviewed and 2 per cent were not located after repeated attempts. Demographic data were gathered about the 10 per cent of persons who refused or were not located, and variations from the characteristics of those interviewed were judged not sufficiently large to introduce significant bias into the results (1).

Except for certain morbidity-related questions, information on the use of particular categories of medicine was obtained in response to the questions "Yesterday or the day before that did you take or use any of the following medicines, pills, or ointments? How many different kinds? How many different kinds were prescribed or suggested by a doctor?" Thus, for purposes of the analysis a prescribed medicine includes medicines that may be sold over-the-counter but that have been suggested by a physician.

A morbidity index combines two indices: one formed from responses to questions about the presence of impairment and chronic illness that limit the respondent's ability to perform usual activities, and the other formed from responses to questions inquiring about the presence of health problems resulting in bed days or restricted activity days or the presence of any other health problem in the two weeks prior to interview, and the extent these caused bother, hurt, or worry to the respondent.

The economic class index based on family income and size is a modification of one used by Bice (1) who adapted the cutting points of a 1963 poverty index for nonfarm families deveoped by Orshansky (10) to the closest $1,000 intervals available in this survey.

When vitamins are excluded from the analysis leaving morbidity-related nonprescribed medicines only, the two day rate of use falls from 36 per cent to 30 per cent. Because the concern of this paper is primarily the relationship of nonprescribed medicine use to use of physicians and prescribed medicines, the analysis is confined to morbidity-related medicines only.

RESULTS

Substantial variation by age and sex occurs among persons using morbidity-related nonprescribed medicine in the population (Fig. 1). The rates vary from a low of 14 per cent for males <2 and 65+ years to a high of 42 per cent for females 15–44 years. Use rates are higher for adults than for children; about two-fifths of adults are users compared to one-fifth of children. Nonprescribed medicine use is not well correlated with assumed morbidity. While illness rates increase for both sexes over age 44 years, rates of nonprescribed medicine use decline. Females have higher rates of nonprescribed medicine use than males in five of the six age groups. Except for ages 2 to 14 years when morbidity and nonprescribed medi-

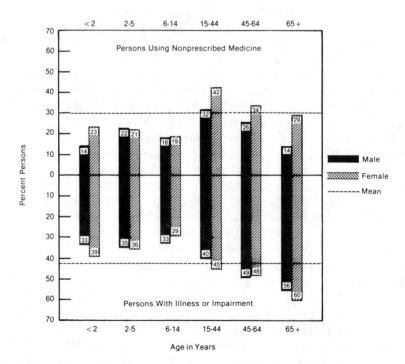

Figure 7.1.   Percentage of persons using nonprescribed medicine in two days and persons with illness or impairment by age. Baltimore SMSA, 1968–69 (N = 3481). Nonprescribed medicines are morbidity-related only (vitamins are excluded).

cine use rates are similar by sex, female rates of use are greater than can be accounted for by greater female rates of perceived morbidity. The mean use rate for females is 33 per cent compared with 26 per cent for males.

Most of the sex related difference in use is accounted for by nonprescribed pain relievers. Both adult and child females are one-third more likely to use them than are males. Other commonly used nonprescribed medicines, those for coughs or colds and skin ointments or salves, vary little by age and sex; laxatives and stomach remedies are more likely to be used by adults (2).

Rates of use of nonprescribed medicine by economic class and morbidity are shown in Table 1. The healthy in each economic class category except the poor are less likely to be users than are those reporting some illness. While rates of use are highest among those with any illness as compared with those chronically ill or impaired only, for only the poor and high economic classes do they increase with increasing severity of acute illness. Economic class alone appears to have little effect on rates of use, which are nearly the same for all classes. By morbidity category, the poor but healthy have a higher rate of use than other healthy persons, but in the rest of the morbidity categories, the rates of use of the poor are lower than average. Of the study population, 58 percent perceive themselves to be without acute or chronic illness, yet almost one-fourth used a nonprescribed morbidity-related medicine. Thus, nonprescribed medicine use is not confined to those experiencing only mild acute illness but is used by the healthy and those who experience severe levels of illness.

Nonwhites (26%) are less likely to be nonprescribed medicine users than whites (31%) ($\chi^2 = 8.43$, df $= 1$, p$< .01$). This difference persists throughout economic classes.

Because prescriptions require contact with physicians, prescribed medicine use is highly correlated with physician visits (9). Thus, if nonprescribed medicines substitute for prescribed medicines, they likely do so by substituting for physician visits. Since use of morbidity-related medicines is a function of perceived morbidity, the question of substitution is posed by asking if nonprescribed medicines substitute for physician visits and thus for the prescribed medicines resulting from those visits at similar levels of perceived morbidity. If the hypothesis is true, we would expect to find the following: persons using prescribed medicine will be less likely to use nonprescribed medicine than will those who are not using prescribed medicine; persons using nonprescribed medicine will be less likely to use prescribed medicine than will those who are not using nonprescribed medicine; persons using nonprescribed medicine will have lower physician visit rates than those who are not using a nonprescribed medicine, and persons who do not visit a physician will be more likely to use a nonprescribed medicine than those who do.

As shown in Table 2, persons using nonprescribed medicine are slightly more likely to be using prescribed medicine (28%) than those who are not using nonprescribed medicine (25%). However, the pattern differs by morbidity category. The similarity in use rates results from opposite patterns of prescribed and nonprescribed medicine use in the healthy and the ill. Healthy persons using nonprescribed medicines are more likely to be using a prescribed medicine (17%) than those without nonprescribed medicine use (13%). However, in all four illness categories the opposite is observed. Persons reporting illness and using nonprescribed medicines are less likely to be using prescribed medicine during the same two-day period than those who are not using any nonprescribed medicine. All of the difference could occur by chance less than 0.1 per cent of the time if rates of use were the same in the population. Thus, the hypothesis is supported for persons reporting morbidity but not for the healthy. The obverse situation supports the hypothesis for ill persons as well: that is, in all four of the morbidity categories relating to illness, persons using prescribed

Table 1. Number and percentage of persons using nonprescribed medicine* in two days by economic class and morbidity (Baltimore SMSA, 1968–69)

| Morbidity | Persons using nonprescribed medicine* by economic class† | | | | | | | | All economic class categories | |
| | Poor | | Low | | Medium | | High | | | |
	No.	(%)	No.	(%)	No.	(%)	No.	(%)	No.	(%)
Healthy	75	(30.7)	106	(21.9)	141	(24.1)	135	(22.7)	457	(23.9)
Mild acutely ill only	12	(30.7)	35	(46.1)	39	(48.1)	36	(38.7)	122	(41.8)
Severe acutely ill only	20	(39.2)	33	(33.8)	27	(37.5)	46	(51.5)	126	(42.3)
Chronically ill or impaired only	18	(25.0)	23	(22.5)	36	(35.3)	49	(31.2)	126	(29.1)
Acutely ill and chronically ill or impaired	31	(35.6)	40	(41.2)	29	(41.4)	56	(48.7)	156	(42.3)
All morbidity categories	156	(31.5)	237	(28.0)	272	(29.9)	322	(30.7)	987	(29.9)

* Nonprescribed medicine is morbidity-related only (vitamins are excluded).
† One hundred eighty persons were not classifiable.

Table 2. Percentage of nonprescribed medicine* users using prescribed medicines* in two days by morbidity (Baltimore SMSA, 1968–69)

	Persons using medicine by morbidity (N = 3477)											
	Healthy		Mild acutely ill only		Severe acutely ill only		Chronically ill or impaired only		Acutely ill and chronically ill or impaired		All categories	
	Non-prescribed		Non-prescribed		Non-prescribed		Non-prescribed		Non-prescribed		Non-prescribed	
Medicine*	No	Yes	No	Yes	No	Yes	No	Yes	No	Yes	No	Yes
Prescribed No	87%	83%	73%	83%	53%	61%	58%	67%	37%	49%	75%	72%
Yes	13%	17%	27%	17%	47%	39%	42%	33%	63%	51%	25%	28%
	100%	100%	100%	100%	100%	100%	100%	100%	100%	100%	100%	100%

*Prescribed and nonprescribed medicines are morbidity-related only (vitamins and oral contraceptives are excluded).

Table 3. Rate of physician visits in two weeks per 100 persons by morbidity and prescribed and nonprescribed medicine* use in two days (Baltimore SMSA, 1968–69)

Medicine*	Physician visits/100 persons by morbidity (N = 3476)					
	Healthy	Mild acutely ill only	Severe acutely ill only	Chronically ill or impaired only	Acutely ill and chronically ill or impaired	All categories
Nonprescribed						
No	17	47	100	25	72	31
Yes	16	21	71	25	44	30
Prescribed						
No	12	18	55	15	34	17
Yes	54	97	128	37	80	72

*Prescribed and nonprescribed medicines are morbidity-related only (vitamins and oral contraceptives are excluded).

medicine are less likely to use nonprescribed than are those who are not using prescribed medicine.

Further evidence to support the hypothesis that nonprescribed medicines substitute for prescribed ones is in Table 3 referring to physician visits. For the population, the rate of physician visits per 100 persons in the two weeks prior to interview is not different for those who use nonprescribed medicines (30) than for those who do not (31). Nor is there any difference for healthy persons. However, for those who have some degree of acute illness or impairment, physician visits are higher for those who do not use nonprescribed medicine than for those who do, while the rates of visits for those with only chronic illness or impairment are the same. This suggests that there is some substitution of nonprescribed medicines for physician visits in the acutely ill group. As expected, physician visit rates are higher for persons using prescribed medicines in all morbidity categories.

Furthermore, the proportion of persons using a nonprescribed medicine (28%) is less among persons having a physician visit than the proportion of persons using a nonprescribed medicine who have not had such a visit (43%) ($\chi^2 = 47.74$, df $= 1$, p<.001). Differences are marked in the acute illness categories and are small in the healthy and chronically ill or impaired only categories.

Respondents were asked about the specific categories of medicine they had used in the past two days. As shown in Table 4, persons report using a prescribed or a nonprescribed medicine in a specific category but rarely both. When both prescribed and nonprescribed medicines are used, they are used for different purposes. Clearly, persons differentiate among categories of medicines and regard a nonprescribed medicine in a specific category as not an adjunct but a substitute for a prescribed medicine in the same category.

In the study group, persons who pay none or only some of the cost of prescribed medicines (13% of the population) are less likely to be users of nonprescribed medicines (31%) than are those bearing all out-of-pocket costs of prescribed medicines (37%) ($\chi^2 = 7.16$, p<.01). Persons without financial help for prescribed medicines have higher rates of use of nonprescribed medicines than those with help in all but the high economic class. However, rates of nonprescribed medicine use are not higher among those who must pay all out-of-

Table 4. Number and percentage of persons using categories of prescribed or nonprescribed medicine in two days (Baltimore SMSA, 1968–69)

Category of medicine	Prescribed No.	(%)	Nonprescribed No.	(%)	Both No.	(%)
Pain relief	203	(5.8)	687	(19.7)	1	(0.0)
Vitamin	322	(9.3)	263	(7.5)	3	(0.1)
Cough or cold	137	(3.9)	200	(5.7)	9	(0.2)
Skin ointment or salve	95	(2.7)	174	(4.9)	2	(0.1)
Laxative or stomach	95	(2.7)	148	(4.2)	0	(0.0)
Tranquilizer or sedative	137	(3.9)	8	(0.2)	1	(0.0)
Sleeping	75	(2.2)	4	(0.1)	1	(0.0)
Other	356	(10.2)	30	(0.8)	11	(0.3)
Heart or blood pressure*	195	(8.2)	0	(0.0)	0	(0.0)
Allergy†	27	(2.4)	1	(0.1)	0	(0.0)
Oral contraceptive‡	105	(13.2)	0	(0.0)	0	(0.0)

*Adults only.
†Children under 15 years only.
‡Females 18 to 50 years only.

pocket costs for physician visits. Thus, insurance that covers prescribed drugs but not insurance that covers physician visits is associated with lower rates of nonprescribed medicine use.

DISCUSSION

Many persons use medicines that are neither prescribed nor suggested by a physician both in the absence and presence of illness. While morbidity-related nonprescribed medicines are more likely to be used by persons perceiving themselves to be ill, a surprisingly high number (almost one in four) who report neither bed nor reduced activity days, nor chronic illness or impairment, nor anything else wrong with their health, are users of such medicines. One can understand why persons who are bothered by symptoms of ill health seek relief through self-medication. It is less easy to understand persons reporting use of morbidity-related medicines and not reporting morbidity. Some persons using antacids, laxatives, and sedatives may use them preventively or for chronic symptoms such as occasional vague gastrointestinal distress or insomnia that they do not view as a health problem. However, the most frequently used category of medicine is for pain relief, suggesting that minor acute symptoms such as head, muscle, or back aches are so common persons may not perceive themselves as deviating from a state of health even when they seek relief through self-medication.

Almost one quarter of healthy persons and almost 40 per cent of ill persons use self-prescribed medicines. In view of these high rates, it is advisable for physicians to inquire into the nonprescribed medicine use of persons they see for preventive checkups and immunizations, but it is most important to do so for ill patients, particularly when prescribing. Patients appear to differentiate between prescribed and nonprescribed medicines of the same category, but they surely do not appreciate the potential for interaction between different types of medicine. Aspirin, the most common nonprescribed drug related to hospitalization in the previously mentioned University of Florida Hospital study (2), has wide ranging interaction effects which modify the pharmacologic activity of prescription drugs. Examples are altered coagulation when used with an anticoagulant and potentiation of hypoglycemia when used with chlorpropamide. Similarly, antihistamines, widely used nonprescription drugs, should not be used with CNS depressants, and antacids, which may modify the absorption of prescribed medicines as diverse as tetracycline and quinidine, should be used cautiously with digitalis and thiazides (5).

Results suggest there is a continuum of care for certain symptom states. Almost all nonprescribed medicine use is accounted for by the following categories: pain relief, vitamins, skin ointment, cough or cold, and laxatives. Nonprescribed medicine is less likely to be used as the severity of acute and chronic disorders increases and is least likely for persons with both acute and chronic disorders. While almost two-fifths of persons using a prescribed medicine in this study also self-medicated, the concomitant use of prescribed and nonprescribed medicines for the same purpose is negligible. When these results, and those reported with respect to substitution, are considered with Knapp and Knapp's findings that 70 per cent of all illness episodes were treated with nonprescribed drugs (8), it seems likely that persons perceive that it is appropriate to use a nonprescribed medicine for certain symptoms but when satisfactory relief is not obtained, a physician may be consulted who is likely to prescribe. Upon consultation, persons are likely to discontinue the nonprescribed medicine that failed to alleviate the symptoms that led them to the physician, although they may use a nonprescribed medicine for different symptoms. However, it is possible that different symptoms are manifestations of the same condition. Thus, while persons are unlikely to use both nonprescribed and prescribed medicines for the same symptoms, they may be using them for the same illness.

Persons reporting similar levels of illness have different tendencies to use nonprescribed medicine depending on their demographic characteristics. In this study, the greater use of nonprescribed medicines by whites and females can neither be explained by greater morbidity (whites do not perceive more illness than nonwhites, and when morbidity is nearly the same in early and late years, females are more likely to be users than males) nor by economic class or lower rates of prescribed medicine use. Thus, use of nonprescribed medicine may be a learned response to illness that is more socially acceptable for whites and females. The learned behavior may begin early; almost one-fourth of female children less than two years old were given a morbidity-related nonprescribed medicine.

Society provides many behavioral options for persons who have health concerns. Personal experiences and situational factors determine which of these options will be considered, and which will be acted upon. Thus, at any one time, persons with similar levels of perceived morbidity will be following different courses of action, some doing nothing, some using folk remedies, some self-medicating, etc. In this sense, one activity is a substitute for another within a population.

Results supporting the hypothesis that nonprescribed medicine use may substitute for physician visits for persons perceiving themselves to be ill, and in particular those who are acutely ill, suggest that measures that would increase access to physicians may decrease the use of self-prescribed medicines relative to prescribed ones. In spite of increased access to the formal system, some substitution may persist. Substitution of nonprescribed medicines for physician visits at similar symptom levels was found in England where no financial barriers exist to physician visits (4).

Substitution is not inappropriate. It would severely strain the existing medical care system in terms of personnel and expense if all health problems were brought to the physician. The problem lies in finding methods to increase the likelihood that persons will treat their minor and transient discomforts with appropriate nonprescribed medicines. While the number of symptoms for which persons perceive it is appropriate to self-medicate appear to be limited the present distribution system of nonprescribed medicines contains few incentives to assure rational use or to decrease use. Both advertising and the retail marketing system encourage use. At its best, irrational use is wasteful of resources and at its worst it is dangerous (6). Of 400 over-the-counter drugs reviewed by the National Academy of Sciences–National Research Council, 15 per cent were found effective, 27 per cent probably effective, 47 per cent possibly effective, and 11 per cent ineffective. To date, panels investigating the safety and efficacy of 26 categories of nonprescribed drugs for the Food and Drug Administration have severely criticized the marketing of antacids, sleep aids and stimulants. Of the latter, all except caffeine were found to be unsafe or inappropriate.

In addition to the risk of adverse interaction effects and direct toxic effects—for example, phenacetin may cause renal disease and salicylates may cause gastric bleeding—nonprescribed medicines are associated with poisonings. In a six-month period, 19 percent of ingestions reported to a poison information center were due to nonprescribed medicines (6).

Efforts to provide consumers with adequate and truthful information through labeling and advertising should be supported as should similar efforts to provide physicians with knowledge of interaction and toxic effects of nonprescribed drugs.

The physician should inquire into medicine use when evaluating symptoms and before prescribing; he should encourage patients to discuss the implications of using self-prescribed with physician-prescribed medicines. In addition, he should point out the risk of having medicines located in the home where the young or the foolish can poison themselves through accidental ingestion.

This study finds that nonprescribed medicines, part of the informal health care system, are perceived as alternate ways to resolve health problems, and that use is a function of personal characteristics. While much nonprescribed medicine use is probably harmless or useful to help with minor and transient injury and illness, our present system contains little to increase, let alone assure rationality. The physician can and should accept some responsibility in assuring that no harm results from their use.

REFERENCES

1. Bice, T. W.: Medical Care for the Disadvantaged. Department of Medical Care and Hospitals, The Johns Hopkins University, Nov., 1971.
2. Caranasos, G. J., Stewart, R. B., and Cluff, L. E.: Drug-induced illness leading to hospitalization. JAMA 228:713, 1974.
3. Cost and Acquisition of Prescribed and Nonprescribed Medicines, United States, July 1964–June 1965. National Center for Health Statistics, Vital Health Statistics, Series 10, No. 33.
4. Dunnell, K., and Cartwright, A.: Medicine Takers, Prescribers and Hoarders. London, Routledge and Kegan Paul, 1972.
5. Evaluation of Drug Interactions, American Pharmaceutical Association, Washington, D.C., 1973.
6. Hodes, B., and Fonaroff, A.: Injurious effects of the drug use process: an analysis of ingested nonprescribed drug products. Presented at the 122nd Annual Meeting of the American Pharmaceutical Association, San Francisco, April 22, 1975.
7. Jefferys, M., Brotherston, J. H. F., and Cartwright, A.: Consumption of medicines on a working-class housing estate. Br. J. Prev. Soc. Med. 14:64, 1960.
8. Knapp, D. A., and Knapp, D. E.: Decision-making and self-medication: preliminary findings. Am. J. Hosp. Pharm. 29:1004, 1972.
9. Kohn, R., and White, K. L., Eds.: Use of Health Services: An International Collaborative Study: Main Report of the World Health Organization/International Collaborative Study of Medical Care Utilization. London, Oxford University Press, 1976.
10. Orshansky, M.: Counting the poor: another look at the poverty profile. Soc. Sec. Bull. 28:3, 1965.
11. Rabin, D. L., and Bush, P. J.: Who's using medicines? J. Commun. Health 1:106, 1975.
12. Stewart, R. B., and Cluff, L. E.: Studies on the epidemiology of adverse drug reactions. VI: Utilization and interactions of prescription and nonprescription drugs in outpatients. Hopkins Med. J. 129:319, 1971.
13. Wadsworth, M. E. J., Butterfield, W. S. H., and Blaney, R.: Health and Sickness: The Choice of Treatment. London, Tavistock, 1971.
14. World Health Organization/International Collaborative Study of Medical Care Utilization. Manual 7: Analysis Manual Baltimore, The Coordinating Committee, 1970.

PHYSICIAN AND PHARMACIST ATTITUDES
TOWARD MEDICATION USE[b]

J. Lyle Bootman
Peter D. Hurd
John A. Gaines

Physicians vary in the extent of their use of medications for therapy and in the quality of their drug prescribing (1-3). Studies have attempted to differentiate and evaluate the many social and economic factors that may influence prescribing behavior. Investigators have attempted to identify factors that correlate with prescribing behavior, including age, training, experience, general conditions of practice, size of practice, average amount of time spent with patient, physician attitudes, sources of drug information, group versus solo practice, institutional versus private practice, and specialist versus general practice (4, 5). In addition, researchers have examined the influence of product promotion, social pressures, demands and expectations of the patient, pressure groups, and the patient's personal characteristics with regard to the mechanics and quality of the prescribing process (2, 3, 6-8). In essence, studies are in agreement with the following conclusions: there is significant variation in the prescribing practices of physicians (2), physicians with higher educational qualifications write fewer prescriptions (9), and "better prescribers," those who prescribe more appropriate therapy by predetermined criteria, also write fewer prescriptions (1, 2, 5, 10). These conclusions indicate that "a better knowledge of drugs leads to a more conservative use of them" (10). Drug prescribing which follows established principles and leads to the minimization of risk to the patient was defined as conservative.

In 1970, Linn et al. (11, 12) attempted to examine the extent to which physicians' attitudes toward the use of drugs varied. Physicians with a more conservative attitude were more likely to rely on professional sources of new drug information than were physicians with a less conservative attitude. More recently, Linn (13) expanded his work to physician use of medications for controversial medical situations. He found that physicians with a more conservative attitude toward the use of medications were younger, tended to be specialists, belonged to a group practice, and relied more heavily on professional sources for new drug information. Linn's method served as the model for an examination of pharmacist versus physician prescribing in this study.

The primary purpose of this study was to assess the attitudes of both physicians and pharmacists with regard to the use of medications in selected situations. A second research question investigated whether a consistent pattern, reflecting a propensity to prescribe, existed within the samples of physicians and pharmacists across the controversial situations presented in the survey. These research questions are especially interesting because the pharmacist's role has expanded to include counseling patients, providing therapeutic advice, and prescribing in various practice settings (14).

METHODS

The survey instrument included two separate sections, one to measure attitudes toward drug use and one to measure characteristics of the respondents. The first section of the question-

[b]Edited and reprinted with permission from Bootman JL, Hurd PD, Gaines JA. Physician and pharmacist attitudes toward medication use. Am J Hosp Pharm 1982;39:818-821.

Table 1. Pharmacist and Physician Responses[a] to 25 Situations.

No.	Situation	Pharmacist Response (n = 217) Mean ± S.D.	Physician Response (n = 198) Mean ± S.D.
1	Medications are now very helpful in handling the social demands and stresses of every day living.[b]	2.9 ± 1.2	2.6 ± 1.2
2	A person is better off taking a sedative than missing a good night's sleep.[c]	3.4 ± 1.1	3.4 ± 1.0
3	A person should take pills only as a last resort.[c]	2.8 ± 1.2	2.9 ± 1.0
4	It is not very legitimate for a truck driver to take an amphetamine in order to get through a long period of driving.[c]	1.8 ± 1.1	1.1 ± 1.0
5	A person is better off taking a tranquilizer than going through the day nervous and tense.[c]	3.2 ± 1.1	3.1 ± 1.1
6	College students would be better off doing poorly on their exams than taking drugs which help them stay awake at night to study.[d]	2.3 ± 1.1	2.7 ± 1.0
	culture.[e]		
13	Some over-the-counter time-release decongestants are just as effective as prescription decongestants.[c]	2.4 ± 1.0	2.3 ± 0.9
14	During high-risk months it is strongly advisable for most people to receive flu vaccines.[c]	3.3 ± 1.1	3.3 ± 1.0
15	The use of cyclamates in diet drinks a few years ago did constitute a serious health hazard.[c]	3.7 ± 1.1	3.5 ± 1.0
16	In spite of the recent ban, saccharin in normal amounts is no more harmful than sugar.[b]	2.2 ± 0.9	2.5 ± 0.9
17	Marijuana is less harmful than many of the drugs which physicians prescribe.[c]	2.9 ± 1.1	2.9 ± 1.1
18	Laetrile probably ought not to be given to any cancer patient who	2.9 ± 1.2	2.6 ± 1.2

No.	Statement		
7	Drugs are rarely helpful in weight control.[c]	2.1 ± 1.1	2.2 ± 1.1
8	Professional athletes who take medications to boost their stamina before games should be disqualified.[c]	1.8 ± 0.9	1.9 ± 0.9
9	The use of small doses of tranquilizers on a daily basis is often effective in treating chronic low-back pain.[e]	3.2 ± 0.9	3.0 ± 0.9
10	Much of the time, prescribing medication is about the only thing a physician can do to help his patients feel better.[d]	3.1 ± 1.2	3.5 ± 1.1
11	No one who has had sexual contact with someone who develops syphilis should be given antibiotics unless their blood is tested and is positive.[d]	2.9 ± 1.2	3.3 ± 1.2
12	It is not acceptable to give patients with cold symptoms antibiotic treatment without doing a	2.6 ± 1.1	2.8 ± 1.2
	wants to buy it.[b]		
19	There is probably little difference between heroin and methadone maintenance.[c]	3.1 ± 1.1	3.2 ± 1.0
20	Vasodilators are not very effective in treating symptoms of recent memory loss in elderly patients.[d]	3.0 ± 0.9	2.5 ± 0.9
21	Injections of Vitamin B_{12} on a regular basis are quite effective.[d]	3.3 ± 1.0	3.8 ± 1.1
22	The use of vitamin C in treating a cold will have no significant effect on how long the cold will last.[c]	2.5 ± 1.0	2.5 ± 1.0
23	Vitamin E in large doses will not increase sexual responsiveness.[e]	2.3 ± 0.9	2.1 ± 0.9
24	Because of the dangerous side effects of aspirin, Tylenol should always be substituted as the casual drug for treatment.[b]	4.0 ± 0.9	3.7 ± 1.0
25	It is not appropriate to treat adolescent onset acne with daily systemic doses of antibiotics.[d]	3.1 ± 1.1	3.5 ± 1.0

[a]The responses were coded as strongly agree = 1, agree = 2, uncertain = 3, disagree = 4, and strongly disagree = 5.
[b]Pharmacist and physician response significantly different at $p < 0.01$.
[c]No significant difference.
[d]Pharmacist and physician response significantly different at $p < 0.001$.
[e]Pharmacist and physician response significantly different at $p < 0.05$.

naire, which solicited demographic information, was designed specifically for the physician or the pharmacist sample. The second section of each instrument was identical for both physicians and pharmacists and measured attitudes toward the use of medication in various situations. This section consisted of 25 statements that asked the participants whether they agreed or disagreed with the use of medications in a given controversial situation (Table 1). The situations have been reported in studies by Linn (11–13).

The respondents were asked to rate the degree to which they agreed or disagreed with each statement. A five-point Likert scale was used. The following directions were given:

> Listed below are a number of different kinds of statements about the use of medications. Based upon your experience, knowledge, and beliefs, rate how much you agree with each statement. Circle one of the numbers on each line to indicate whether you *strongly agree* (SA) with the statement, *agree* (A) with it, or are *uncertain* (UN), *disagree* (DA), or *strongly disagree* (SD). Although for some statements you may want to say that "it depends on the situations," please think in more general terms and circle one of the responses listed. Again, there are no right or wrong answers. We just want your opinion.

The physician sample was selected from the list published by the Arizona State Board of Medical Examiners 1977–1978. The population included 3514 Arizona-licensed physicians who were practicing and residing in Arizona. The pharmacist sample was drawn from the Directory of Arizona Professional Pharmacists, 1978–1979, published by the Arizona State Board of Pharmacy, which listed 1839 registered pharmacists practicing in Arizona. A sample of 300 physicians and 300 pharmacists was randomly selected from the lists.

RESULTS

Response Rate

The overall response rate was 69%. Sixty-six percent of the physicians responded, and 72% of the pharmacists responded.

Attitude Survey

To reduce the 25 questionnaire items to a single summary score or to at least some small number of summary indices, the responses of the physicians and pharmacists were factor analyzed using principal-axis factoring with varimax rotation. However, neither set showed inter-item correlations of sufficient magnitude to justify such a reduction. The largest correlation for the physician respondents was 0.53, and 62.7% of the inter-item correlations were below 0.10. Among the pharmacists, the largest correlation was 0.37, with 51.7% below 0.10. Thus, a single summary score would have very low reliability. Moreover, for either respondent group, no conceptually inherent subset of the 25 items was identifiable as a usable subscale. Thus, it was decided to examine differences between the respondent groups on each of the original 25 items, rather than on empirically unsupported summary indices.

Table 1 provides the mean response for each situation for the physician and pharmacist samples. Significant differences between pharmacists and physicians were found in 13 of the 25 items using the two-tailed Student's *t* test. Pharmacists tended more toward medication use in situations 1, 10, 16, 18, 20, 21, and 23 than did physicians. Physicians had more favorable attitudes regarding medication use in situations 6, 9, 11, 12, 24, and 25. While statistical significant differences were found, the magnitude of these differences was no greater than 0.5 on a 5-point scale. Additionally, means were always on the same side of the midpoint except for situations 11 and 20.

Table 2 provides a summary of responses for both physician and pharmacist samples,

Table 2. Percent of Pharmacist and Physician Responses in Each Category for 25 Situations

Situation No.	Pharmacist Response [a] (%) (n = 217)			Physician Response [a] (%) (n = 198)		
	Agree	Uncertain	Disagree	Agree	Uncertain	Disagree
1	47	8	45	59	6	35
2	31	12	57	26	21	53
3	49	10	41	46	14	40
4	81	7	12	78	12	10
5	35	17	48	32	26	42
6	67	15	18	49	24	27
7	76	5	19	68	13	19
8	81	11	8	81	11	8
9	30	29	41	35	31	34
10	43	10	47	31	9	62
11	49	12	39	32	13	55
12	59	9	32	50	8	42
13	74	6	20	73	13	14
14	33	13	54	27	18	55
15	18	18	64	16	27	57
16	73	15	12	58	28	14
17	39	26	35	42	25	33
18	45	16	39	57	18	25
19	35	22	43	28	33	39
20	33	34	33	54	33	13
21	30	23	49	19	11	70
22	63	14	23	58	23	19
23	71	15	14	76	14	10
24	10	5	85	18	7	76
25	37	13	50	22	17	61

[a]The strongly agree and agree categories were combined, as were the strongly disagree and disagree categories.

displaying the percent of respondents for three categories of Agree, Uncertain, and Disagree for each situation.[a] In the pharmacist sample, 21 of 25 situations indicated a bimodal distribution[b] and in the physician sample 17 of 25 situations were bimodal. In other words, in both samples a large number of respondents either agreed or disagreed with the situation. To further illustrate the bimodal distribution, in 15 of 25 situations more than 25% of the pharmacists agreed and more than 25% disagreed with the situation. In the physician sample, this was true for 13 of 25 situations. These findings reveal a degree of polarization for both physician and pharmacist respondents.

DISCUSSION

The results of this study indicated that more research is needed to develop an instrument to adequately measure physician and pharmacist attitudes regarding given drug-use situations. Past research has suggested that there are physicians who are relatively cautious in their attitude regarding the use of medication and those who are relatively less cautious (12, 13). It seems logical to assume that one's attitude regarding the use of medication in one treatment situation would be consistent across comparable treatment situations. Since the survey instrument consisted of 25 drug-use situations, we thought that at least some of the variables should be highly intercorrelated. As a result of the factor analysis, there were insufficient intercorrelations among the variables to warrant data reduction to a set of underlying dimensions. It appeared from these analyses that in each of the 25 situations we measured independent dimensions. The results from the factor analysis could be interpreted in several ways. One interpretation is that the items regarding the situations were poor, but they do have strong face validity. Therefore, we suggest that neither the physicians nor the pharmacists have developed an integrated attitude structure with regard to these situations. It appears that their response to these items were based upon factors not yet identified, rather than on an underlying "propensity to prescribe."

The results also indicated a degree of polarization in the responses for both the physician and pharmacist samples across several of the situations. This finding is very interesting because one might expect that respondents would, as a group, tend to agree or disagree with a given situation. However, this was not true. Both the responses of pharmacists and physicians were bimodal. It should be kept in mind that this observed polarization was unpatterned. In other words, the respondents did not consistently agree or disagree across situations. This observed polarization, coupled with an unpredictable pattern in response, illustrates the need to investigate what factors predict response. Bush (7) has suggested that the appropriateness of medication prescribing may be based upon many intervening social factors, such as patient expectations and prescriber values or ethics, as opposed to experience in therapeutics. These social factors possibly could explain the results of this study and deserve further investigation.

Finally, it should be pointed out that the situations used in this study represent situations frequently encountered by the physician that are not only controversial in nature but are rarely addressed during professional training in therapeutics. We expect that the professions of pharmacy and medicine would be uncomfortable with the implications of these results in that there is no consensus within the decision-making process regarding the use of medications in these situations. We suggest that educators concerned with the training of future pharmacists and physicians begin to address some of these controversial issues so that the use of medication in such situations may be more consistent.

CONCLUSION

Both the pharmacists and physicians reported a wide range of unpatterned attitudes regarding medication use in controversial situations. More research is needed to improve the instrument used to measure attitudes in this study.

REFERENCES

1. Becker MH, Stolley PD, Lasagna L et al. Correlates of physicians' prescribing behavior. *Inquiry.* 1972; 9:30-42.
2. Hemminki E. Review of the literature on the factors affecting drug prescribing. *Soc Sci Med.* 1975; 4:111-5.
3. Stolley PD, Becker MH, Lasagna L et al. The relationship between physician characteristics and prescribing appropriateness. *Med Care.* 1972; 10:17-28.
4. Hemminki E. Factors influencing drug prescribing: inquiry into research strategy. *Drug Intell Clin Pharm.* 1976; 10:321-9.
5. Stolley PD, Lasagna L. Prescribing patterns of physicians. *J Chronic Dis.* 1969; 22:395-405.
6. Miller RR. Prescribing habits of physicians: a review of studies on prescribing of drugs. *Drug Intell Clin Pharm.* 1973; 7:492-500.

7. Bush PJ. Prescribing is a social process. *Pharm Int.* 1980; 1:8–10.
8. Staudenmayer H, Lefkowitz MS. Physician-patient psychosocial characteristics influencing decision-making. *Soc Sci Med.* 1981; 15E:77–81.
9. Joyce CB, Last JM, Weatherall M. Personal factors as a cause of differences in prescribing by general practitioners. *Br J Prev Soc Med.* 1968; 22:170–7.
10. Miles DL. Multiple prescriptions and drug appropriateness. *Health Serv Res.* 1977; 12:3–10.
11. Linn LS. Physician characteristics and attitudes toward the legitimate use of psychotherapeutic drugs. *J Health Soc Behav.* 1971; 12:132–8.
12. Linn LS, Davis MS. Physicians' orientation toward the legitimacy of drug use and their preferred source of new drug information. *Soc Sci Med.* 1972; 6:199–203.
13. Linn LS. Some aspects of medical practice and the tendency to favor medication. Los Angeles, CA: Health Services Research Center, University of California at Los Angeles; 1978.
14. Department of Health, Education, and Welfare. Task Force on the Pharmacist's Clinical Role. Washington, DC: U.S. Government Printing Office; 1971.

8
Determinants of Medication Use

MICKEY C. SMITH

Why do people use medicines? That question is the reason for this chapter. In the previous chapter, we were introduced to the sociology of drug use and in many ways provided some answers to the question. In this chapter we will proceed from that well-prepared base to some practical specifics about the use of medication.

There are many reasons to study and to understand the determinants of medication use, for such behavior is not as simple and straightforward as logic might suggest. That logic would tell one that an intelligent rational individual suffering from disease, illness, sickness or any combination of these (Ref. 1, p. 16) who knows the existence of appropriate medication and has access to that medication would take it. The facts, however, suggest that there is many a slip between the medication cup and the lip. Who cares?

When medication is used inappropriately—too much *or* too little—it is important to the patient's well-being, certainly. There are others who have a stake in the process, too: the patient's family, his/her physician, any third party payer that might be involved, the manufacturer of the medication, regulatory agencies such as the Food and Drug Administration, and most assuredly the practicing pharmacist involved.

The reasons that people *do* and *do not* use medication properly are important to discover for, as in the isolation of an infective bacterium, once the cause is discovered, action can be taken.

What do we know and what can be done about it? Let us respond with a rather curious bit of research data.

CASE OF LAXATIVES

As part of a large study of medication use among a sample of noninstitutionalized elderly, Juergens, Smith, and Sharpe (2) focused especially on the use of laxatives. Although older people appear to use laxatives in greater proportions and more frequently than do the rest of the population, not *all* use them. That is consistent with the findings of the study under discussion.

Statistical analysis of the data from this study produced a profile of the elderly laxative users that suggests that they tended to live alone in a rural setting and reported using a single pharmacy that did not deliver medication as a source of over the counter (OTC) drugs. They were not likely to ask a pharmacist questions about OTC medicines and perceived the availability of pharmacy services as low. Laxative use was equally likely among men and women. In terms of health perceptions, the use of OTC laxatives was associated with lower perceptions of general health and a higher degree of perceived morbidity. Users also were more likely to report signs of anxiety and use more prescription medication than nonusers of laxatives. So what?

Gerbino and Gans (3) describe the management of patients with chronic constipation as "one of the most frustrating problems in geriatric medicine." Especially troublesome are patients who are laxative dependent or abuse laxatives. Cummings (4) has estimated that women constitute 90% of this group.

Poe and Holloway (5) suggest that laxatives are "the most overused and abused of all drugs." They posited that advertising might be a major reason but also suggested custom and the lay referral system as factors. "Hundreds of thousands, if not millions, of people have adopted laxatives lore as a matter of faith. For many people the use of laxatives has been a lifelong custom, passed on from generation to generation." They suggest that "isolation and depression cause people to become self-conscious" and therefore constipated. Certainly other explanations suggest themselves. What kind of cooking and eating habits are practiced by people (whatever their ages) who live alone? Maybe they really need a laxative, although what may be needed is a better diet.

Eve and Friedsam (6) reported on a sample of more than 8000 over-60 north Texans and their use of vitamins and laxatives. Vitamins were selected as evidence of preventive health behavior and laxatives as evidence of curative behavior. Although the methods of analysis were somewhat different and each study collected data not duplicated in the other, there were some striking similarities in results between that study and the one reported here with regard to laxative use.

Eve and Friedsam found laxative use to be related positively to age, feelings of loneliness, being single, being dissatisfied with social interaction, having less education, having lower incomes, having less access to medical care, and having a lower level of perceived health. Although not identical with the results of the current studies, none of these results is inconsistent with it.

The picture of the laxative user as a relatively lonely, socially isolated "sick" person is reinforced by the findings of this study. Eve and Friedsam suggest as explanation:

- Poor health contributes to social isolation through lack of opportunity.
- Social isolation creates hypochondriasis, with self-medication for the somatic complaints an alternative to other solutions.

They do not suggest which is the more compelling.

Laxatives, indeed the entire process of evacuation, have been trivialized through jokes, television commercials, and jokes about television commercials. Yet laxatives are serious medicine. When used regularly, even daily, laxatives can have adverse physiological consequences, result in changes in drug effects, and, through fluid and electrolyte loss, affect or aggravate other problems.

It is apparent that long-term, chronic use of laxatives may be a problem, although data are sparse. In a Florida study among more than 3000 elderly, nearly 15% reported using laxatives. Further, nearly two-thirds of the laxatives had been used by the respondents for longer than 2 years, and nearly half were used on a daily basis (7).

More than 25 years ago Ernest Dichter (8), then "guru" of motivation research, found deep meaning in constipation.

In a psychological sense, irregular elimination is disturbing because the body is not functioning; control has been lost over it. It is not illness, but it is disquieting; it resembles impotence. On the other hand, bowel movements are accompanied by essentially pleasant feelings that ally it to sexual gratification. There is in elimination, as in sex, a relationship of tension and relief. However, as with sex, there are also feelings of inhibition, guilt, sin, and embarrassment.

A 1969 national survey (9) jointly sponsored by seven different government agencies shed some light on laxative use patterns. Among the findings:

- Forty-two percent of the respondents over the age of 65 (compared with 31% of the total sample) agreed with the statement, "People should do something regularly to help with bowel movements."
- Forty-seven percent of those over 65 (compared with 30% of the total sample) "Ever (did) anything to help with bowel movements."
- Fourteen percent of the over 65 (compared with 5% of the total) did something daily to help with bowel movements.
- People over 65 were nearly twice as likely as the total sample to overrely on bowel movement aids (i.e., do something daily or nearly daily to help with bowel movements, not on the advice of a physician).
- Although age breakdowns were not provided for this item, it appeared that the overreliers did not view daily laxative use as treatment, but rather as something more akin to hygiene.

The results of the studies referred to above suggest that not all of the reasons for the use of laxatives are necessarily medical or physiological. The same could be said for virtually all medications. Discovery of the reasons for medication use and appropriate action following these discoveries make a worthy future professional agenda for pharmacists—individually and collectively. We will suggest a framework for doing that and provide examples in the remainder of this chapter.

The framework for analysis flows from the work of Anderson and Newman (10) who propose a model of medical care utilization consisting of a three-stage sequence of: (*a*) predisposing, (*b*) enabling, and (*c*) need for care variables that interact in various ways to produce a continuum of utilization rates for the several components of medical care.

Our adaptation of the Anderson-Newman model is shown in general form in Figure 8.1, which requires some comment. First, the variables identified are exemplary rather than exhaustive. Indeed, variable identification is an ongoing process. Second, some variables are identified as more than one kind of factor. For example, Third Party Coverage can be both a predisposing and an enabling factor. In the first instance the patient who knows that his medication costs will be covered in whole or in part by a third party may be "predisposed" to think of medication when a health problem arises. Then, clearly, the existence of such coverage will "enable" some patients to acquire medication who might not otherwise be able to afford it. Finally, although logic and professional intuition suggest some of the relationships shown, not all have been demonstrated empirically.

UTILIZATION DECISIONS

Let us begin the discussion of the model at its *end*—the utilization decisions. Data on medication use ultimately reflect the results of these decisions. It is notable that the first decision that must be made is that of the patient (or his surrogate) that something is wrong. Nothing happens in the field of medication use until that decision is made (see Ref. 11).

The first drug-related decision is comparatively simple: "Will medication help or is some other action (diet, exercise, surgery) indicated?" Nearly all serious research suggests

	Predisposing factors →	Enabling factors →	Need for care factors →	Utilization decisions
Patient variables	Doctor Pharmacist Age Sex Race Prior experience Marital status Media exposure Family Psychographics Residence	Doctor Pharmacist Relationship Family Education Symptoms Income Residence Third party coverage	Diagnosis Symptoms Perceived morbidity	Use a drug (versus other therapy) Use a specific drug Use a specific drug product Acquire the drug Whether and how to administer the drug Discontinue use
Medication variables	Cost Legal status		Legal status Dosage form Dosage schedule Therapeutic class Effectiveness Safety	
Delivery system variables	Pharmacy services Marketing practices Medical practices Third party coverage Institutionalization	Pharmacy services Marketing practices Medical practices Third party coverage Institutionalization	Diagnosis Marketing practices Medical practices Third party coverage Institutionalization	

Figure 8.1. Model for the study of determinants of medication use. Adapted from Anderson R, Newman J. Societal and individual determinants of medical care utilization. Milbank Mem Fund Q 1973;51:91–124.

that people confronted with some kind of symptom are more likely *not* to use medications than to use them. Indeed, a recent nationwide study found that people with everyday health problems used a prescription drug only 11% of the time and an OTC drug only 35% of the time—a total of less than half.

What of those who do decide to use a medication? They must still decide whether to self-medicate (with an OTC product or with an on-hand prescription drug) or enter the medical care system leading, in the majority of cases, to the use of a prescription drug. In either of these cases someone, or some combination of persons, must yet decide which drug to use, which product containing that drug to use, how to use the drug, and when to stop using the drug. Entangled with these decisions and complicating them are such factors as: patient compliance, physician-prescribing capabilities, coverage by third party formularies, promotional activities of the manufacturers, and decisions about need for care.

NEED FOR CARE

The most rational view of medications would suggest that sick people would use them and people who are not sick would not. The fact is that not every sickness lends itself to easy diagnosis. Thus, even though morbidity is comparatively highly correlated to medication use in most studies, the morbidity is frequently perceived and often not medically confirmed. Verbrugge (12) recognizes this issue in her model of legal drug use (see Fig. 8.2 and her article in the reading that follows this chapter).

ENABLING FACTORS

Many factors make it easier to use medications. (Their absence constitutes barriers to use, of course.) From the patient's perspective one must consider:

- The doctor-patient relationship and the pharmacist-patient relationship as well as the patient's satisfaction with each
- The family structure and medication-taking practices of the family members
- The education of the patient as well as his/her socioeconomic class
- Residence (i.e., rural or urban) as a measure of accessibility of care
- Third party coverage, especially as this factor interacts with income

The medications themselves may vary in their effects on use. Variables to be considered include:

- Legal status: prescription, OTC, narcotics
- Brand name versus generic issues
- Dosage forms that affect portability, compliance
- Comparative effectiveness
- Comparative safety
- Cost-benefit ratios and effects on such patient concerns as quality of life

The marketing activities of the pharmaceutical industry are just one group of variables in the medication delivery system that help determine whether medication will, in fact, be used. Some of these activities are directed at the prescribing physician (and at the pharmacists). The complexities of the simple act of prescribing are described in cogent fashion in the accompanying paper by Hepler, Segal, and Freeman (p. 000).

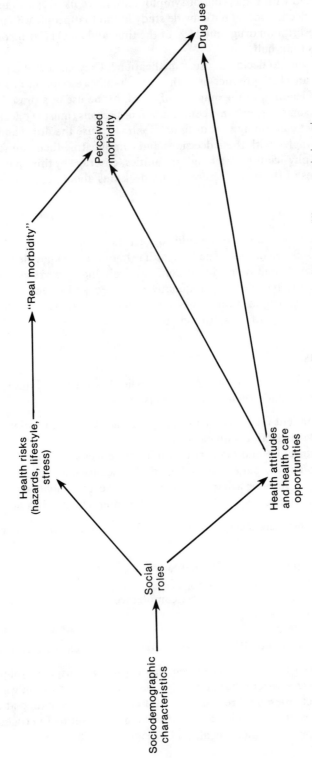

Figure 8.2. Model of legal drug use. Adapted from Verbrugge LM. Sex differences in legal drug use. J Soc Issues 1982;38:59–76.

PREDISPOSING FACTORS

In the list of predisposing factors are such "mundane" factors as the age and sex of the patient. Mundane perhaps, but definitely important. We have added three readings (by Verbrugge, by Smith and Sharpe, and by Bush and Davidson) to demonstrate that age (such as being a child or being an elder) and sex, especially being female, may make a difference in medication use that cannot be totally explained by illness experience.

There are many factors that may be predisposing but have not been explored and/or quantified through research. How much effect do television commercials have? What are the consequences of education in the schools about drug abuse on use of the legitimate medications? Are some medications overvalued while others are thought of as something less than medicine? What has been the effect of sales of medications in grocery stores and quick stops?

We cannot hope to explore all of the factors that go into determining use of medications here. Indeed, there is hardly room even to identify them. Rather, let us examine another case study, the most widely prescribed class of medications in modern times, the minor tranquilizers. Even here, we can hope only to demonstrate, rather than explicate, the complexities of the medication use process.

CASE OF MINOR TRANQUILIZERS[a]

In 1982, the health research group of Ralph Nader's organization, Public Citizen, published a 108-page book entitled *Stopping Valium* (13). The book charged, among other things, that:

- Thousands of people are addicted to Valium and other benzodiazepines.
- Many of the 1.5 million people who have taken the drugs continuously for more than 4 months may be addicted and not know it.
- The drugs present special dangers to the elderly, to pregnant women, and to drivers.

In early 1983, it was announced that the recipient of the 1982 John Scott Medal Award for research was Dr. Leo H. Sternbach, the retired Roche chemist who invented Valium and its precursor, Librium. Sternbach was in good company, as previous winners of the award included Madame Curie, Thomas Edison, and James Salk.

How does it happen that a prestigious award is accorded the inventor of substances that a major consumer organization is committed to eliminating? Such an event is, in fact, a typical example of the ambivalence with which our society views the minor tranquilizers. The drugs are more than medicines. They are a social fact. Indeed, these drugs may be more social than medical. Both their use and the prescriptions for such use have been extensively studied and criticized.

Prescribing Studies

A number of studies of prescribing patterns for psychotropic drugs have been conducted. Unfortunately, many of these studies failed to distinguish between major and minor tran-

---

[a]Some materials in this section adapted from: Smith MC. Small comfort, a history of the minor tranquilizers. New York: Praeger Publishers, 1985.

quilizers, sedatives, antidepressants, and other drugs. Consequently, comparisons are often difficult. In this section, we will review the reports of a few of the studies.

Shapiro and Baron (14) were among the first to study the prescription of psychotropic drugs in a noninstitutionalized population. Their study was conducted in 11 of the 32 medical groups that then participated in the Health Insurance Plan of Greater New York. Even then, the data showed women receiving more psychotropic drugs at more than twice the rate of men. This class of drugs represented 12% of all prescriptions studied. Of all psychotropic drugs prescribed, 22% were minor tranquilizers. A notable finding, even in this early work, was that only one-third of the prescriptions for minor tranquilizers were written for diagnoses of mental, psychoneurotic, and personality disorders. The percentage so prescribed for all psychotropic drugs was only 18%.

Why do some psychiatrists prescribe drug therapy for their patients more than others? That was the question posed by Klerman (15) early in the tranquilizer era. Specifically, he tested the hypothesis that the degree of drug use was related to the degree of "authoritarianism" of the psychiatrist and found such a relationship in this study of one mental hospital. The confirmation of this link, suggested by others, was enriched by discussion of some potential implications of the findings. For example, the author constructed a summary of the treatment orientations and value preferences of the study group with the higher rate of drug use.

The psychiatrists in this group, to a greater extent than their colleagues in the "low" group, were found to value assertiveness, self-control, and forceful leadership. Holding these values, they were willing to assume a moderate degree of authority and exercise their medical responsibility in treating and caring for their patients. According to Klerman (15), "They consider it their obligation as physicians to use every reasonable means to promote symptom reduction, to relieve the patient's distress, and to maintain a relatively stable ward atmosphere." Such attempts at insight into physician drug-prescribing behavior have been extremely rare, and it should be noted that this study did not focus on minor tranquilizers.

Linn, in two related papers (16, 17), examined attitudes of a sample of 235 Los Angeles physicians toward use of Librium in certain situations. Physicians' general attitudes toward the use of medications were ascertained on the basis of their agreement with the following statements:

Statement	Percentage Agreeing
1. Certain medications are often very helpful in handling the social demands and stresses of everyday living.	79
2. A person should take pills only as a last resort.	17
3. A person is better off taking a sedative than missing a good night's sleep.	45
4. A person is better off taking a tranquilizer than going through the day tense and nervous.	57

Physicians in the sample were then asked to respond to a number of situations in which Librium was used. As a group, they were not in agreement over what constitutes legitimate use of the drug (see Table 8.1).

In the companion publication, Linn and Davis (17) added data on physicians' preferred sources of drug information. They reported that physicians preferring professional sources were significantly more likely to express conservative attitudes toward when drugs should be

Table 8.1.   Physician Evaluations of Legitimate Use of Librium from a Medical Point of View (n = 114)[a]

Drug-using Situation	Assessment of Legitimacy	(%)
A middle-aged housewife having marital trouble takes 15 mg of Librium daily to settle her nerves.	Very legitimate	34
	Somewhat legitimate	53
	Not very legitimate	7
	Illegitimate	6
		100
A college student takes 15 mg of Librium occasionally when the stresses and demands of college life become too great.	Very legitimate	20
	Somewhat legitimate	41
	Not very legitimate	21
	Illegitimate	18
		100
A physician takes 15 mg of Librium occasionally when the stresses and demands of his practice become overbearing.	Very legitimate	17
	Somewhat legitimate	38
	Not very legitimate	25
	Illegitimate	18
		100
A college student, highly anxious, takes 15 mg of Librium daily to combat anxiety.	Very legitimate	22
	Somewhat legitimate	31
	Not very legitimate	25
	Illegitimate	22
		100

[a]Reprinted with permission from Linn L. Physician characteristics and attitudes toward legitimate use of psychotherapeutic drugs. J Health Soc Behav 1971;12:132–139.

used than physicians preferring commercial sources, and they were significantly less likely to feel that medical advice from sources other than a physician was acceptable. Linn and Davis suggested that the medical professional contains "rather diverse philosophies of medication."

Williams (18) has reviewed this use of "mental" drugs for "body" ailments and suggests three factors relating to why psychotropic (mainly minor tranquilizer) drugs are prescribed for physical illness:

1. Secondary properties of the drugs. Examples include reserpine in cardiovascular disease and diazepam as a muscle relaxant in arthritis/rheumatism.
2. Coexistence of physical and psychiatric disease. This is purported to be a function of (a) increased likelihood of physical morbidity among the psychiatrically ill; (b) increased likelihood of psychiatric morbidity among the physically ill; (c) existence of some individuals who are prone to both types of illness.
3. Psychic component of somatic disease. (The evidence cited in support of this type of use is reported to be weak.)

It is, of course, more likely that a general practitioner will see the patient with some kind of mind/body problem.

Near the end of the first 25 years with the minor tranquilizers, T. Donald Rucker (19), a health economist, essayed a quantitative opinion about the causes of "irrational" prescribing of minor tranquilizers. His estimates, which appear in Table 8.2, reflect rather well the themes that have emerged, although the proportions hardly constitute a consensus.

Table 8.2.   Factors Leading to Irrational Prescribing Classified by Quartile of Probable Level of Importance [a]

Proportion of Problem		
50%	I.	Promotional activities sponsored by pharmaceutical manufacturers that are designed, directly or indirectly, to influence practitioner prescribing and dispensing
		Limitations in the medical record system
		Casual empiricism-practitioner interpretation of evidence regarding patient response to drug therapy
About 30%	II.	Drug product proliferation without significant therapeutic contribution
		Practitioner attitude toward treatment options in general and drug therapy in particular—the subjective component
		Patient behavior—designed to influence prescribing patterns and subvert coordination of care
About 20%	III.	Formal education received by practitioners
		Practitioner postgraduate education (excluding promotional activities identified in I but including all other inputs or lack thereof)
		Practitioner proficiency in diagnosis and selection of optimum modality within treatment model
Nearly 10%	IV.	Various characteristics of practice environment
		Conflict of interest situations
		Posture of professional associations toward drug use and drug industry

[a]Adapted from Rucker T. Production and prescribing of minor tranquilizers: a macro view. Paper presented to the American Orthopsychiatric Association, 1980.

Utilization Studies

In addition to studies of prescribing and prescriptions, some researchers have used the patient as the unit of analysis, i.e., what proportion of a population used the drug under study? Parry (20) was one of the first to present extensive data on the utilization rates for psychotropic drugs. Parry noted that psychotropic drugs accounted for 14% of all prescriptions in the period 1963–1965 and pointed out that two-thirds of these prescriptions were refills, compared with about 50% for other drugs. "The preponderance of refills" Parry wrote, "[tended] to operate against any sharp decline of consumption."

Manheimer and his associates (21), in a paper published at about the same time as that by Parry, studied psychotropic drug use by adults in California. Based on a sample of just over 1000, the study showed that about 30% had used some type of psychotropic drug in the previous 12 months. About one in six used the drugs frequently, with women users outnumbering men by about two to one.

As with many utilization studies, the results are clouded by the combination of several types of psychotropic drugs, both prescription and nonprescription. One interesting finding with regard to use of prescription drugs (particularly tranquilizers) by lower income groups was that while they were less likely overall to use them, their use, when it occurred, tended to be frequent. Manheimer et al. suggested that only those with substantial need in this group actually get the drugs.

Prevalence of use, however, varied greatly by sex and age of the person, by therapeutic class, and by intended and actual source of drug. Persons between 45 and 59 years old were more likely than others to use prescription drugs from medical sources. Use of OTC drugs and prescription drugs obtained from nonmedical sources was most prevalent among persons aged 18–29. Overall, prevalence of psychotherapeutic drug use was highest among persons under 30 years. Persons who obtained prescription drugs from nonmedical sources were more likely than others to use a variety of drugs, but were less likely to use any drug regularly.

In the first quarter century of the minor tranquilizers, only one truly national study of utilization was conducted. A number of researchers were involved in this project, which was conducted under joint sponsorship of the National Institute of Mental Health (NIMH), the Social Research Group (George Washington University), and the Institute of Research in Social Behavior (22). The research resulted in a considerable number of publications, some of which contained similar data. Because theirs was the only one of this magnitude in the 25-year history of the minor tranquilizers, it deserves special attention.

The comprehensive report of this collaborative study sppeared in the *Archives of General Psychiatry* in June 1973 (22). The data were based on extensive personal interviews (60–90 minutes each) with 2552 adults selected through "rigorous probability sampling methods" throughout the 48 contiguous states in late 1970 and early 1971.

As with many other studies, this one included a variety of psychotherapeutic agents. Because of our focus on the minor tranquilizers, and in the interest of space, we list below some of the specific findings based on the survey relative to this class of drugs.

- Most current users felt they were helped by them.
- The percentage using minor tranquilizers/sedatives during the previous year is shown below.

			Age		
	18–29	30–44	45–49	60–74	All
Men	5	7	9	11	8
Women	12	21	22	25	20

		Region		
	Northeast	North Central	South	West
Men	7	7	7	13
Women	18	17	21	25

- Women were more likely than men to say they would take a tranquilizer in advance of a possibly unpleasant event.
- The United States would rank about in the middle of western countries in level of use of minor tranquilizers, and the male-to-female use ratio is similar.
- About 5% of users used minor tranquilizers daily for at least 2 months (defined in the study as "high" use).
- Among users whose use level of minor tranquilizers was "high," the following characteristics appeared important:
  1. Greater proportion in middle age
  2. Greater proportion in the West
  3. Greater proportion in lower socioeconomic class (similar to Parry's findings)
- There was little overlap between prescription and nonprescription tranquilizer use.

Using a symptom checklist and a social readjustment scale, it was possible to classify persons in terms of emotional distress and life crises. One of the principal findings was that 60% of the men and 70% of the women who used psychotherapeutic drugs in the year preceding the interview scored high on one or both indexes, psychic distress and life crises. Among the relatively small group of persons who used the drugs daily for 2 months or longer, the figures were somewhat higher: 70% of the men and 80% of the women.

A majority of the remaining drug users who were not classified as high on one index achieved a rating of at least moderate on the other. Only 2–3% of those who used drugs daily for 2 or more months were classified as low on both indexes, as compared with 16% of persons who used no psychotherapeutic drugs in the preceding year.

Why these differences in prescribing and utilization of this fascinating group of drugs? The reasons discovered to date are many and affect and are affected by both the patient and his physician.

Throughout their history, the minor tranquilizers, their use and prescription, have been studied in efforts to determine reasons for their popularity. Various hypotheses, resulting mainly from research, are presented here.

In 1970 and 1972, Pflanz and colleagues (23) conducted a survey in Hannover, West Germany, among 1251 subjects. They found that 14.7% of the men and 27.1% of the women took tranquilizers "regularly" and "presently" (sic). Consumption was higher in the upper and middle classes, particularly for men. They also found a strong relationship between drug consumption and mental health (as assessed on a 22-item scale). Drug use was shown to be related to subjective ill health and unrelated to objective indicators of health status. The researchers saw the data as supporting a psychiatric medical model rather than a sociological one.

This last issue was at the core of the study. Pflanz et al. reviewed the literature of sociological studies of tranquilizer use and found that although a variety of cultural and social variations were reported, the one unanimous finding was a higher rate of use in women— and this finding was not dependent on the respective status of women in the various counties. In the Pflanz study, some of the findings were:

- Users were more "health conscious."
- Homemakers were not found to be heavier users than employed women.
- There was no relationship between drug use and role status inconsistency.
- Some 29 questions about "mental health" distinguished between users and nonusers, which was "true for mainly somatic symptoms, for psychosomatic symptoms, and for purely psychological symptoms" (perhaps most significant).

Pflanz and colleagues made a special effort to isolate the factors involved in the consistently higher use of tranquilizers by women. They found it appropriate to assume that women have more psychological symptoms and therefore take tranquilizers more often than men. They also found support for the hypothesis that women perceive and express more symptoms of ill mental health than do men. They finally raised an interesting reverse question: Is the question why do women take more, or why do men take less? Again, the assumption appears to be that less is better.

According to Cooperstock and Lennard (24), the people who are most likely to receive prescriptions for minor tranquilizers fall into three groups:

1. Those who describe their problem to the physician in psychological or social terms.
2. Those who describe a physical complaint (insomnia, stomach pains, backache), but who are discovered to experience "problems of living." (For women these tend

to relate to structural strains in the nuclear family. For men they are more likely to be job related.)

3. Those with chronic somatic illness for whom the drugs may be prescribed to diminish stress generally and in reaction to the illness particularly.

They noted also that "since the legitimation of a personal problem as a 'disease' affords considerable advantages, it is readily 'traded' for a medical diagnosis."

Publication of such studies culminated in one of the strongest attacks on the increased prescribing of Valium, Librium, and other drugs. Waldron (25) presented a plethora of arguments (some supported, others not supported) to the effect that these and many other drugs are often prescribed for nonmedical (i.e., social) reasons. She referred to the "extremely rapid" increase in the use of Valium and Librium, referring especially to the advance of Valium, from its introduction in 1963 to a position as top seller in 1972. (In fact, that is not "rapid" by drug industry standards and suggests, instead, a steady rise based on positive experiences.)

Quoting drug advertisements for such conditions as a major discord in parent-child relations, she noted (25) that they appear

to offer a resolution for a common and difficult dilemma for doctors, namely, how to respond to a patient who is distressed by psychological and social problems, given that both the doctor and the patient expect the doctor to do something to relieve the patient's distress in an appointment that averages less than 20 minutes.

Such prescribing for social and psychological problems, Waldron noted, "appears to satisfy substantial needs of both doctor and patient." Indeed, even she agreed that the period of increasing use of Valium and Librium was also a period of increasing social problems.

Waldron also argued that the vaunted effect of the major tranquilizers on mental hospital discharges was greatly overstated. Whether her arguments are correct or not, the fact is that many people in the 1950s believed in this relationship and that belief must certainly have contributed to the ultimate acceptance of the minor tranquilizers.

It has been hypothesized that in achievement-oriented societies, illness may be used as justification for a culturally induced sense of personal failure to fulfill socially prescribed role obligations. Prince (26) has produced data that were consistent with this hypothesis, which had been formally proposed by Cole and Lejeune (27). In a study with admitted limitations of previously hospitalized patients, Prince found that welfare recipients were more likely to consider their health as fair/poor than those not on welfare. Cornely (28), in a commentary, denounced not only the study itself, but studies of the genre, urging social scientists to study such factors as employment, housing, nutrition, environmental sanitation, and personal accountability.

Other researchers continued to search for determinants of tranquilizer use in a variety of places.

Webb and Colette (29) examined a hypothesis that urban crowding might be associated with a higher incidence of use of stress-alleviative drugs. They found the reverse relationship and also that such drug use increases directly with the number of persons living alone.

Radelet (30) set out "to identify health beliefs and social networks that distinguish users from nonusers." His population consisted of only 181 university students (46 of whom used tranquilizers), but his findings were interesting. He found the users, in comparison with nonusers, to be:

- More reluctant to admit unpleasurable feelings

- More likely to define anxiety as a biophysical problem
- Less critical of OTC drug advertisements
- More likely to have friends and relatives who use tranquilizers (especially the father)
- More anxious as measured by Spielberger's State-Trait Anxiety Inventory

Radelet acknowledged that symptoms of anxiety play a role in tranquilizer use but argued that they are only part of the picture. He wrote, "The extensive prevalence of tranquilizer use in American Society is therefore not indicative simply of high levels of anxiety, but also is associated with a general cultural framework that tends to define anxiety as an individual biophysical reality that warrants and necessitates drug treatment."

Such cultural definitions of medical situations present dilemmas for the prescribing physician.

PRESCRIBING DILEMMAS

In 1980, Dr. Louis Lasagna published a collection of "point/counter-point" papers under the broad title, *Controversies in Therapeutics.* Dr. John Morgan drew the challenge of the position that perhaps our society is not overmedicated. The benzodiazepines were one class of drugs that he discussed in a cogent and pragmatic fashion:

> Everyone seems to know that we are an overmedicated society, and one imagines editors of publications small and large, common and arcane, swallowing benzodiazepines while rushing to meet a deadline with an article on the overmedicated society.

Lasagna's book exemplifies well the proposition that physicians face many dilemmas in their choice of drug therapy. Further, the use of the term "controversies" in the title illustrates the divergence of opinion that often exists. Among the controversial types of therapy were blockers, antacids, aspirin, opium derivatives, and, of course, benzodiazepines.

Morgan's Chapter 6 specifically addressed the issue of Valium use. He noted that Valium has an ample supply of both critics and defenders, and that, curiously, both sides tend to buttress their arguments with the same findings and data. Some of Morgan's comments offer an appropriate staging for our brief discussion of the dilemmas that the minor tranquilizers have brought to the prescribing physician.

> One reason we stumble over questions of "appropriate" drug utility is our lack of understanding of the cultural context of drug use. We are asked to define a "proper" level of medication in society when we do not understand the social utility of powerful chemicals.

> It is presumptuous—even preposterous—to define appropriateness solely from a clinical view.

> Until we make more progress in defining the social utility of drugs and the social utility of health and well-being, it behooves us to be a bit more humble about appropriateness.

> Diagnosis and conventional medical thought have essentially nothing to do with the usual use of benzodiazepines.

Morgan refers to a "somewhat tattered army of academics" caught between those who argue, forcefully, both sides of the overmedicated issue. Equally tattered, certainly, must be the practicing physician trying to make prescribing decisions while awaiting some resolution of the conflict between the political and medical leadership. The foregoing surely demonstrates some of the physicians' dilemmas, a few which will be reviewed briefly here.

"Do Something" Dilemma

In his book *Profession of Medicine,* sociologist Eliot Friedson (31) argued for the activist orientation of the medical practitioner: "The aim of the practitioner is not knowledge but action. Successful action is preferred, but action with very little chance of success is to be preferred over no action at all." He further noted that sociologist Talcott Parsons had observed that activism is, in fact, a basic part of the American value system.

Physicians, themselves action-oriented, are thus faced with an "anxious" patient who also expects something to be done. Further, given the notoriety of the minor tranquilizers, the patient is likely to know that something can be done. On what basis can physicians withhold antianxiety therapy?

Definition/Diagnosis Dilemmas

Although there are paper and pencil anxiety tests and clinical algorithms for diagnosis of clinical anxiety, these are relatively recent developments. Physicians have had no mental sphygmomanometer with which to measure mental pressure as with blood pressure. They do what they can, but rather well.

A recurring medical problem is the difficulty in diagnosing and treating depression. Although this may seem removed from the present subject, it is not, for depression is apparently often misdiagnosed and consequently treated as anxiety. Kline (32) has called depression the "most misunderstood of all major diseases," advising that "any case of anxiety that does not respond to appropriate treatment within 1 or 2 months should be reconsidered as possibly having an underlying depression. Many patients with such depression develop anxiety *secondarily* and do not respond to treatment until the primary depression is relieved."

The laboratory test, so helpful in other forms of illness, has not had much impact in this area. By 1980, however, some promise of progress had appeared. Gold et al. (33) reported in 1981 that the use of a combination of the dexamethasone suppression test and the thyrotropin-releasing hormone test had high diagnostic value, although they warned against use "without regard for the entire clinical presentation or as a substitute for medical observation and judgment."

Information Dilemma

How much of the information supplied by the drug manufacturers should physicians accept? How much should they believe? What are their alternatives?

Clearly, commercial information is biased, although the Food and Drug Administration (FDA) has considerable authority to require a certain balance and to correct misleading messages. In any case, the information is palatable, convenient, and omnipresent. Further, the "scientific" information is often conflicting and sometimes unscientific.

Medicalization Dilemma

In 1971, Lewis (34) reported that nearly two-thirds of his (nonscientific) sample of physician respondents felt that other physicians were prescribing too many tranquilizers. He made clear, through the example of a Valium advertisement, his belief that a major reason for overprescribing was the "medicalization of human problems," noting that "once daily living is defined as disease, how logical it is for us to attempt to treat that disease."

Again, if one looks to Friedson's exposition on medicine, one finds an explanation, if not an excuse, for the medicalization of human problems. As he observes (and supports by argument), "The medical profession has first claim to jurisdiction over the label of illness and anything to which it may be attached, irrespective of its capacity to deal with it effectively." In fact, people come to physicians because there is anxiety in their lives. By the simple act of seeking medical assistance, the patient has medicalized the problem. Of course, by treating the patient, the physician confirms that this medicalization was appropriate. If the drug works, even if only briefly, the actions of both patient and physician are reinforced, and the drugs have worked. Criticism of the effectiveness of the benzodiazepines, at least, has been rare.

One may argue (and many do) that the drugs do not cure the anxiety and do not eliminate the cause. True enough, but the same can be said of antihypertensive medication, antiarthritics, and even aspirin. Should the patient be denied relief of mental discomfort when it is caused by problems of daily living?

Unless and until society is provided with an acceptable alternative to the physician in dealing with their personal problems, as long as they continue to seek relief from this source, it is unrealistic to expect the physician to turn them away because they have a problem with which he or she should not deal.

Society has medicalized human problems, it appears. Medicine has, perhaps, been an accessory, and the pharmaceutical industry, certainly, has provided both with the means. To expect either of the latter parties to do, or have done, otherwise bespeaks a considerable naiveté.

Friedson (31) pointed out that "while medicine is hardly independent of the society in which it exists, by becoming a vehicle for society's values it came to play a major role in the forming and shaping of the social meanings imbued with such a role." He argued that physicians became "moral entrepreneurs," seeing "mental illness" in cases in which the layperson has come to the physician for help. If the physician eschews treatment (with drugs), the patient is likely to be disappointed (the activism value), and the physician becomes equally a moral entrepreneur, saying, in effect, "You were wrong to come to me. Pull yourself together and get your life in order." However correct that judgment may be, the personal burden on the physician can be enormous.

LOOK AHEAD

Our struggles to deal with the role of the minor tranquilizers, very real in its own right, is also part of several other social concerns including the future role of the physician. Many of the issues that these drugs have caused to surface have yet to be resolved. Each of us will be involved in that resolution.

Mary Davis (35) has described the kind of problem we face:

> The role of the physician, according to Webster, is to "treat disease"; a physician is one "skilled in the art of healing." This seems a clear enough statement, one which should occasion little controversy, and yet many people today are confused as to exactly what duties a physician is to perform. It is widely accepted that one's life-style and environment may be etiological factors in diseases such as ulcers and hypertension (as well, of course, as many psychiatric diseases). Does it then become the physician's responsibility to modify the life-style or environment of the patient? Each physician must, finally, answer this question for himself, deciding where lies the dividing line between medical practice and unwarranted interference in another's life. Society, however, has not yet drawn this line clearly; until it does so, physicians and patients alike will continue to be confused regarding the physician's role.

It is an intentional oversimplification to describe the minor tranquilizers as drugs used to treat the symptoms of minor mental irregularity—not so different from a laxative, antacid, or cold tablet, except that they affect the mind. Although certainly not innocuous, they are also not as dramatically dangerous as, for example, lysergic acid diethylamide (LSD). Yet we have dealt with these drugs in an emotional, sometimes irrational, fashion. Kline (36) said, "There seems to be a icebox built somewhere into our skulls which is the seat of cold logic and rational thought, and next to it is a hothouse of irrational, affect-based beliefs," and the two do not interact. Indeed, that seems often to have been the case with our views of the minor tranquilizers.

But what next?

Nearly 15 years ago, Kline (36) suggested that the year 2000 would see drugs that, inter alia,

- Provide safe, short-acting intoxication
- Prolong or shorten memory
- Provoke or relieve guilt
- Control affect and aggression
- Shorter or extend experienced time

These and other predictions were not idle futuristic exercises, but rather serious predictions of a knowledgeable scientist.

Surely it is time to review our performance with the comparatively simple drugs we have had for a quarter century or more to attempt to discover how better to deal with those that are to come, especially if pharmacists are to exercise a greater and more responsible role in the rational use of medication.

REFERENCES

1. Smith M, Knapp D. Pharmacy, drugs and medical care. 4th ed. Baltimore: Williams & Wilkins, 1987.
2. Juergens J, Smith MC, Sharpe TR. Determinants of nonprescription laxative use among an elderly population. J Soc Admin Pharm 1984;2:174–179.
3. Gerbino PP, Gans JA. Antacids and laxatives for symptomatic relief in the elderly. J Am Geriatr Soc 1982;30(Supplement):581–587.
4. Cummings JH. Laxative abuse. Gut 1979;15:578.
5. Poe WD, Holloway DA. Drugs and the aged. New York: McGraw-Hill, 1980, pp 39–40.
6. Eve SB, Friedsam HJ. Factors influencing older persons' use of nonprescription medicines for prevention and cure. Paper presented to the XII International Congress of Gerontology. Hamburg, 1981.
7. Stewart RB. Laxative use among an elderly population: a report from the Dunedin Program. Contemp Pharm Prac 1982;5:166–169.
8. Dichter E. Handbook of consumer motivations. New York: McGraw-Hill, 1964, pp 202–203.
9. Anonymous. A study of health practice and opinions. Final Report, FDA Contract. Philadelphia: National Analysts, 1972.
10. Anderson R, Newman J. Societal and individual determinants of medical care utilization. Milbank Mem Fund Q 1973;51:91–124.
11. Twaddle A, Hessler R. A sociology of health. St. Louis: CV Mosby, 1977.
12. Verbrugge LM. Sex differences in legal drug use. J Soc Issues 1986;38:59–76.
13. Bargmann E, Wolfe S, Levin J. Stopping valium. Washington, DC: The Public Citizen Health Research Group, 1982.
14. Shapiro S, Baron S. Prescriptions for psychotropic drugs in a non-institutional population. Pub Health Rep 1961;76:481–488.
15. Klerman G. Sociopsychologic characteristics of drug therapy. Am J Psych 1960;117:111–117.
16. Linn L. Physician characteristics and attitudes toward legitimate use of psychotherapeutic drugs. J Health Soc Behav 1971;12:132–139.

17. Linn L, Davis M. Physicians' orientation toward the legitimacy of drug use and their preferred source of new drug information. Soc Sci Med 1972;6:199-203.
18. Williams P. Physical ill—health and psychotropic drug prescription—a review. Psych Med 1978;8:683-693.
19. Rucker T. Production and prescribing of minor tranquilizers: a macro view. Paper presented to the American Orthopsychiatric Association, 1980.
20. Parry H. Use of psychotropic drugs by US adults. Pub Health Rep 1968;83:799-810.
21. Manheimer D, Mellinger G, Balter M. Psychotherapeutic drugs. Calif Med 1968;109:445-451.
22. Parry H, Manheimer D, Mellinger G, Balter M. National patterns of psychotherapeutic drug use. Arch Gen Psych 1973;28:769-783.
23. Pflanz M, Basler H, Schwoon D. The use of tranquilizing drugs by a middle aged population in a West German city. J Health Soc Behav 1972;18:194-205.
24. Cooperstock R, Lennard H. Some social meanings of tranquilizer use. Soc Health Illness 1979;1:331-347.
25. Waldron I. Increased prescribing of Valium, Librium and other drugs. Intern J Health Serv 1977;1:37-62.
26. Prince E. Welfare status, illness and subjective health definition. Am J Pub Health 1978;68:865-871.
27. Cole S, Lejeune R. Illness and legitimation of failure. Soc Rev 1972;37:347-356.
28. Cornely P. Comments on welfare status, illness and subjective health definition. Am J Pub Health 1978;68:870-871.
29. Webb S, Colette J. Urban ecological and household correlates of stress—alleviative drug use. Am Behav Scientist 1975;18:750-770.
30. Radelet M. Health beliefs, social networks, and tranquilizer use. J Health Soc Behav 1981;22:165-173.
31. Friedson E. Profession of medicine. New York: Dodd, Mead, 1970.
32. Kline N. Antidepressant medications. JAMA 1976;227:1158-1160.
33. Gold M, Bennett G, Keller B, Tharp C. Diagnosis of depression in the 1980s. JAMA 1981;245:1562-1564.
34. Lewis D. The physician's contribution to the drug abuse scene. Tufts Med Alum Bull 1971;30:36-39.
35. Davis M. Disease and its treatment. Comp Psych 1977;18:231-233.
36. Kline N. Psychotropic drugs in the year 2000. Springfield, IL: Charles C Thomas, 1971.

SUGGESTED READINGS

Predisposing Factors

1. Jackson JD, et al. An investigation of prescribed and nonprescribed medicine use behavior within the household context. Soc Sci Med 1982;16:2009-2015.
2. Kaufert PA, Gilbert P. The context of menopause: psychotropic drug use and menopausal status. Soc Sci Med 1986;23:747-755.

Enabling Factors

1. Juergens JP, Smith MC, Sharpe TR. Mothers' anxiety and medication use in rural families on welfare. Am J Hosp Pharm 1983;40:103-106.
2. Fincham JE, Wertheimer AI. Using the health belief model to predict initial drug therapy. Soc Sci Med 1985;20:101-105.
3. Hadsall RS, Norwood GT. Differences in drug usage patterns between medicaid and private-pay population. Med Market Media 1977;12:52-57.

Need For Care Factors

1. Smith MC, Sharpe TR, Banahan BF. Patient response to symptoms. J Clin Hosp Pharm 1981;6:267–276.
2. Anonymous. Health care practices and perceptions. Washington DC: Harry Heller Research Corporation (for the Proprietary Association), 1984.

SELECTED READINGS

MEDICINES AND "DRUGS": WHAT DO CHILDREN THINK?[b]

Patricia J. Bush
Frances R. Davidson

Taking medicine during childhood is a common activity (1-4). Minor ailments such as colds, stomach aches, headaches, and muscular discomforts, are usually treated in the home with medicines available locally, both with and without prescriptions. The underlying assumption with regard to children's medicine use is that parents play the major role in deciding what kind of ailments the child has, and whether medication is needed. If it is, then the adult provides it. Studies of rates of children's medicine use (1-4), and children's noncompliance (5) have been based solely on interviews with parents. In this, as in other areas of behavior, children are assumed to be passive recipients of parent-initiated action. There is little or no information about children's autonomy in medicine use, or the development and sources of their beliefs in this potentially confusing area, where medicines both help and harm, where drugs are sometimes medicines and sometimes abusable substances, and where medicines are sometimes given to treat problems caused by abusable substances.

This article reports some of the findings of the exploratory study, specifically information about how much autonomy children say they have in medicine use, children's perceptions of their own and their mothers' probabilities of taking medicines for selected illnesses, and some examples of how children's thought processes in an area which has great potential for misunderstanding lead them to errors in beliefs about medicines and abusable substances.

The rate of medicine use reported among the exploratory study group of 64 elementary school children was consistent with that found in prior studies (1-4) where adults were asked about their children's use of medicines and vitamins.

The responses of the children to the series of questions about their autonomy in medicine use—taking it by themselves, asking for it, getting it for themselves and others, buying it—indicate that, for most school-aged children, the medicine cabinet is unlocked. Most children do not view themselves as passive recipients of medicines, but as actively involved in the process. Thus, for many children, perceptions of appropriate behavior relative to medicine use may be formed through their own decision making, and not merely observing what others do to them and for themselves. More than two-fifths of the children said they had asked someone specifically for aspirin at some time. Of interest was that some children called aspirin only by its brand name, most often Bayer, although other proprietary analgesics, such as Tylenol and St. Joseph's, were also mentioned. It is possible that these children were not aware that some of these products were aspirin. When asked to name all of the

[b]Edited and reprinted with permission from Bush PJ, Davidson FR. Medicines and "drugs": what do children think? Health Educ Q 1982;9:113–128. A follow-up study, more technical in its presentation, appears as "A longitudinal study of children and medicines" in Brenner DD, Speiser P, eds. Topics in Pharmaceutical Sciences. Amsterdam: Elsevier Publishers, 1985.

medicines they could, children often listed both brand and generic names of aspirin. The impression given was that proprietary drug advertising has been very successful, and that this is an area where children might profit from educational programs designed to teach them, for example, that Bayer works no better than other, less expensive, house brands of aspirin. This type of information may be particularly appropriate for children who are most likely to be buying proprietary medicines on their own, older children, and children living in neighborhoods where there are many commercial establishments selling proprietary medicines.

The degree of independence in medicine use of children suggests that, when physicians are prescribing medicines for children, and when pharmacists are dispensing or selling medicines to children, their efforts to ensure that the medicines are taken appropriately be addressed at the children, and not only at the adult who has come with the child. As noted by Lewis et al., "while the child is the object of pediatric care, few physicians—to our knowledge—treat the child . . . as co-equal participants in the process of care" (6).

Although finding that children differentiated between their and their mothers' probabilities of taking medicines, was consistent with Campbell's work, the patterns were unexpected. Campbell (13) found that hospitalized children were more likely to define symptoms as indicating illness in their mothers than themselves, and this suggested that children might also say their mothers were more likely to take medicines than themselves. Also, surveys have found rates of medicine use during childbearing years to be higher than that of schoolage children (1-4). Thus, children may observe medicine use by their mothers more often than they use medicines themselves. However, for six of eight health problems, the responses indicated that children saw themselves as more likely than their mothers to take medicines. Except for toothache, the health problems for which children saw themselves as more likely to take medicines are common childhood illnesses. Lack of familiarity, however, did not account for children finding that mothers were more suitable candidates for medicines than themselves for trouble sleeping and nervousness. The average child's perceptions of medicine use probabilities may be objectively based. Indeed, it seems likely that mothers' nerves are more often treated than children's, and that children's colds are given more attention than mothers'.

An extention of Campbell's suggested explanation of his findings may fit the medicine situation as well, however. Campbell (7) suggested that children may protect themselves from perceptions of their own vulnerability, commenting that differences relate to objective appraisals, but that ascription of illness is subjectively as well as objectively determined. The pattern in Campbell's data was consistent with a tendency for children to maintain adequate self-images in their

> perception of and response to the social world; the self is perceived as a valued object to be protected and enhanced. If the symptoms themsleves are not too overwhelming, it may be both easy and important to deny illness, to preserve the image of health as a valued attribute of the self. To see illness in other person may not be as threatening.

These needs to perceive themselves as not ill may also account for children's greater willingness to see themselves engaged in activities that will return them to states of health when they are ill. Children may thus both be less willing to define themselves as ill when interpreting symptoms, but more likely to see themselves as taking action for specific illnesses.

Bibace and Walsh (8) have reviewed approaches to the development of causal thinking in children and concluded that theories cannot lead to predictions about how the form of children's cognitions will be manifested in a particular content area. That is, prior knowledge that a child was in a preoperational developmental stage, would not lead to predictions about what, for example, a child would respond to questions about how medicines help or abusable substances harm. As these authors show, however, explanations in a particular area such as health, can usually be classified into broad Piagetian categories and associated with children's age groups. Although it was not a goal of the research reported here to classify children's responses to questions about medicines and abusable substances into developmental categories, it was expected that the combination of children in the concrete operational stages of cognitive development, and questions about medicines and abusable substances—a potentially extremely confusing area of health beliefs—would lead to responses showing considerable misinformation in children's minds. As was shown for two children, age seven and nine, their literal approach to things they heard, e.g., "drugs mess up your mind," led them to reason that drugs must then be taken out of the head, for the drug taker to get back to normal. For these children, drugs were substances that are shot in the arm, and medicines were pills that, along with booster shots, can fix up problems caused by drinking and drugs. It is easy to understand why some children said that bad drugs come from drug stores.

Although expectations about children's misinformation were borne out, one may note that adults also have a great deal of misinformation about medicines and abusable substances, and in their behaviors provide children with mixed messages and sources of anxiety. Not only do children appear to need more knowledge about medicines and abusable substances, but they may need a forum in which to discuss the beliefs that cause them stress, and to deal with misinformation that may cause them physical or economic harm.

The study reported here should be regarded as exploratory only. Data limitations did not permit extensive analyses by demographic or other characteristics. Data from the larger study which is currently underway should provide much more information on children's knowledge, and the development of their orientations toward medicines and abusable substances.

REFERENCES

1. Haggerty RJ, Roghmann KJ: Noncompliance and self medication. *Pediatr Clin N Am 19*:101-115, 1972.
2. Bush PJ, Rabin DL: Who's using nonprescribed medicines? *Med Care 14*:1014-1023, 1976.
3. Rabin DL, Bush PJ: Who's using prescribed medicines? *Drugs Health Care 3*:89-100, 1976.
4. Gagnon JP, Salber EJ, Greene SB: Patterns of prescription and nonprescription drug use in a Southern rural area. *Pub Health Rep 93*:433-437, 1978.
5. Sackett DL, Haynes RB (Eds): *Compliance with Therapeutic Regimens.* Baltimore, Johns Hopkins University Press, 1976.
6. Lewis CE, Lewis MA, Lorimer A, et al: *Child-Initiated Care: A Study of the Determinants of the Illness Behavior of Children.* National Technical Information Service, U.S. Department of Commerce, Springfield VA, p. 309.
7. Campbell JD: Attribution of illness: another double standard. *J Health Soc Behav 16*:114-126, 1975.
8. Bibace R, Walsh ME: Developmental stages in children's conceptions of illness. In G Stone, F Cohen and N Adlert (Eds), *Health Psychology.* Washington DC: Jossey-Bass, 1979.

SEX DIFFERENCES IN LEGAL DRUG USE[c]

Lois M. Verbrugge

In recent years, popular and scientific articles have paid much attention to women's greater use of psychotropic drugs than men's. Yet this is not an unusual phenomenon, since in general women use more legal drugs than do men. Is this because women are sicker than men and need more drugs? Or are women more willing to use drugs to cure and prevent illness? Or do women have greater access to prescription drugs, either because of more contact with physicians or because physicians offer them drugs more readily? Some of the reasons for women's higher drug use may be perfectly benign, but some may point to aspects of health services and medical practice that need modification.

This paper examines how morbidity, health attitudes, and several other personal characteristics influence drug use, and how these factors help account for women's higher use. It examines total number of drugs used and use of certain types (curative, preventive, prescription, nonprescription). It uses data for white adults in the Detroit metropolitan area to address the following questions: Do women or men use more drugs? How do morbidity, social roles, stress, health attitudes, and opportunities for health care influence adults' use of drugs? Which of these factors is most important? Do the same factors explain high drug use for women as for men? What factors account for sex differences in drug use?

The paper focuses on personal characteristics of women and men that influence drug use. But some structural factors, including aspects of medical care, health insurance and health services, and some features of the drug industry, will be considered in drawing conclusions. The paper studies drugs used for medical purposes, not for recreational purposes. The term "drugs" will mean legal pills, medications, and treatments taken for one's physical health.

THE HEALTH IN DETROIT STUDY

The Health In Detroit Study was a population-based survey of white adults (18+ years of age) living in the Detroit metropolitan area in 1978. It generated extensive data on drug use for chronic conditions, acute conditions, and preventive health.

A probability sample of households in the Detroit SMSA was selected; in each household, one adult was chosen as the study respondent. An Initial Interview was conducted at the residence, covering such topics as current health status, health services use, health attitudes, life style behaviors, stress, social roles, time constraints, and other sociodemographic items. Respondents then kept Daily Health Records (a health diary) for six weeks following the interview. Each day they answered questions about their general health status, symptoms, curative and preventive health actions (including drug use), mood, and special events of the day.

The Initial Interview asked about drugs being taken for chronic conditions and also drugs taken regularly for preventive reasons. Respondents named the specific drugs they were taking. The Daily Health Records had information about all drugs taken during the six-week diary period. Each day respondents filled out a Drug Chart. They wrote down the

---

[c]Edited and reprinted with permission from Verbrugge LM. Sex differences in legal drug use. J Soc Issues 1982;38:59–76.

name of each drug taken that day, then checked reasons for taking it (to treat symptoms bothering you today, for other health problems not bothering you today, to prevent illness or to become more healthy in general, other reasons), and finally stated any symptoms that prompted use of the drug.

The following hypotheses were tested: 1. People with active social roles (employment, marriage, parenthood) use fewer drugs than other people. Active people experience less morbidity than others (Verbrugge, 1981), so their need for drugs is less. 2. As stress increases, so does drug use. Drugs are one strategy for coping with stress. 3. The more health problems a person has, the more drugs he or she uses. 4. People who feel they have control over their lives use fewer drugs than other people. The same is true for people who can ignore physical discomforts and those who value their health highly. Such people probably have low psychological needs for drugs, and also high confidence in their body's ability to maintain and restore health. 5. People who find it difficult to restrict their usual activities or to see a physician when ill use more drugs. Drugs may be an alternative to other kinds of curative care, and they are used more when opportunities to rest or have medical care decrease. In the analysis, sociodemographic items were used as control variables, so no hypotheses were stated for them.

Sex Differences in Drug Use

Women use notably more curative drugs than men do. On the average, these women currently take 1.7 drugs for chronic problems, compared to 1.0 for men. Women also have more drugs on hand in case of flareups (1.2 vs. 0.9). During the diary period, women report taking, on the average, 17.0 drugs to alleviate symptoms and 14.3 to control asymptomatic chronic conditions, compared to 9.6 and 9.3 for men respectively.

Women also use more preventive drugs. In the Initial Interview, almost half (43%) of the women say they take something regularly to stay healthy, compared to 28% of the men. Among users, however, women and men take the same average number of "other regular medicines" (1.8). Female products such as contraceptives, menstrual products, and vaginal therapeutics are excluded here, so we are considering drugs appropriate for both sexes (vitamins, tonics, laxatives, etc.). During the diary period, women also used more preventive drugs: 24.8 vs. 19.2 to prevent illness or to become more healthy in general, and 4.6 vs. 1.6 for "other reasons."

Overall, women used more drugs during the six-week diary period (60.3 vs. 37.7 for men). They use drugs on more days (25.7 days vs. 17.6 days for men). Both prescription and nonprescription uses are greater for women (26.0 prescription drugs vs. 17.3 for men; and 24.4 nonprescription drugs vs. 15.3 for men).

WHAT PREDICTS HIGH USE OF LEGAL DRUGS?

Sociodemographic Characteristics

Curative drug use rises sharply with *age*. Preventive drug use also rises until age 75+, after which it drops. Whether this is a cohort effect (due to specific features of people now aged 75+) or an age effect (due to needs and preferences of elderly people in general) is unclear. There is no overall relationship between drug use and *education*. But one group does stand out: People with 8 grades of school or less have low drug use during the diary period, compared to others. *Ethnicity* is weakly related to drug use. People of Balkan or Mediterranean background sometimes (but not always) have lower drug use than other groups.

Social Roles

Nonemployed people use more curative drugs than currently employed people. They also use more preventive drugs during the diary period (but not in the Initial Interview). For *domestic status,* one group stands out: Nonmarried parents have very low curative drug use, especially during the diary period. Nonmarried parents also have low morbidity during the diary period, compared to other domestic statuses. Why these men and women appear so healthy is perplexing, and it is contrary to prior research (Berkman, 1969) and to popular beliefs about their health. Women who are nonmarried parents also take fewer preventive drugs than other women; but nonmarried fathers take substantially more than other men. These women and men face high emotional and time demands; the men seem to respond with health-promoting behaviors while the women do not. (The number of men is small (8), but the data are very strong and consistent so they are worth noting.) How marital and parent status are each related to drug use is reported in another paper (Verbrugge, 1981): Being married and being a parent are each associated with low drug use.

Stress

Acute stress is usually unrelated to drug use. When a pattern does appear, it shows that drug use increases with stress, as hypothesized. *Stressful life events* and *special daily events* show clearer ties to drug use. The more such events people experience, the more they use curative and preventive drugs. Both "positive" and "negative" events boost drug use during the diary period; only negative ones boost it in the Initial Interview. These results suggest that disruptive events trigger drug use more than general upset feelings do.

Morbidity

As the number of *chronic conditions* and *daily symptoms* increase, so does drug use. Both preventive and curative drug use rise with morbidity. *General ratings of health status* show a different situation: The worse someone thinks his or her health is, the more curative drugs are used, but the fewer preventive ones (Initial Interview). The health diaries show a parallel result: People who feel terrible most of the six weeks take more curative drugs but fewer preventive ones than other people. Do people with "poor" or "terrible" evaluations of their health think that preventive health actions are useless?

Attitudes

Feeling helpless about life increases curative drug use, but it decreases preventive use. People who feel most helpless ("strongly agree") have an especially sharp profile of high curative and low preventive use. With little sense of control over life, they may feel that preventive health habits are useless; and when sick, they need to rely on some external agent to restore health rather than trust the healing capabilities of their own bodies. The more people can *ignore symptoms,* the fewer curative and preventive drugs they take. People who say they can always ignore symptoms stand out sharply with very low drug use. There is no overall relationship between *value of health* and drug use. But one group stands out; contrary to expectations, people who place very low value on health take very few drugs.

Health Care Opportunities

Difficulty in restricting activity or in seeing a doctor when ill is seldom related to drug use. When there is a link, it shows the hypothesized substitution effect between drugs and doctors: People who have trouble seeing a doctor take more curative and preventive drugs. But there is a compatibility effect for activity restriction: People who have no trouble restricting their usual activities tend to take more drugs. Possibly, drug use is viewed as a self-care activity, and it may often be combined with bed rest or reduced activities.

DISCUSSION AND CONCLUSION

Women use more drugs of all kinds than men do—to cure health problems, to control asymptomatic conditions, and to prevent illness. Women use more prescription and nonprescription items. For most variables about drug use, women's use is 50–80% greater than men's.

What personal characteristics are linked with high drug use? As hypothesized, drug use increases with morbidity, age, lack of active social roles, disruptive life events, acute stress, inability to ignore physical discomforts, and difficulty in seeing a doctor when ill. The relation with morbidity is easy to understand; "need" generates use. The relation with age reflects people's increasing need for drug assistance during illness as they grow older. People in nonactive social roles may focus more on their symptoms and try to relieve them with drugs. (One exception was noted—unexpectedly low use of curative drugs by nonmarried parents, and of preventive drugs by nonmarried mothers. We expected lowest drug use among married parents.) Unusual events—whether good or bad—are disruptive and may lead to more drug use as people attempt to cope with change. Feelings of tension and anxiety also sometimes boost drug use; again, drugs may be a coping strategy. People who cannot ignore symptoms easily are likely to turn to drugs for relief. Finally, drugs sometimes act as a substitute for medical care.

Some results that do not fit the hypotheses are intriguing and interpretable: First, negative health attitudes and perceptions inhibit people from using drugs. As subjective health status worsens and feelings of helplessness increase, preventive drug use drops. People who feel terrible most of the time and those who put low value on health have exceptionally low drug use. Some of these people may feel that drugs are useless, and others may simply pay little attention to their health. Second, people who have trouble cutting down their activities when ill also use few drugs. These are both self-care behaviors, and people who have difficulty doing one seem to have trouble with the other too.

Overall, morbidity is the strongest predictor of drug use, and age ranks second. Understandably, "need" is the driving force behind curative use. But it is interesting that morbidity and age also spur more preventive drug use. Possibly, people with health problems try to ward off further health problems by taking these drugs.

When we look at men and women separately, the same relationships between predictors and drug use appear. In other words, both sexes respond to morbidity, age, disruptive events, and so forth, in the same way in their use of legal drugs.

When predictors (sociodemographic characteristics, social roles, stress, morbidity, attitudes, and health care opportunities) are statistically controlled, sex differences in drug use become much smaller. In other words, women tend to have personal characteristics that boost drug use, especially curative use: They are slightly older than men, have less active social roles, experience more disruptive events and more morbidity, consider their health worse, feel more helpless about life, and are unable to ignore symptoms as easily.

The most important "reason" for sex differences in use is morbidity. It differs sharply by sex, and it also has a strong link to drug use. Evidence suggests that women have more symptoms from acute and chronic conditions than men do, although their conditions are probably less life-threatening than men's (Verbrugge, 1982). Women's more frequent symptoms lead to more drug use. But we still do not know the physical and psychosocial factors that lie behind women's greater morbidity. Hypotheses are discussed in Mechanic (1976), Nathanson (1977), and Verbrugge (1979, 1982). There is now active research to test some of those hypotheses.

In the final regression model, sex differences in drug use have narrowed for all variables, especially curative ones. The gap between men and women decreases by 50% or more for many variables. This means that the personal characteristics included in this analysis are indeed important "reasons" for differential use of drugs by men and women.

What might explain the sex differences that remain? Some important health attitudes and health care opportunities may not be included in this analysis; for example, attitudes specifically about drugs, frequency of contact with doctors, or income available for drug purchases. The importance of doctor visits for prescribed medicine use has been demonstrated by Bush and Osterweis (1978). By including more attitude and access variables, we might reduce the sex differences still further.

Overall, this analysis shows that drug use depends mainly on need (morbidity and age), next on attitudes about life and health, then on stress, and least on social roles and one's ability to take other health actions besides drugs. In other words, on a day-to-day basis people are using drugs mainly because they feel sick or want to prevent future illness. This is not a simple-minded or obvious finding. There has been little prior research on actual use of drugs by the general population. It is reassuring to document that, when people take drugs, their personal health needs and attitudes are the key factors.

This does not deny the importance of structural factors such as access to health services (and thus to drug prescriptions), health insurance coverage, employer rules about sick leave, physicians' drug-prescribing behavior, or the impact of drug industry advertisements on physicians. These structural factors may greatly influence aspects of men's and women's drug behavior. In particular, how often they *receive prescriptions* and the *frequency and cost of drug purchases* depend greatly on the structural factors named. Getting prescriptions and purchasing drugs certainly do affect whether people have drugs to use on a day-to-day basis.

Public discussions have focused on how structural factors may differ for men and women; for example, how physicians may prescribe drugs more readily to women than to men, or how employed women may have less flexible sick-leave options. These are certainly important issues, and scientific research on them is needed to determine when women, or men, receive inappropriate or inadequate health care. This analysis of drug use does not discount such public policy issues; the Detroit data are simply not directed toward studying them. Instead, the study's focus is on day-to-day drug use by men and women in the general population, and personal factors that are responsible for women's more frequent use. We find that actual drug use depends closely on health needs and attitudes for both men and women. Structural factors lie at greater distance, probably influencing whether people get drugs at all more than how they use drugs on a day-to-day basis.

REFERENCES

Berkman, P. L. Spouseless motherhood, psychological stress, and physical morbidity. *Journal of Health and Social Behavior,* 1969, *10*(4), 323–334.

Mechanic, D. Sex, illness behavior, and the use of health services. *Journal of Human Stress*, 1976, 2(4), 29–40.

Nathanson, C. A. Sex, illness, and medical care: A review of data, theory, and method. *Social Science and Medicine*, 1977, *11*, 13–25.

Verbrugge, L. M. Female illness rates and illness behavior: Testing hypotheses about sex differences in health. *Women and Health*, 1979, *4*(1), 61–79.

Verbrugge, L. M. Multiple roles and physical health of women and men. (Submitted for publication), 1981.

Verbrugge, L. M. Sex differentials in health. *Public Health Reports*, July/August, 1982.

MEDICATION USE AMONG A NON-INSTITUTIONALIZED RURAL ELDERLY POPULATION[d]

Mickey C. Smith
Thomas R. Sharpe

Despite the importance of medicines to the elderly and the consistent finding that the elderly consume substantially more medication than the rest of the population, there still remain relatively few descriptive studies of the medication-taking practices of this population group. Data are especially sparse among the rural elderly.

The present study examined medication use among a sample of elderly individuals all of whom resided in a single, rural Mississippi county. In this paper we report on the health characteristics of that sample and their medication-taking practices.

The sample consisted of a total of 300 individuals aged 60 or older, residing in Tupelo, Mississippi, and in the surrounding Lee County. Tupelo is a town with a population of more than 25,000 which serves as a medical center for northern Mississippi. Its hospital, now over 600 beds, is the largest in the state and is staffed by every major medical specialist.

Data were gathered via an instrument which consisted of eight sections, two of which are relevant to the present paper. These were:

- The Health Status Section, which asked for an assessment of general health as well as reports of bed days, limited activity days, and days when some other health problem existed, each within the two weeks prior to the interview. Chronic illnesses were also covered in this section.
- The Medication Use Section, which specifically identified all prescription and over-the-counter nonprescription (OTC) drugs taken by the respondent in the preceding two weeks.

Extent and Nature of Medication Use. Within the previous two weeks 262 (87%) of the respondents said they had taken a prescription drug, and 277 (92%) indicated that they were "generally satisfied" with the results of their overall prescription drug use. Fewer (178: 59%) had taken an OTC drug in the previous two weeks and 244 (81%) indicated general satisfaction with the results of their OTC drug use generally. The range for numbers of different prescription drugs taken in the two week period was 0–13. For OTC drugs the range was 0–6.

Table I provides data on drug use with race and sex comparisons. The data show that

---

[d]Edited and reprinted with permission from Smith MC, Sharpe TR. Medication use among a non-institutionalized rural elderly population. J Clin Exper Gerontol 1984;6:207–230.

Table I.   Sex and Race of Drug Users Vs. Non-Users

Respondent Characteristics	Used No Drugs	Used RX But Not OTC	Used OTC But Not Rx	Used Both Rx and OTC
	Frequency (Per cent)*			
White				
Male (N = 72)	5 (6.9)	29 (40.3)	8 (11.1)	30 (41.7)
Female (N = 134)	3 (2.2)	38 (28.4)	7 (5.2)	86 (64.2)
Black				
Male (N = 33)	2 (6.1)	14 (42.4)	7 (21.2)	10 (30.3)
Female (N = 61)	3 (4.9)	28 (45.9)	3 (4.9)	27 (44.3)
All Whites (N = 206)	8 (3.9)	67 (35.5)	15 (7.3)	116 (56.3)
All Blacks (N = 94)	5 (5.3)	42 (44.7)	10 (10.6)	37 (39.4)
All Males (N = 105)	7 (6.7)	43 (41.0)	15 (14.3)	40 (38.1)
All Females (N = 195)	6 (3.1)	66 (33.8)	10 (5.1)	113 (57.9)
All Respondents (N = 300)	13 (4.3)	109 (36.3)	25 (8.3)	153 (51.0)

*Percent of number of persons in that category.

males were more likely to use prescription or OTC drugs, but not both. Females, especially white females, were more likely to use both. Males were more likely than females to use no medications.

OTC drugs were seldom used in response to respondent identified morbid episodes (Table II). When this did occur the medication was usually already on hand. It should be noted that the OTC usage reported in this context is considerably less than that reported on the section of the questionnaire devoted exclusively to drug use. It appears from this that there is considerable OTC drug use in cases in which the individual does not perceive himself to be ill. Indeed, OTC drugs tended to be "on hand" with only 10 percent of uses reported to be purchased specifically for an illness episode.

Prescription drug use was more often associated with morbid episodes (Table II), than was OTC use. Refills or prescription medications already on hand were used predominantly, when such medications were used at all.

Table II.   Use of Drugs for Morbid Episodes

Type of Morbid Episode	Number (%) Using OTC Drugs: By Source			
	New OTC	OTC on Hand	No OTC Drug Used	Total
Bed Days	2 (5.5)	4 (11.1)	30 (83.3)	36 (100.0)
Limited Activity	1 (1.9)	10 (19.2)	41 (78.8)	52 (100.0)
"Anything Else"	3 (10.0)	4 (13.3)	23 (76.7)	30 (100.0)

	Number (%) Using Prescription Drug: By Source				
	Prescription	Refill	Prescription on Hand	No Prescription Used	Total
Bed Days	7 (20.6)	20 (29.4)	9 (26.5)	8 (23.5)	34 (100.0)
Limited Activity	16 (28.6)	10 (35.7)	6 (10.7)	14 (25.0)	56 (100.0)
"Anything Else"	2 (8.7)	5 (21.7)	6 (10.7)	10 (43.5)	23 (100.0)

SUMMARY

It has been recognized that for some of the elderly drugs become an important part of their physical and psychosocial survival (1). The presence of multiple chronic physical and mental conditions in this age group has been offered as one explanation for increased drug consumption among the aged (4). The assertion is logical, since chronic illness can often be alleviated through long term management and symptomatic control. The present study provides further support for this line of reasoning.

The results of the present study are reasonably consistent with other investigations showing the existence of a variety of physical and mental maladies and a remarkable range of medications used to treat them. It provided further evidence of sex and race differences in level of drug consumption and some suggestions that OTC drugs may not be perceived as "real medicine." Some differences, although not dramatic ones, were noted between rural and urban residents. Continued study of drug use phenomena, especially as they relate to social and psychological determinants of such use are certainly warranted.

REFERENCES

1. Chien C, Townsend E, Ross-Townsend A. Substance use and abuse among the community elderly: the medical aspect. Addict Dis 1978;3:357–372.

HOW PHYSICIANS CHOOSE THE DRUGS THEY PRESCRIBE [e]

Charles D. Hepler
Richard Segal
Robert A. Freeman

For economic and humanitarian reasons, prescription drug use in the United States is an object of mounting concern among professionals and administrators. Typically, health care professionals and administrators, especially governmental program administrators, do not leave problems unsolved. Programs will continue to be developed to improve prescription drug use. Many people inside and outside pharmacy recognize the pharmacist's potential value in such programs but are not sure how pharmacists might fit in.

Meanwhile, various other factors in health care are combining to offer pharmacists the opportunity to participate. To accept this opportunity, three prerequisites must be met. First, the pharmacist—especially the pharmacy program manager—must recognize the need to improve prescribing quality. Second, he or she must be able to accept such participation as a legitimate part of pharmacy practice. Third, as for anyone who would influence any process as complicated as prescribing, a set of models, concepts or theories for prescribing is needed to guide practical interventions.

Several reviews of drug-prescribing studies are available in the literature (1–3). Generally, these reviews categorize the drug-prescribing studies into two major approaches: (1) studies of factors associated with appropriate or inappropriate prescribing and (2) studies of the diffusion and adoption of new drugs. Both approaches are sociological and operate at a level that ignores psychological variables like a prescriber's beliefs. More recently, sev-

ᵉEdited and reprinted with permission from Hepler CD, Segal R, Freeman RA. How physicians choose the drugs they prescribe. Topics Hosp Pharm Management 1981;1:23–44.

eral studies have been published that use a psychological approach that assumes that a prescriber's behavior is determined by a set of beliefs at the moment of prescribing.

PSYCHOLOGICAL STUDIES

In contrast to large numbers of prescribing factors and information-diffusion studies, only five psychologically based prescribing studies have appeared in the literature. If information diffusion and adoption research operate at the group level, then psychological prescribing research operates at the individual level. Prescribers are viewed as autonomous actors whose position in a group is not of primary importance. A prescriber may exchange information with colleagues in a group, but in the psychological view he or she acts alone to choose drugs.

Behavioral Theory

There are two general classes of psychological theory relevant to prescribing. The oldest—and perhaps still best known—is called stimulus-response or behavioral theory. In the behaviorist view behavior results from a momentary stimulus and past reward or punishment experience. Behavior is habitual in this view, in the sense that no cognition (e.g., conscious knowledge or belief) is presumed (4). For example, in a strict behaviorist view the drug-choice process does not involve a prescriber's awareness of the consequences of various alternatives. Many behaviorist terms (e.g., *operant conditioning, positive reinforcement, behavior modification*) have become familiar in education and management, illustrating the recent importance of the behaviorist view. No studies of prescribing that used a behaviorist model have appeared, although some terminology (*prescribing habits*) suggesting a behaviorist view is occasionally seen (2, 5) and implicitly behaviorist interventions are commonplace.

Cognitive Theory

The second general class of psychological theory relevant to prescribing is called stimulus-cognition-response or cognitive theory. In the cognitive view cognition is presumed to occur between the receipt of a stimulus and the response to it. In this view behavior is the result of active conscious problem solving. The theories that guided the research described later all consider the prescriber's drug choice to be a function of an interaction of prescriber's beliefs about the consequences of various drug choices for a specific patient and the values attached to those consequences by the prescriber. The beliefs are termed *expectancies* or *instrumentalities* and can most easily be understood as subjective probability estimates ("If I choose A, then the chance of consequence B is 95 percent").

Psychological prescribing studies operate at the individual level, where prescribing actually occurs, in contrast to sociological prescribing studies at more aggregated levels such as groups or whole societies. This seems a more specific and precise approach, because it allows the interplay of variables to be observed within subjects.

It has the disadvantage, however, of being somewhat obtrusive. Prescribers are usually questioned directly about their beliefs and behaviors (or behavioral intentions). This raises the risk that a prescriber's attention may be directed to facts that he or she might not notice or outcomes that he or she might not consider when prescribing outside of the study. A series of questions could lead a prescriber to a different conclusion from what he or she would have drawn if the questions had not been asked. In short, the psychological approach is specific and individualized, but it raises philosophical issues concerning the effect of its observation methods on the subjects observed.

Interventions Suggested by Psychological Studies

All published psychological prescribing studies use a model that includes cognitions (conscious knowledge, beliefs and other mental constructs). Some have shown that these models have the ability to predict prescribing intention. No work that formally studied prescribing as habitual behavior has appeared, and no comparison of the two views has been attempted. There is evidence therefore to support a cognitive view but none to support a behaviorist (habitual behavior) view. The practical importance of this distinction lies in designing and timing interventions that are intended to change prescribing behavior.

The Behaviorist View

In the behaviorist view behavior results from a stimulus and past experience. No cognition is presumed. In behavior modification, for example, desired behavior is rewarded and undesired behavior is not. The important points are that (1) the intervention (giving or withholding the reward) occurs *after* the behavior and (2) no explanation or other operation on the actor's cognitions is necessary. A behaviorist-prescribing intervention therefore would occur after a prescribing decision had been made, would tend to emphasize reward giving or withholding and would tend to deemphasize (or omit) an explanation to the prescriber of why the prescribing decision resulted in a reward or an intervention.

Operation of a restrictive formulary policy is an example. After the prescriber has chosen a drug and written a drug order, he or she either receives a reward (the patient obtains the drug without effort from the prescriber) or the reward is withheld (the prescriber receives a communication explaining that the drug was withheld in accordance with formulary policy).

In gentler versions the prescriber may receive a personal visit from the pharmacist, who explains the situation, offers alternative suggestions and helps get the drug if necessary. In harder versions the prescriber may be mildly punished by being asked to justify his or her order or to complete a special nonformulary drug request (perhaps in triplicate with countersignature by the chief of service). Little emphasis is placed on explaining why the formulary drug would have been a better choice or on reeducating the prescriber about the pharmacologic issues involved. The prescriber's behavioral intention is in effect blocked; frustration is possibly a frequent result. Presumably, the prescriber eventually becomes conditioned to choose formulary drugs.

The Cognitive View

In contrast, a cognitive intervention preferably occurs before the prescriber chooses a drug, and emphasizes explanations of the consequences of various choices. For example, a clinical pharmacist may become aware of a particular prescribing stimulus (for example, a patient with a cardiac arrhythmia) and decide to influence the drug choice made. The pharmacist approaches the prescriber and offers information before the prescriber has chosen a drug, if that timing is possible.

Like behaviorist interventions, cognitive interventions can range from gentle (e.g., oral suggestions from a pharmacist) to hard (e.g., compulsory formal consultation with a clinical specialty service) (68). Cognitive interventions are also possible after the fact; their major characteristic is their emphasis on explaining the consequences of various choices: changing cognitions rather than providing or withholding a "positive reinforcement."

Because psychological theories of prescribing refer to the individual prescriber, their greatest practical contribution is in suggesting personal interventions. In the psychological view an intervention directed at a group of prescribers is really a set of identical interventions directed at each individual in the group. Unfortunately, the interventions may be inappropriate for some individuals in the group. Cognitive theory stresses the importance of an individual's beliefs and values in directing his or her behavior and implies interventions that are specifically adapted to the individual.

Physician Attitude about Outcome

The research summarized above suggests that the practical importance of a prescriber's instrumentality belief (connecting a drug choice and an outcome) depends on his or her attitude about the outcome. For example, if a particular prescriber cares little about colleague opinion, then his or her belief that colleagues would agree or disagree with a particular drug choice would not be a factor in his or her choosing that drug. If the same prescriber strongly disvalues side effects, then a belief that a particular drug would cause side effects in a patient would be an important deterrent from choosing that drug. Knowing what outcomes a physician feels most strongly about might increase the effectiveness of a clinical pharmacist who wishes to advise that physician about drug therapy.

Pharmacists are recognizing that a complete set of pharmaceutical services to inpatients must include (1) impersonal, production-oriented goods and services (e.g., the materials distribution system) and (2) personal, patient-specific services (e.g., discharge counseling, therapeutic monitoring). In an analogous manner, a complete set of influences to encourage better drug prescribing must include (1) distribution of reliable information through a stable influence network (perhaps involving the P&T committee and its appendages) and (2) personal, patient-specific advice from a therapeutic advisor (e.g., a clinical pharmacist). A complete drug-use control system should weld these activities into a unified whole.

REFERENCES

1. Hemminki, E. "Factors Influencing Drug Prescribing—Inquiry into Research Strategy." *Drug Intelligence and Clinical Pharmacy* 10:6 (1976) p. 321–329.
2. Miller, R. "Prescribing Habits of Physicians: A Review of Studies on Prescribing of Drugs." Parts I–III. *Drug Intelligence and Clinical Pharmacy* 7:11 (1973) p. 492–500; Parts IV–VI, 7:12 (1973) p. 557–564; Parts VII–VIII, 18:2 (1974) p. 81–91.
3. Worthen, D. "Prescribing Influences: An Overview." *British Journal of Medical Education* 7:2 (1973) p. 109–117.
4. Skinner, B. cited in W. Hammer and D. Organ. *Organizational Behavior* (Dallas: Business Publications 1978) p. 42.
5. Stolley, P. et al. "The Relationship between Physician Characteristics and Prescribing Appropriateness." *Medical Care* 10:1 (1972) p. 17–28.

9
Nonmedical Uses of Drugs

BERNARD SOROFMAN
TOMAS L. GRIEBLING

If asked to describe the functions of drugs, most people would probably place the treatment of disease at the top of the list. Indeed, therapeutic use is the primary function for which most drugs are developed. However, as Chapter 8 has described, drugs fulfill a wide variety of other functions in contemporary society.

In order to guide a discussion on the nonmedical uses of drugs, the question must be asked: "What is a drug?" By definition a drug is a chemical that is intended to affect the structure and function of some physiological component of the body (1). It is not there to specifically cure or even treat abnormal physiological conditions.

This chapter focuses on the nonmedical uses of drugs in humans. For discussion purposes, these uses have been divided into six categories. The therapeutic area covers medical, diagnostic, and research uses of drugs. Social uses include recreation, performance enhancement, and social control. Economic, political, and religious uses are all considered as nonmedical functions of drugs in society. And last, personal uses of drugs for abuse, dependence, cosmetic purposes, and contraception will be considered.

REVIEW OF THE MEDICAL USES OF DRUGS

The most commonly known uses of drugs are for the mitigation of illness and/or the cure of disease. Collectively these are known as therapeutic uses. There is a generally accepted theory, most would say fact, that a chemical substance, given in the correct quantities, dosage form, and at the right time, will return the body to a normal or nearl normal condition. Traditionally, medicine in the United States evolved from two major philosophical orientations. Allopathic medicine approaches the medical event as a battle between opposites. Suppose a person has a fever. From the allopathic point of view the fever needs to be counteracted by a drug that will under normal conditions decrease the temperature of the body. Therefore, aspirin or acetaminophen is prescribed to lower the fever. In contrast to allopathic medicine, homeopathic medicine works through a different set of principles. Within this health care philosophy, a drug that produces a fever under normal, healthy conditions is used in minute quantities to balance a fever in abnormal conditions. In either case, the drug is used for therapeutic reasons.

Drugs not only assist in the amelioration of an existing acute health care problem, they have therapeutic functions as well. Chronic illnesses are long-term and usually incurable. Medications are used in these conditions to create a nearly normal physiological environment for the stricken individual. A person who is not producing insulin will, in all likelihood, eventually be diagnosed as diabetic (2). The treatment, insulin, will be injected into the body on a daily basis. This action is not intended to cure the disease but rather to replace the missing chemical. Medications in the form of drug therapy also may be used to prevent disease and illness. Calcium is given to women who are known candidates for osteoporosis, a disease that results from demineralization of the bones. Calcium supplements are provided to prevent the loss of calcium and, therefore, to prevent the onset of the disease (3).

Drugs also are used in health care for nontherapeutic, medical reasons. Diagnostic tests assist health providers in the recognition of the presence or absence of a disease. These tests may be performed by the use of specific drugs. Edrophonium is used to terminate cardiac arrhythmias. However, because it inhibits the breakdown of acetylcholine in the nerves, edrophonium also is used to diagnose a serious neuromuscular disease known as myasthenia gravis.

Finally, it can be said that medicine is founded on, and improved by, scientific investigation. Nathan Kline has sarcastically referred to a drug as ". . . a chemical substance which, when brought into contact with a living organism, produces a paper" (4). Research is now the cornerstone of drug development. Many drugs are used exclusively for research purposes. Perhaps, for one reason or another, the drug did not make it through the process that ends in federal approval as a commercially available therapeutic entity.

SOCIAL USES OF DRUGS

One nonmedical use for drugs in society is consumption for personal or social enjoyment. Recreational drug use may be described as the utilization of psychoactive substances for euphoria or the decrease of social inhibitions. In recent years the United States has witnessed an overwhelming increase in recreational drug use. Like alcohol, marijuana has been used in situations to create an environment that enhances social interaction (5). Cocaine has been shown to establish a similar setting (6). Other recreational examples include amyl nitrite, used by some individuals for sexual enjoyment (7), and lysergic acid diethylamide (LSD) for out-of-body experiences (8).

Like the "soma" described in Huxley's *Brave New World* (9), drug use in the United States may, in selected cases, be a form of social control. Social and economic problems may be medicalized and treated with drugs. Diazepam, for example, has been reported as the drug of choice for loneliness and marital problems (10, 11). Some authors would argue that the normal condition of being young and female is a sufficient reason, for a significant portion of the medical profession, to prescribe tranquilizers (12).

In the quest for excellent maximizing performance is often everything. The only goal is to be the best—to win. Nowhere is this more evident than in sports. The saying goes something like this: "Winning is not everything; it is the only thing." The ethical use of drugs in sports varies considerably among the various sporting activities. Both illicit and licit drugs may be accepted and used. Football and baseball players, golfers, and other sports enthusiasts (professional and amateur) have different ethical standards regarding the use of drugs for performance (13). These standards not only reflect what is socially acceptable among the athletes of each sport, they also reflect the needs within each sport for physical conditioning for flexibility, strength, and endurance. Patterns of use also vary by the setting in which the sport is played. For example, in college football the use of legally available prescription steroids is unacceptable; this is not true in professional sports.

Several pharmacological categories of drugs are abused by athletes. Stimulants, for example amphetamines and sympathomimetic amines such as ephedrine, hide fatigue and increase cardiac output. Analgesics, both narcotic (meperidine) and nonnarcotic (aspirin), are used to decrease inflammation and/or the sensation of pain. Muscle relaxants relieve spasms, and depressants, barbiturates for example, aid in sleep and relaxation. Pure oxygen in high doses provides rapid, short-term relief to muscle cells that are being pushed for endurance. This procedure is known as "blood doping" (14). The most commonly known class of enhancers are steroids. Anabolic and androgenic steroids are used by athletes to increase lean body mass and muscular strength. These drugs are developed from derivatives of testosterone.

Performance can be enhanced in artistic areas as well. A well-known story among health professionals is that single doses of a β-blocking drug will help to calm an individual who is nervous about performing a specific activity. Research may prove this true. Whether it is due to nervousness or other physiological conditions, musical performance may indeed be enhanced by β-blockade. In a double-blind, placebo-controlled trial, nadolol was studied to determine whether there was an improvement in performance anxiety. Low doses did indeed enhance performance, higher doses impaired performance (15). Another study showed that high school students given β-blockers prior to taking a college entrance exam scored higher than those who had not taken the drug (16).

An area of drug use that may become more popular in the future is the chemical enhancement of daily social performance. A womam who is old and frequently forgetful is diagnosed with Alzheimer's disease. The solution may be as simple as a drug—vasopressin 3 times a day (17). The drug will enhance her ability to remember. Does forgetfulness fall within the realm of disease? Maybe. If there is a drug that improves the memory of a person with Alzheimer's disease, perhaps it will improve memory in other individuals, for example the mentally retarded (thioridazine is being tested) (18). However, organic disease does not need to be present to want to enhance one's memory. College students need to retain large quantities of facts in order to pass qualifying exams. Pharmacists need to retain facts to properly counsel patients. The limits may be bounded only by ethical standards.

Performance enhancers are as common as coffee, tea, and soda pop. Caffeine, that "pick-me-upper" and "morning-eye-opener," is ever present in our society. Used to maintain alertness and decrease fatigue, caffeine provides the energy many feel they need to accomplish their daily tasks (19).

ECONOMIC USES OF DRUGS

For most of the approximately 170,000 pharmacists in the United States, the pharmacy profession revolves around the sale of pharmaceuticals. These are bought and sold daily in pharmacies all across the nation. Drugs are an economic commodity with an intrinsic value and a large infrastructure to facilitate their sale. The pharmaceutical industry discovers, develops, studies, and markets chemical entities as medicinals. Their primary goal is to sell the product, a drug, for a profit. Wholesale pharmaceutical firms buy drugs in order to sell them to distribution sites such as pharmacies and hospitals. Pharmacists buy drugs to sell to patients. In each case, one would expect a profit to be generated in real dollars.

Drugs are sold through three major distribution channels in the United States. The first is by prescription. A licensed prescriber authorizes the distribution of a socially controlled substance by a licensed dispenser to a patient/consumer. The second method for drug sales is an unrestricted open market. Nonprescription drugs (over-the-counter) may be sold by any vendor and are available for direct purchase by a consumer. The third major channel of drug distribution is best described as the organized illegal drug trade. This method of sale, although illegal, is no different from a business or economic standpoint than the legal channels (20). The idea of cash crops is not restricted to wheat and corn but can be applied to marijuana and poppy plants as well.

Certainly a unique twist on the above classification is the "designer drug" business. This enterprise concerns itself, like the major pharmaceutical industry, with the research and development of new chemical entities. The goal of a designer drug operation is to discover legal chemical moieties that mimic the psychoactive properties of similar, illegal chemical entities. The market life of these products is relatively short. They are quickly regulated or legislated as illegal substances (21, 22).

POLITICAL USES OF DRUGS

Most of us have read mystery novels at sometime in our lives. Agatha Christie carefully crafts a story about a lover whose sudden death appears unusual. The plot quickly thickens when it is determined that she was murdered. And then, slowly and with great detail, the detective discovers that the death was the result of an assassination plot founded upon greed and jealousy. The murder weapon was an overdose of a prescription medication. This is not unusual in real life. Drug substances are used to commit murder. There is the case of a nurse who injected lethal doses of digoxin, a cardiovascular drug, into neonates and infants (23). After a meticulous investigation, the deaths were discovered to be the result of a premeditated act. In the early 1980s there was a well-publicized trial about a man who was accused of systematically overdosing his rich invalid wife with insulin (24). The prosecution contended that he had done this to acquire his wife's great wealth. After months of front page news, he was acquitted.

As in the above examples, drugs can and have been used as a weapon for murder. On a grander scale, chemical and biological agents can be used to facilitate the deaths of many individuals. The purpose is war. Chemical weapons were first used in World War I. Generally, these agents attack the nervous system causing tremendous morbidity and mortality (25). In the mid-1980s there were several reported incidences of both chemical and biological warfare with one country attacking another.

The defense of an ideological position is one argument in support of war. However, there are other ways to use drugs to protect ideologies. The medical literature is filled with articles on the use of drugs for the torture of human beings. Sodium thiopental, often used as an anesthetic, has been used to interrogate prisoners. Restrained and drugged, these persons are forced to comply with the wishes of their captors. Occasionally, reports are received from a politically turbulent corner of the world that someone has been institutionalized against his or her will (26). Incarcerated and chemically restrained through the use of psychotherapeutic agents such as chlorpromazine, trifluoperazine, or haloperidol, these persons are held prisoner.

Society also sanctions the use of drugs for killing. Originated in Oklahoma and adopted by other states, conventional medications may be used to carry out state-mandated executions. This form of capital punishment has evolved because it is inexpensive and reportedly humane. A combination of thiopental and tubocurarine, succinylcholine chloride, or potassium chloride (often used in therapeutic medical procedures) is administered in lethal doses as a means of execution (27). The role of a health professional in the administration of these drugs is controversial. Actions that promote death are the antithesis of health professional goals. The American Pharmaceutical Association and the American Society of

Hospital Pharmacists have both responded by saying that the pharmacist should not be forced by his or her employer to participate in such activities (28). In a "strong" act of social consciousness the American Pharmaceutical Association denounced the use of the term drug for chemicals used in capital punishment, a head-in-the-sand approach at best (29).

RELIGIOUS DRUG USE

The practice of religion is a cultural institution in which the use of drugs is common. In this case drugs may be used to assist in the creation of an appropriate environment for a religious experience. Although not primarily concerned with religion, a graphic example of this concept can be seen through the writings of Carlos Castaneda (30, 31). His books depict the period in his life when he apprenticed with a fortune teller/shaman called "Don Juan." Don Juan and Castaneda used the chemical components of plants and the spirits of animals to project themselves into a plane of reality that allowed them to seek spiritual and curative powers. The case of Don Juan is sensational and may be difficult to accept as a religious experience.

In the United States today there is a religious organization known as the Native American Church. This religion represents many North American Indians who practice a spiritual and religious teaching associated with their ancestors. The religion was established to link the contemporary Native American culture to the ancestor's religious beliefs prior to the strong advent of Christianity in North America (32). In order to reach the "Great Spirit" the practitioners use the peyote plant to attain a specific state or trance. Biochemically, we as pharmacists may say that they are ingesting alkaloids including mescaline. The hallucinatory effects of the peyote assist the individual in achieving a spiritual plane. This enables someone with proper training to have a religious experience. Symbolically, the use of this illicit drug represents Native American independence from the federal government.

Strange as this may seem, drug use is common in popular contemporary religions as well. The communion wine of Christianity symbolizes the blood of Christ (33). Yet alcohol can be considered both a food and a drug. Societal mores governing religious drug use are quite different from those for other types of use. Behavior that may be viewed as inappropriate in other contexts, such as the consumption of alcohol, is considered an integral and accepted part of religious practice.

PERSONAL USES OF DRUGS

Drugs are frequently used for mood alteration. Such ego-disrupting functions have intense psychological dimensions. One of the drugs commonly used for ego-disruptive purposes is alcohol. Alcohol, a central nervous system depressant, may cause severe personality shifts if consumed in sufficient quantities (34). Other drugs often used for ego disruption include amphetamines, barbiturates, tranquilizers, hallucinogens, and psychedelics.

The personal abuse of licit and illicit drugs is one of the most devastating problems now facing American society. In the United States tranquilizers are one of the most popularly prescribed classes of drugs (35). Experts contend that 10% of all Americans either are or will be affected by alcoholism. Although no age group can be excluded, statistics indicate that the young are especially susceptible to the negative effects of drug use. The routine and habitual use of drug substances (drug abuse) is a major social problem. Heroin addicts number in the hundreds of thousands. It is estimated that up to 20% of all Americans use marijuana daily. Tranquilizer use is estimated at approximately 20% of the United States population as well (36).

Because of the destructive effects of substance abuse on an individual, attempts to control illicit drug use now dominate public policy and legislative decisions. Public service announcements about the dangers of drug and alcohol use regularly appear both on television and in printed media, and educational programs for youth are common. Currently the campaign is "Just say no to drugs." Numerous toll-free hotlines have appeared that offer easily accessible counseling. Alcoholics Anonymous, originally founded in 1935, has recently been joined by dozens of other national self-help and awareness organizations such as Mothers Against Drunk Driving (MADD), Students Against Drunken Driving (SADD), and others.

Researchers have long contemplated why some people become addicted to drugs. Numerous theories have been proposed with varying degrees of acceptance by the academic community. These theories fall along three basic lines. One theoretical perspective focuses on the stages of human development (37). Another explains the influences of social development, family, and peers on the tendency to abuse drugs (38). A third theoretical approach is to look at drug abuse as developing in stages: from tobacco, to beer, to liquor, to marijuana, to "harder" drugs (depending on the accessibility of these substances for the individual) (39). A great deal of research in the field of addiction has recently focused on the similarities between addiction to psychoactive substances and other types of addictive behavior such as gambling and overeating. Many factors have been identified that affect drug and alcohol usage. Sociocultural factors and social customs are very important (40). It should be remembered that any given drug has risks and benefits that vary with the context of use.

In current society, body image is very important. Obesity or even the perception of being slightly overweight is thought by some to be unattractive and unacceptable. For young women in the United States, this sense of body image is especially important. Often, in order to maintain or achieve an acceptable body image, they abuse laxatives and emetics (41). Bulimia is a serious health problem that is associated with this behavior. The drugs used in these cases prevent the absorption of food and decrease caloric intake without necessarily decreasing food consumption. Laxative "abuse" may be defined as laxative use several times a week to simply remove food from the intestinal tract (42).

Personal drug use extends far beyond drug abuse. Drugs are used as aphrodisiacs. For centuries, people have sought to chemically improve their sexual functioning (43). Although some substances may appear to have aphrodisiac qualities, none is known to actually work. They probably perform more of a psychological than a physiological function.

Drugs are used to enhance personal beauty. A cosmetic is by definition something that is applied in some manner (rubbed, poured, sprinkled, sprayed) to the skin in order to promote attractiveness or beauty. Cosmetics also can be used for cleansing or, in some unspecified way, to enhance appearance (44). Major research and development pharmaceutical manufacturers are getting into the vanity business in a big way. An antihypertensive medication has been developed and marketed by one of them. Therapeutically, the medication worked well in persons with certain hypertensive symptomatology. It had, however, one drawback. The use of the drug caused hirsuitism—abnormal hair growth. Some women became bearded, some men had to trim the hair on the backs of their hands. The drug was aesthetically displeasing, a reason for therapeutic failure. Turning the "side effects" of a drug into a benefit is common practice in the pharmaceutical industry. The chemical was recognized for its potential in the treatment of that great social disease—alopecia (baldness). Now under a new name, the antihypertensive applied topically will cosmetically improve the appearance of hair in some cases (45). Similarly, acne (the noncystic, teenage version) is socially unpleasant. Tetracycline, a bacteriostatic antibiotic, is an effective treatment (46). One can only speculate at the range of cosmetic options open to us with "cosmeceuticals." Will the future bring drugs that can enlarge or reduce body parts, color skin, and dentition, or change other personal characteristics? The options are boundless.

The above discussion raises an interesting point. What disease is treated by the use of oral contraceptives—pregnancy? Is pregnancy a disease or a normal physiological condition? Pharmacists dispense millions of cycles of oral contraceptives each year to prevent pregnancy. It is by volume the largest mass-marketed pharmaceutical for nonmedical, personal control of a normal physiological condition.

A final area of personal drug use is euthanasia. Everyone could probably name a major public figure who has committed suicide by using a drug. Marilyn Monroe, once an internationally known actress, is often cited as the classic example of a person who, for some reason known only to her, overdosed on pharmaceuticals (47). In 1985, the Brown University student body passed a referendum that would "stockpile suicide pills for optional use by students only after a nuclear war" (48). One may argue that the option was a joke; it was not. "Students for Suicide Tablets," as the grassroots organization was called, wanted to show that their fear of a nuclear war had forced them to consider euthanasia by drug consumption. It was to them an important symbolic act—another use for a drug.

SUMMARY

Nonmedical drug use, for a variety of purposes, is common in modern society. Pharmacy plays an important role in the distribution of drugs for both medical and nonmedical use. Considering that drugs serve more than merely therapeutic functions (see Chapter 8), pharmacists must, from time to time, recognize that even though they are working within a health care/medical system, some of the drugs that they dispense may not be used for the mitigation of illness or the cure of disease.

REFERENCES

1. Benet LZ, Sheiner LB. General principles. In Gilman AG, Goodman LS, Rall TW, Murad F, eds. The pharmacologic basis of therapeutics. 7th ed. New York: Macmillan, 1985, pp 1–2.
2. Foster DW. Diabetes mellitus. In Braunwald E, Isselbacher KJ, Petersdorf RG, Wilson JD, Martin JB, Fauci AS, eds. Harrison's principles of internal medicine. 11th ed. New York: McGraw Hill, 1987, pp 1778–1797.
3. Krane SM, Holick MF. Metabolic bone disease. In Braunwald E, Isselbacher KJ, Petersdorf RG, Wilson JD, Martin JB, Fauci AS, eds. Harrison's principles of internal medicine. 11th ed. New York: McGraw Hill, 1987, pp 1889–1894.
4. Kline N. Manipulation of life patterns with drugs. In Evans WO, Kline NS, eds. Psychotropic drugs in the year 2000: use by normal humans. Springfield IL: Charles C Thomas, 1971, p 69.
5. Richards LG. Perspectives on Drug Use in the United States. Drugs Soc 1986;1:111–126.
6. Weil A. The natural mind: a new way of looking at drugs and the higher consciousness. Boston: Houghton Mifflin, 1972.
7. Centers for Disease Control Task Force on Kaposi's Sarcoma and Opportunistic Infections. Epidemiologic aspects of the current outbreak of Kaposi's sarcoma and opportunistic infections. N Engl J Med 1982;306:248–252.
8. Lilly J. The center of a cyclone: an autobiography of inner space. New York: Crown, 1985.
9. Huxley A. Brave new world and brave new world revisited. New York: Harper & Row, 1965.
10. Caplan RD, Andrews FM, Conway TL, Abbey A, Abramis DJ, French JRP Jr. Social effects of diazepam use: a longitudinal field study. Soc Sci Med 1985;21:887–898.
11. Koumjian K. The use of valium as a form of social control. Soc Sci Med 1981;15E:245–249.
12. Marinier RL, Phil RO, Wilford C, Lapp JE. Psychotropic drug use by women: demographic, lifestyle, and personality correlates. Drug Intell Clin Pharm 1985;19:40–45.

13. Cowart V. Road back from substance abuse especially long, hard for athletes. JAMA 1986;256:2645-2649.
14. Voy R. Illicit drugs and the athlete. Am Pharm 1986 S26:763-769.
15. Gates GA, Saegert J, Wilson N, Johnson L, Shepherd A, Hearne EM III. Effect of [beta] blockage on singing performance. Ann Otol Rhinol Laryngol 1985;94:570-574.
16. Hutchinson S. A drug to lessen test anxiety? Newsweek on Campus. October, 1987, p 7.
17. Legros JJ, Gilot P, Seron X, Claessens J, Adam A, Moeglen JM, Audibert A, Berchier P. Influence of vasopressin on learning and memory. Lancet 1978;71(8054):41-42.
18. Breuning SE, Ferguson DG, Davidson NA, Poling AD. Effects of thioridazine on the intellectual performance of mentally retarded drug responders and nonresponders. Arch Gen Psych 1983;40:309-313.
19. Murry TH. The coercive power of drugs in sports. Hastings Center Rep August 1983;13:24-30.
20. Ricks TA. Inside dope. The cocaine business: big risks and profits, high labor turnover. Wall Street Journal. June 30, 1986, p 1.
21. Schulman R, Sabin M. The losing war against designer drugs. Business Week. 24 June 1985, pp 101, 104.
22. Anon. Clandestine chemists crank out new drugs. Quad-City Times. 24 March, 1985, p 16A.
23. Buehler JW, Smith LF, Wallace EM, Heath CW, Kusink R, Herndon JL. Unexplained deaths in a children's hospital. N Engl J Med 1985;313:211-216.
24. Friendly J. Von Bulow jury issues acquittal on all charges. New York Times 1985;134(46437):1, B8.
25. Anonymous. Chemical and bacteriological weapons in the 1980s. Lancet 1984;2(8395):141-143.
26. Kirschner RH. The use of drugs in torture and human rights abuses. Am J Foren Med Pathol 1984;5:313-315.
27. Curran WJ, Casscells W. The ethics of medical participation in capital punishment by intravenous drug injection. N Engl J Med 1980;302:226-230.
28. Perchak G. Capital punishment and the responsible pharmacist. Am Pharm 1985 S25:406-407.
29. Anonymous. 1985 APhA Policy Actions. Am Pharm 1985 S25:307.
30. Castaneda C. Journey to Ixtlan: the lessons of Don Juan. New York: Simon & Schuster, 1972.
31. Castaneda C. The fire from within. New York: Simon & Schuster, 1984.
32. Stewart OC. Peyote religion. Norman OK: University of Oklahoma, 1986.
33. Briggs CA. Theological symbolics. New York: Charles Scribner's Sons, 1914, p 133.
34. Fleischhacker WW, Kryspin-Exner K. The psychopathology of alcoholism. Drug Alcohol Depend 1986;17:73-79.
35. Helman CG. "Tonic," "fuel," and "food": social and symbolic aspects of the long-term use of psychotropic drugs. Soc Sci Med 1981;15B:521-533.
36. Zozicki Z. Why do adolescents use substances (drugs/alcohol)? J Alcohol Drug Educ 1986; 32:1-7.
37. Huba GJ, Bentler PM. The role of peer and adult models for drug taking at different stages in adolescence. J Youth Adolesc 1980;9:449-465.
38. Needle R, McCubbin H, Wilson M, Reineck R, Lazar A, Mederer H. Interpersonal influences in adolescent drug use—the role of older siblings, parents, and peers. Int J Addictions 1986;21:739-766.
39. Kandel D. Stages in adolescent involvement in drug use. Science (Wash DC) 1975;190:912-914.
40. Stimmel B, ed. Cultural and sociological aspects of alcoholism and subst abuse. Adv Alcohol & Substance Abuse 1984;4(1).
41. Mitchell JE, Boutacoff LI. Laxative abuse complicating bulimia: medical treatment implications. Int J Eating Disord 1986;5:325-334.
42. Mitchell JE, Boutacoff LI, Hatsuakami D, Pyle RL, Eckert ED. Laxative abuse as a variant of bulimia. J Nerv Mental Dis 1986;174:174-176.
43. Gottlieb A. Sex drugs and aphrodisiacs. New York: High Times/Level Press, 1974.
44. Kanof NM. Cosmetics: proposal for redefinition. J Am Acad Dermatol 1979;1:67-69.
45. Anonymous. Unapproved use of minoxidil. FDA Drug Bull 1985;15:38.
46. Shalita AR. Acne vulgaris and rosacea. In Rakel RE, ed. Conn's current therapy. Philadelphia: WB Saunders, 1986, pp 609-611.
47. Anonymous. Marilyn Monroe dead, pills near. New York Times. 1962;106(38180):1,13.
48. Salsman J. The suicide-pill option. Newsweek on Campus. March 1985, p 36.

SELECTED READINGS

ANATOMICALLY CORRECT [a]

Laurence J. Purdy

Walking to the morgue, I couldn't help thinking of a friend of mine who recently lost a child at term, a tragedy for him and his wife. For weeks the effects of this loss worked on him and changed him; he buried himself deeper in his work and lost, along with the child, his remarkable sense of humor that formerly had made work for everyone in the lab that much more enjoyable. As I opened the door of the morgue, I was struck hard by the thought of the pain that another set of parents must be suffering at this very moment.

Before beginning the autopsy, I played out the scenario that happens all too often in these circumstances, that the child will appear perfectly normal and no anatomic defect will be seen to explain the intrauterine death, leaving the parents with the burden of resolving their own private guilt, of asking themselves what it was that they did wrong. While unwrapping the infant from its white cloth, I expected to see in its pristine nakedness a perfect little form that never had a chance, and nothing more. But I was stunned by the horror that I uncovered. The fetus had a face deformed by a severely cleft lip and palate and a nose that was a flap of skin hanging like a veil from the center of the brow ridge. Inside, there was a set of pelvic, cystic kidneys and a hypoplastic left lung. I vicariously applied my own feelings to this situation and thought how fortunate it really was that this child didn't live and hoped that the parents didn't get a glimpse of it. Had it been normal, I would have stared at it a minute, briefly caressed its soft skin, and wondered what the parents were thinking at that very moment and what the infant might have grown to become.

It happens all the time, as one theory has it, that severe genetic abnormalities are taken care of by Mother Nature through spontaneous abortions, often occurring before the would-be mother knows she is pregnant. Any part of the complex genetic code can go awry and trigger such abortions. Medical science now has the skill to detect certain genetic mistakes prenatally, alerting the parents to problems their newborn may have, thus offering them the option of abortion. This prenatal diagnosis averts anxiety in some parents of a conceptus that is not normal and in a few who are worried that theirs might not be so. It is a marvelous advance against one small realm of human suffering.

Throughout my years as a pathologist, I have seen strikingly bizarre genetic monsters who resisted the urgings of Mother Nature and dodged the careful scrutiny of medical science only to face the impossibility of life outside the womb. Siamese twins joined by a single heart, anencephalics, infants with hypoplastic lungs, and a variety of others unequipped for life are conceived and delivered daily. We cringe at the sight of the genetic misfits who survive, trying not to look twice, and our hearts go out to the parents of these unfortunates, parents who would spend their entire lives caring for these offspring, parents compelled by a guilt most people will never know. Standing on the outside of this arena of suffering, it is hard to avoid sympathy for the parents and not to consider it fortunate that many can look

[a] Reprinted with permission from Purdy LJ. Anatomically correct. *JAMA* 1987;257(12):1648.

forward to old age unbridled from their children; many of them simply do not make it past childhood. But we have all seen that resigned and stoic expression on the face of an old, graying woman waiting outside a men's restroom, waiting until her middle-aged Down's syndrome child comes bouncing out with the typical eternal smile carved on his face. They walk off together, one happy and carefree, the other almost as if weighed down by a scarlet letter.

The genetic aberrancies are just a visual reminder of a much larger problem. When I finished the autopsy, I thought it best to gather all the data I could before dictating the case. Maybe it was a form of voyeurism passed off as the need for better documentation that made me look at the mother's chart. She was a 35-year-old drug addict—cocaine, PCP, heroin—who did not know who the father was and who had had no prenatal care. She took her last "fix" the morning of the delivery; perhaps the fetus died of a drug overdose. I reassessed my sweeping empathy for the parents of stillborn infants when I considered the kind of life this child was likely to have had, even if she had been perfectly normal, anatomically.

CAPITAL PUNISHMENT AND THE RESPONSIBLE PHARMACIST [b]

George J. Perchak

Lethal injection as a particular method of capital punishment first started in Oklahoma, and other states followed soon after. Since the Federal government is not constitutionally delegated the power to specify the method of capital punishment to be employed, the states have reserved this power for themselves.

Acting under this doctrine of federalism, the various states presently use five different methods of administering capital punishment: hanging, firing squad, electric chair, gas chamber, and now, lethal injection (1).

The reason for using new technology—whether injection or something else—to execute convicted criminals is generally the same as it has always been—to provide a humane method of killing condemned prisoners, one that is presumably less painful than a previous method.

It was for humane reasons that a physician invented the guillotiné (2), that New York gave us the electric chair, and Nevada contributed the gas chamber (3). Curiously, however, Oklahoma justified its lethal injection program with the twin arguments that it would be both more humane and a cost-effective alternative to reconstructing its electric chair or building a gas chamber.

INCONSISTENCIES

A closer look at the history of these macabre innovations, however, reveals that there have been some inconsistencies in the arguments about which particular method should be considered the most humane.

In the past, an 1887 commission definitely favored electrocution over chemical methods (4). Even Thomas Edison supported the use of electricity for executions (5).

---

[b]Reprinted with permission from Perchak GJ. Capital punishment and the responsible pharmacist. Am Pharm 1985;25:406–407.

Today, lethal injection appears to have made a comeback as the most humane method: electricity no longer enjoys the popularity it once had.

Nonetheless, the import of all this has been to try and somehow make the killing of condemned criminals reasonably acceptable. Socially, the less the act of capital punishment horrifies the public, the greater likelihood of it continuing. And, constitutionally, the less violation there is of the Eighth Amendment's ban on cruel and unusual punishment, the less fear of interference from the courts.

But regardless of which method of execution may be currently considered more humane, or the social and constitutional impact of that method, capital punishment essentially remains what it has always been from a moral viewpoint—a condemnable system of legalized retribution. Variations in the means employed to reach the same end do not appreciably alter an insoluble moral dilemma: that taking any convicted criminal's life only adds a second wrong to the first wrong committed by the criminal.

No one has the moral authority to execute a human being. When one kills killers, it is still murder.

It does not stand to reason that, as one commentator has put it, "Capital punishment is . . . a controversial issue itself, but the question of using 'prescription drugs' to carry out the process of execution is a completely separate and distinct matter" (6).

SPECIAL CONCERNS

However, lethal injection per se does pose special concerns to pharmacists, since the procedure entails requesting—or conscripting—their services. There have already been notable attempts at involving pharmacists in capital punishment via injection, as though the pharmacist were some kind of "death-care provider" whose expertise should be integrated into the process.

Cases in point include the proposed legislation requiring the Dean of the Arkansas College of Pharmacy to provide appropriate consulting services to the director of the department of corrections, and the Connecticut department of corrections' attempt to get professional advice on the agents to be used in lethal injection from the Drug Information Center at the University of Connecticut Health Center.

OFFICIAL POLICIES

Some pharmacy organizations have responded by adopting official positions on the issue. The American Pharmaceutical Association adopted the following policy in 1985:

1. *The American Pharmaceutical Association opposes the use of the term "drug" for chemicals used in lethal injections.*
2. *The American Pharmaceutical Association opposes the laws and regulations which mandate the participation of pharmacists in the process of execution by lethal injection.*

The American Society of Hospital Pharmacists' policy states:

1. *A decision by a pharmacist to participate in the use of drugs in capital punishment is one of individual conscience.*
2. *Pharmacists, regardless of who employs them, should not be put at risk of any disciplinary action, including loss of their jobs, because of refusal to participate in capital punishment.*

Both these policy statements do not prevent an individual from availing himself of his personal liberty to participate in capital punishment, nor do they have the wisdom to morally condemn such participation.

PERSONAL RESPONSIBILITY

However, individual pharmacists can still personally condemn lethal injection, and all of the other methods of capital punishment. For my part, moral law dictates that human life must be our highest value, and since capital punishment clearly negates that value, it is a moral atrocity. The legalization of this punitive process does not in any way redeem it.

In addition to not providing consultation or information services for this process, or actually participating, pharmacists need to be more aware of the less obvious ways that they might inadvertently become a party to an act of capital punishment.

For example, the medical director of Oklahoma's correction department can order his supplies from a pharmacy near the state prison, and those supplies may become the lethal tools of an execution (3). A responsible pharmacist must consider that what he dispenses might be the means by which an execution takes place, and therefore, by natural extension, the pharmacist could in some way figure in that execution.

One must safeguard against the practice of indiscriminately dispensing products without giving thought or care as to how they will be used. Not taking those safeguards invites involvement, tacit approval, and blame.

Likewise, it would be unethical to author an article on, say, the toxicokinetics involved with an execution, or any other subject that might lend itself to promoting the act, even if it is done in the belief that such work will result in a humane execution.

The same prohibition applies to research in this area that would have similar negative consequences. The probable results of one's work should always be given consideration before it is initiated. If the foreseeable outcome of that research is not very likely to be used in the service of mankind, and will instead be abused, then it should be abandoned.

MAINTAINING INTEGRITY

Pharmacy is a life-giving profession. To maintain the integrity of that heritage, pharmacists need to consider their actions carefully and confer moral character to their professional responsibilities. Lesser standards of conduct are unacceptable, and the profession must be maintained at the highest level possible.

It may be that the lethal injection issue in particular has sensitized pharmacists to capital punishment. Reflecting on only that single issue, however, is not enough.

While particular care should be given to all the immediate professional considerations, condemning the whole notion of capital punishment is also justifiably a part of our obligation, as is warning other pharmacists away from any involvement whatsoever. If policy statements fall short of this obligation, then individuals must rise to the occasion and speak out.

REFERENCES

1. T. O. Finks, *The Journal of Legal Medicine, 4,* 384 (1983).
2. D. B. Weiner, *Journal of the American Medical Association, 220,* 85 (1972).
3. P. Malone, "Death Row and the Medical Model," The Hastings Center, vol. 9, 1979.

4. J. M. Bleyer, *Medical Legal Journal, 5,* 425 (1887).
5. N. P. Brown, *Medical Legal Journal, 6,* 386 (1888).
6. E. G. Feldmann, *Journal of Pharmaceutical Sciences, 73,* 1189 (1984).

THE MEANING OF MEDICATIONS: ANOTHER LOOK AT COMPLIANCE[c]

Peter Conrad

Compliance with medical regimens, especially drug regimens, has become a topic of central interest for both medical and social scientific research. By compliance we mean "the extent to which a person's behavior (in terms of taking medications, following diets, or executing lifestyle changes) coincides with medical or health advice" (1). It is noncompliance that has engendered the most concern and attention. Most theories locate the sources of noncompliance in the doctor-patient interaction, patient knowledge or beliefs about treatment and, to a lesser extent, the nature of the regimen or illness.

This paper offers an alternative perspective on noncompliance with drug regimens, one situated in the patient's experience of illness. Most studies of noncompliance assume the centrality of patient-practitioner interaction for compliance. Using data from a study of the experience of epilepsy, I argue that from a patient-centered perspective the meanings of medication in people's everyday lives are more salient than doctor-patient interaction for understanding why people alter their prescribed medical regimens. The issue is more one of self-regulation than compliance. I develop the concept of medication practice to aid in understanding patient's experiences with medication regimens. This perspective enables us to analyze 'noncompliance' among our sample of people with epilepsy in a different light than the usual medically-centered approach allows.

EPILEPSY, MEDICATION AND SELF-REGULATION

The common medical response to a diagnosis of epilepsy is to prescribe various medications to control seizures. Given the range of types of epilepsy and the variety of physiological reactions to these medications, patients often see doctors as having a difficult time getting their medication 'right.' There are starts and stops and changes, depending on the degree of seizure control and the drug's side effects. More often than not, patients are stabilized on a medication or combination at a given dosage or regimen. Continuing or altering medications is the primary if not sole medical management strategy for epilepsy.

Medications are important to people with epilepsy. They 'control' seizures. Most take this medication several times daily. It becomes a routine part of their everyday lives. Although all of our respondents were taking or had taken these drugs, their responses to them varied. The effectiveness of these drugs in controlling seizures is a matter of degree. For some, seizures are stopped completely; they take pills regularly and have no seizures. For most, seizure frequency and duration are decreased significantly, although not reduced to zero. For a very few of our respondents, medications seem to have little impact; seizures continue unabated.

[c]Edited and reprinted with permission from Conrad P. The meaning of medications: another look at compliance. Soc Sci Med 1985;20:29–37.

Nearly all our respondents said medications have helped them control seizures at one time or another. At the same time, however, many people changed their dose and regimen from those medically prescribed. Some stopped altogether. If medications were seen as so helpful, why were nearly half of our respondents 'noncompliant' with their doctors' orders?

Most people with illnesses, even chronic illnesses such as epilepsy, spend only a tiny fraction of their lives in the 'patient role.' Compliance assumes that the doctor-patient relationship is pivotal for subsequent action, which may not be the case. Consistent with our perspective, we conceptualize the issue as one of developing a *medication practice*. Medication practice offers a patient-centered perspective of how people manage their medications, focusing on the meaning and use of medications. In this light we can see the doctor's medication orders as the 'prescribed medication practice' (e.g. take a 20 mg pill four times a day). Patients interpret the doctor's prescribed regimen and create a medication practice that may vary decidedly from the prescribed practice. Rather than assume the patient will follow prescribed medical rules, this perspective allows us to explore the kinds of practices patients create. Put another way, it sees patients as active agents rather than passive recipients of doctors' orders.

Although many people failed to conform to their prescribed medication regimen, they did not define this conduct primarily as noncompliance with doctors' orders. The more we examined the data, the clearer it was that from the patient's perspective, doctors had very little impact on people's decisions to alter their medications. It was, rather, much more a question of regulation of control. To examine this more closely we developed criteria for what we could call self-regulation. Many of our respondents occasionally missed taking their medicine, but otherwise were regular in their medication practice. One had to do more than 'miss' medications now and again (even a few times a week) to be deemed self-regulating. A person had to (1) reduce or raise the daily dose of prescribed drugs for several weeks or more or (2) skip or take extra doses regularly under specific circumstances (e.g. when drinking, staying up late or under 'stress') or (3) stop taking the drugs completely for three consecutive days or longer. These criteria are arbitrary, but they allow us to estimate the extent of self-regulation. Using this definition, 34 of our 80 respondents (42%) self-regulated their medication.†

To understand the meaning and management of medications we need to look at those who follow a prescribed medications practice as well as those who create their own variations. While we note that 42% of our respondents are at variance with medical expectations, this number is more suggestive than definitive. Self-regulators are not a discrete and separate group. About half the self-regulators could be defined as regular in their practice, whatever it might be. They may have stopped for a week once or twice, or take extra medica-

---

† Reports in the medical literature indicate that noncompliance with epilepsy regimens is considered a serious problem (2–6). One study reports that 40% of patients missed the prescribed medication dose often enough to affect their blood-level medication concentrations (7); an important review article estimates noncompliance with epilepsy drug regimens between 30 and 40%, with a range from 20 to 75% (8). Another study suggests that noncompliant patients generally had longer duration of the disorder, more complicated regimens and more medication changes (9). Attempts to increase epilepsy medication compliance include improving doctor-patient communication, incorporating patients more in treatment programs, increasing patient knowledge and simplifying drug regimens. Since noncompliance with anti-convulsant medication regimens is deemed the most frequent reason why patients suffer recurrent seizures (10), some researchers suggest, "If the patient understands the risks of stopping medication, he *will not stop*" (11). Yet there also have been reports of active noncompliance with epilepsy medications (12). In sum, epilepsy noncompliance studies are both typical of and reflect upon most other compliance research. In this sense, epilepsy is a good example for developing an alternative approach to understanding how people manage their medications.

tion only under 'stressful' circumstances; otherwise, they are regular in their practice. On the other hand, perhaps a quarter of those following the prescribed medical practice say they have seriously considered changing or stopping their medications. It is likely there is an overlap between self-regulating and medical-regulating groups. While one needs to appreciate and examine the whole range of medication practice, the self-regulators provide a unique resource for analysis. They articulate views that are probably shared in varying degree by all people with epilepsy and provide an unusual insight into the meaning of medication and medication practice. We first describe how people account for following a prescribed medication practice; we then examine explanations offered for altering prescribed regimens and establishing their own practices. A final section outlines how the meaning of medications constructs and reflects the experience of epilepsy.

A TICKET TO NORMALITY

The availability of effective seizure control medications early in this century is a milestone in the treatment of epilepsy (Phenobarbital was introduced in 1912; Dilantin in 1938). These drugs also literally changed the experience of having epilepsy. To the extent the medications controlled seizures, people with epilepsy suffered fewer convulsive disruptions in their lives and were more able to achieve conventional social roles. To the extent doctors believed medications effective, they developed greater optimism about their ability to treat epileptic patients. To the degree the public recognized epilepsy as a 'treatable' disorder, epileptics were no longer segregated in colonies and less subject to restrictive laws regarding marriage, procreation and work (24). It is not surprising that people with epilepsy regard medications as a 'ticket' to normality. The drugs did not, speaking strictly, affect anything but seizures. It was the social response to medication that brought about these changes. As one woman said: "I'm glad we've got [the medications] . . . you know, in the past people didn't and they were looked upon as lepers."

For most people with epilepsy, taking medicine becomes one of those routines of everyday life we engage in to avoid unwanted circumstances or improve our health. Respondents compared it to taking vitamins, birth control pills or teeth brushing. It becomes almost habitual, something done regularly with little reflection. One young working man said: "Well, at first I didn't like it, [but] it doesn't bother me anymore. Just like getting up in the morning and brushing your teeth. It's just something you do."

But seizure control medications differ from 'normal pills' like vitamins or contraceptives. They are prescribed for a medical disorder and are seen both by the individual and others, as indicators or evidence of having epilepsy. One young man as a child did not know he had epilepsy "short of taking [his] medication." He said of this connection between epilepsy and medication: "I do, so therefore I have." Medications represent epilepsy: Dilantin or Phenobarbital are quickly recognized by medical people and often by others as epilepsy medications.

Medications can also indicate the degree of one's disorder. Most of our respondents do not know any others with epilepsy; thus they examine changes in their own epilepsy biographies as grounds for conclusions about their condition. Seizure activity is one such sign; the amount of medications 'necessary' is another. A decrease or increase in seizures is taken to mean that epilepsy is getting better or worse. So it is with medications. While two may be related—especially because the common medical response to more seizures is increased medication—they may also operate independently. If the doctor reduces the dose or strength of medication, or vice versa, the patient may interpret this as a sign of improvement or worsening. Similarly, if a person reduces his or her own dose, being able to 'get along' on this lowered amount of medication is taken as evidence of 'getting better.' Since for a large portion of people with epilepsy seizures are considered to be well-controlled, medications become the only readily available measure of the 'progress' of the disorder.

TAKING MEDICATIONS

We tried to suspend the medical assumptions that people take medications simply because they are prescribed, or because they are supposed to control seizures, to examine our respondents' accounts of what they did and why.

The reason people gave most often for taking medication is *instrumental:* to control seizures, or more generally, to reduce the likelihood of body malfunction. Our respondents often drew a parallel to the reason people with diabetes take insulin. As one woman said, "If it does the trick, I'd rather take them [medications] than not." Or, as a man who would "absolutely not" miss his medications explained, "I don't want to have seizures" (although he continued to have 3 or 4 a month). Those who deal with their medication on instrumental grounds see it simply as a fact of life, as something to be done to avoid body malfunction and social and personal disruption.

While controlling body malfunction is always an underlying reason for taking medications, psychological grounds may be equally compelling. Many people said that medication *reduces worry,* independent of its actually decreasing seizures. These drugs can make people feel secure, so they don't have to think about the probability of seizures. A 20 year-old woman remarked: "My pills keep me from getting hysterical." A woman who has taken seizure control medication for 15 years describes this 'psychological' function of medication: "I don't know what it does, but I suppose I'm psychologically dependent on it. In other words, if I take my medication, I feel better." Some people actually report 'feeling better'—clearer, more alert and energetic—when they do not take these drugs, but because they begin to worry if they miss, they take them regularly anyhow.

The most important reason for taking medication, however, is to insure 'normality.' People said specifically that they take medications to be more 'normal': The meaning here is normal in the sense of 'leading a normal life.' In the words of a middle-aged public relations executive who said he does not restrict his life because of epilepsy: "Except I always take my medication. I don't know why. I figure if I took them, then I could do anything I want to do." People believed taking medicine reduces the risk of having a seizure in the presence of others, which might be embarassing or frightening. As a young woman explained:

> I feel if it's going to help, that's what I want because you know you feel uncomfortable enough anyway that you don't want anything like [a seizure] to happen around other people; so if it's going to help, I'll take it.

This is not to say people with epilepsy like to take medications. Quite the contrary. Many respondents who follow their medically prescribed medication practice openly say they 'hate' taking medications and hope someday to be 'off' the drugs. Part of this distaste is related to the dependence people come to feel. Some used the metaphor of being an addict: "I'm a real drug addict"; "I was an addict before it was fashionable"; "I'm like an alcoholic without a drink; I *have* to have them [pills]"; and "I really don't want to be hooked for the rest of my life." Even while loathing the pills or the 'addiction' people may be quite disciplined about taking these drugs.

The drugs used to control seizures are not, of course, foolproof. Some people continue to have seizures quite regularly while others suffer only occasional episodes. Such limited effectiveness does not necessarily lead these people to reject medication as a strategy. They continue, with frustration, to express "hope" that "they [doctors] will get it [the medication] right." For some, then, medications are but a limited ticket to normality.

SELF-REGULATION: GROUNDS FOR CHANGING MEDICATION PRACTICE

For most people there is not a one-to-one correspondence between taking or missing medications and seizure activity. People who take medications regularly may still have seizures, and some people who discontinue their medications may be seizure-free for months or longer. Medical experts say a patient may well miss a whole day's medication yet still have enough of the drug in the bloodstream to prevent a seizure for this period.

In this section we focus on those who deviate from the prescribed medication practice and variously regular their own medication. On the whole, members of this subgroup are slightly younger than the rest of the sample (average age 25 vs 32) and somewhat more likely to be female (59–43%), but otherwise are not remarkably different from our respondents who follow the prescribed medication practice. Self-regulation for most of our respondents consists of reducing the dose, stopping for a time, or regularly skipping or taking extra doses of medication depending on various circumstances.

Reducing the dose (including total termination) is the most common form of self-regulation. In this context, two points are worth re-stating. First, doctors typically alter doses of medication in times of increased seizure activity or troublesome drug 'side effects.' It is difficult to strike the optimum level of medication. To people with epilepsy, it seems that doctors engage in a certain amount of trial and error behavior. Second, and more important, medications are defined, both by doctors and patients, as an indicator of the degree of disorder. If seizure activity is not 'controlled' or increases, patients see that doctors respond by raising (or changing) medications. The more medicine prescribed means epilepsy is getting worse; the less means it is getting better. What doctors do does not necessarily explain what patients do, but it may well be an example our respondents use in their own management strategies. The most common rationales for altering a medication practice are drug related: the medication is perceived as ineffective or the so-called side effects become too troublesome.

The efficacy of a drug is a complex issue. Here our concern is merely with perceived efficacy. When a medication is no longer seen as efficacious it is likely to be stopped. Many people continue to have seizures even when they follow the prescribed medication practice. If medication seemed to make no difference, our respondents were more likely to consider changing their medication practice. One woman who stopped taking medications for a couple of months said, "It seemed like [I had] the same number of seizures without it." Most people who stop taking their medicine altogether eventually resume a medication practice of some sort. A woman college instructor said, "When I was taking Dilantin, I stopped a number of times because it never seemed to *do* anything."

The most common drug-related rationally for reducing dose is troublesome 'side effects.' People with epilepsy attribute a variety of side effects to seizure control medications. One category of effects includes swollen and bleeding gums, oily or yellow skin, pimples, sore throat and a rash. Another category includes slowed mental functioning, drowsiness, slurred speech, dullness, impaired memory, loss of balance and partial impotence.* The first category, which we can call body side effects, were virtually never given as an account for self-regulation. Only those side effects that impaired social skills, those in the second category, were given as reasons for altering doctors' medication orders.

Social side effects impinge on social interaction. People believed they felt and acted differently. A self-regulating woman described how she feels when she takes her medication:

> I can feel that I become much more even. I feel like I flatten out a little bit. I don't like that feeling. . . . It's just a feeling of dullness, which I don't like, almost a feeling that you're on the edge of laziness.

If people saw their medication practice as hindering the ability to participate in routine social affairs, they were likely to change it. Our respondents gave many examples such as a college student who claimed the medication slowed him down and wondered if it were affecting his memory, a young newspaper reporter who reduced his medication because it was putting him to sleep at work; or the social worker who felt she 'sounds smarter' and more articulate when 'off medications.'

Drug side effects, even those that impair social skills, are not sufficient in themselves to explain the level of self-regulation we found. Self-regulation was considerably more than a reaction to annoying and uncomfortable side effects. It was an active and intentional endeavor.

SOCIAL MEANINGS OF REGULATING MEDICATION PRACTICE

Variations in medication practice by and large seem to depend on what medication and self-regulation mean to our respondents. Troublesome relationships with physicians, including the perception that they have provided inadequate medical information (13), may be a foundation on which alternative strategies and practices are built. Our respondents, however, did not cite such grounds for altering their doctors' orders. People vary their medication practice on grounds connected to managing their everyday lives. If we examine the social meanings of medications from our respondents' perspectives, self-regulation turns on four grounds: testing; control of dependence; destigmatization; and practical practice. While individual respondents may cite one or more of these as grounds for altering medication practice, they are probably best understood as strategies common among those who self regulate.

Testing

Once people with epilepsy begin taking seizure-control medications, given there are no special problems and no seizures, doctors were reported to seldom change the medical regimen. People are likely to stay on medications indefinitely. But how can one know that a period without seizures is a result of medication or spontaneous remission of the disorder? How long can one go without medication? How 'bad' is this case of epilepsy? How can one know if epilepsy is 'getting better' while still taking medication? Usually after a period without or with only a few seizures, many reduced or stopped their medicine altogether to test for themselves whether or not epilepsy was 'still there.'

---

*These are reported side effects. They may or may not be drug related, but our respondents attribute them to the medication.

People can take themselves off medications as an experiment, to see 'if anything will happen.' One woman recalled:

> I was having one to two seizures a year on phenobarb . . . so I decided not to take it and to see what would happen . . . so I stopped it and I watched and it seemed that I had the same amount of seizures with it as without it . . . for three years.

She told her physician, who was skeptical but 'allowed' her this control of her medication practice. A man who had taken medication three times a day for 16 years felt intuitively that he could stop his medications:

> Something kept telling me I didn't have to take [medication] anymore, a feeling or somethin'. It took me quite a while to work up the nerve to stop takin' the pills. An one day I said, "One way to find out. . . ."

After suffering what he called drug withdrawal effects, he had no seizures for 6 years. Others test to see how long they can go without medication and seizures.

Testing does not always turn out successfully. A public service agency executive tried twice to stop taking medications when he thought he had 'kicked' epilepsy. After two failures, he concluded that stopping medications "just doesn't work." But others continue to test, hoping for some change in their condition. One middle-aged housewife said:

> When I was young I would try not to take it . . . I'd take it for a while and think, "Well, I don't need it anymore," so I would not take it for, deliberately, just to see if I could do without. And then [in a few days] I'd start takin' it again, because I'd start passin' out . . . I will still try that now, when my husband is out of town . . . I just think, maybe I'm still gonna grow out of it or something.

Testing by reducing or stopping medication is only one way to evaluate how one's disorder is progressing. Even respondents who follow the prescribed medication regimen often wonder 'just what would happen' if they stopped.

Controlling Dependence

People with epilepsy struggle continually against becoming too dependent on family, friends, doctors or medications. They do, of course, depend on medications for control of seizures. The medications do not necessarily eliminate seizures and many of our respondents resented their dependence on them. Another paradox is that although medications can increase self reliance by reducing seizures, taking medications can be *experienced* as a threat to self reliance. Medications seem almost to become symbolic of the dependence created by having epilepsy.

There is a widespread belief in our society that drugs create dependence and that being on chemical substances is not a good thing. Somehow, whatever the goal is, it is thought to be better if we can get there without drugs. Our respondents reflected these ideas in their comments.

A college junior explained: "I don't like it at all. I don't like chemicals in my body. It's sort of like a dependency only that I have to take it because my body forced me to. . . ." A political organizer who says medications reduce his seizures commented: "I've never enjoyed having to depend on anything . . . drugs in particular." A nurse summed up the situation: "The *drugs* were really a kind of dependence." Having to take medication relinquished some degree of control of one's life. A woman said:

> I don't like to have to *take* anything. It was, like, at one time birth control pills, but I don't like to take anything *everyday*. It's just like, y'know, controlling me, or something.

The feeling of being controlled need not be substantiated in fact for people to act upon it. If people *feel* dependent on and controlled by medication, it is not surprising that they seek to avoid these drugs. A high school junior, who once took medicine because he feared having a seizure in the street, commented:

> And I'd always heard medicine helps and I just kept taking it and finally I just got so I didn't depend on the medicine no more, I could just fight it off myself and I just stopped taking it in.

After stopping for a month he forgot about his medications completely.

Feelings of dependence are one reason people gave for regulating medicine. For a year, one young social worker took medication when she felt it was necessary; otherwise, she tried not to use it. When we asked her why, she responded, "I regulate my own drug . . . mostly because it's really important for me not to be dependent." She occasionally had seizures and continued to alter her medication to try to 'get it right':

> I started having [seizures] every once in a while. And I thought wow, the bad thing is that I just haven't regulated it right and I just need to up it a little bit and then, you know, if I do it just right, I won't have epilepsy anymore.

This woman and others saw medications as a powerful resource in their struggle to gain control over epilepsy. Although she no longer thinks she can rid herself of epilepsy, this woman still regulates her medication.

In this context, people with epilepsy manipulate their sense of dependence on medications by changing medication practice. But there is a more subtle level of dependence that encourages such changes. Some reported they regulated their medication intake in direct response to interventions of others, especially family members. It was as if others *wanted* them to be more dependent by coaxing or reminding them to take their medications regularly. Many responded to this encouraged greater dependence by creating their own medication practice.

A housewife who said she continues regularly to have petit mal seizures and tremors along with an occasional grand mal seizure, remarked:

> Oh, like most things, when someone tells me I have to do something, I basically resent it. . . . If it's my option and I choose to do it, I'll probably do it more often than not. But if you tell me I have to, I'll bend it around and do it my own way, which is basically what I have done.

Regardless of whether one feels dependent on the drug or dependent because of others' interventions around drug taking, changing a prescribed medication practice, as well as continuing self-regulation serve as a form of *taking control* of one's epilepsy.

Destigmatization

Epilepsy is a stigmatized illness. Sufferers attempt to control information about the disorder to manage this threat (14). There are no visible stimata that make a person with epilepsy obviously different from other people, but a number of aspects of having epilepsy can compromise attempts at information control. The four signs that our respondents most frequently mentioned as threatening information control were seizures in the presence of others, job or insurance applications, lack of a driver's license and taking medications. People may try to avoid seizures in public, lie or hedge on their applications, develop accounts for not having a driver's license, or take their medicine in private in order to minimize the stigma potential of epilepsy.

Medication usually must be taken three or four times daily, so at least one dose must be taken away from home. People attempt to be private about taking their medications and/or develop 'normal' pill accounts ("it's to help my digestion"). One woman's mother told her to take medications regularly, as she would for any other sickness:

> When I was younger it didn't bother me too bad. But as I got older, it would tend to bother me some. Whether it was, y'know, maybe somebody seeing me or somethin', I don't know. But it did.

Most people develop skills to minimize potential stigmatization from taking pills in public.

On occasion, stopping medications is an attempt to vacate the stigmatized status of epileptic. One respondent wrote us a letter describing how she tried to get her mother to accept her by not taking her medications. She wrote:

> This is going to sound real dumb, but I can't help it. My mother never accepted me when I was little because I was "different." I stopped taking my medication in an attempt to be normal and accepted by her. Now that I know I need medication it's like I'm completely giving up trying to be "normal" so mom won't be ashamed of me. I'm going to accept the fact that I'm "different" and I don't really care if mom gives a damn or not.

Taking medications in effect acknowledges this 'differentness.'

It is, of course, more difficult to hide the meaning of medications from one's self. Taking medication is a constant reminder of having epilepsy. For some it is as if the medication itself represents the stigma of epilepsy. The young social worker quoted above felt if she could stop taking her medications she would no longer be an epileptic. A young working woman summed up succinctly why avoiding medications would be avoiding stima: "Well, at least I would not be . . . generalized and classified in a group as being an epileptic."

Practical Practice

Self-regulators spoke often of how they changed the dose or regimen of medication in an effort to reduce the risk of having a seizure, particularly during 'high stress' situations. Several respondents who were students said they take extra medications during exam periods or when they stay up late studying. A law student who had not taken his medicine for 6 months took some before his law school exams: "I think it increases the chances [seizures] won't happen." A woman who often participated in horse shows said she "usually didn't pay attention" to her medication practice but takes extra when she doesn't get the six to eight hours sleep she requires: I'll wake up and take two capsules instead of one . . . and I'll generally take it like when we're going to horse shows. I'll take it pretty consistently." Such uses of medication are common ways of trying to forestall 'possible trouble.'

People with epilepsy changed their medication practice for practical ends in two other kinds of circumstances. Several reported they took extra medication if they felt a 'tightening' or felt a seizure coming on. Many people also said they did not take medications if they were going to drink alcohol. They believed that medication (especially Phenobarbital) and alcohol do not mix well.

In short, people change their medication practice to suit their perceptions of social environment. Some reduce medication to avoid potential problems from mixing alcohol and drugs. Others reduce it to remain 'clear-headed' and 'alert' during 'important' performances (something of a 'Catch-22' situation). Most, however, adjust their medications practically in an effort to reduce the risk of seizures.

CONCLUSION: ASSERTING CONTROL

Regulating medication represents an attempt to assert some degree of control over a condition that appears at times to be completely beyond control. Loss of control is a significant concern for people with epilepsy. While medical treatment can increase both the sense and the fact of control over epilepsy, and information control can limit stigmatization, the regulation of medications is one way people with epilepsy struggle to gain some personal control over their condition.

Medication practice can be modified on several different grounds. Side effects that make managing everyday social interaction difficult can lead to the reduction or termination of medication. People will change their medication practice, including stopping altogether, in order to 'test' for the existence or 'progress' of the disorder. Medication may be altered to control the perceived level of dependence, either on the drugs themselves or on those who 'push' them to adhere to a particular medication practice. Since the medication can represent the stigma potential of epilepsy, both literally and symbolically, altering medication practice can be a form of destigmatization. And finally, many people modify their medication practice in anticipation of specific social circumstances, usually attempting to reduce the risk of seizures.

It is difficult to judge how generalizable these findings are to other illnesses. Clearly, people develop medication practices whenever they must take medications regularly. This is probably most true for long-term chronic illness where medication becomes a central part of everyday life, such as diabetes, rheumatoid arthritis, hypertension and asthma. The degree and amount of self-regulation may differ among illnesses—likely to be related to symptomatology, effectiveness of medications and potential of stigma—but I suspect most of the meanings of medications described here would be present among sufferers of any illness that people must continually manage.

In sum, we found that a large proportion of the people with epilepsy we interviewed said they themselves regulate their medication. Medically-centered compliance research presents a skewed and even distorted view of how and why patients manage medication. From the perspective of the person with epilepsy, the issue is more clearly one of responding to the meaning of medications in everyday life than 'compliance' with physicians' orders and medical regimens. Framing the problem as self-regulation rather than compliance allows us to see modifying medication practice as a vehicle for asserting some control over epilepsy. One consequence of such a reframing would be to reexamine the value of achieving 'complaint' behavior and to rethink what strategies might be appropriate for achieving greater adherence to prescribed medication regimens.

REFERENCES

1. Haynes RB, Taylor DW, Sackett DL (eds). Compliance in Health Care, Johns Hopkins University Press, Baltimore, 1979.
2. Trostle J, et. al. The logic of non-compliance: Management of epilepsy from a patient's point of view, Cult Med Psychiat 1983;7:35–56.
3. Lund M, Jurgensen RS, Kuhl V. Serum diphenylhydantoin in ambulant patients with epilepsy, Epilepsia 1964;5:51–58.
4. Lund M. Failure to observe dosage instructions in patients with epilepsy, Acta Neurol Scand 1975;49:295–306.
5. Browne TR, Cramer IA. Antiepileptic drug serum concentration determinations, In Epilepsy: Diagnosis and Management (Edited by Browne TR and Feldman RG). Little, Brown, Boston, 1982.

6. Pryse-Phillips W, Jardine F, Bursey F. Compliance with drug therapy by epileptic patients, Epilepsia 1982;23:269–274.
7. Eisler J, Mattson RH. Compliance with anticonvulsant drug therapy, Epilepsia 1975;16:203.
8. The Commission for the Control of Epilepsy, and its Consequences. The literature on patient compliance and implications for cost-effective patient education programs with epilepsy. In Plan for Nationwide Action on Epilepsy, Vol. II, Part 1, pp. 391–415, U.S. Government Printing Office, Washington, D.C., 1977.
9. Bryant SG, Ereshfsky L. Determinants of compliance in epileptic conditions, Drug Intel Clin Pharmac 1981;15:572–577.
10. Reynolds EH. Drug treatment of epilepsy, Lancet 1978;11:721–725.
11. Norman SE, Browne TK. Seizure disorders, Am J Nurs 1981;81:893.
12. Desei BT, Reily TL, Porter RJ, Penry JK. Active non-compliance as a cause of uncontrolled seizures, Epilepsia 1978;19:447–452.
13. Becker MH, Maiman LA. Sociobehavioral determinants of compliance with health and medical care recommendations, Med Care 13:10–24.
14. Schneider J, Conrad P. In the closet with illness: epilepsy, stigma potential and information control, Soc Probl 1980;28:32–44.

ROAD BACK FROM SUBSTANCE ABUSE [d]

Virginia Cowart

It is not hard to see why athletes feel comfortable with Forest Tennant, MD, the California physician who has treated many athletes for substance abuse. In looks, speech, and actions, he is one of them. There is more than just a hint of the late University of Alabama football coach Paul (Bear) Bryant in Tennant, who would look perfectly at home striding up and down the sidelines turned out in a houndstooth check hat.

To watch him with a patient in end-stage liver disease as a by-product of alcoholism is a study in benevolent paternalism. The patient's eyes betray his confusion, and his anxiety is manifest in a flickering smile that gradually becomes more genuine as Tennant gives him the game plan of treatment.

"Paternalism is needed in treating addiction," Tennant says calmly, "and I really believe that most doctors are not comfortable with that. Fortunately, we see most substance abusers today before they are in as grave physical condition as this patient [who died within the month]."

NATIONAL FOOTBALL LEAGUE

Tennant has been thrust even more into the public eye lately because he is the physician who would have overseen the National Football League drug testing and treatment program announced last summer by Commissioner Pete Rozelle, if the plan had been upheld in arbitration.

Although his approach is upbeat and team-oriented, ask Tennant about the prospects for addicted athletes and the very sober physician appears.

"We know what will work," he says thoughtfully, "but it's a labor-intensive program. I got into the sports part of this because of false promises to athletes; they were being sent to

[d] Reprinted with permission from Cowart V. Road back from substance abuse. JAMA 1986;256(19):2645–2649.

the hospital for 28 days and called cured [by their teams and the public]. It just isn't that simple."

Actually, the outlook for an athlete with drug addiction is poorer than average, according to Tennant, who says, "They cannot be expected to do well. You have to have certain elements in your treatment program, self-help groups, counseling, urine testing, monitoring, social supports. An athlete is on the road all the time. Most of the time, he can't obtain what he needs to stay clean. Not that many athletes don't do well in spite of this," he hastens to add. "It's just more difficult for them."

That is also the view of Joseph A. Pursch, MD, who has treated many famous people for substance addiction. He outlined two things he has learned in a quarter century of treating substance abuse problems: "Don't believe anything the user tells you about the problem. Don't wait for an athlete to volunteer for testing or treatment; he can't make that kind of decision and the people around him will protect him."

He also noted that even when an athlete's performance is affected enough to command attention, it does not necessarily mean he will be tested or treated. The team may want him to finish the season or appear in the playoffs.

Additional hazards are that drugs are readily available wherever professional athletes gather, and pushers know who is vulnerable. Athletes have the money to purchase drugs and many of them fall into a population subgroup that he says is especially vulnerable to substance abuse; that is, males, age 20 to 50 years, upwardly mobile, and superficial in their attachments. (Some athletes are unable to form lasting emotional attachments simply because their jobs require almost constant travel during the season.)

Several investigators have noted that adolescents who are most likely to use illicit drugs are more alienated from parents, more critical of society, more adventuresome and thrill-seeking, more extroverted, less traditional, and less oriented to religion than their peers (*Comp Therapy* 1986;12:44–50).

IMPAIRMENT SYNDROME

Based on his experience with athletes, Tennant believes that some who are substance abusers (and this includes marijuana) may suffer harm to their careers, even if they cease using drugs, by developing what he calls Post Drug Impairment Syndrome (PDIS) and which he characterizes as a permanent chemical imbalance of the brain.

"I see it primarily in persons who take drugs in their early teen years," he continues, "but it can happen to anyone exposed to certain drugs for a long enough time."

The syndrome is characterized by inability to concentrate, maintain attention, hold a job, maintain personal relationships, achieve financial stability, handle stress, or physically remain in one location very long. It may also include fits of temper and antisocial behavior.

Tennant is executive director of Community Health Projects, Inc, which operates 23 medical clinics in 13 California cities. This system includes the largest drug abuse program in the western United States. He is associate professor at the University of California at Los Angeles School of Public Health, and a consultant to the National Football League, the Los Angeles Dodgers, the California Department of Justice, and the California Highway Patrol.

An athlete participating in an individual sport often is at less risk of becoming a substance abuser than one who is part of a team, according to both Tennant and Pursch, who was interviewed on the eve of his departure for England where he was the team physician for the United States men's tennis team which was competing at Wimbledon.

Pursch spent 20 years in the US Navy, many of them as a flight surgeon on aircraft carriers, and the last seven as director of the alcohol and drug program, Long Beach Naval Hospital. From 1980 through 1986, he was medical director of Careunit Hospital, Los Angeles. Currently, he treats patients with substance abuse problems at Family Care Clinic in Orange, Calif, and at South Coast Medical Center in Laguna Beach, Calif.

"Tennis is different," he said. "There are no contracts; if you don't work, you don't get paid. You're a solo performer but you don't even know the exact hours when you will give your performance—it depends on how long the match before yours runs."

Drug testing was done at Wimbledon this year for the first time and also at the US Open in September, but Pursch said recreational drug use among top level tennis players is minimal.

Tennant agrees that the solo player is less apt to take drugs: "In a professional football game, you could have as many as 70 people on the field in one afternoon. Just because a linebacker takes amphetamines on the day of the game, the outcome is not likely to be affected. There are too many people involved. But if it's an Olympic cyclist, he's out there alone and whatever he does will have performance impact."

REACHING A PEAK

Both physicians think a current peak of drug use in professional sports has been reached and Tennant thinks there are two aspects to this: "Players have seen too many of their fellow players go under to drugs, and professional teams have learned that their ability to rehabilitate a true addict is not good."

Treatment of an athlete is complicated by the fact that many of the professional sports figures are one-person corporations, not just a person with a substance abuse problem.

"When I have a sports star in my office for the first time, I can expect all the buttons on my telephone to be lit up," says Pursch, whose famous patients have included such well-known persons as Betty Ford, who now is actively engaged in helping others.

"His agent is on one line to tell me he has a beer commercial lined up for his client that can't be shot if it's known he is an alcoholic and the income loss will be multiple thousands of dollars. The coach wants to know how soon he can play, the hospital administrator wants to make a public announcement, and the star's lawyer wants it quiet. A TV network demands a full report. Agents for the players' association and the team have their interests, and his wife and ex-wife (and maybe a girl friend) want to be assured his income will continue. And all this," he sighs "is before I have ever taken his blood pressure."

What does Pursch think about the outlook for such a patient? "If you can find out who loves him and who pays him, then you can treat him."

Some of his better-known athlete patients have included baseball stars Vida Blue and Steve Howe, football players Thomas (Hollywood) Henderson and Charles White, and Olympic and professional boxer Tyrell Biggs.

Pursch himself has the lean build and fit look of the former Navy doctor and the often cynical but very funny wit of one who has seen the human condition at its worst. He thinks alcohol addiction may be the hardest substance abuse problem to treat in athletes "because of team spirit, which has alcohol use embeded in it."

In the locker room after the game when interviews are shown, many times the beer or champagne is flowing. When the team gets on the plane to go home after an out-of-town game, says Pursch, there will be a six-pack in each seat. The environment is such, he continued, that an athlete almost can't function as a teetotaler and some give up trying during their playing years. Because full-blown alcoholism may not be recognized for 15 to 20 years, many athletes are past their active sports participation when their addiction to alcohol can no longer be hidden.

"However, it's a different story with cocaine," Pursch continued. "Things go faster with coke."

Both Pursch and Tennant became interested in treating substance abuse in the military when it was more widespread than today. Since then, military education, treatment, and deterrent programs have been successful.

Tennant said he was so uniformed about drug use when he first went to Vietnam that when his commanding officer asked what he was going to do about the "hash problem," he thought first of food contamination.

"Often there would be other diagnoses on the charts," said Pursch of his early Navy years, "but alcoholism was the real problem. What offended me was that, since it was covered up, the patient never got well because the real problem was never addressed."

HUMAN FAILINGS

That exact situation—which has been successfully handled by the Navy—often prevails now in professional sports where even the public has a vested interest in not recognizing that the idol has clay feet. Often given privileges and accolades foreign to the general public, some athletes find it difficult to admit a human failing, particularly when fellow players, the coach, management, family, and even the public would rather not hear about it.

"The athlete gets sicker and sicker," says Pursch, "and we still offer excuses to explain away his drinking or drug addiction. Not until he is arrested or injured is there a push for treatment and, if he is killed, everybody says: How could this have happened?"

For an example of alcohol-related personal tragedy, one has to look no further than National Hockey League star Pelle Lindbergh who was killed when his automobile crashed at high speed into a wall. Lindbergh reportedly was intoxicated at the time.

Both Tennant and Pursch agree that drug use would surface much faster with a competent system of random testing. Drug testing was performed on a group of college football players who attended an NFL scouting camp last January (and who had reason to believe they would be tested) and 55 had positive results for cocaine or marijuana. Twenty-six were later picked in the NFL draft.

While many college students still equate alcohol and marijuana use, Tennant thinks that athletes cannot do so. He believes that marijuana use is particularly harmful to athletes and can permanently impair their visual perception and their ability to do fine muscle or mental tasks. The timing sense so critical in many sports may be affected just enough to make the small difference between success and failure in professional sports participation.

There is evidence, both in amateur and professional sports, of a management response to the dangers of drug taking. For example, the National Football League implemented a program in the early 1970s to monitor all prescription drugs given by the clubs. Don Weiss, executive director of the NFL, said that teams must give periodic reports (from the team physician) on what drugs have been dispensed and what the teams have on hand.

"We have a pretty good handle on what drugs are being prescribed legitimately," he says, "but trying to cut off all sources is very difficult."

RANDOM TESTING

Weiss thinks both amphetamine and steroid use have decreased in football, but adds that the only way to define the extent of drug problems in the NFL is with random testing.

Professional athletes themselves have not taken the idea of drug testing to their collective bosom, particularly random testing. When NFL commissioner Rozelle announced his drug plan, which included random testing at least twice a year for each player, the NFL Players Association set up an immediate howl.

Gene Upshaw, the executive director, said he favors stronger penalties for drug offenders but that the union is adamantly against random drug testing (a position that has found expression in Home Box Office's series on a fictional football team and where the good guy resisted testing after drugs were planted in his locker. That fiction has no foundation in fact since clubs already have the right to require a urine test "for reasonable cause.")

"I don't agree with him [Rozelle] that random testing is the answer," Upshaw said. "If we put teeth into the 'reasonable cause' argument, I could sell that to the players easily. I could sell harsher penalties easily. But the biggest problem for us is random testing and confidentiality. That I can't sell."

Yet testing is exactly what many team physicians think must be done to preserve the integrity of sports.

"I find it ironic that the team and their physicians are trying to help the professional athletes get off and stay off drugs while the players' union is fighting the effort," Bertram Zarins, MD, team physician for the New England Patriots football team, said at a conference. "It's crazy. We're trying to save their careers, maybe their lives, and they want a perk [perquisite] or two to let us do it," he continues.

Rozelle's plan for organized football calls for one announced preseason test and two random in-season tests for cocaine, marijuana, opiates, phenylcyclohexyl piperidine (PCP), amphetamines, and alcohol. Amphetamine use would not lead to punishment, according to the commissioner, but high alcohol levels would. Anabolic steroids would have been added to the list of prohibited drugs, possibly by 1987. Tennant said the reason steroids were not included in the original plan was the difficulty in arranging for the type of laboratory support he desired.

Tennant has done a number of videotapes for players on drug use and says that widespread drug education will be necessary to alert athletes to the hazards of recreational drug use, and Rozelle agreed with him in his news conference to announce the drug testing plan.

"We are going to continue education and counseling," Rozelle said, "but there has to be a bottom line. Without becoming theatrical about it, there has to be an end. There has to be testing."

BASEBALL'S PROGRAM

That evidently is also the belief of Major League Baseball Commissioner Peter Ueberroth, although he refused to answer questions submitted in writing for this article. Last June, Ueberroth announced penalties (ranging from mandatory random drug testing for the future to suspensions) against 21 baseball players who had been involved in drug use.

A news release from Ueberroth's office said: "Drug testing is a proven deterrent to use and an effective tool to be employed where job performance is critical or where obvious problems exist. It is definitely not a sole solution. It should be used in conjunction with a total program including penalties, where appropriate, and education."

Tennant said that Ueberroth "inherited a bad drug situation in baseball" and that he is so far behind that anything done at the moment is only catch-up.

If drug testing comes, the next big hurdle will be what to do with the results, and Upshaw is on solid ground in expressing concern about confidentiality. The Patriots had a humiliating public lesson on handling drug information after the Super Bowl last year when specific players were identified as having drug problems. (These were not current drug users, but players who either had been or were in treatment for past drug use.)

When the names of the six players were published, player representative Brian Holloway grimly promised: "I can guarantee you, with the release of those players' names, you have seen the end of the voluntary program with the Patriots."

One of the players publicly identified said it would be difficult for him to continue playing football for the Patriots, that he could no longer trust the coach or the owner.

"They should trade me, release me, waive me—anything," he said. "I can't play for an organization I don't respect and a coach I don't respect." (It should be noted, however, that neither he nor any other player actually left the team for that reason.)

Team physician Zarins said that the Patriots' drug rehabilitation program had been very successful but, with the public disclosure, "our whole voluntary program is up for grabs."

Patient confidentiality is probably at the heart of any successful drug treatment program and, while physicians have no trouble with the concept, some segments of the media believe that a public figure has no right to privacy. Well known athlete (or any other public figure) will be well aired in the public press well before any treatment is sought.

Tennant and Pursch see this as another argument in favor of early detection programs, so an athlete can get help before he staggers on the field, makes a fool of himself in public, gets arrested, or is killed while under the influence of drugs.

PRIVACY PRIMARY

Privacy is a key feature of the recently adopted drug testing program of the Association of Tennis Professionals (which is only the men; there is ?????????? sional tennis players). Each player signs an agreement to be tested whenever it is done. The tests will not be performed at every tournament, but will be on a random, unannounced basis. A player who refuses testing will be disqualified and cannot play in tournaments sanctioned by the Men's International Professional Tennis Council, the international sports governing body. A player whose test is positive will be contacted privately by Pursch and must talk with him about evaluation. Treatment is mandatory or the player is disqualified from further competition; however, so long as the player is treated, the matter rests entirely between the athlete and Pursch.

"Not even the association knows if a player tests positive," Pursch said, adding that even if it seems that privacy is carried to an extreme, the players consented to the program on that basis. With that in mind, Pursch would not say if there were any positive tests at Wimbledon or the US Open.

Pursch, who has treated athletes from every sport except horse racing (jockeys), makes a strong case for mandatory random testing. "Pro tennis has been the only one so far to make it mandatory and unannounced," he said. "Other sports won't have it mandatory or they announce them, say when they report for spring training. Only a severe addict who can't stay off the stuff even for a day, or a person who is so brain damaged he doesn't know what is going on, or a person who has total and flagrant disregard for the organization, will be caught on that type of test, and if he's like that, he won't be in professional sports long anyway."

RECREATIONAL USE

He believes that player unions in sports where there is considerable drug use have a vested interest in opposing measures that would decrease that use. He also notes that addicts often tell him that they have a right to use illegal drugs recreationally.

"Most addicts say this in the beginning," he continued, "whether they are athletes, board chairmen, military personnel, physicians, or housewives. They feel that they are able to handle it and that they have a right to use them."

There are special considerations in inpatient treatment of addicted athletes, Pursch says.

"We as therapists have to be aware that people will want to do something they do extremely well and avoid doing things they don't do well. Athletes perform well physically and like to, and often don't perform so well emotionally and intellectually in the sense of being open and honest in group therapy or with spouses or lovers. They don't do well in talking, sharing, and taking emotional risks."

For that reason, he will not allow an athlete unlimited exercise time, in the same way, he says, that he tells physician addicts under treatment that the medical library is off limits to them.

"If you leave the schedule open, the jocks will be in the gym all day. If physical exercise helped these people, they wouldn't be in here in the first place. They have to learn what it is that is defective about their life-style. A well-known jock has to be watched or the minute he gets on the running track, he takes over and everybody gravitates around him and treatment is just that much more difficult," Pursch says.

THE USE OF VALIUM AS A FORM OF SOCIAL CONTROL[e]

Kevin Koumjian

INTRODUCTION

Use of the minor tranquilizer diazepam (better known by its trade name Valium) is now a widespread phenomenon in American society and has raised questions concerning medicine's position as an institution of social control. Critics point out that treatment with antianxiety drugs such as Valium provides only symptomatic relief from anxiety and does not address the social origins of stress. One major cause of this 'medicalization' of anxiety and tension has been attributed to the attitudes and beliefs promoted by drug company advertising and the conditions of modern medical practice. These attitudes and beliefs could influence patients to:

1. Define social problems related to family, work and other spheres of social life, as medical problems;

[e]Edited and reprinted with permission from Koumjian K. The use of valium as a form of social control. Soc Sci Med 1981;15:245–249.

2. Seek the medical solution for such problems (i.e. Valium), which is often merely treatment of symptoms, and
3. Become dependent upon the medical solution because the social problem is not addressed and symptoms recur.

This article attempts to provide an analysis which will elucidate the social process outlined above.

THE EXTENT OF VALIUM USE AND SOME PROBLEMS IT PRESENTS

Diazepam (trade name Valium) is one particular drug among a larger class of drugs known as the minor tranquilizers. It has been chosen as the focus of this study because it is a prototype of its class, and it is the most widely prescribed drug in American medicine today (1). Although this study concerns one particular drug, most issues presented here concern the entire group of minor tranquilizers, especially Valium's immediate class, the benzodiazepines.

The first benzodiazepine marketed was chlordiazepoxide (trade name Librium) in 1960 and this was soon followed by the introduction of Valium in 1963. The benzodiazepines and especially Valium were promoted as specific 'anti-anxiety' or 'anxiolytic' drugs which brought drug treatment of anxiety into a new era. In comparison with earlier forms of sedative drugs, Valium was welcomed because: (1) it showed less of a sleep producing effect, (2) it was clearly safer in overdose; (3) it was thought to be less prone to the development of tolerance in users, (4) it was thought to be less liable to induce dependence, and (5) it was found to be effective in reducing certain parameters of symptoms associated with anxiety.

In the years following the arrival of the benzodiazepines, prescriptions for the drugs rose at such a high rate that by 1972 Valium had become the most frequently prescribed drug in the United States, and Librium (Valium's sister drug) had become the third leading prescription drug (1). (America was not alone; statistics from Western European nations showed similar results (2).) In 1978, approximately 68 million prescriptions were filled for the minor tranquilizers, of which 44.6 million were for Valium (1).

The extent of the use of minor tranquilizers in American society has been studied through national surveys and prescription drug data. Based on these studies it has been estimated that one in ten adults in the United States use Valium or Librium during any 3 month period (3). During a typical year it is estimated that 15% of Americans use a minor tranquilizer of some kind (4). A more conservative estimate maintains that ten million Americans used benzodiazepine anti-anxiety drugs in 1978 (5).

The typical user take minor tranquilizers for a period varying from a few days to a few months. However, the use of these drugs on a chronic basis has become an occurrence of great magnitude. In a national survey reported in 1973 it was estimated that 4% of the general American adult population had used a minor tranquilizer on a daily basis for longer than 6 months during the previous year. An additional 1% used a minor tranquilizer for periods varying from 2 to 5 months (4).

Chronic use of Valium has only recently been recognized as a major health problem. For many years it was commonly believed that Valium had a very low addictive potential, however this belief in recent years has been disputed by addiction researchers and by the U.S. Food and Drug Administration.

THE SOCIAL IMPACT OF VALIUM FROM A PERSPECTIVE WHICH RECOGNIZES MEDICINE AS AN INSTITUTION OF SOCIAL CONTROL

Medicine as an Institution of Social Control

The social process involved in the prescription and use of Valium forms a particular subsystem within the larger institution of medicine. Therefore, in order to understand the social effects of anti-anxiety medication, it is necessary to outline the broad social activities performed by American medicine.

As a social institution, medicine performs activities within the sphere of life which a particular society defines as relevant to health and illness. Recently a number of social scientists have recognized that the institution of medicine has taken on functions of social control (6-10). Thus, often moral and value-laden issues are judged by whether they are 'healthy' or 'unhealthy' under the presumption that medical science offers an expert and objective position. However, medical decisions often do carry moral and value laden judgments and as a social institution, the judgments usually reinforce the norms of society.

The notion of social control is often mistakenly dismissed as an overly simplistic concept. However, it should be clear that medicine is not a narrowly defined institution (8, pp. 7-8) and that it has become involved in social control as a result of a web of social changes. These changes include people's attitudes towards health and illness, new medical technologies and information, and economic and political factors which influence health issues. As I. K. Zola states:

> This [expansion of medicine] is not occurring through the political power physicians hold or can influence, but is largely an insidious and often undramatic phenomenon accomplished by 'medicalizing' much of daily living by making medicine and the labels healthy and ill relevant to an ever increasing part of human existence (9, p. 487).

The Use of Valium as a Form of Social Control

The prescription and use of Valium can be viewed as a form of social control by demonstrating, first, a redefinition of social problems as medical problems and, second, the social effects of treating anxiety in a medical context.

The Process of Redefinition

Anxiety is a term which has broad applications in the sense that there are both 'normal' states of anxiety which everyone experiences and 'psycho-pathological' states of anxiety which are considered to be indications of poor mental health. Generally, anxiety is thought of on a scale in which 'normal' or 'healthy' anxiety is less than 'unhealthy' anxiety but there is no clear point at which either the doctor or the patient can draw a line between the two states. Even with objective scales developed to measure signs and symptoms of anxiety (11) there is a fundamental problem. These scales tend to measure rather non-specific and superficial items which ignore the origins of anxiety. The clinician often recognizes that a significant level of anxiety exists yet must rely upon subjective impressions in determining whether the level of anxiety is healthy or unhealthy for a particular patient. This unclear middle ground requires that the definition of healthy versus unhealthy anxiety be made by a consideration of the individual's social functioning. Thus, the individual's abilities to live up to personal ideals, social expectations, or the physician's judgment are factors in a pseudo-objective diagnosis, which leads to the prescription and use of Valium.

The evidence that this redefinition process has taken place is based on the increased number of people who go to a doctor with frankly social problems such as loneliness or marital discord, the increased use of minor tranquilizers observed during periods of increased social stress (12), and the distribution of users of minor tranquilizers among different social groups (discussed below).

Social Effects

The possible social effects of treating anxiety through medical sedation have been outlined by Ingrid Waldron:

> It [prescription of Valium] focuses attention on individual malfunction and alleviations of symptoms of distress, rather than on seeking to understand and deal with the problems and their causes. As a consequence, social and economic problems are dealt with in the framework of a medical model of the relief of individual distress rather than in the social and political context of cooperative efforts for social change. Medicalization of these problems reduces pressures for social change and this outcome is advantageous for those who profit from the existing order (12, p. 43).

In considering the social effects of anti-anxiety medication it is imperative to identify variations in the rate of use among different social groups. One concrete example of Waldron's argument applied to a particular social group is the case of nursing homes for the elderly in which "oversedation has long been recognized as a service to the caretaker and a disservice to the patients" (13). In relation to broader social groups, minor tranquilizers are used more commonly among women than men and among older compared to younger people. Regarding socioeconomic status, significant differences have not been found in the prevalence of use. If a person is a user of a psychotherapeutic drug, however, the probability of frequent and long term use is greater in lower socioeconomic groups (4).

How the use of drugs such as Valium might affect social interactions is another important question. The subtle effects on social life produced by regular use of a minor tranquilizer like Valium are difficult to assess. These effects are difficult to measure because the observer must witness the actual social interactions as they take place rather than relying on subjective interpretation of drug effects.

The difficult nature of such research has left us with little documented evidence of the social effects of Valium. In 1971, Dr. Henry L. Lennard called for research into "the whole array of drug effects upon the individual, his family, and all of the social networks within which the drugged individuals interact" (14). At the present, this important field of research has not yet received adequate attention.

Attitudes and Beliefs which Support the Use of Valium in Social Control

A system of attitudes and beliefs exists which supports the use of Valium as a form of social control. Critics of this system challenge the validity of three pervasive assumptions which may promote the use of the drug: (1) that anxiety originates from individual malfunction and that treatment of symptoms of anxiety therefore alleviates the problem; (2) that many different problems can be reduced to a single category, which is then treatable with Valium; (3) that treatment with Valium has a specific effect in reducing anxiety without altering other aspects of physiology, subjective experience and social interaction. These beliefs contribute to the medicalization of anxiety because they define anxiety as a medical problem and leave the diagnosis and treatment of anxiety in the hands of medical professionals. These three beliefs will be analyzed below.

Anxiety as an Individual's Problem

People who use anti-anxiety drugs usually are experiencing very high levels of psychic stress (15, 16). The fact that intrapsychic stress is a very important clinical problem is not in question. However, problems of stress are often construed to be completely intra-psychic at the exclusion of recognizing the social relations which contribute to the problem. Thus often when the primary cause of stress is a social condition in which the person lives, it is interpreted to be a personal shortcoming either in terms of the individual's responsibility for self care or as a physiological problem which he or she cannot alter.

When primary origins of stress are investigated, one finds that patients taking tranquilizers have very difficult social problems characterized in part by isolation and frustrating, unfulfilled life situations (12, p. 41; 25, pp. 163–164). From this point of view, stress is only a word to connect the direct effects of social agents on the person's body and mind (17).

One reason why social origins of stress are often overlooked is because people take their social problems to doctors. The doctor may then concentrate on the symptoms of anxiety, thereby reinforcing the belief that the origin of anxiety is within the individual (15, p. 164).

A Reductionist View of Non-Specific Symptoms

The indications for the use of Valium are very broadly stated on the product label. There are some specific uses of Valium (for example, in the treatment of status epilepticus), but the very non-specific uses proposed are:

> . . . for the symptomatic relief of tension and anxiety states resulting from stressful circumstances or whenever somatic complaints are concomitants of emotional factors. It is useful in psychoneurotic states manifested by tension, anxiety, apprehension, fatigue, depressive symptoms, or agitation (18).

This implicit belief that Valium can be effective in so many varieties of human experience is probably a result of an emphasis on finding specific medical causes of disease. The tendency to attempt to define a specific agent of disease is one which has permeated scientific medicine, and led to many successful discoveries. The doctrine of specific causation has befuddled physicians and patients who are faced with 'psychosomatic' or 'non-specific' medical symptoms. This void in the practice of medicine is often filled by the readily available use of Valium. In effect, non-specific diagnoses are legitimized by a specific form of treatment. Statistics on the indications for which Valium has been prescribed reflect this phenomenon. They are: mental disorders, 30%; musculoskeletal, 17%; circulatory, 16%; geriatric, 8%; medical/surgical aftercare, 7%; gastrointestinal, 6%; genito-urinary, 3%; and others, 7% (19).

The most striking effect of this process of reducing non-specific complaints to treatment with a particular agent is provided by research which shows that doctors tend to change diagnoses to match the diagnoses for which new drugs are available (19). Clearly, the belief in Valium as effective in so many non-specific diseases legitimizes its frequent use. The following report illustrates this process:

> It appeared that the patients who were given these drugs [Valium and Librium] did not have specific illnesses, but were usually treated for situational or chronic unchanging problems. When asked specifically, the prescribing doctors admitted that they were giving the medication in a spirit of "what else can you do, you have to give them something (20)."

Belief in Valium's Specificity

The belief that Valium has a specific effect in reducing anxiety without inducing any significantly undesirable changes in physiology, subjective experience, or social interaction would also contribute to the abundant use of Valium. This belief, although not held by sophisticated observers of drug action, is often implicit in the way drugs are advertised and in the remnants of the traditional conception of drug action as a 'magic bullet' wherein a given chemical agent is believed to seek out a specific target in the organism (21). This notion has recently been strengthened by a report that 'Valium receptors' have been identified in the brain (22). Another factor which has helped Valium to achieve its commonly held recognition as a safe drug is in its comparison with earlier sedative drugs, including the barbiturates and meprobamate, which were both clearly unsafe and addictive.

However, reports are now mounting concerning the insidious effects which Valium has upon its users. The most significant are tolerance and addiction. Other common adverse effects include drowsiness (which is dose related), muscular incoordination, slurred speech, and spotty memory. Additional, but less common effects are excitement, hostility, hallucinations and delusions, depressed feelings with suicidal ideas, headache, dizziness, decreased sex drive, dry mouth, constipation, and slow urination (23). The fact that Valium is not a 'magic bullet' is shown by this array of adverse effects. Even Valium's impact on anxiety is not a clearly defined action. Much of its effect is accomplished by influences other than the drug. A study of patients with minor emotional problems displayed a placebo response of 50% and an active response of 75% (24). Furthermore, the effects of Valium are so diffuse that one authority stated that "to make a single 'yes' or 'no' statement as to drug efficacy in some situations may boil down to the clinician's judgment of the relative value of various modes of evaluation (25)."

It is unknown what other effects Valium may have upon the individual's social interaction and subjective experiences. It is, however, easy to speculate that the response will vary from individual to individual since Valium is a drug which leaves much leeway for cognitive interpretation. Since it is difficult to generalize about cognitive effects, research on Valium has generally ignored in-depth reports of subjective experiences in favor of more easily quantifiable measures. The danger in this approach is that other important factors, such as whether the patient feels dependent upon the use of Valium and whether he or she has been able to identify or work to change the sources of stress, may be ignored.

Factors which Promote the Use of Valium in Social Control

In 1972 the state of South Carolina banned benzodiazepines from the state Medicaid formulatory for budgetary reasons. In six months 35% of the benzodiazepine users had received an alternative sedative prescription but 65% of the users were no longer on medication (and no significant changes in the health of patients was reported (26). In another case, a rigorous information campaign on the problems in using tranquilizers reduced the number of prescriptions by 33% in one clinic (27). These experiences raise an important question—if Valium is not fundamental to the care of many patients, what promotes the beliefs, outlined earlier, which lead to the frequent use of Valium?

Drug Company Promotion

Hoffmann-La Roche, the producer of Valium and Librium, depends heavily upon the successful marketing of minor tranquilizers. By 1971, it was estimated that Valium and Librium had been worth over $2 billion in sales. Approximately, one fifth of this revenue was reinvested in sales promotion through drug detail men, advertising and 'public service projects' (18). The effectiveness of drug advertising is evident in the following statistics: 50% of doctors reported that their first source of drug information was a drug company sales representative, and 25% reported that their first source was drug house mail and periodicals (29). Finally, most doctors rely on the *Physician's Desk Reference* for drug information which contains descriptions of drugs paid for by the companies (30).

Advertising for minor tranquilizers has been very explicit in its message to use drugs in controlling social conflict. One example, which appeared in 1969, was an ad promoting the use of a minor tranquilizer for producing a "less demanding and complaining patient" (12, p. 41). Another pictures a worried young college woman and conveys the message that Librium can be of some help in solving the problems created when "exposure to new friends and other influences may force her to reevaluate herself and her goals," and "newly stimulated intellectual curiosity may make her more sensitive to and apprehensive about unstable national and world conditions" (21, p. 31).

Today the drug companies are much more subtle in their promotion of drugs for social problems. One such subtle campaign is an educational program entitled, 'Consequences of Stress' and sponsored by Hoffmann-La Roche. This program drew the following response from J. Richard Crout, Director, Bureau of Drugs, of the U.S. Food and Drug Administration:

> We are not entirely comfortable about this program [because it is difficult to distinguish between drug promotion and legitimate support of medical education]. The program is aimed at stress, and it has the potential of subtly conveying the message that tranquilizers should be prescribed for many patients whose internal discomfort is much closer to that accompanying the normal pressures of life rather than the medical disorders for which tranquilizers are indicated.

The Conditions of Modern Medical Practice

The doctor makes the final judgment about whether to prescribe Valium and is therefore the principal object of attention for the drug company, the government agencies which hope to control overuse, and the patients who often want 'something' for their distress. Yet two major factors which often determine the physician's decision to prescribe more than these external influences are lack of time and lack of training in the social context of medicine. According to one survey, 50% of medical visits lasted less than 15 min, with only 20% lasting over 30 min (15, p. 164). One easy way for a doctor to end an interview is to write a prescription. The evidence that lack of training in the social aspects of medicine and a hesitancy to use time consuming psychotherapy contribute to increased prescription writing can be inferred from statistics which show that psychiatrists account for less than 17% of all of the prescriptions for minor tranquilizers (3). These statistics are explained by the tendency for psychiatrists to use psychotherapy and to hold a less symptom oriented view of anxiety.

CONCLUSION

This article has presented an analysis of the use of Valium as a means of social control, some attitudes and beliefs which may work to support the use of Valium, and two factors which promote the use of Valium. It is essential to understand that these components all interact within one social system. Therefore, it becomes clear that the use of Valium as a form of social control is not usually done in an overtly coercive fashion. Rather, dominant attitudes and beliefs concerning the realm of medicine (which in American society includes anxiety) and the strategy of treatment (Valium) pervade both ends of the doctor-patient relationship as well as the larger systems within which individuals act. Furthermore these attitudes and beliefs are strengthened by interests which benefit from this social arrangement. Therefore drug companies (which reap profits) and doctors (whose practice is simplified by this process) actively promote the use of Valium. Also patients, as members of a technologically oriented society, may demand Valium due to their acceptance of the pervading assumption that anxiety is a medical problem requiring a technological remedy.

The result of this approach to anxiety is that human conflicts arising from the relation between individuals and the social system become objectified and are controlled without a resolution of the structural conflicts involved. This mechanism preserves the existing social order but at several costs. It may harm individuals due to adverse side effects, addition and/ or the continuation of a living situation in which the person is not satisfied. Also alternative modes of therapy and social changes which address the more fundamental causes of anxiety are discouraged by this more direct and specific cure provided by medical science.

REFERENCES

1. Despite these high levels of use reported in 1978, it should be pointed out that between 1973 and 1978 total prescriptions for all minor tranquilizers including Valium fell somewhat. The reasons for this decline are not entirely clear but may involve concern about addiction. *National Prescription Audit,* Therapeutic Category Report, 1964–1978, IMS America, Ambler, PA 19002.
2. Balter M. B. *et al.* Cross-national survey of the extent of anti-anxiety sedative drug use. *N. Engl. J. Med.* **290,** 769, 1974.
3. Weise C. E. and Price S. F. *The Benzodiazepines: Patterns of Use.* Addiction Research Foundation, Toronto, Canada, 1975.
4. Parry H. J., *et al.* National patterns of psychotherapeutic drug use. *Archs gen. Psychiat.* **28,** 769, 1973.
5. *National Disease and Therapeutic Index.* Drug File, Jan.–Dec., 1979, IMS America, Ambler, PA 19002.
6. Conrad P. The discovery of hyperkinesis: notes on the medicalization of deviant behavior. *Soc. Probl.* **23,** 12, 1975.
7. Ehrenreich B. and Ehrenreich J. Medicine and social control. In *The Cultural Crisis of Modern Medicine* (Edited by Ehrenreich J.). Monthly Review Press, New York, 1978.
8. Waitzkin H. and Waterman B. *The Exploitation of Illness in Capitalist Society.* Indianapolis, Bobbs-Merril, 1974.
9. Zola I. K. Medicine as an institution of social control. *Sociol. Rev.* **20,** 487, 1972.
10. Zola I. K. In the name of health and illness: on some socio-political consequences of medical influence. *Soc. Sci. Med.* **9,** 83, 1975.
11. Hartlage L. C. Common approaches to the measurement of anxiety. *Am. J. Psychiat.* **128,** 1145, 1972.
12. Waldron I. Increased prescribing of Valium, Librium, and other drugs—an example of economic and social factors in the practice of medicine. *Int. J. Hlth Serv.* **7,** 41, 1977.
13. Butler R. N. Overuse of tranquilizers in older patients. *Int. J. Ag. Hum. Dev.* **7,** 2, 1976.
14. Lennard H. L. *Mystification and Drug Misuse,* p. 76. Jossey-Bass, San Francisco, CA, 1971.
15. Lader M. Benzodiazepines—opium of the masses? *Neuroscience,* **3,** 161, 1978.
16. Mellinger G. D. *et al.* Psychic distress, life crisis and use of psychotherapeutic medications. *Archs gen. psychiat.* **35,** 1045, 1978.
17. Berliner H. S. and Salmon J. W. The holistic health movement and scientific medicine. *Soc. Rev.* **9,** 31, 1979.
18. Product label for Valium, Hoffmann-La Roche, 1979.
19. Blackwell B. Psychotropic drugs in use today, the role of diazepam in medical practice. *J. Am. Med. Ass.* **225,** 1638, 1973.

20. Pursch J. A. (testimony), Subcommittee on Health and Scientific Research, U.S. Senate, Sept. 10, 1979.
21. Lennard H. L. *et al.* Hazards implicit in prescribing psychoactive drugs. *Science* **169,** 438, 1970.
22. Iverson L. Anti-anxiety receptors in the brain? *Nature* **266,** 678, 1977.
23. Goldberg M. and Egleston G. *Mind Influencing Drugs.* p. 179. P.S.G., Littleton, MA, 1978.
24. Wheatley D. Evaluation of psychotherapeutic drugs in general practice. *R. Soc. Med.* **65,** 317, 1972.
25. Greenblatt D. J. and Shader R. I. *Benzodiazepines in Clinical Practice,* Chap. 4. Raven Press, New York, 1974.
26. Keller M. H. and McCurdy R. L. Medical practices without anti-anxiety drugs. Read before the 125th convention of the Am. Psychiat. Ass., Dallas, May 3, 1972.
27. Kaufman A. *et al.* Tranquilizer control. *J. Am. Med. Ass.* **221,** 1504, 1972.
28. Ball R. The secret life of Hoffmann-La Roche. *Fortune,* pp. 130–134, 162–171, 1971.
29. Miller R. R. Prescribing habits of physicians. *Drugs Intell. Clin. Pharm.* **7,** 492 and 557, 1973, and **8,** 81, 1974.
30. *Examination of the Pharmaceutical Industry, 1973–74.* Subcommittee on Health, Committee on Labor and Public Welfare, U.S. Senate, U.S. Gov. Print. Office. Wash., D.C., 1974.

10
Health Environment

JACK E. FINCHAM

INTRODUCTION

Change has always been an underlying force of the American health care system. Although at present the health care system seems burdened with new impacts and forces of change, many current dilemmas when examined closely have been present for a long period of time (1). The problems may not be new, but certainly specific facets have forced a revolution in United States health care delivery. Questions of access, turf, payment, and allocation of scarce resources have been forces for change in the past, just as they are today and most certainly will be tomorrow. The ultimate paradox of increasing technology coupled with decreasing resources allocated for payment has inserted political, social, and philosophical aspects into health care delivery as never before.

Changing Face of American Health Care

The functions, provision, and utilization of United States health care are rapidly changing as never before. With the advent of governmental entitlement programs in the 1960s (Medicare and Medicaid), political and economic overtones were thrust upon the health care system. Perceived shortages of physicians, pharmacists, and other health care professionals in the 1960s and 1970s led to capitation grants from the United States government to health professional schools. The results of this capitation in addition to the emergence of new health professionals [physician assistants (PAs) and nurse practitioners (NPs)] have led to a projected surplus of physicians and others in the 1990s and beyond. Patterns of utilization will surely be affected by increasing technology and possible finite resources for payment for services delivered. Issues of indigent care, prospective payment for hospital services, and competition have revolutionized the activities of hospitals in the past decade (2). Patients have changed as well. Expectations from health care in some cases exceed possibilities. There is still only so much that can be done for patients even in the technologically intensive health care system of today.

Impacts upon Health Care Components

The impacts affecting the health care system have included social, economic, professional, political, and structural factors. The United States system perhaps as no other system has been affected by, and subject to, political influence. Despite spending approximately 10% of the United States Gross National Product (GNP) on health care, the resultant expectation of "the best" health in the world has not come to pass.

Indices such as the neonatal birth rate have indicated the United States lags behind several Western European countries in estimating the health of the health care system. This crude measure of the health of the health care system is an indication of the improvement needed in the health care system. Despite the enormous expenditures for health care in the past century, rising income levels and advances in public health practices have been the most important reasons for the fall in infant mortality (3).

Reactive versus Proactive Considerations of Health Care Impacts

Planning for health care needs of the future was an emphasis of the political climate of the 1970s (4). There were many enabling legislative and regulatory efforts to institute a system of planning for future needs and regulating the health care industry to make sure any brick and mortar changes (buildings, hospitals, etc.) and/or equipment in the health care delivery system were truly needed in any one geographic area. Certificate of need (CON) approval was required for expansion of existing structural components or completion of new structural components. The intent of such efforts was to curtail expenditures in the entire system and thus save money, as well as to ensure that additions to the delivery system were truly necessary.

In the 1980s, this enabling legislation and regulatory thrust was dismantled in favor of competition. Competition was felt to be a more suitable way to deal with the costs of care in a much more appropriate fashion. This laissez-faire approach to health care may have succeeded in reducing the tide of expense outlays of the United States health care system, however, without planning for the future. Many efforts in the current health care climate are indeed reactionary rather than proactionary. Satisfaction of current needs takes precedence over any planning for the future. The situation for the future must be considered now, or the potential for trouble in the future will grow. The current system is just not structurally or financially able to deal with the future needs of providers or recipients of health care.

The influence of these competitive impacts upon pharmacy and pharmacists has been enormous. One need only consider preferred provider organizations (PPOs), health maintenance organizations (HMOs), mail order pharmacy, physician dispensing, and drug diversion to realize the scope and magnitude of the current health care delivery disorganizational status. We are where we are in the current system because of the lack of a continuous degree of proper planning for future health care needs and practice functions.

Multidimensional Nature of Change, Present and Future

Although the United States health care system has been characterized as a nonsystem, or as an amalgamation of entities without an organization structure, the components are definitely interrelated. Any impact affecting one segment or professional body has ramifications and reverberations affecting the entire system. This multidimensional interrelationship of the various health care system components leads to change that is also multidimensional in nature.

Examples abound to support this multidimensional nature of change. When the diagnosis related group (DRG) system of prospective reimbursement for inpatient Medicare patient care was instituted, hospitals sought methods of increasing revenues in ways previously not pursued. Outpatient services took on added importance for hospitals because they were excluded from DRG reimbursement regulation. Thus outpatient prescription departments became potential areas for marketing for institutions. As well, and for the same reasons, home health care departments became prominent in institutions.

Involvement in these two areas of nontraditional marketing involvement on the part of hospitals placed hospitals in direct competition with community and chain pharmacies in an open fashion for the first time at a competitive level hitherto unknown. Hospitals certainly had these departments in place earlier, however, marketing efforts could best be characterized as passive.

Other examples of the dimension of change and subsequent effects upon many segments of the health care system are physician dispensing and pharmacist prescribing. Pharmacists are averse to physician dispensing but view pharmacist prescribing in a favorable light (5). On the other hand, some physicians view dispensing as a function suitable for their practice repertoire and view pharmacist prescribing as a threat to their practice roles. Who is right? It depends upon whom you talk with. Regardless of who is right or justified, both pharmacist prescribing and physician dispensing have roots in several facets of health care components—economics, practice responsibilities, numbers of professionals in the discipline, and future desires for expanded role possibilities. Each of the previously mentioned components has been and will be subject to many changes affecting many points in the health care system in the future.

Mergers

One aspect of health care delivery and structure that has taken on added importance recently and on into the near and long-term future is mergers. Whether it is the merging of brand name and generic drug companies, hospitals, purchasing groups, academic health centers with hospital chains, various practitioners (physicians, pharmacists, etc.), or any or all of the above, mergers have made an impact upon the health care system. All of the above have the potential to influence many other points in the system. However, the merging and combination of structural components have the potential to dramatically affect all in the health care system (6).

Scenarios have been suggested whereby a few very large conglomerates will be the major providers of United States health care on a nationwide basis (7). Under this tier of large producers will be a segment of smaller conglomerates with a lower level of a larger group of individuals and groups that feed into the system above them. Another scenario involves the formation and success of integrated health care clusters (IHCs) (8). This integrated system would contain any and all of the services a defined population would need—from wellness to acute and long-term care. Also, this system would effectively lock out nonparticipating providers. Which of these scenarios will succeed is debatable, what is significant is they are discussed and the subsequent attention the discussion garners. What of the patient and practitioners in such a system? Time will tell, but the system will be irrevocably different if such scenarios play out.

QUALITY VERSUS COST IN HEALTH CARE

What should the paramount issue in health care be? Should quality be the goal or should cost play the dominant role in assigning or assessing options? Perhaps the combination of quality and cost should be the major objective. The patient, the provider, or someone else may desire input. But, who should decide?

Economics of Health Care

The purse strings of the health care system are controlled by many forces. These forces include private insurance, personal funds, state and local governments, and the federal government. A description of health care economics is beyond the scope of this chapter, however, certain key points need to be addressed. Beyond the payment issue alone lies perhaps an even more pressing concern for the future. Namely, what should be paid for, and for whom?

Expending resources to secure health benefits is engaging in a game of chance. What works and what does not is not often easy to summarize. Zeckhauser and Shepard (9) analyzed age-specific death rates for adult males from 1930 to 1970. Findings showed the older age group reduction in mortality was one-fourth as large as for the younger age groups. The dramatic differences in mortality could perhaps be attributed to changes in sanitation, public health efforts, or medical care. The implications are that all segments are aided by health improvements, however, there are risk factors present in certain age groups not present in others. The interaction of risk factors and improvements in nutrition, medicine, public health, etc. has benefited some, but because of the larger number of risk factors in older individuals the benefits may not have accrued in this age group as with younger individuals.

With increasing levels of technology present and projected in the future, it is possible that more and more health care will be available for fewer and fewer individuals. Funds available to cover all interventions, both expensive and inexpensive will be sparce (10). Currently in the health care system, deductibles and coinsurance force many needy individuals to delay or postpone care.

The financing of health care became a publicly debated topic in the 1930s with the emergence of the private insurance industry and discussion of health care as a right similar to rights to police protection and public education. In the 1960s, with the passage of Medicare and Medicaid, millions of poor and elderly Americans were eligible for unrestricted medical care for the first time. Public discussion of the financial impact of this legislation was negligible while tax coffers overflowed. However, when recession and inflation became simultaneously prominent in the 1970s, discussion of public financing of medical care became commonplace. Virtually every legislative impact upon health since the early 1970s has sought to reduce expenditures for health, either through recipient benefit reduction, curtailing of covered services, or institution of beneficiary copayment for certain services (medical visits, prescriptions, etc.). What has characterized these past impacts upon the financing and payment for health care has been their reactive nature. An impending crisis must loom on the horizon before appropriate action is instituted. For example, DRG prospective reimbursement came into play in the mid-1980s after the financial solvency of the Social Security system was questioned. Dire forecasts of a bankrupt Social Security program occurred in the late 1970s and early 1980s. What the next crisis will be is uncertain, the ramifications of the crisis most certainly will be more clear—more cutbacks and/or decreases in funding.

Quality of Care

The quality of medical care delivered has ramifications for all involved in health care, from user to provider to payer. Despite the ramifications, the determination of what constitutes quality has been mercurial (11). However, care suspect in quality can profoundly affect the health care system. These potential ramifications have led to governmental efforts to develop a method of ascertaining quality of care standardization. Although the face of quality assurance has changed with the demise of health planning regulations in the 1980s, other requirements associated with the Tax Equity and Fiscal Responsibility Act, and subsequent DRG regulations (12) have put into place peer review organization (PRO) assessments of quality of care (13). Despite the mercurial nature of quality of care assessment, the need and importance of assessing quality of care will no doubt continue in the future as governmental payment for health care services continues at present or enhanced levels in the years to come.

Corporate or managed health efforts at ensuring quality of care also have been recently enhanced. Managed systems have determined the best method of attracting new subpopulations of patients is that which provides health care that is cost-effective, stable, and of an ascertained certain level of quality. Health Maintenance Organizations have had quality assurance components built in their infrastructure from the onset of governmental regulation and involvement in the HMO movement.

Reimbursement Issues

The payment for health care in general, and for prescription drugs specifically, has never been more complicated. Pharmacists are faced with an elaborate maze of payers, beneficiary limitations, formulary and reimbursement restrictions, and ever-changing guidelines. These impacts affect institutional as well as community and chain pharmacists. Even though not necessarily an exciting topic, pharmacy reimbursement issues affect how pharmacists are paid and the scope of practice roles and responsibilities. Roles and responsibilities are exciting topics.

A small sampling of current reimbursement-related issues of note include prospective reimbursement, resource limits, and who is and is not insured.

Prospective Reimbursement

Prospective reimbursement has had a dramatic impact upon hospital pharmacy practice. Formerly hospitals were reimbursed on a retrospective basis for Medicare services provided. Because of this after-the-fact billing, pharmacy services were viewed as a revenue-generating component of services provided. However, now that rates of hospital services are predetermined for Medicare patients, all expenses incurred are considered as costs as opposed to revenues. Thus, the lower the costs, the higher the amount hospitals can garner as the "above cost-below payment level" profit buffer. Because of the short-term success of DRG reimbursement in the Medicare program, it will no doubt be retained for Medicare and perhaps instituted for other government programs such as Medicaid. In addition, private insurers see prospective reimbursement as a way to decrease costs associated with the care they purchase.

Resource Limits

How much health care can and should governmental programs purchase? What limits should be placed upon recipients' use of health care services? These are questions previously not often asked in the United States. The enormous increase in technology has been utilized by those who can afford it through their own payment or through their insurer. This technology does the uninsured or underinsured patient no good whatsoever. Do the limits of the collective ability to pay for health care adversely affect one segment of society? Jonas (14) suggests the situation has always existed with regard to resource utilization.

Who Shall Be Insured?

If there are limits on how much technology can be purchased, who decides who gets what? Disadvantaged segments will no doubt increase in the future. Bovbjerg (Ref. 15, p. 403) has noted: "People on their own or in small groups, as well as increasing numbers of dependents of workers in large groups, are disadvantaged in comparison with workers in large groups." Is it the insurer, the provider, or the government who decides on coverage? The questions, although not easily answered, must nonetheless be addressed. Limits placed upon health care utilization have been in place in the past, but never to the extent they will be in the future. The experience of Great Britain sheds light on the problem and potential ways to manage the situation (16). British patients and providers have perhaps expected less in the way of technology as opposed to their American counterparts. Through this lowered expectation, the British have coped with the issue of technology and its use better than Americans have. Patients and provider alike understand the limits of the British system and as such do not place heroic demands related to what can and cannot be obtained.

THE PROFESSIONS

The United States health care system is a personnel-intensive system. The array of specialists, subspecialists, technicians, technologists, consultants, and attending individuals seems to expand yearly as technology and expectations for care expand. Despite different titles and hierarchical breakdown of assignment of duties within a professional component, there is an overlap of responsibilities and duties that will no doubt increase in the future. How the professions interact, overlap, or challenge each other's efforts affects not only health care delivery, but also utilization. In fact, the degree of cooperation or lack thereof will determine the future direction and control of the health care system.

Physicians

The practice of medicine has changed rapidly in the past decade. One aspect of change has been the dramatic shift from solo practice to group practice as the norm. Coupled with the change in practice location is the expansive increase in the number of practicing physicians. From the 1970s to the present, the scenario has changed from a projected lack of physicians to a projected surplus. If the glut has occurred, are there still underserved areas in desperate need of physicians? The answer is an explicit yes (17). Despite the increase in numbers of physicians and specialties, there remain underserved populations in need of basic primary care practitioners, namely internists, general practitioners, obstetrician-gynecologists, and pediatricians. To further complicate the picture, the liability crisis in medicine has forced many physicians from their chosen specialty in the profession they worked so diligently to attain rank in. So, in examining the so-called physician glut, expansion of numbers, responsibilities, and liability concerns must be factored in.

The physician glut disappears if you live in a small community devoid of a physician. It conversely expands if you live in a major metropolitan area with hundreds of individuals listed in the yellow pages from which you are to select one for your needs. The divergence of points of view pertaining to practice sites will continue as long as physicians are free to choose when and where they will practice. This freedom has the potential to be impacted upon by many factors which may include: changing demographic shifts, payment for service alterations, future liability concerns, actual practice expansion due to technology, or practice compression due to the expansion of other professionals' roles or responsibilities.

Nonphysician Providers

The so-called physician shortage of the 1960s and 1970s led to exploration of the concept of a physician extender. The concept was proposed that an individual with requisite skills in patient triage, clinical assessment, and patient education would ease the strain the lack of physicians had created. It was generally felt these physicians extenders with proper training could serve the patient and the system through easing the shortage of physicians and resultant effects.

Physician assistant and nurse practitioner training programs were inaugurated and have flourished. The PA profession is male dominated and the NP profession is female dominated. This differentiation has led to interesting confrontations between the two physician extender components. Apart from disagreements between themselves, NPs and PAs must potentially deal with the notion they both may compete for patients with physicians in the years to come. Physicians may view these extenders as potential replacements. Pharmacists may view these professions as potential unwelcome dispensers (18).

As long as the shortage of physicians coupled with a lower medical school enrollment was perceived, the issue of overlap of services provided by physicians, NPs, and PAs was not a major issue. As long as physicians were in short supply, any new health worker was a welcome addition to the team. Whereas the key words in the late 1960s were "shortage," "crisis," and "expansion of training capacity," in the 1980s the components of note included "oversupply," "overtaining," and "costs." However, as medical school enrollment and graduates increase, the overlap of services rendered will become a major issue for all health professions in the future (19).

Who shall perform what tasks will be a question to be answered in the years to come. Who prescribes, dispenses, and administers may not be an easily definable series of questions.

PATIENTS

The patients treated in the health care system collectively are aging. Pharmacists will be dispensing drugs in the future to a clientele on the average older than any age group previously served by the profession. Current planning for future health and pharmacy needs for the elderly is lacking to say the least. We as a society, health care system, and profession are not prepared to deal with the elderly population that awaits us in the future. One in eight Americans is currently age 65 or older. Projections are staggering for the future as well—one in three Americans will be age 65 in the year 2030. According to the American Association of Retired Persons (AARP) (Ref. 20, p. 1): "The old themselves are also getting older. In 1985, the 65–74 age group (17 million) was nearly 8 times larger than in 1900, but the 75–84 age group (8.8 million) was 11 times larger, and the 85+ age group (2.7 million) was 22 times larger." Because of age-related complications of growing old, the amount of drugs consumed by the elderly at the turn of the century will be staggering. Vestal has suggested the figure will be 40% of medications, up from a projected 25% in 1986 (21).

Subpopulations

Certain subpopulations of the elderly will require the use of tremendous amounts of health care services and pharmaceuticals because of resultant morbidity associated with the aging process. Chronic treatment for chronic diseases and multiple pathologies will challenge the pharmacy practitioner of the future. If and when provision of services becomes problematic because of resource scarcity, then the allocation of resources becomes a crucial concern. At this point the issues raised earlier regarding rationing will require attention. Will different subpopulations be in competition for health care? At present, 40% of the Medicaid budget for the poor of all ages is consumed by the elderly (22). Competition between generations for health care services will challenge the moral and ethical fiber of the health care system and professional components (23).

Despite the common sense assumption that the elderly of the future will be sicker with more and more infirmities, we may as a profession be providing more and more preventive or wellness-based care for the well elderly subpopulation. These patients will be normal in every sense of the word; the only remarkable fact about them may be their advanced age. How we as a profession deal with this subpopulation will undoubtedly affect how we succeed as a profession and as professionals in the years to come.

Changing Sociogeographic Patterns

Often Americans are referred to as a mobile population. This overall assessment is particularly applicable to a number of facets of society, including the health care delivery system. It is particularly important from service provision, resource utilization, and health professional training points of view. It is also important from an analysis of the age of patients standpoint.

Consider that in 1985, about 49% of persons 65 years and older lived in eight states. California, New York, and Florida had over two million each, and Illinois, Michigan, Ohio, Pennsylvania, and Texas had over one million each (20). Even though previously the elderly have been less likely to change residence than any other group, in 1985 about 800,000 persons 65 and over had moved to a different state since 1980. Of these, over 35% had moved from the Northeast or Midwest regions to the South or West (20). If indeed the "well old" grow in numbers in the years to come, they may be more willing to move than their contemporaries of previous times. American society and the health care system are not currently prepared to deal with these future projected continuations of patient mobility and geographic change from a delivery, financing, and structural standpoint.

REGULATORY ASPECTS

Health care decisions have always had political ramifications. But, with the portion of health care consumed by governmental payers exceeding 40% of total payments, the interjection of politics into health care decisions has increased and will continue to do so. An example of increased political activity has been the formation and prominence of political action committees (PACs). The lobbying and financial contributory efforts of PACs cannot be underestimated. If financial input equates with decision outputs, does the greater contributor win? What if competing contributors have drastically different policy perspectives? Will pharmacy, medicine, consumer, or manufacturing PACs have equivalent expectations for support from legislators, regardless of level of input (state or federal)? Chances are that the concerns and views may be quite different.

And what of the issues? From a regulatory or policy perspective, any number of "hot" topics will be debated, acted upon, or possibly changed from the status quo in the years to come. One such area of potential change is the drug milieu.

Drug Milieu

Aspects pertaining to all components of medication consumption will be malleable in the future. These aspects include the switching of drugs from prescription to over the counter (OTC) status, the approval time and process for new drugs, the drug lag, and orphan drugs. What follows is a brief listing of each of these items and discussion pertaining to their importance in the health environment.

Prescription to OTC Classification of Drugs

Certainly the switching of medications from prescription to OTC status has impacted pharmacists and patients (24). Pharmacists decry on the one hand the lack of information consumers have with regard to the prescription drugs consumed and yet are faced with more and more prescription drugs being switched from prescription to OTC status. The crucial consideration pertaining to appropriateness of the switching may revolve around consumer ability to self-medicate with these drugs. Self-monitoring of body functions is necessitated with the use of many of these drugs. Certainly different points of view may be espoused by OTC drug manufacturers, consumer groups, and health professionals.

Drug Approval

The United States Food and Drug Administration is placed under tremendous pressure concerning the drug approval process. On the one hand, efforts may be seen as stringent if a pharmaceutical company considers the length of the drug approval process and the resultant number of years of patent protection remaining on a product. Consumers and their physicians desperate for the release of a product may see the extended process as also being too lengthy. Other groups may view postmarketing emergent side effects (not discovered in clinical trials) as an indication that the drug approval process needs further scrutiny from the sense of allowing drugs on the market too easily. Any effort to speed the approval process along for drugs for one group of patients (eg., AIDS patients) may be resented by other groups of patients requiring a miraculous drug but also required to wait for a longer period of time.

Drug Lag

If a particular drug is available overseas before available in the United States, reference is made to the problem of a drug lag for United States patients. Arguments are voiced relative to the therapies United States patients are being deprived of in relation to patients abroad. Thus, the line between prudent patience before release of a drug and the notion of a drug lag is a fine one indeed. The drug lag also can refer to prescription to OTC switched drugs that are made available in other countries before being made available as OTC drugs in the United States. These deliberations are all the more interesting when political and economic impacts are factored in the scenario.

Orphan Drugs

Drugs of importance in treating rarely occurring exotic diseases are referred to as orphan drugs. Often the costs associated with producing such drugs are prohibitive. The potential to recapture investment dollars often is limited, and as such treatable diseases may be left untreated. Recently, the orphan drug issue has been partially diffused, and the burden of the manufacturers has been reduced (25). However, with costs skyrocketing throughout the health care system, orphan drugs and diseases may increase as resources to cover many health needs become stretched.

PRESENT AND FUTURE CONSIDERATIONS

Current issues of note in the health environment will also be issues of note in the future. What the professions provide to patients and what patients do for themselves will ultimately converge and allow for determination of how good the health of the system is or will be. Each practitioner must decide how to fit into the system and ultimately help patients achieve what they can in the health environment.

Self-Care

What role will self-care play in the years to come? With many more drugs available for self-medication and the promotion of self-care activities, more and more individuals will use self-managed treatments. The bombardment of consumers with advertisements promoting self-selection of products and therapies will undoubtedly stimulate further marketing of more products. The advertising, marketing, and labeling of OTC products is complex and, in some cases, confusing. In addition, and to further compound the situation, more and more products will be targeted for switching from prescription to OTC status. There are debatable issues surrounding the switching process. This debate will not lessen in intensity in the years to come. What individuals should be allowed to do to, or for, themselves is not an issue likely to be resolved in the present or short-term future.

Prevention versus Treatment

Where should money be spent in the health care system? Is money better spent in treating the outcomes, sequelae of chronic disease, or prevention of the disease? Certainly money will always need to be spent for acute and chronic care. There can be no question of the importance of the treatment of acute and chronic disease. But, is it better to spend enormous amounts of money in treating the outcomes of sometimes preventable conditions—hypertension for example in some cases—or in educational or other preventive programs aimed at reducing cigarette smoking, hypercholesteremia, or obesity. Individuals have suggested preventive efforts would be more cost-effective in the long run (26). Still, there will always be a demand for technology to undue what it is we do to ourselves.

Elaborate Technology versus Basic Needs

The United States health care system contains the most elaborate and technologically advanced health care available anywhere in the world. Whether this technology is too elaborate is a debatable issue. The elaborate technology serves only those who can afford it; if unaffordable, it is unusable. Questions have been raised surrounding the spending of money on technology that by its design has limited applicability to a broad spectrum of society, as opposed to expenditures for basic needs (1). To a patient without access to a physician, access to elaborate medical devices and interventions becomes a secondary consideration.

FUTURE

No one can predict with certainty what the future will bring. An uncertain future should not prohibit the pharmacy professional from reaching his or her own potential in the years to come. The profession as well as individual pharmacists must plan for the future and be prepared to deal with changes that will inevitably occur.

The high drug use consumption trends in the 1980s should continue to increase in the future. This projected increase is based upon projected morbidity that is chronic in nature, coupled with a population growing older and consuming ever more medications. The drugs of the future may or may not be of the shape and form of today. But, there can be certainty that more medications will continue to be consumed by more and more of us.

The switching of drugs from prescription to OTC status will increase in the future. The subsequent counseling as to proper use of the medications will challenge future pharmacists from both a content and delivery standpoint. The potential for misuse of OTCs will increase parallel to the potential for increased use. Pharmacists can impact upon both the use and misuse of OTC drugs in a positive fashion. Pharmacists must become better managers of the drugs patients consume. Aggressive management of patients' therapies needs to be undertaken in the ambulatory environment, just as it has been accomplished in the institutional setting (hospital and long-term care facilities).

The health of the health environment rests with the health of all components—financing, delivery, professionals, and patients. The future of pharmacy can be bright, however, the hue and intensity of this brightness rests where it always has—with the individual practitioner.

REFERENCES

1. Jonas S. Health care delivery in the United States. 3rd ed. New York: Springer Publishing Company, 1986.
2. Merrill JC, Somers SA. The changing health care system: a challenge for foundations. Inquiry 1986;23:316–321.
3. Fuchs VR. How we live. Cambridge, MA: Harvard University Press, 1983.
4. Tierney JT, Waters WJ. The evolution of health planning. N Engl J Med 1983;308:95.
5. Angorn RA. Florida legalizes pharmacist prescribing. Legal Aspects Pharm Pract 1986;9(3):1,3,9.
6. Ginzberg E. The monetarization of medical care. N Engl J Med 1984;310:1162–1165.
7. Hagness JR. The corporatization of health care. AACP Newsletter, June 1987, pp 6–7.
8. McManis GL. The integrated healthcare system of the future. Healthcare Exec 1987;2(1):60.
9. Zeckhauser RJ, Shepard DS. The choice of heal policies with heterogenous populations. In Fuchs VR, ed. Economic aspects of health. Chicago: The University of Chicago Press, 1982.
10. Schramm CJ, ed. Health care and its costs. New York: W. W. Norton and Company, 1987.
11. Einthoven AC. Cutting costs without cutting the quality of care. N Engl J Med 1978;298:1229–1238.
12. Prospective Payment System-Hospitals, Social Security Amendments of 1983. Prospective Payments for Medicare Inpatient Hospital Services. Public Law 98-21. April 20, 1983.
13. Dans PE, Weiner JP, Otter SE. Peer review organizations. N Engl J Med 1985;313:1131–1137.
14. Jonas S. Health care delivery in the United States. 3rd ed. New York: Springer Publishing Company, 1986, p 5.
15. Bovbjerg RR. Insuring the uninsured through private action: ideas and initiatives. Inquiry 1986;23:403–418.
16. Aaron HJ, Schwartz WB. The painful prescription. Washington, DC: The Brookings Institution, 1984.
17. Fruen MA, Cantwell JR. Geographic distribution of physicians: past trends and future influences. Inquiry 1982;19:44–50.
18. Keith B. Court upholds dispensing by PAs. Drug Topics 1987;131(12):82.
19. McTernan EJ, Leiken AM. A pyramid model of health manpower in the 1980s. J Health Politics Policy Law 1982;6(4):739–751.
20. AARP. A profile of older Americans, 1986. Washington, DC: AARP, 1987.
21. Vestall R. Drugs in the elderly. Boston: Adis Press, 1985.
22. Avorn J. Medicine, health, and the geriatric transformation. Daedalus 1986;115(1):211–225.
23. Clark PG. The social allocation of health care resources: ethical dilemmas in age-group competition. Gerontologist 1985;25(2):119–125.
24. New resources in self-medication. Washington, DC: The Proprietary Association, Rx-OTC, 1982.
25. Althuis TH. Contributions of the pharmaceutical industry. In Karch FE, ed. Orphan Drugs. New York: Marcel Dekker, Inc, 1982.
26. Chobanian AV. Treatment of the elderly hypertensive patient. Am J Med 1984;77(2B):22–27.

SELECTED READINGS

THE RX TO OTC SWITCH[a]

Peter Temin

THE ROLE OF GOVERNMENT

The 1938 Federal Food, Drug, and Cosmetic Act was intended to improve and facilitate, not to hamper, the availability of drugs for self-medication. But before the end of 1938 the FDA had already sharply curtailed the selection of drugs available directly to the consumer. The agency had appointed doctors as the consumers' agents in selecting drugs. The 1951 Durham-Humphrey Amendments codified those distinctions which the FDA had developed through the 1940's between Rx and OTC drugs.

It is important to remember that doctors do not have complete information about drugs; therefore, prescription-only status does not guarantee that a drug will be used in an optimal fashion. Current drug policy recognizes this fact. Law and regulation have moved to separate doctors and consumers, reserving relevant medical information to doctors. But it is also recognized that much information has to be supplied by the government. In practice, the difference between doctors and consumers is not between knowledge and ignorance, but between different degrees of knowledge.

If the thrust of regulation were altered, the levels of doctors' and consumers' knowledge might be brought closer together. As the major health problems in the United States are becoming chronic conditions affected by general living styles, as opposed to medical therapy alone, involvement of consumers in their health becomes more important.

COST-BENEFIT ANALYSIS

Cost-benefit analysis is often used to help decide if a public policy should be undertaken. For example, costs are those of constructing, maintaining and operating a dam or bridge, the costs of equipment to clean up the atmosphere, or other expenditures including social or "external" costs, such as damage to the environment or public health. The benefits are the net gains expected to flow from these expenditures.

This framework is useful in the analysis of switching drugs from Rx to OTC, but it needs some tailoring to fit this subject. **There are limited investment costs involved in switching drugs—mainly those of gathering data and spending time on deciding whether to switch. The initial action is an administrative one of changing the terms under which a drug is sold. However, there may be additional costs to switching drugs. Any adverse drug reaction, for example, would be a loss of satisfaction by consumers and a cost to society to treat. There also may be external costs—the development of bacterial resistance to antibiotics, for example, if these agents become more widely used.** While these costs normally are treated as deductions from benefits, it is preferable here to list them as costs.

---

[a]Edited and reprinted with permission from The Proprietary Association. Costs and benefits in switching drugs from Rx to OTC. Presented at the Symposium, New Resources in Self-Medication. Washington, DC, November 1982.

The benefits of using a drug can be measured in two quite separate ways. The more orthodox method is to start from the preferences of consumers as indicated by the demand curve for a drug. This demand curve illustrates the various quantities of drugs that consumers are willing and financially able to buy at different prices at a given time. The benefit from a price reduction is that area under the demand curve above a new price, reflecting the value to consumers of each additional unit of drugs, known as the "consumer surplus."

This method, however, assumes that people have a thorough understanding of the drugs they are taking—that their demand for drugs takes into account the risk of adverse drug reactions, and that these reactions are not surprises. They therefore should not be counted as costs. If people do *not* make allowances for the possibility of unfavorable outcomes when they purchase drugs, then the adverse reactions are a cost. But in that case, the demand curve is not an accurate measure of consumer benefit because it is based on incomplete information about the product.

When effects of a drug are subtle, therefore, benefits and costs should be calculated by valuing the expected outcomes of using the drug without reference to the observed demand curve. The outcomes can be predicted from epidemiological evidence, and it is not necessary to assume that consumers have read and understood the literature. This procedure constructs the demand curve for a fully-informed consumer from epidemiological evidence, as opposed to inferring it from the market behavior of actual consumers.

Conventional cost-benefit analysis counts all people equally. And the normal deduction of costs from benefits to get a single total implicitly assumes not only that people are weighted equally, but also that it does not matter that some people lose while others gain. If the benefits outweigh the costs, then the gainers can pay compensation to the losers and still be better off than before the policy was undertaken. The losers have the satisfaction of knowing that they could be compensated for their losses without destroying all the gains of the gainers—for whatever comfort that is—but they are still worse off.

This approach weights the increase in efficiency more than the change in the fortunes of those unlucky people hurt by the policy. It is justified—when it is noticed at all—either by an overriding concern with efficiency or by the assertion that any political decision to alter the distribution of income can be and should be separated from the decision whether to undertake the policy in question. I will comment on a few implications of this approach in the examples.

Penicillin

Penicillin has been used widely for over 30 years and remains the drug of choice for many infections, notably upper respiratory infections (URIs). It is widely regarded as one of the least toxic of prescription drugs and seems a promising candidate for switching to over-the-counter status.

While the analysis of the other drugs indicated that much of the gain from the switch would derive from added use of the drugs, the gain from switching penicillin would come primarily from a reduction in doctor visits. Consumers gain more than the doctor's fee; they also save the time used to go to the doctor. Society gains the use for other purposes of both the patient's and the doctor's time.

The first question to ask is whether a consumer can self-diagnose a URI for which penicillin is appropriate. Common infections are easy to spot, particularly by people who get recurrent ones. URIs typically are treatable with penicillin if they are bacterial, and the problem in diagnosing them is to decide if they are viral or bacterial. **In concert with switch-**

ing penicillin, it should be made easier for individuals to get a culture of their infection, either by opening laboratories to consumers or by making cultures available through the mail, as they already are for doctors. Increased diagnostic tools would help consumers accurately assess their condition.

However, accurate diagnosis may not be crucial. A recent study of "pharyngitis management" compared the cost-effectiveness of three strategies: treating everyone (who was not allergic) with penicillin, treating only those with positive cultures, and treating no one. The analysis showed that it was preferable to culture before treating only when the proportion of positive cultures (that is, cultures with bacterial infections) was between five and twenty percent. And in that range the difference in costs between this policy and the policy of treating everyone was less than ten percent. The implication is that a widespread use of penicillin without reference to culture results would not be such a bad thing.

There are risks in taking penicillin. One is that the dosage may be insufficient to kill the infecting bacteria. If the penicillin were not working at all, the fever would not be reduced, and the consumer would know within hours. The cost to him or her would be any delay in seeking medical help while waiting to see if the penicillin worked. Given the rapidity with which penicillin reduces fever, this is unlikely to be large. The more serious problem comes after the fever is reduced. Some people will stop using the drug before the infection is eliminated, running the risk of reinfection. This risk can be stated clearly on the label and—like the risk of inappropriate use in the first place—is also present with prescriptions.

Another risk is of an adverse reaction. There are many mild reactions, such as rashes, which can be limited by ceasing to use the drug. But one serious reaction, that of anaphylactic shock, may be fatal. The risk of dying from penicillin-induced anaphylaxis has been estimated as one in 50,000 uses.

This risk needs to be factored into any policy decision about penicillin. Unlike many drug risks, this one is well known, and the responsibility of dealing with this risk already rests with the consumer. Rarely is a doctor or hospital expected to be aware of a patient's penicillin allergy. Instead, it is the patient who is expected to respond to a question about a previous allergic reaction to penicillin or in some other way to inform the medical personnel of his or her allergy. Switching penicillin to over-the-counter status would not shift this responsibility at all.

Unlike the previous drugs considered in this paper, there is a clear external cost in using penicillin. Use of this drug has encouraged the growth of bacteria resistant to its effects. If switching penicillin increased its use, it would also increase the likelihood that resistant strains would grow. Eminent physicians have been warning of this danger for twenty years, but the latest review of the evidence of penicillin-resistant bacteria concludes that the alarm of some years ago was premature.

Resistant strains grow most frequently in locations of high antibiotic usage, such as hospitals. The environment there gives a clear edge to the resistant strains. OTC penicillin, however, would be taken in the home, where the concentration of antibiotic usage is very low. An increase in low-density use would not have much impact on the overall ecology of infective bacteria.

It is likely, therefore, that almost every consumer who used OTC penicillin would gain. A small proportion would lose, possibly in much greater proportion than any single individual could gain. In the aggregate, the gains would outweigh the costs, but the inequitable distribution of those gains may make them hard to realize.

CONCLUSIONS

These three very diverse examples suggest the following principles for a policy of switching drugs to over-the-counter status. First, the policy is likely to be most effective when the benefit of the drug can be seen immediately and monitored by the consumer. The consumer then has an incentive to use the drug properly and can seek medical help if there is any problem. While it is true that the effect of a diuretic on blood pressure can be monitored easily, the benefit is in the reduction in morbidity and mortality, which is impossible to observe on an individual level. Second, side effects should either be minor or at least partly avoidable. The fatal reaction to penicillin is both rare and—at least in part—foreseeable, so that there is little added danger from a switch. Third, there should be little damage to the environment.

Many more drugs than are now over-the-counter fit these requirements, but careful study is needed to see which ones do. Each candidate for a switch should be scrutinized carefully with the aid of the most recent medical knowledge, and more information about the actual use of OTC drugs is needed.

CURRENT AND FUTURE PHARMACY INITIATIVES IN INSTITUTIONAL AND CORPORATE PRACTICE[b]

Joseph A. Oddis

Although currently there are hundreds of issues affecting hospital pharmacists to some extent, I am going to concentrate on six areas in which extraordinary developments have taken place. I will attempt to show how these developments are influencing and will continue to influence hospital pharmacy as we now know it.

The issues that I foresee as having a strong impact on institutional pharmacists during the next several years are as follows:

- Health-care financing,
- Clinical pharmacy services,
- Institutional outreach programs,
- Consolidation of hospitals and corporate restructuring,
- Use of pharmacy manpower,
- Product selection.

HEALTH-CARE FINANCING

Allow me to introduce health-care financing by giving a bit of its history. With the inception of Medicare and Medicaid in the mid-1960s, the philosophy that health-care benefits were a human right, regardless of social or economic class, took hold as a widely held national premise. The result was a dramatic increase in demand for health care, coupled with a growing perception that not only was health care a right, but it was also "free." Consumers of health care had virtually no incentive to be prudent buyers. As a matter of fact, because of the nature of reimbursement schemes, there were actually instances when the more eco-

[b]Edited and reprinted with permission from Oddis JA. Current and future pharmacy initiatives in institutional and corporate practice. Am J Hosp Pharm 1984;41:279-284.

nomic route was discouraged. Throughout the 1970s, each Administration attempted to stem the tide of rising health-care costs through a labyrinth of regulation that, on the one hand, mandated programs and services and, on the other hand, whittled away at the extent to which government would pay for them.

As we are all aware, earlier this year Congress enacted the Social Security Act Amendments of 1983 that incorporates prospective pricing by diagnosis-related groups (DRGs). The effect of that legislation is to change the incentives and payment mechanisms for health care for the elderly and, ultimately, the substance of what health care is for all Americans. I believe we are on the brink of dramatic and revolutionary change in the delivery of health care. With health-care financing as the driving force, during the next several years we will see unprecedented change regarding where care is provided, how it is provided, who provides it, and perhaps even to whom it is provided.

The implications of the new federal reimbursement scheme, the first phase of which began October 1, will reach far beyond the Medicare population and inpatient hospital setting at which it is aimed. A chain of events has been set in motion that will influence the decisions of private carriers, like Blue Cross, Travelers, and Aetna; other providers, such as health maintenance organizations, home health-care agencies, long-term care facilities, and preferred provider organizations; and, perhaps most important, employers and business coalitions. Their decisions may be based first on issues of cost and then on issues of relative quality.

William A. Zellmer (1), editor of the *American Journal of Hospital Pharmacy*, aptly described the potential impact of the new reimbursement scheme:

> Heretofore, physicians have dictated the level of hospital care provided to patients with little or no regard to cost. Now for the first time, cost will become a part of the equation, at least for Medicare patients, because hospitals will have an incentive to minimize expenditures. If the system works—and there is no guarantee that it will—it could be adopted by other third-party payers.

Indeed, this adoption by third parties is already beginning to happen.

The shift of primary emphasis to cost issues clearly presents health-care professionals, including pharmacists, with conflict. We have spent two decades or more focusing attention on quality of care. We have "sold" pharmaceutical services primarily on that basis, and much of the documentation we have gathered to justify systems and services relies on the perspective that more is better when it comes to health care. Congress has told us that now not only is more not better, but even if it were, we probably could not afford it. The challenge to pharmacy will be to maintain and continue to improve the quality of care made possible through good, comprehensive pharmaceutical services while refocusing attention on the relative cost of providing those services.

In my opinion, the success of institutional pharmacists in dealing with this refocused decision-making process based on cost will be determined by how effectively they develop clinical skills and services so that they can show how clinical services can reduce costs. A solid base of distributive and administrative services, including strict formulary controls and strict purchasing and inventory-control measures, is virtually a prerequisite to controlling cost and quality creatively and innovatively. From that base, clinical skills have the potential to improve therapeutic patterns by decreasing the incidence of iatrogenic illness, length of stay, cost of therapy, and inventory—all of which further decrease the total cost of care. Therefore, the goals of rational drug use and reduction of health costs are not incompatible; rather, they are complementary.

Critical to the successful transition from cost-based reimbursement to prospective pricing by diagnosis will be the ability of institutional pharmacists to understand the challenges facing them on both the philosophical and implementation levels. ASHP stands ready to assist its members in coping with present and future challenges of health-care financing, but the successful transition to DRGs will depend upon all professionals involved in health care, from those in academia to those in the pharmaceutical industry, from the hospital administrator to the physician (whose cooperation is essential to the pharmacist) to the pharmacy faculty member. Everyone has a personal responsibility to contribute to the collective effort to understand and cooperate with changes in health-care financing. We all have a stake in the outcome of these changes.

CLINICAL PHARMACY SERVICES

Pharmacists in institutions have made major progress in implementing up-to-date clinical services in hospitals. This statement is built upon facts drawn from the most recent ASHP-conducted national survey of hospital pharmaceutical services (2). Compared with surveys done by us in 1975 and 1978, remarkable gains in the implementation of contemporary pharmaceutical services are evident. For example, the 1982 survey shows the number of hospitals with complete unit dose and complete i.v. admixture programs has increased dramatically, jumping from 9.2% in 1975 to 45.1% in 1982. Approximately 72% of all hospitals in the United States covered some portion of their beds with a unit dose drug distribution system in 1982, which is triple the amount in 1975. Two thirds of the hospitals had at least a partial i.v. admixture program last year; this is more than double the percentage in 1975. Such programs are intrinsic to maintaining quality patient care while controlling costs.

When reviewing this survey I found it reassuring to note that the number of hospital pharmacies using computers has doubled in the past four years, and nearly half of all pharmacies have plans to purchase a major piece of equipment this year. Clearly, computerization is becoming a necessary component of contemporary pharmacy practice. These data indicate that members of our profession are gathering the skills and expertise needed in various technologies to thrive in the future.

Since the last survey conducted in 1978, we have also seen a doubling of the number of hospitals in which pharmacists assume an active role in counseling patients, monitoring drug therapy, and attending rounds with physicians. Implementation of such contemporary clinical services is the key to cost containment and improved patient care.

INSTITUTIONAL OUTREACH PROGRAMS

Just as changes in the area of health-care financing offer an opportunity to advance clinical services, so also do we observe changes in a third area, institutional outreach programs. These programs should present similar opportunities for pharmacy. I am using the phrase "institutional outreach programs" as an umbrella for various ambulatory-care programs, including free-standing physician group practice clinics, emergency-care centers, and general patiet counseling programs. Additional delivery modes for institutional outreach programs include hospital-based clinics, emergency rooms, and community and hospital outpatient pharmacies.

The whole area of institutional outreach programs has burgeoned from the traditional ambulatory-care clinic. Much progress has been made in this area, and, because the concept of institutional outreach programs is compatible with the previously described emphasis on cost containment and clinical services, I believe that the near future holds much progress here.

By the mid-1960s, ambulatory-care clinics associated with hospitals were a well-established part of health care in this country. As these clinics were built, some hospital pharmacists found themselves poorly equipped to take care of their growing outpatient population and simultaneously maintain a good level of service to inpatients. Very frankly, when hospital pharmacists had to make a choice, outpatients came out on the short end. It was not too long ago—in the 1950s—when most outpatient pharmacies issued drugs in coin envelopes and recycled glass bottles, frequently with handwritten labels. Patient-pharmacist communication did not exist, and, in general, outpatient services were crude. But we have come a long way since then, and we are still going. In 1970, 37% of the hospitals in the U.S. operated ambulatory-care programs; by 1980 that figure rose to 46% (3, 4). During that 10-year period the total number of annual outpatient visits rose from 114.8 million to 135 million. Annual visits to hospital emergency departments also rose during this period from 52 million to 82 million. Most dramatically, outpatient revenue now averages about 12% of total revenue for hospitals and is growing at a rate faster than inpatient revenue.

We are now seeing the development of emergency-care centers based upon the same concept as legal clinics and no-frills airlines. In 1979 there were about 80 such centers in the U.S.; by the beginning of next year 750 will be in operation. Supporters of these centers claim that they fill the gap between what could be costly emergency-room treatment and private physician consultation. Critics and investment advisors refer to them as a "Medical McDonald's" or "Doc-in-the-Box." Regardless of viewpoint, such options are now available to outpatients, and some physicians have admitted to extending their hours and even to making house calls to meet the competition from such centers. Whatever the outcome, the message is obvious: Ambulatory care is changing at such a rapid rate that we cannot assume an institution's ambulatory-care philosophy is the same today as it was just six months ago. Certainly the next few years will be even more telling.

What does all this mean in relation to hospital pharmacy departments? It means that if a hospital is committed to overall ambulatory-care expansion—and most of them are—pharmacy must be an integral part of that development. Pharmacy departments initiate involvement in such areas as dialysis programs, home total parenteral nutrition services, oncology chemotherapy, diabetes management programs, pain management programs, home antibiotic injection programs, and general patient counseling programs. We are seeing and will continue to see an increase in such programs because pharmacies in hospitals must adapt to the changing roles and needs of the institutions they serve.

This issue of institutional outreach programs points to an inescapable conclusion and that is as follows: The future of institutional pharmacists is being shaped by some very positive factors that are allowing them to enhance their role as true health professionals and providers of quality care. As we advance through the 1980s, we are seeing a time when institutional pharmacists are able to provide a continuum of care to ambulatory patients who continue to consider the hospital as their source of health care. This is exciting, challenging, and is happening now. And one of the ways in which we see it enforced is through what I view as the fourth dynamic issue influencing the profession of institutional pharmacy: hospital corporate restructuring and consolidation.

CONSOLIDATION OF HOSPITALS AND CORPORATE RESTRUCTURING

The consolidation and corporate restructuring of hospitals permit diversification of services in a highly competitive environment. Currently, large corporations operate approximately 15% (about 1000) of America's 7000 hospitals. This is nearly double the number since 1976, and this number is increasing. Certainly such a change in ownership will have tremendous impact on the mix of hospital services.

According to Thomas Frist, Jr., president of Hospital Corporation of America, which is the largest of the investor-owned hospital chains, one of his primary concerns is to keep Wall Street happy by maintaining an upward slope in HCA's earnings per share. Frist said that he hopes to have 500 hospitals by 1985 or 1986, and he wants HCA to be the country's largest health-care company, topping Johnson & Johnson, by 1990. (Remember, HCA had 328 hospitals in 1981 and only 186 in 1980.) His plan is that by the year 2000 HCA will have attained the stature of General Electric and IBM and will be one of the country's top five companies. Paul M. Frison, president of Lifemark Corporation, believes that the investor-owned sector will possess between 25% and 30% of the country's hospitals within the next 10 years. Lifemark, which operates 35 hospitals in 10 sun belt states, as well as ancillary contract management business, plans on having between 40 and 45 hospitals by 1986. Clearly, with such shifting of management structures, hospital departments and services will be affected.

An interesting trend has developed within various multihospital systems. Not only are we noticing similarities in services such as the development of free-standing clinics (many of which contain pharmacies), but both profit and nonprofit systems are now quite similar.

According to Donald Wegmiller, president of the nonprofit Health Central System, nonprofit multihospital corporations will increase their margins in existing lines of business. This will be done through reductions in personnel, energy, and materials consumption and an increase in management efforts aimed at cost containment. Wegmiller believes that the shift toward prospective pricing will benefit nonprofit hospital systems because they have more room to improve productivity. Meanwhile, aggressive pricing of services by nonprofit corporations will lead to better profit margins, which are needed to build equity and win the support of bond buyers. In the short run, however, nonprofit corporations will be forced to examine their patient mix and compare that with services offered. In the long run, though, corporate restructuring of hospitals will provide the ability for hospitals to attract the best people, and training programs will be implemented to produce not only better quality health care, but eventually to create lower-cost health care as well. And because multihospital corporations are already supporting programs such as quality assurance, fiscal management, and information systems, they are well equipped to meet the future.

USE OF PHARMACY MANPOWER

As a direct outgrowth of the issue of corporate restructuring of hospitals comes another issue that I believe will have a great impact on hospital pharmacy. This issue is one of manpower.

Samuel J. Tibbitts, president and chief executive officer of Lutheran Hospital Society of Southern California and chairman of Health Network of America, Inc., states that by the year 2000 more than 90% of all U.S. hospitals—profit and nonprofit alike—will belong to multihospital systems. And, as described previously, trends now are showing this to be true.

This consolidation is resulting in a re-evaluation of manpower, and we do not have to wait until the year 2000 to see this. Already hospital pharmacists are acting in executive and managerial positions in multihospital systems and corporations. Where once these people were only responsible for the function of one institution's pharmacy, now they are overseeing the function of pharmacies in consolidated systems. One of the selling points of clinical pharmacy is its cost-containment aspect, and it is the clinical pharmacist with good management background who may be selected for pharmacy management positions within multihospital systems. During the next several years, we will see these pharmacist managers stress productivity, efficiency, energy conservation, systems review and design, and purchase practices. In many hospitals, already we are seeing pharmacy personnel learning all facets of operations to maximize their versatility and improve their skills.

This retraining and refocusing of pharmacy personnel has resulted in some interesting statistics. For instance, the total number of individuals completing ASHP-accredited hospital pharmacy residency programs in 1973 was 143; this year we anticipate 375 pharmacists will complete these postgraduate programs. In other words, within 10 years we have seen more than a 250% increase in the annual number of practitioners successfully completing residency programs. One of the primary reasons for this jump in numbers is that graduates of ASHP-approved residency programs are better equipped to face the changes now being encountered by the profession, and because of this preparation they are more attractive to employers. I should also add that there are 154 accredited residency programs now available across the country in both general and specialized practice areas; 20 years ago, the accreditation program was just being launched.

The use of technicians in hospital pharmacies will continue to grow as more and more pharmacists become good managers and develop the savvy about what it takes to succeed in the hospital environment of the next several years. In a study published last year in the *American Journal of Hospital Pharmacy*, the proportion of time pharmacists spent in professional versus nonprofessional activities was shown to be directly related to the number of technicians in the pharmacy (5). As staffing patterns varied, differences occurred in the ratio of professional to nonprofessional activities, with the greatest percentage of professional activity recorded when a pharmacist worked with more than one technician. This is certainly a manpower issue to ponder.

PRODUCT SELECTION

Twenty years ago, ASHP and the American Medical Association, the American Hospital Association, and the American Pharmaceutical Association worked out an agreement on the principles of the hospital formulary system. This agreement placed the responsibility for the authorization and implementation of the formulary system in the hands of the hospital pharmacy and therapeutics (P & T) committees. We have seen over the ensuing years that the formulary system has spawned pharmacy's most effective programs for ensuring the quality and the cost of institutional patient care. Now that hospitals have become extremely aware of the need for cost containment, the formulary system will become increasingly important over the next several years.

According to contemporary hospital formulary systems, the pharmacist has the authority to select the supplier or the brand of medication dispensed unless the prescriber makes a specific notation to the contrary. The results of the 1982 survey of hospital pharmaceutical services demonstrate that this practice occurs in 90% of all short-term hospitals in the

United States. Additionally, in 40% of short-term hospitals the medical staff has given the pharmacy authority to dispense a particular drug entity in place of a therapeutically similar but chemically different drug.

As we witness the changes happening in the health-care arena today, especially the drastic changes in the system of health-care financing, it is imperative that medicine and pharmacy cooperate to retain professional control over drug therapy. ASHP believes that a formulary system, within which the medical staff may authorize and place conditions upon use of therapeutic equivalents, is a means under which health professionals can control costs without compromising patient care.

FUTURE OF INSTITUTIONAL PHARMACY PRACTICE

As we ponder the future of health care in general, and of institutional pharmacy in particular, we must first ponder the future of health-care financing. Whether or not prospective pricing and DRGs will survive is not the issue. Rather, what we must realize is that we cannot afford to perpetuate a health-care system that stimulates growth in costs at three times the general rate of inflation. Zellmer (1) identified four implications of the changing health-care financing milieu for hospital pharmacists. Paraphrased somewhat, these implications are as follows:

1. We will see that strategic planning is more important than ever for hospital departments. The trend toward increased competition among hospitals was apparent well before DRGs entered the picture. A hospital that had a formal plan to deal with this factor would not have had to adjust much to accommodate DRGs. As one pharmacist put it, "DRGs have not changed any of my goals for pharmacy. . . . What DRGs have done, however, is compelled us to move more quickly—we no longer have the luxury of time."
2. We will also witness an intensification of initiatives by pharmacy and therapeutics committees, including drug-use review and prescribing restrictions. Formulary systems in general, and pharmacists' product-selection prerogatives in particular, will be strengthened. P & T committees are likely to give special attention to the use of antibiotics. Any expensive new drug product can expect closer scrutiny than ever before.
3. Department directors will need to keep closer tabs on operational expenses. Within the next few years, administrators will probably expect pharmacy departments to determine their average costs per DRG. This will escalate the need for computerization and the demand for a pharmacy work-measurement system such as the one ASHP is developing.
4. Institutional pharmacists will have to sharpen their political skills. Competition will be keen not only among hospitals but also among hospital departments. Pharmacists will have to position themselves for appointment to key committees that will be reviewing the cost and quality of patient care and developing corrective programs. Also, pharmacy managers will have to be flexible to move into new areas (such as home health care) to help institutions meet their objectives.

Other changes in institutional practice that are likely to occur include the following:

1. Institutional pharmacy can expect to see a decrease in the size and dollar value of drug inventories, an increase in the use of bid prices, prescribing sanctions established by P & T committees, physician education on the relative costs of alternative therapies, and certainly an increase in drug-use reviews.

2. It is not unreasonable to anticipate the physician oversupply, which is predicted to reach 70,000 by the year 1990, to influence institutional pharmacists' responsibilities and prerogatives. However, the increasing number of salaried physicians, which is now estimated to be 30–50% of all physicians, may provide incentives for physicians to become active partners in the effort to control hospital costs because reduced expenditures will mean greater hospital income. This can be translated into increased benefits and salaries for all hospital personnel, including salaried physicians.

3. In spite of our best efforts to control costs, health care will continue to be a growth industry during the next decade, possibly reaching 15% of GNP. New "partners" on the health-care team will be technology and educated consumers who will be increasingly involved in their own wellness scenarios.

CONCLUSION

Although we are seeing many changes in the health-care industry that will have an impact on institutional pharmacists, such changes in the long run will have a very positive effect on our profession. The word "change" can be intimidating, but we must remember that each time one door closes, another opens.

We are seeing institutional pharmacists equipping themselves to provide the leadership within their institutions to balance the pharmaceutical needs of health-care consumers with the financial constraints of the times. The future of institutional pharmacists is being shaped by factors that ultimately will enable practitioners to enhance their roles as health professionals and providers of economical quality care. Our responsibility is to respond to this challenge.

REFERENCES

1. Zellmer WA. Preparing for prospective pricing. *Am J Hosp Pharm.* 1983; 40:1479. Editorial.
2. Stolar MH. National survey of hospital pharmaceutical services—1982. *Am J Hosp Pharm.* 1983; 40:963-9.
3. American Hospital Association. Hospital statistics: 1971 edition. Chicago: American Hospital Association; 1971.
4. American Hospital Association. Hospital statistics: 1981 edition. Chicago: American Hospital Association; 1981.
5. Dostal MM, Daniels CE, Roberts MJ et al. Pharmacist activities under alternative staffing arrangements. *Am J Hosp Pharm.* 1982; 39:2098-101.

THE "RATIONING" OF MEDICAL CARE [c]

Victor R. Fuchs

"The United States will soon have to begin rationing medical care." Although we hear this warning with increasing frequency (1), taken literally the statement is sheer nonsense. It is nonsense because the United States has always rationed medical care, just as every country always has and always will ration care. No nation is wealthy enough to supply all the care

---

[c] Reprinted with permission from Fuchs VR. The "rationing" of medical care. N Engl J Med 1984;311:1572–1573.

that is technically feasible and desirable; no nation can provide "presidential medicine" for all its citizens. Moreover, medical care is hardly unique in this respect. The United States "rations" automobiles, houses, restaurant meals—all the goods and services that make up our standard of living.

The dictionary says that to ration is to apportion or to distribute. The suggestion that until now this country has not apportioned or distributed medical care can hardly be taken seriously. What, then, is all the fuss about? Is anything changing? Indeed, there are changes under way—not from no rationing to rationing, but rather in the way rationing takes place—who does the rationing and who is affected by it.

The basic method of rationing goods and services in this country is through the market. The willingness and ability of consumers to pay for goods and services, and of producers to supply them, determine how they are apportioned or distributed. As recently as 20 years ago, more than half of all personal health-care expenditures were paid for directly by patients. Did this ration care? Of course it did. Consider, for instance, surgery rates among urban whites 65 years of age and over before the introduction of Medicare. In 1963 the rate was 66 operations per 1000 for persons with below-average incomes and 86 per 1000 for those whose incomes were above average. It is not likely that the poorer elderly were less in need of surgery than their wealthier counterparts. The "system" was rationing care even though individual physicians may not have been. Medicare changed this distribution dramatically. By 1970 the rate for persons with below-average incomes was up 85 per 1000, whereas the rate for those with above-average incomes had actually fallen to 80 per 1000 (2).

The growth of federal insurance programs substantially diminished the role of income as a rationing device, but large differences in the availability of care remain, frequently as a result of geographic location. For instance, in short-term-care hospitals in Massachusetts there is one registered nurse for every patient, but in Arkansas there is only one for every two patients. In the average American community there are 2 physicians to care for every 1000 persons, but in San Francisco there are approximately 5. Thus, even with widespread third-party payment, the amount and kind of care that physicians provide is still constrained by how busy they are, what facilities, equipment, and auxiliary personnel are available, how much training the physicians have had, and the informal messages that they receive from peers about what constitutes "appropriate" care in any particular situation.

To the extent that the spread of private and public insurance has relieved the economic pressure on patients and physicians, it has also been a major factor in the expansion of expenditures. Now, questions are being raised about the benefits of additional care relative to its cost. In the American economic system, expenditures for most goods and services are determined by consumers, who balance the benefits expected from an additional purchase against the additional cost. By and large, this balancing results in a reasonably efficient allocation of resources, given the distribution of income and the preferences of consumers.

Expenditures for medical care are different. Because most Americans want to be insured against large medical bills and most do not want to see the poor dying for lack of care, the bulk of medical care is paid for by third parties, private or public. But when a third party is paying, the patient will want additional care and the conscientious physician will provide it, even though its cost to society exceeds the benefit to the patient.

This divergence between what is good for the patient (given insurance) and what is efficient for society as a whole is a key element in current concerns over health-care spending. Deductibles and coinsurance can reduce this divergence a little, but the basic problem remains: how to provide insurance without pushing the use of resources to the point at which the additional cost far exceeds the additional benefit.

Increasingly, physicians are being asked to resolve this problem; that is one reason why the issue of "rationing" takes on a new urgency. The pressure to be more economical in the provision of care will force physicians to make decisions that are contrary to the best interests of individual patients, even though these decisions may make a great deal of sense from the viewpoint of society as a whole. Moreover, pressure to control costs will raise explicitly the question of who gets how much care. In the past this question was often answered implicitly by where the patient lived and whether he could pay. In the future, in the interest of maintaining equity while controlling costs, it may be necessary to withhold care from patients who have ample income or complete insurance and who therefore believe that they are entitled to "everything possible." Reimbursement methods, such as Medicare's Prospective Payment System plan, that pay a uniform amount for each admission in a diagnosis-related group will tend to redistribute resources away from hospitals that have been providing a great deal of care to those that have been providing less.

A major concern is whether attempts to control the use of health-care resources will affect the health of the population. Opinions differ concerning this question, and no one knows the answer with certainty. Some health experts contend that it is possible to cut expenditures substantially without seriously affecting health. They claim that some care—say, 10 per cent—is actually harmful to patients, that they would be better off without it. It is not difficult to believe that another 10 per cent has a relatively low yield even though there may be a slight benefit. Thus, *if* cuts were concentrated on the 20 per cent that had a negative or low yield, the overall effect on health would be small. But that is a big "if." Two major problems stand in the way of such an outcome. First, much of medical practice lacks a firm, quantified, scientific base; therefore, no one can be certain just which care should be cut. Second, even as clinical experience and systematic research reveal which hospital admissions, operations, x-ray procedures, prescriptions, and the like can be forgone without harm (or even possible benefit) to patients, there is no guarantee that medical practice will be modified accordingly. Media hype, irrational patient preferences, distortional insurance coverage, and perverse incentives for health-care professionals and institutions may result in a pattern of care that is far different from the ideal.

What needs to be done? First, the nation's practitioners, hospitals, and academic medical centers must launch a major effort to identify the benefits that patients receive from the various components of the $400 billion that is spent annually for health care. Second, experts on health-care policy need to continue to press for reforms in organization and finance that will lead patients to want, and health professionals to deliver, more cost-effective care.

Even with more knowledge and better incentives, however, limitation of resources will eventually mean worse health for some patients, even if it changes the probability of complications or survival by only a small fraction. "Low-yield" medicine is not "no-yield" medicine. For physicians to have to face these trade-offs explicitly every day is to assign to them an unreasonable and undesirable burden. The commitment of the individual physician to the individual patient is one of the most valuable features of American medical care. It would therefore be a great mistake to turn each physician into an explicit maximizer of the social-benefit/social-cost ratio in his or her daily practice.

But the trade-offs must be made. Usually the best time for making such decisions is during the evaluation of the costs and benefits of new facilities, the development and diffusion of new technologies, and the training of personnel. As I suggested at the beginning of this article, physicians have always practiced within constraints, but as long as the "rationing" is implicit, it is tolerable.

In the past, the "system" produced the constraints without a great deal of analysis or a conscious policy choice. In the future, there will be considerably more systematic analyses regarding the location of facilities, investment in equipment, training of specialists, and designing of screening programs and treatment protocols. Health-plan managers, hospital administrators, insurance-company executives, and government officials will use these analyses to help them make difficult decisions about the allocation of scarce resources. This shift in the locus of decision making will inevitably reduce the power of practicing physicians. To the extent that these decisions set the constraints within which individual practitioners function, however, there will be less need for them to ration care to their patients explicitly.

REFERENCES

1. Schwartz WB, Aaron HJ. Rationing hospital care: lessons from Britain. N Engl J Med 1984; 310:52-6.
2. Bombardier C, Fuchs VR, Lillard LA, Warner KE. Socioeconomic factors affecting the utilization of surgical operations. N Engl J Med 1977; 297:699-705.

11
Ethics

ROBERT A. BUERKI
LOUIS D. VOTTERO

INTRODUCTION

Through the systematic application of ethical principles professionals may reflect upon their ordinary actions, judgments, and behaviors and compare them with accepted standards. Professional ethics are designed to illuminate and affirm the professional as an independent, responsible, and accountable individual who respects the rights of those individuals who are served by the profession. Applying such standards to everyday specific situations encountered daily in the contemporary practice of pharmacy, however, is difficult to do and sometimes can be achieved only through choosing the least objectionable course of action among a bewildering array of choices, each of which may have profound consequences for patient care.

Throughout their centuries of service to mankind, pharmacists have expressed their individual and group concern for the need to practice their profession in an ethical manner. A number of commissioned studies have reported on the broad aspects of pharmacy as a profession and upon the professional behavior of pharmacists. These studies report the belief that pharmacy is an honorable and respected profession, as intoned in *Basic Material for a Pharmacy Curriculum* (1927), and that pharmacists are responsible and autonomous decision makers. "After all has been said and done," concluded the deeply probing *General Report of the Pharmaceutical Survey* (1950), "the outstanding factor determining the future of the profession of pharmacy is fundamentally moral in nature" (1).

Pharmacist as a Professional Person

In addition, a number of studies have attempted to ascertain and confirm the professional status of pharmacy. These studies typically conclude that pharmacy falls short of meeting an idealized list of professional characteristics developed by sociologists and others and hence is less "professional" than the "ideal" profession (see, for example, Ref. 2). The Report of the Study Commission on Pharmacy, *Pharmacists for the Future* (1975), however, although acknowledging that pharmacy has been recently characterized as "obsolete," "obsolescent," or "peripheral," prefers to speak of the "process" of pharmacy, pointing to gaps in health services involving drugs and urging that pharmacists undertake new duties to fill them (3). Nevertheless, since nearly all professions that are subjected to such scrutiny are usually found to be deficient in at least a few areas, pharmacy seems to be no worse off than most other professions, and better off with respect to perceived public attitudes about pharmacy practice.

Regardless of these comparisons, pharmacy does have a legitimate claim to professional status through its heritage, knowledge base, socially sanctioned decision-making authority, and the generally laudable behavior of its practitioners. Pharmacists, in responding to the unique societal privileges extended to them through the licensure process, have demonstrated a level of personal and group behavior that meets and often exceeds the expectations of society. In Chapter 2, Mrtek and Catizone carefully state the case for the pharmacist being a professional person.

Importance of a Professional Ethic

Self-regulation and self-discipline are generally viewed by the public as essential requisites for a profession, especially when a professional assumes duties that are linked to the personal health of the individual, involving life-and-death decisions in a literal sense. Furthermore, despite the increasing sophistication among segments of the American public, very few individuals are able to judge the quality of the professional services they receive. As a result, a professional ethic is one of several generally accepted criteria that serve to distinguish a profession from other occupations or business endeavors.

Professionals are given certain legal prerogatives by society, such as a license to practice and a quasimonopoly to operate in a certain professional arena. In return for these prerogatives, a profession accepts responsibility to maintain a standard of conduct beyond conformity to law or technical skill. This standard of conduct, this common concern for collective self-discipline, this control of a profession from within, is known as ethics.

In philosophy, *ethics* is usually defined as "the science of rightness and wrongness of human conduct as known by natural reason." *Professional ethics,* however, may be defined as "rules of conduct or standards by which a particular group regulates its actions and sets standards for its members." Ethics controls a particular group in society, not society at large; control of this group is from the group itself.

The system of ethics is closely related to and overlaps with two other systems designed to control society, law, and morals. *Law* refers to regulations established by a government applicable to people within a certain political subdivision. Law controls all people within a certain political subdivision, not a particular group in society; control of the people is external to any group within society. By contrast, *morals* are generally accepted customs of right living and conduct, and an individual's practice in relation to these customs. Morals control individuals within society by means of internal, personal controls. These distinctions are summarized in Table 11.1.

Of the three systems, law would seem to have the greatest payoff to society, because sanctions for noncompliance include not only fines but imprisonment. Nevertheless, the system of law does not cover all areas of professional endeavor or all potential risks a professional encounters. Thus, no matter how broadly laws and regulations are written or how detailed they might seem, there are still areas that must be covered by a system of voluntary self-discipline, the system of ethics.

Table 11.1. Comparison between systems of ethics, law, and morals

System	Application	Control Source	Form
Ethics	Specific group	Within the group	Codes of ethics
Law	Political subdivision	Outside the group	Legislation
Morals	Individuals	Religious beliefs, conscience	Religious writings

Society also expects a profession, through its collective members, to generate its own statement of acceptable and unacceptable behavior, usually in the form of a *code of ethics,* a detailed, explicit operational blueprint of norms of professional conduct, a recital of desirable and undesirable actions having an impact on the character of a profession and its functional reliability. The behavior pattern established in a code of ethics is generally enforced through a peer-review mechanism associated with a professional academy, organization, or association. One measure of professionalization is the extent to which such a peer-review mechanism actually works to control a profession.

Structure also can affect the utility of a code of ethics. If a code is too long, it becomes unwieldy and unusable. Overly long codes are not easily changed and require a very complicated process in order to be updated, generally through a standing or special committee on ethics impaneled by a professional association. If a code of ethics is too short, it may be too abstract or idealized to be useful and may avoid dealing with sensitive areas. Such codes are designed for their public relations value and are usually described as "suitable for framing and display in your place of practice." The ideal code of ethics usually consists of a concise, generalized code supplemented by a manual of interpretations or case histories. Both medicine and law use this latter approach, an approach that has yet to be attempted in pharmacy.

EVOLUTION OF TRADITIONAL ETHICAL PRINCIPLES

The professional heritage of American pharmacy draws its roots from the highly structured English tradition that relied, perhaps too heavily, on the tensions created by overlapping segments of medical and pharmaceutical practices. English physicians, surgeons, and apothecaries of the eighteenth century were unencumbered for the most part by royal decrees and statutes governing their professions. To function effectively in this laissez-faire environment, each burgeoning speciality developed rigid codes of conduct based upon those developed by medieval guilds.

The English apothecaries who emigrated to the American colonies, therefore, carried with them a sense of self-directed behavior in the English laissez-faire tradition without the rigid professional structure that had allowed the English medicopharmaceutical system to function. An undistinguished practice of medicine and pharmacy appropriate to a frontier-like colonial society worked well for nearly two centuries, but as America emerged as a young and increasingly complex republic, practitioners sought a new professional structure combining the strengths of the English system with the multinational potpourri of the American experience.

This structure first emerged in Philadelphia during the mid-eighteenth century as physicians organized educational institutions and professional associations to distinguish their practice from an alarming array of self-styled medical practitioners. By the early nineteenth century, this structured profession of medicine had acquired both the organizational strength and the political power to pose a threat to all unorganized or unorthodox related practitioners, including pharmacists. For example, the founding of the Philadelphia College of Pharmacy in 1821 reflected in part a perceived threat from a local medical school that proposed to educate and certify pharmacy practitioners as "Masters of Pharmacy." Those who were unable or unwilling to submit to this certification process were to be characterized as "neglectful or indifferent" (4). Yet by midcentury, the Philadelphia College of Pharmacy and the handful of other local pharmaceutical associations that had emerged had established a standard of professional practice that reflected the collective values and aspirations of a self-selected membership of dedicated practitioners committed to raising the overall standards of pharmacy by example rather than relying upon the more stringent and less desirable effects of legislation and societal sanctions. The circumstances surrounding the founding of the American Pharmaceutical Association in 1852 also reflected a similar threat to professional autonomy as the newly formed American Medical Association sought to assume responsibility for controlling the flood of adulterated drugs that threatened the health of the American public. Both of these examples serve to underline the importance that professional associations place upon *exclusivity* as conferred by association membership.

This exclusivity is also reflected in the early professional codes promulgated by these same associations. Both the code of ethics for the Philadelphia College of Pharmacy (1848), which attempted to advance "professional conduct and probity" to correspond to the "standard of scientific attainments" it felt it had achieved, and the 1852 code of the American Pharmaceutical Association (APhA), modeled after the Philadelphia example, which asked those who honored it to "protect themselves and the public from the ill effects of an undue competition, and the temptation to gain at the expense of quality," established guidelines for professional practice far beyond the realities of everyday practice (5, 5a). In doing so, the associations created a pattern of lofty professional expectations that persists to this day.[a] Ironically, the obligation to subscribe to the APhA code as a condition of membership was dropped in 1855, and the code itself disappeared from the pharmacy literature until 1921 when former APhA President Charles H. LaWall wrote a new and comprehensive code for the Association (6).

This new code, and its subsequent revisions, continued to reflect societal concerns as organized pharmacy attempted to extract an ever-expanding standard of practice from its membership, and by implication, from American pharmacists at large. For example, the rapidly expanding enrollments in American schools and colleges of pharmacy by students of questionable motivation in the years following the enactment of prohibition prompted a detailed reference to the "dispensing and sale of narcotic drugs and alcoholic liquors" in the 1922 code of the Association. By the same token, the 1952 revision reflected the emergence of brand-name pharmaceutical products and subsequent state-based antisubstitution legislation, as it urged pharmacists to recognize the "significance and legal aspects of brand names and trade-marked products," while remaining silent upon the then moot "alcoholic liquor" issue.

By the mid-1960s, it became apparent that although a reactive approach to developing an ethical code resulted in increasingly detailed standards of practice, no mechanism existed within the Association for either interpreting the code or securing adherence to its principles. Consequently, in 1966, the Association established a Judicial Board empowered to "discipline members and render advisory opinions and interpretative statements, reprimanding, suspending or expelling a member in any category . . . for unprofessional conduct" (7). The following year, the Association convened a conference on ethics to reconsider the code, which was judged no longer suitable for guiding pharmacists in their expanded role in the modern health-care system.

The code that eventually emerged from these discussions was not only more streamlined but also focused more upon the protection of the public rather than upon proscriptive

---

[a] The best single source for comparing the various versions of the code of ethics of the American Pharmaceutical Association may be found in Buerki RA, ed. Challenge of Ethics in Pharmacy Practice. No. 8, new series. Madison WI: American Institute of the History of Pharmacy, 1985, pp 55-64.

guidelines for pharmacy practitioners. For example, the new code placed a positive duty upon the pharmacist to "render to each patient the full measure of his ability," removing the traditional restriction to "not discuss the therapeutic effects or composition of a prescription with a patient," thus encouraging the development of a patient-oriented, clinical practice of pharmacy. Another provision, aimed at discouraging arrangements that could interfere with the patient's free choice of pharmacy services, had an unhappy legacy. The provision, which required that the pharmacist "not solicit professional practice by means of advertising," led to a complaint to the Judicial Board regarding advertising of prescription services by two pharmacy chains in Michigan. In its attempt to enforce the ban of the code on advertising, the Board became embroiled in a lawsuit that resulted in a temporary injunction prohibiting the Board to take further action against the chains, effectively nullifying the Board's power to enforce this provision of the code of ethics of the Association. Moreover, the publicity surrounding the lawsuit also drew the attention of federal agencies to the dispute, causing the Association to revise this portion of the code to be more circumspect of federal antitrust laws. Finally, a number of state boards of pharmacy have enacted statutes or regulations in an attempt to secure so-called "ethical" behavior under the vague legal umbrella of "unprofessional conduct." These attempts to enforce ethical behavior through the force of law have not withstood judicial scrutiny and have met with little success (8).

The most recent revision of the code (1981) places the pharmacist-patient relationship on a new plane of shared responsibility for health-care outcomes, encouraging the pharmacist to "provide information to patients regarding professional services truthfully, accurately, and fully," a provision that has been interpreted as not only permitting but requiring pharmacists to take an active role in counseling their patients concerning the proper use of both prescription and over-the-counter medications. As a result, thoughtful practitioners of pharmacy today often feel uneasy as they search for more authoritative guidance in their professional practice, guidance that more closely reflects the values that underlie the traditional professional codes of ethics.

NEWER PRINCIPLES IN A PHARMACY ETHIC

Framers of the earliest codes of professional practice presumed that their codes would reflect their patients' best interests. Primarily based upon the ancient Hippocratic principle of doing good and avoiding evil, these codes essentially reflect paternalistic attitudes that pose challenges to patient autonomy, question professional veracity, and raise other potentially disturbing questions. For example, the basic principle that underlies the Hippocratic Oath enjoins physicians to work for the benefit of the sick according to their "ability and judgment" without necessarily including patients in the decision-making process surrounding their therapy.

Recently, this somewhat exclusive focus for a pharmacy ethic has been examined and challenged as self-serving. In 1985, pharmacist-ethicist Robert M. Veatch brought this concern to the attention of a symposium of pharmacists during a national meeting and challenged them to "respond to the critical questions of the day," especially as they moved "beyond the traditional conception of our profession" (9). Veatch argues persuasively that several additional ethical principles beyond *beneficience*—"doing good" in Hippocratic terms—must be considered in developing an ethic for the current practice of pharmacy. Such principles include *autonomy, veracity,* and *justice.*

The principle of *autonomy* is considered paramount in formulating a contemporary code of professional conduct. The autonomous person has the right to decide what—if any—medical treatment he or she will accept, based upon the advice of a practitioner. The ethical value associated with this principle may be expressed through the patient's right to *informed consent*, the knowledge base upon which a patient may rationally choose or refuse treatment. Given the sophistication of our current medical system and its complex modern pharmaceuticals, many practitioners unintentionally violate this right by assuming their patients would not understand the technical details underlying their treatment plan. Other practitioners assume that their patients are not interested in such details. Still other practitioners, sadly, are guided by the traditional paternalistic view that they know what is in the best interest of their patients, with or without their consent, informed or otherwise. The resistance by organized medicine and pharmacy to the proposed inclusion of patient package inserts with all prescription drugs dispensed was argued on the bases of increased cost and decreased efficiency in the dispensing process rather than on the right of patient to have access to complete and relevant information concerning their medications.

The principle of *veracity*, or truth-telling, is reflected in the APhA code of ethics statement encouraging the pharmacist to "strive to provide information to patients regarding professional services truthfully, accurately, and fully." Curiously, the code seems to fall short in its endorsement of truth-telling only as it applies to a pharmacist's professional services, but in Veatch's words, is the closest that the code comes to "acknowledging moral obligations that potentially may have harmful consequences" (10). Even within the professional arena, pharmacists are often torn between conflicting values: Full disclosure of all possible harmful side effects of a potent prescription medication may seriously interfere with a patient's compliance with the drug regimen or result in refusal to even take the medicine. Certainly, the pharmacist is obliged to warn his or her patients of potentially life-threatening side effects, but may use professional judgment and discretion in discussing side effects that may not be clinically significant. By the same token, the use of placebo therapy, as ordinarily defined, relies upon the violation of this principle for its successful effect.

The principle of *justice*, as applied to the practice of medicine and pharmacy, is primarily associated with the allocation of goods and services. The questions associated with allocating access to a kidney dialysis machine provides an intellectual challenge to students of professional ethics, but the allocation of professional services to an ever-increasing aged population provides a less dramatic, but equally pressing need for applying the principle of justice. Drug compliance among the marginally indigent population often depends upon pharmacists extending credit or making other special arrangements for providing expensive maintenance drugs. The principle applies to the pharmacist's relationships with patients at all levels of the socioeconomic scale, ranging from the wealthy to those receiving public assistance. To selectively deny professional services to Medicaid recipients or other "undesirable" patients based on their inability to pay or upon a misanthropic dismissal of all public assistance programs is to violate or flaunt the principle of justice in its fullest sense.

Each of these principles is independent and of equal importance in establishing the basis for more concrete ethical rules and guidelines. In many cases, however, two or more of these principles may apply to a single complex moral dilemma. Thus, in attempting to solve such a dilemma, the practitioner should recognize that each principle may not be totally binding in and of itself and must be tempered by reason and personal judgment. Many practitioners, inured by years of study in the objective world of pharmaceutical sciences, find it difficult to resolve these dilemmas based upon unfamiliarity with the principles of professional ethics as well as their uneasiness with the subjective nature of ethical decision making. For this reason, many pharmacists find it useful to employ a formal process of *conflict resolution* to assist them in balancing the conflicts between ethical principles.

Veatch proposes four possible strategies: (*a*) *rank-ordering the principles* according to one's perceived priorities (which may prove impossible in practice); (*b*) *balancing the competing principles* according to one's personal beliefs (which is "discomfortingly" vague); (*c*) *collapsing the principles* into one larger all-encompassing principle (which may result in the loss of specificity); and (*d*) *balancing beneficence and nonmaleficence* (the so-called "consequentialist" principles) *against autonomy, veracity, and justice* (the so-called "non-consequentialist" principles), using the former to break any resulting "ties" (11). Nevertheless, many pharmacists ultimately behave in a manner reflecting their individual commitment to specific values and attitudes. For this reason, we should examine the values and attitudes that are associated with the professionalization process.

Values and Attitudes of the Pharmacist

In his recent analysis of the shift of moral values over time, Daniel Callihan envisioned "a resurgence in social ethics and an emphasis on community, on the common good, on the hazards of an excessive dependence on the language of rights and on an exultation of individual over community" (12). Character and virtue are coming back, according to Callihan, and some survey research data show that there is at least some resistance to the value system that prizes the individual over the community and exalts duty to self over duty to society.

Values may be considered as beliefs or ideals to which an individual is devoted and which ultimately guide that individual's behavior. A closely held value system will be contin-

Table 11.2. Essential values and behaviors for professional pharmacists [a]

Essential Values	Attitudes	Professional Behavior
Altruism (concern for the welfare of others)	Commitment Compassion Generosity Perseverence	Gives full attention to patient Assists other health personnel Sensitive to social issues
Equality (having the same rights, privileges, or status)	Fairness Self-esteem Tolerance	Provides services based on needs Nondiscriminatory relations Provides leadership in improving access to health care
Esthetics (qualities of objects, events, and persons that provide satisfaction)	Appreciation Creativity Sensitivity	Creates salubrious patient care environments
Freedom (capacity to exercise choice)	Openness Self-direction Self-discipline	Respects each individual's autonomy
Human dignity (inherent worth and uniqueness of an individual)	Empathy Kindness Trust	Respects the right of privacy Maintains confidentiality
Justice (upholding moral and legal principles)	Integrity Morality	Acts as a health care advocate Allocates resources fairly Reports incompetent, unethical, and illegal practice
Truth (faithfulness to fact or reality)	Accountability Honesty Rationality	Documents actions accurately Protects the public from misinformation about pharmacy

[a]Adapted from Essentials of College and University Education for Professional Nursing: Final Report. Washington DC: American Association of Colleges of Nursing, 1986, pp 6–7.

ually reflected through an individual's attitudes, personal qualities, and a consistent pattern of behavior. Unfortunately, value identification and acceptance are not included to any great extent in our schools and colleges of pharmacy or in the programs of its professional pharmaceutical associations (13). Periodic attempts to recharge the professional psyche of American pharmacists have usually been self-congratulatory and self-serving and thus limited in consequence.

Table 11.2 depicts a set of essential values that might be acceptable to professional pharmacists. The table was adapted from a set of values and behaviors that were intended to guide educational programs for professional nursing. It is clear that the same set of values prevails for all of the health professions, although some professions may need to stress some areas in different ways.

In practice, professional pharmacists assign priorities to these values as they encounter their patients or when they engage in specific decision-making situations. The individual pharmacist, relying on and guided by these values, will demonstrate a behavior that is consistent with the strength of conviction that he or she holds for these values. It is often during these "testing" periods that the individual novice pharmacist will grope for a suitable, satisfying response. Experience may provide some guidance, yet many pharmacists who are unfamiliar with either ethical concepts or are unable to act based upon a consistent, internalized value system, will attempt to deal with each problem in an ad hoc manner and may not approach similar problems in a consistent manner. For this reason, professional pharmacists need to both identify the basic values that impinge upon their professional practice as well as utilize a process of values clarification to guide them to make rational and consistent professional judgments when faced with ethical dilemmas.

REFERENCES

1. Elliott EC. The general report of the pharmaceutical survey, 1946–49. Washington DC: American Council on Education, 1950, p 4.
2. Thorner I. Pharmacy: the functional significance of an institutional pattern. Am J Pharm Educ 1942;6:3:305–319, and the response by Urdang G, 319–329.
3. Millis JS. Pharmacists for the future: the report of the study commission on pharmacy. Ann Arbor, MI: Health Administration Press, 1975, p 2.
4. Sonnedecker G. Kremers and Urdang's history of pharmacy. 4th ed. Philadelphia: JB Lippincott Company, 1976, p 190.
5. A code of ethics adopted by the Philadelphia College of Pharmacy. Am J Pharm 1848;20:2:148.
5a. LaWall CH. Pharmaceutical ethics: a historical view of the subject with examples of codes adopted or suggested at different periods, together with a suggested code for adoption by present-day associations. J Am Pharm Assoc 1921;10:11:900.
6. Griffenhagen GB. Our code of ethics. J Am Pharm Assoc 1963;NS3:2:65.
7. Resolutions—1966. J Am Pharm Assoc 1966;NS6:6:294.
8. Brushwood DB. Grounds for revocation or suspension of a pharmacist's license. Am Pharm 1982;NS22:11:574–576.
9. Veatch RM. Ethical principles in pharmacy practice. In Buerki RA, ed. The challenge of ethics in pharmacy practice. No. 8, new series. Madison, WI: American Institute of the History of Pharmacy, 1985, pp 18–19.
10. Veatch RM. Ethical principles in pharmacy practice. In Buerki RA, ed. The challenge of ethics in pharmacy practice. No. 8, new series. Madison, WI: American Institute of the History of Pharmacy, 1985, p 16.
11. Veatch RM. Ethical principles in pharmacy practice. In Buerki RA, ed. The challenge of ethics in pharmacy practice. No. 8, new series. Madison, WI: American Institute of the History of Pharmacy, 1985, pp 18–19.
12. Callihan D. Ethics and health care: the next twenty years. In Bezold C, Halperin J, Binkley HL,

Ashbaugh RA, eds. Pharmacy in the 21st Century: Planning for an Uncertain Future. Bethesda, MD: Institute for Alternative Futures and Project HOPE, 1985, pp 82-83.
13.   Smith MC, Smith MD. Instruction in ethics in schools of pharmacy. Am J Pharm Educ 1981;45:1:14-17.

SUGGESTED READINGS

1.   Abram MB. The private ethic—the public ethic: the role of the law. Proc Fourth Ann Arnold Schwartz Memorial Program 1983, pp 8-18.
2.   Arras J, Hunt R. Ethical theory in the medical context. In Arras J, ed. Ethical Issues in Modern Medicine. 2nd ed. Palo Alto, CA: Mayfield Publishing Company, 1983, pp 1-31.
3.   Banner S, Levine C. Medicaid boycotts: economics and ethics in conflict. US Pharm 1979;4:3:71-72.
4.   Brushwood DB. The pharmacist and execution by lethal injection. US Pharm 1984;9:9:25-28.
5.   Brushwood DB. Is there a pharmacist-patient privilege? Law, Med Health Care 1984;12:2:63-67.
6.   Callahan D. Ethics and health care: the next twenty years. In Bezold C, Halperin JA, Binkley HL, Ashbaugh RR, eds. Pharmacy in the 21st Century. Bethesda, MD: Institute for Alternative Futures and Project HOPE, 1985, pp 79-86.
7.   Dasco CC, Rodning CB. A physician/medical industrial ethos. Am J Med 1985;79:6:675.
8.   Fedo DA, Richardson JD. Applying ethics to community pharmacy practice. Apothecary 1979;91:6:18-30.
9.   Fink JL, III. Applied ethics in pharmacy ethics. In Buerki RA, ed. The challenge of ethics in pharmacy practice. Madison WI: American Institute of the History of Pharmacy, 1985, pp 23-30.
10.   Grapes ZT, Smith MC, Sharpe TR. Mississippi pharmacists and tobacco: why they might stop selling cigarettes. Miss Pharm 1985;11:6:8-9.
11.   Knapp DA. Ethical pharmacy practice: prospects for the future. In Buerki RA, ed. The challenge of ethics in pharmacy practice. Madison WI: American Institute of the History of Pharmacy, 1985, pp 33-38.
12.   Myers MJ, Grieshaber LD. Ethics. In Gennaro AR, ed. Remington's pharmaceutical sciences. 17th ed. Easton, PA: Mack Publishing Company, 1985, pp 19-28.
13.   Pellegrino ED. Moral choice and the good of the patient: the relationship of duties, rights and virtues. Proc Fourth Annual Arnold Schwartz Memorial Program. 1983, pp 44-68.
14.   Perchak GJ. Capital punishment and the responsible pharmacist. Am Pharm 1985;NS25:7:406-407.
15.   Shuler J. Indirect Rx advertising to consumers. Pharm Exec 1984;4:11:10.
16.   Smith MC, Knapp DA. Control of the practice of pharmacy. Pharmacy, drugs and medical care. 4th ed. Baltimore: Williams & Wilkins, 1987, pp 209-235.
17.   Smith WE. Ethical, economic and professional issues in home health care. Am J Hosp Pharm 1986;43:3:695-698.
18.   Sonnedecker G. Kremers and Urdang's history of pharmacy. 4th ed. Philadelphia: JB Lippincott Company, 1976, pp 200-202.
19.   Szasz TS. The moral physician. Center Mag 1975;8:2:2-9.
20.   Vaught DV, Cardoni AA. Should pharmacists take part in executions: Drug Topics 1985;129:12:12-13.
21.   Veatch RM. A draft medical ethical covenant. A Theory of Medical Ethics. New York: Basic Books Inc, 1981, pp 324-330.
22.   Veatch RM. Ethical principles in pharmacy practice. In Buerki RA, ed. The challenge of ethics in pharmacy practice. Madison WI: American Institute of the History of Pharmacy, 1985, pp 8-20.
23.   Veatch RM. The ethics of generic drug use. US Pharm 1982;7:3:62-64.
24.   Veatch RM. Informed consent: the emerging principles. US Pharm 1981;6:3:78-80.
25.   Veatch RM. Placing a $ on human life. US Pharm 1984;9:7:53-55.
26.   Zellmer WA. Ethics and integrity of the drug supply. Am J Hosp Pharm 1985;42:8:1715.

SELECTED READINGS

INFORMED CONSENT: THE EMERGING PRINCIPLES [b]

Robert M. Veatch

THE PURPOSE OF INFORMED CONSENT

There is real confusion about why health professionals are expected to obtain consent from their patients. Traditionally, health professionals have been committed to the principle that their moral obligation was to do what they thought would benefit their patient, according to their ability and judgment. This is the core of the Hippocratic Oath and is reflected in the codes of the pharmacist and other health professionals. Some have, therefore, assumed that the real purpose of obtaining consent was that it would benefit the patient. It cannot be denied that if patients know about the actions and side effects of the drugs they are taking, they are likely to be better off. For example, in the now famous aspirin study, a patient with an ulcer and another with eczema, both of which are contraindications for aspirin, were able to refuse to participate in the projected study.

It is often the case that a patient may know of some peculiar medical problem that is a contraindication of a drug being prescribed. For example, a neurologist prescribed amitriptyline for a patient with trigeminal neuralgia. Unknown to the neurologist, the patient also suffered from carcinoma of the prostate. The patient was not told of the drug's side effect of urinary retention. When this effect appeared, urinary catheterization was required in order to rule out the possibility of a recurrence of a tumor. Had the patient been informed of this side effect, and the peculiar problems it would create for patients with prostate problems, perhaps the neurologist would have been able to choose a different drug. At least the patient would have been relieved of the fears generated by the occurrence of this particularly threatening side effect.

Although informed consent will often be beneficial for patients, many have concluded that this is not the primary justification for informing them. If patient benefit were the basis, then information could justifiably be waived whenever a physician or pharmacist believed that information on balance might be harmful.

Occasionally, informed consent is justified on the basis of total benefits, including those to the broader society as well as to the patient. For example, in a research project where hospital researchers wanted to obtain human placentas from the delivery room, a requirement to get consent of the women giving birth in that delivery room was defended, in part, on the grounds that if word gets out into the general community that some research is being done in the hospital without getting consent, there might be a general hostility and suspicion against the hospital, thus doing more harm in the long run.

If the ethical foundation for getting consent is rooted in this general notion of social consequences, however, consent would not realistically be often required. In fact, research on therapy without consent would be justified whenever the greater good were served. This would justify potentially serious violations of individual rights and interests.

---

[b] Edited and reprinted with permission from Veatch RM. Informed consent: the emerging principles. US Pharmacist 1981;5(3):78–80.

A third and more forceful reason for getting informed consent is rooted in the principle of autonomy. According to this theory, a patient has a right to the information necessary to make choices about his or her own behavior. The women in the delivery room have a right to know that their placentas may be used for research simply because that is their right. In 1914, Justice Cardozo articulated forcefully the patient's right to self-determination when he said, "Every human being of adult years and sound mind has a right to determine what shall be done with his own body."

IMPLICATIONS FOR PHARMACISTS

The implications are enormous. It means that, in principle, no professional can determine what to disclose to a patient by introspecting and asking himself or herself what he or she would want to know in that circumstance. It means, further, that the question cannot be answered by turning to one's colleagues or examining what is normally disclosed in similar circumstances. If the principle of self-determination is the foundation of the informed consent doctrine, then the patients will have to be told whatever they would reasonably want to know, even if it is not normal practice for any particular health professional group to disclose that information.

It is unclear the extent to which the pharmacist bears responsibility for obtaining informed consent and assuring that the patient has adequate knowledge of the medications being taken. It is also unclear whether the right to consent implies a right of access to written documents such as the PDR or patient package inserts prepared for the physician and pharmacist. It is clear, however, that we are entering into a new era of informed consent, and the traditional answers will no longer apply. Some pharmacists are beginning to take greater responsibility for assuring that the patient has adequate information and education about medications being taken.

The principle of informed consent is built on the notion that the relationship between the health professional and the patient is a fiduciary one, that is, one of trust and confidence, rather than a mere business transaction conducted under the attitude of "let the buyer beware." If the pharmacist is to be a health professional in the full sense of the word, it may be that he or she will bear some of the responsibility for educating the patient and assuring that the patient's consent for the use of medication is adequately informed. It seems unreasonable, however, to assume that any pharmacist, no matter how competent, can have mastered the full range of content of a volume such as the PDR or any other standard reference. Even if asked about the side effects of a drug, it seems unreasonable to expect the pharmacist to pick out those effects that might be of peculiar significance to the patient, such as the urinary retention, that would be more significant for patients with particular problems. If the foundation of the consent doctrine is the principle of autonomy and the notion that patients are to be treated as respected collaborators in the health care enterprise, then the right of patients to the actual documents may, in certain cases, be essential. Many jurisdictions have now recognized the right of patient access to their medical records (12, 13), in part based on the same reasoning.

It would appear that the physician and the pharmacist together have to take the responsibility for assuring that patients are adequately informed, that is, that they are given information they would want to know in order to decide to participate in the treatment regimen. In some cases, especially those where the physician has not fulfilled the responsibility and the pharmacist perceives that the patients is not adequately informed, it may be at least the ethical responsibility, if not the legal responsibility, of the pharmacist to take a more active role in informing the patient.

A DRAFT MEDICAL ETHICAL COVENANT [c]

Robert M. Veatch

While the drawing up of a covenant between the profession and the rest of society, one containing these principles and rules, necessarily requires full participation by all who can approximate the role of reasonable people capable of taking the moral point of view, it might be fun to close this volume with one person's initial effort to set out what such a covenant might look like. It differs in content, in spirit, and especially in procedure from the traditional codes of professional physician ethics—those from Hippocrates to the AMA's 1980 "Principles." In that spirit then, I present a draft of the covenant I would bring to the bargaining table, if I were part of the group of citizens of the moral community trying to articulate a medical ethical covenant.

A DRAFT MEDICAL ETHICAL COVENANT

We lay people and health professionals realizing the importance of health as an important part of human welfare articulate and affirm the following basic understanding of our mutual responsibility one to another.

The common starting point of our medical ethical commitment is our recognition that we are members of a common moral community of responsible people endowed with reason, dignity, and equality of moral worth. Thus together we recognize the fundamental ethical principles.

- We acknowledge the moral necessity of keeping promises and commitments to one another, including the commitment of this covenant.
- We acknowledge the moral necessity of treating one another as autonomous members of the moral community free to make choices that do not violate other basic ethical requirements.
- We acknowledge the moral necessity of dealing honestly with one another.
- We acknowledge the moral necessity of avoiding actively and knowingly the taking of morally protected life.
- We acknowledge the moral necessity of striving for equality in individual welfare and equality in the right of access to health care necessary to produce an opportunity for health equal insofar as possible to the health of others.
- We acknowledge the moral importance of producing good for one another and treating one another with respect, dignity, and compassion insofar as this is compatible with the other basic principles to which we are bound.

Within this basic moral commitment we grant to certain members of our community the privilege of certification by the society and its agents as health professionals who in turn

---

[c] Reprinted with permission from Veatch RM. A Theory of Medical Ethics. New York: Basic Books, Inc, 1981, pp 327–330.

acknowledge certain responsibilities different from normal moral requirements of the community and certain exemptions from those normal moral requirements. In exchange, the rest of our community acknowledges certain responsibilities for our own health and for responsible treatment of those so certified.

It is our understanding that many important choices to be made by lay people about their own health care and by professionals setting limits on the nature of their practice will be left unspecified by this covenant and that those choices should be spelled out by lay people and professionals in covenants establishing and maintaining individual lay-professional relationships.

The starting point of such relationships shall be a promise made by lay persons and professionals, as members of the moral community, to fulfill the responsibilities of the relationship including those spelled out in this covenant and any other not incompatible with this covenant agreed to by individuals. The professional member of that relationship agrees to maintain competence in his or her certified area of professional service and to serve the health of the patient insofar as that is agreed to by the patient and insofar as that is compatible with the other rights and responsibilities promised in this covenant. The lay person agrees to fulfill his or her responsibilities in the relationship as spelled out in this covenant and in individual mutual understanding with the professional.

Acknowledging the principle of promise keeping, professionals promise to keep in confidence all confided to them by lay people unless breaking that confidence is required by law or becomes necessary to protect another individual from serious, immediate threat to life or grave bodily harm.

Acknowledging the principle of promise keeping, lay people promise to keep in confidence information they should learn about other patients or about the nonprofessional lives of health care providers except when disclosures are necessary to protect another individual from serious, immediate threat to life or grave bodily harm.

Lay people and professionals promise to keep appointment times, monetary arrangements, and other normal commitments of the lay-professional relationship unless emergencies require reformulating these commitments, in which case the other party will be informed expeditiously and compassionately.

Acknowledging the principle of autonomy, the professional will seek the full, active participation of the lay person in his or her own health care and decisions made about that care including reasonably informed consent for all procedures, experimental or otherwise. Unless the individual covenant between the lay person and the professional spells out any other mutually acceptable arrangement based on the fact that the lay person wants more or less information, the lay person will be told what the reasonable lay person would want to know before deciding to participate in a procedure. This consent shall not be excluded because a procedure is routine or because the information may be disturbing, but only on the grounds that reasonable people would not want information before deciding to participate in the procedure. Likewise, the professional shall consent to any special, unusual agendas and goals of the lay person in the relationship, and the lay person shall inform the professional of such agendas or goals. Both lay person and professional may exercise their autonomy at any time to terminate the relationship unless suitable help would not be available for the lay person if the relationship were terminated.

Unless the individual covenant specifies otherwise, the lay person shall have a right of access to his or her medical records as a way of maintaining openness and trust in the lay-professional relationship and autonomy for the lay person in medical decision making.

Lay persons acknowledge that the free pursuit of knowledge is of unique importance to professionals and that they shall be free in such pursuit unless it conflicts with other basic ethical requirements.

Among the things lay people have a right to know are: reasonably complete current information concerning diagnosis, treatment, and prognosis including reasonable alternatives available; the financial, educational, and other ties of his or her providers and their institutions; the identity of the spokesperson for the professionals involved in the relationship; the role various professionals and students will play in the relationship (especially in surgery and other cases where the lay person may not be in a position to observe the relationship directly); the procedures, if any, that are considered experimental.

Subject to the moral requirements of this covenant, lay people shall be free to choose the professionals participating in their medical care from among those professionals willing to enter into such a covenantal relation. Subject to the moral requirements of this covenant, professionals shall be free to choose to enter lay-professional relationships with lay people willing to enter such a covenantal relation.

Both lay people and professionals shall be free to communicate information about medical services in media and other channels of communication, including types of services offered, fees, and the ethical and other values underlying the services. Any such advertising or other communication should be accurate, without any attempt to mislead, and in keeping with the dignity and significance of the lay-professional relationship.

Acknowledging the principle of honesty, both lay person and professional pledge to deal honestly with one another, the professional informing the lay person of all he or she would reasonably want to know and the lay person informing the professional of all he or she would reasonably want to know unless specific understandings are reached to the contrary.

Acknowledging the principles of avoiding killing, professionals pledge to be especially diligent in avoiding the active, knowing taking of morally protected life even for reasons of mercy. They are to be exempt from participation in executions. Lay people pledge to refrain from asking for any such participation.

Acknowledging the principle of justice, lay people and professionals as groups pledge to arrange the health care system so that all have access to the health care necessary to have health equal insofar as possible to the health of others. Professionals, as members of the moral community, accept the moral limit on their compensation in the name of justice. They accept the necessity, in emergencies, for relocating those with needed skills in order to serve human need. They accept the necessity of using incentives in the structuring and financing of medical education to encourage a fair geographical, ethnic, racial, sexual, and disciplinary distribution within the profession. Lay people, in turn, recognize the importance of giving professionals the maximum freedom of choice compatible with the requirements of justice for them to select areas of subspecialization and geographical location as well as type of practice.

Individual practitioners shall be exempt from the general moral requirements of the principles of justice, including their impact on health care planning and cost containment, insofar as they are committed to patients in ongoing lay-professional relationships. However, the needs of one's own patients shall be taken into account in deciding how to allocate one's professional time among patients in need, and the extreme needs of nonpatients shall be taken into account in deciding whether to sacrifice temporarily the marginal welfare of one's patient in order to meet the desperate need of a nonpatient. In cases where this must happen, the professional should, if possible, obtain the permission of the patient before turning to the needs of another.

Lay people and professionals acknowledge the importance of this covenant and pledge to uphold it by exposing illegal or unethical conduct of those deficient in competence or acting in ways not in accord with this covenant.

In this spirit of mutual responsibility we pledge together to establish this covenant as the basis for our medical ethical responsibility.

MERCHANDISING CIGARETTES IN PHARMACIES
A San Francisco Story*

Steven A. Schroeder
Jonathan A. Showstack

There is little doubt that cigarette smoking is injurious to health. The relationship between inhaling cigarette smoke and development of respiratory airway cancers, especially carcinoma of the lung, arteriosclerotic and peripheral vascular disease, and chronic obstructive pulmonary disease has been well established (1-10). Yet, powerful merchandising incentives for the sale of cigarettes are created by the fact that over one-third of the adult population of the United States smokes cigarettes (11).

The problem of patient compliance with pharmaceutical regimens has become recognized as an important variable in determining the outcomes of health care (12). As one solution to this problem, it has been suggested that the role of the pharmacist as health educator be strengthened (13). For example, legislation was recently passed in California calling for mandatory inclusion of educational inserts into every dispensed prescription medication (14). However, the role of health educator can, at times, conflict with the pharmacist's role as merchant. A case in point is the sale of tobacco products in pharmacies. This study documents the prevalence of cigarette merchandising in pharmacies in one large metropolitan area to provide data on the extent of this role conflict.

METHODS

A random sample of 100 San Francisco pharmacies was chosen from the over 200 retail pharmacies listed in the yellow pages of the San Francisco telephone directory. Each of the 100 pharmacies was visited in September 1976, by one of the two authors. It was determined whether cigarettes were sold, where the cigarettes were displayed in relation to pharmaceutical dispensation, whether cigarettes were advertised or promoted on the premises, and the type of pharmacy (chain, independent, clinically affiliated). A "chain" pharmacy is one clearly identified with other stores or pharmacies of the same name, including stores owned outright by the parent company and those which are franchises. An "independent" pharmacy is one not identified with other pharmacies nor affiliated with a clinic. A "clinically affiliated" pharmacy is one located on the premises of a medical office building or clinic. These definitions are thus based on appearances and do not identify the legal ownership of the pharmacy, nor do they specify the relationship of the pharmacist to the ownership of the pharmacy; that is, whether the pharmacist is a paid employee or is an owner.

---

*Reprinted from *American Journal of Public Health*, 68:494-495 (May) 1978.

RESULTS

Table 1 shows the number of pharmacies selling and advertising or displaying cigarettes by type of pharmacy. Eighty-nine pharmacies sold cigarettes; of the 11 which did not, five were affiliated with clinical centers such as doctors' office buildings, while six were independent retail stores. However, only 15 of the pharmacies actually advertised cigarettes, ranging from nine of 24 chain stores to none of 12 clinically affiliated stores. In 52 of the 89 pharmacies which sold cigarettes, they were located at the pharmacist's counter, where prescribed medications were dispensed.

DISCUSSION

At its 1971 annual meeting, the American Pharmaceutical Association House of Delegates passed a set of recommendations regarding the hazards of cigarette smoking. The first recommendation was that tobacco products not be sold in pharmacies. The other three related to developing educational programs for pharmacists, young people, and the student American Pharmaceutical Association. In 1973 and again in 1977, the House of Delegates of the California Pharmaceutical Association adopted a recommendation that, "pharmacists, in the interest of raising the standards of public health and social welfare in the community, shall discourage the sale of tobacco products in the pharmacies in which they practice." In spite of these national and state professional postures, 89 per cent of pharmacies picked at random in San Francisco were selling cigarettes in 1976, a figure that is increased to 93 per cent if clinically affiliated pharmacies are omitted. Although data are not available to explain this conflict between professional recommendations and actual practice, at least two reasons were elicited in informal discussions with retail pharmacists and pharmacy educators. The first, and probably most compelling, is that pharmacists might face the loss of income in highly competitive locales such as San Francisco. Not only is profit derived from the sale of cigarettes, but cigarette products may induce customers into the store, who later purchase other items. Also, many pharmacists feel that a patient should have the ultimate decision as to the purchase of cigarettes, although the pharmacist has a professional responsibility to warn of the health hazards of cigarette smoking.

Even if the sale of cigarettes were banned from pharmacies, it is not clear that any impact on the consumption of cigarettes nationally, or of cigarette-related disease, would ensue. Nevertheless, there is an obvious conflict between the role of the pharmacist as a health professional and as a merchant of injurious substances. For this reason alone, we suggest that pharmacy associations consider the available range of strategies with which they might implement their own recommendation passed at the 1971 annual meeting.

Table 1. Sale and advertising of cigarettes in 100 pharmacies, San Francisco, California, 1976

Type of pharmacy	Cigarettes sold?		Cigarettes advertised?	
	Yes	No	Yes	No
Independent	58	6	6	58
Chain/franchise	24	0	9	15
Clinically affiliated	7	5	0	12
Total	89	11	15	85

REFERENCES

1. Ochsner A. Carcinoma of the lung. Archives of Surgery 42:209, February 1941.
2. Wynder EL, Graham EA. Tobacco smoking as a possible etiologic factor in bronchogenic carcinoma. JAMA 143:329–336, May 1950.
3. Hammond EC, Horn D. Smoking and death rates. JAMA 155:1316–1328, August 1954.
4. Hammond EC, Horn D. Smoking and death rates. JAMA 166:1159, 1294, March 1958.
5. Hammond EC. Smoking in relation to mortality and morbidity. Journal of the National Cancer Institute 32:1161–1187, May 1964.
6. Smoking and Health: Report of the Advisory Committee to the Surgeon General of the Public Health Service. U.S. Department of Health, Education and Welfare, PHS Publication No. 1103, 1964.
7. The Health Consequences of Smoking. A Public Health Service Review: 1967. U.S. Department of Health, Education, and Welfare, PHS Publication No. 1696, 1968.
8. Hammond EC, Garfinkel L. Coronary heart disease, stroke and aortic aneurysm: Factors in the etiology. Archives of Environmental Health 19:168–182, August 1969.
9. Diehl HS. Tobacco and Your Health. New York: McGraw Hill Book Company, 1969.
10. Smoking and Health Now—A New Report and Summary on Smoking and Its Effects on Health from the Royal College of Physicians of London. London: Pitman Medical and Scientific Publishing Co., Ltd., 1971.
11. Adult Use of Tobacco 1975. U.S. Department of Health, Education, and Welfare, Public Health Service, Center for Disease Control, Bureau of Health Education, Atlanta, Georgia, June 1976.
12. Komaroff AL. The practitioner and the compliant patient. Am J Public Health 1976;66:833–835.
13. Mattar ME, Markello J, Yaffe SJ. Pharmaceutic factors affecting pediatric compliance. Pediatrics 1975;55:101–108.
14. California State Assembly Bill No. 939, 1975.

ON BALANCE [d]

Mickey Smith

An April, 1985 issue of **Wall Street Journal** carried a report that should be interesting to all of us, but especially those in community (retail) practice. It's about smoking, and suing the tobacco companies when you suffer from it.

The article notes that cancerous and emphysemic smokers have been going to court for years trying to recover damages from the cigarette companies because they were harmed by smoking. Nobody yet, according to the article, has collected a cent. The reasons the suits have failed included:

- (In earlier cases) Failure to prove that smoking caused the problem.
- Failure to show that a particular brand caused the problem, especially where the plaintiff changed brands.
- (Of course) The fact that the plaintiff knew they were harmful. It says so right on the pack.

Lately, though not in any tobacco cases yet, the courts have begun to decide that if a product is dangerous the plaintiff might collect. Also, they have held that simply offering a product for sale constitutes an implied warranty of safety. Finally, even when the plaintiff was partly at fault, damages have been awarded—reduced, but still awarded.

---

[d] Reprinted with the permission from Smith M. On balance. Miss Pharm 1985;11(7):35.

Now Melvin Belli apparently believes the time is right to take on the giant, R.J. Reynolds. His case involves a deceased 68 year old who smoked three packs of Camels a day and eventually died of cancer and emphysema. This fellow even occasionally removed his oxygen mask to "sneak a smoke." Belli's charge will include that smoking is an addiction.

The tobacco firms, some lawyers say, will argue, both that:

1. You still can't prove that smoking is harmful.
2. We told you on the package it was harmful.

Interesting logic, but I suppose lawyers understand these things.

What's all this got to do with pharmacy? Well, let's just make a few observations:

-   Millions of dollars worth of cigarettes are sold annually in pharmacies.
-   Pharmacists are health professionals. Surely they wouldn't sell anything that would hurt anybody.
-   The most successful new prescription product launch of 1984 was Nicorette, a product to help the smoker break his/her nicotine addiction.

Are we getting any ideas from all this? Here's another little bit of information. According to a letter I received from Druggists Mutual, one of the two largest growing areas of pharmacy liability claims is from patients claiming addiction caused by failure of the pharmacists to provide adequate warnings.

Got any Camel smokers as long time customers?

ARE YOU GEARED TO KILL?[e]

Douglas J. Pisano
James D. Richardson

It's a terrible fall evening, about 8 p.m. The cold rain is coming down in sheets. Your front-store help are busily filling the shelves while you are buried under stacks of computer paper, trying to straighten out some third party billing.

A young man enters. He's wet and looks cold. You look up and flash your "welcome in out of the cold, friend" smile. Then it happens. From under his coat comes a wicked-looking sawed-off shotgun. He announces "this is a hold-up," and fires into the ceiling.

Your head is spinning, but your mind is clear. You are on auto-pilot. As if by radio control, you draw the licensed and registered snub-nosed revolver from its waist band holster under your smock. It seems like an eternity as you hold with both hands, lock your elbows, point with your body, line up your sights, stroke the trigger, and connect with center of mass.

The assailant stands looking at you in disbelief. This wasn't supposed to happen. He feels the burning in his chest where he was hit and thinks "no, no, not me!" He tries to level the shotgun and you react in the same way: "point, sight, stroke, fire."

He drops to one knee, curses, and makes one more futile attempt to punish you. You fire for the third time. He is now on the floor facing you. There is no expression on his face.

[e]Reprinted with the permission from Pisano DJ, Richardson JD. Are you geared to kill? Am Druggist 1987;196(5):58–62.

Denial sets in. Your rational mind takes over again. My God, you think, am I that cold blooded?

You then begin to notice things. Your front-store clerk is screaming and you've lost bladder control. You call the police and request an ambulance. You realize that what has just occurred in the past three to five seconds will have a profound effect on nearly every waking and many sleeping moments for the rest of your life.

Accounts of incidents like the fictitious one above may cause you to think about obtaining and using a firearm to protect yourself and the people in your pharmacy. For some, fantasies of becoming a hero riding off into the sunset may predominate. For others, the killing of another human being by a health care professional may provoke feelings of revulsion. In either case, the pharmacist may make a decision about whether or not to obtain a firearm largely on the basis of uninformed emotion.

What is needed is careful thought prior to making a decision—thought that includes an assessment of the ethical, legal, and personal issues involved with owning a firearm, using that firearm, and coping with the aftermath of its use. What we are trying to do in this article is provide some impetus for that thought by bringing out a number of the issues which need to be considered.

We will be drawing on an ethical theory which is based on the consequences of one's actions—that is, one which claims that the right action to perform in a particular situation is one which produces the greatest net balance of good over evil. In determining the consequences, one must look at the consequences for all affected parties (including the pharmacist in our scenario).

HARD FACTS

Obviously, in applying this theory to specific cases, a person needs factual knowledge—*e.g.*, what will, or is likely to, happen if I attempt to defend myself with lethal force? What alternative actions are open to me? Just as obviously, some sense of the good or evil produced with respect to each affected party is also necessary—*e.g.*, the psychological effects on the clerk in our scenario.

Prior to purchasing a firearm for self-defense, a pharmacist needs to consider a number of issues. How likely am I to be in a position to need it to defend myself or others against the threat of deadly force? Are there less radical ways which are practical in reducing that risk to an acceptable level? (See for example, the discussion of how the 7-11 convenience stores reduced armed robberies in Michael Castleman's *Crime Free,* Simon & Shuster, Inc., 1984.)

How likely am I to be in a situation in which there would be an ethically appropriate opportunity to use the firearm? Do I have the physical and psychological capabilities so that, *with appropriate training and practice,* I would have a reasonable chance of successfully using deadly force? Am I willing and able to devote the time and effort necessary to be trained adequately in the physical skills, decisionmaking and emotional self-control needed?

Firing a weapon in self-defense is not the same as target shooting. Besides the obvious differences in time and position constraints, one's catecholamine levels are likely to be sky-high, especially if one has not trained for this. Furthermore, one needs the ability to make near-instantaneous decisions about whether to attempt to use one's firearm, and if so, when and how. This is no trivial matter, because a poor decision may result in your death or that of an innocent third party. These decisions need to be made under conditions of extreme stress and often incomplete knowledge.

DEADLY FORCE

Since the pharmacist in our scenario was armed, there is still the question of whether he (or she) was ethically and legally justified in using deadly force. By definition, deadly force is "that degree of force that a reasonable person could assume capable of causing death or grave bodily harm." Why are we talking of deadly force? What about just showing the firearm, or firing a warning shot to repel the armed robber? The answer is simple. In the overwhelming majority of cases, such action would merely increase the risk to the pharmacist and innocent third parties. Hence, in the vast majority or cases, *if* the pharmacist employs a firearm ethically, that pharmacist will be using deadly force.

There is a real probability that the result will be the death of the assailant. Legally, the taking of a human life will be classified as a homicide. The key legal question is "What makes any homicide justifiable?" Generally, the law will deem a homicide justifiable (and hence not subject to criminal sanctions) when there is an immediate or otherwise unavoidable danger of death or grave bodily harm to an innocent party or parties.

The pharmacist must consider whether his use of lethal force will put innocent persons at significant risk of harm that they would not have incurred if he had not employed lethal force. This includes both the risk directly attributable to the actions of the pharmacist as well as the response of the assailant. In our scenario, of course, with the store essentially deserted, this was not a difficult decision.

If the responding police officers know you personally, you might be slightly better-off than if they do not. "Slightly better-off" means that when they got their radio call "Shooting at XYZ Pharmacy, man with a gun" the instant recognition of you by the officers can avoid some hairy moments of trying to identify yourself at gunpoint (or worse, if you are still holding the firearm and turn towards them.) Also, be prepared to be arrested. Remember, right or wrong, you have just taken a human life.

NEWS PROMINENCE

There are other consequences. The press and other news media may resort to front-page spreads and six o'clock news-spots. You are likely to suffer a significant short-term loss of privacy. As a result of the deed and its attendant publicity, total strangers will come to have strong evaluative judgments concerning you—some positive and some negative, but generally, with a totally inadequate data base.

Your patients, customers, and friends will almost certainly look at you (and behave towards you) in a different way. Even if their reactions are positive, you may ultimately find all the attention distressful.

There may also be other demons: nightmares, sleep disturbances, flashbacks, appetite disturbances and impotence. You may find yourself unable to stop thinking of the shooting, including seeing the face of the assailant in your mind. The life of the party you may no longer be; even the smallest social function may be an enormous undertaking. Your family will probably suffer also. They may have to bear the harrassment from the family, gang or friends of the deceased assailant, as well as the public at large. Your children may have to learn to deal with the cruel comments of the other children.

WHY ARM?

With all the time, expense, effort and risk associated with the use of deadly force in self-defense, why would any knowledgeable pharmacist even think of obtaining a firearm? For the answer, one must look at the potential negative factors involved in not doing so. Foremost of these is the risk of harm or death to you and others.

Not to be neglected here are other risk-reducing actions which one might take, short of using a firearm. Among these would probably include changing hours, creating an unobstructed view of the store from within or without, and installing a good alarm system.

To the extent that pharmacists are easy marks, their being armed discourages criminals from robbing pharmacies. On the other hand, once it becomes known in the criminal community that a pharmacist is armed, then although the incidence of robbery attempts may drop, the risk to the pharmacist *per robbery attempt* may increase substantially.

Although there is no guaranteed correct answer to each and every situation which might involve the use of lethal force, anyone who enters such a situation without proper training is asking for trouble.

Besides expertise in the various shooting techniques that have been proven under deadly pressure, training should cover decision-making and lethal stress management.

Does this sound as if we advocate proper training? You're right. We hope this article has demonstrated that importance. As in pharmacy, proper education is a basic building block. Keep in mind that even with good education and appropriate actions by the pharmacist there will be situations in which the pharmacist should *not* respond with deadly force to the threat of deadly force. Recognizing these situations is an important part of lethal stress education. On the other hand, there will be situations in which a properly trained and armed pharmacist who takes appropriate action can protect the life of an innocent person.

12
International Comparisons

ALBERT I. WERTHEIMER

INTRODUCTION

Too often, the pharmacy practitioner or pharmacy student assumes that pharmacy practice is at least similar and perhaps identical all around the world. Nothing could be further from the truth. Although the functions served by pharmacists are accomplished in virtually every country, in every society, in every region, and among all ethnic, religious, and other groups, it is not always a person known as the pharmacist who performs these roles. We see pharmacy practice all around us as being very similar to what we have learned and do. Therefore, we make the assumption that because pharmacy practice is virtually identical in neighboring states, other parts of the United States, and in neighboring countries such as Canada, it must be roughly similar everywhere. Also, many if not most individuals have an ethnocentric approach in which they believe that what they know and do is the best way of accomplishing things. It is often said that it is impossible to change another person's opinions or attitudes about politics and religion. Perhaps for the sake of controversy in this chapter we might want to add pharmacy education and practice.

In reality, there are very few similarities in the education and practice of pharmacy around the world. These are the very basic elements that students are taught in professional practice and dispensing courses including chemistry, and that a drug is physically handed to a patient. Beyond this, the similarities diminish rather rapidly. It is only reasonable to understand that most persons have not had a need to consider practice environments outside their own country and therefore, probably have had very little interest in learning more about foreign schemes. In addition, concise information is rather hard to find and where it is found, rarely is it of a comparative nature so that one can make general comparisons and contrasts. It is, therefore, the purpose of this chapter to present a view of the practice of pharmacy in other lands with some slight additional attention devoted to the education of the pharmacy practitioner.

Some assistance to the reader might be found in first being exposed to and considering how pharmacy practice came to be the way it is in the United States today. This did not happen by accident nor was it the plan of one individual or organization. Pharmacy developed around the world in very different formats long before the United States even existed as a nation. During this several thousand year development period, progress was made in the great civilizations of the Far East, the Middle East, and, in more recent times, Europe. Only more recently did pharmacy become established in North America. And this was due, in large part, to the cultural heritage and assets that accompanied the early settler groups to North America.

HISTORY OF PHARMACEUTICAL DEVELOPMENT

Although we know of recorded pharmacy materials dating back to nearly 2000 BC, the ancient development of pharmacy will not be the focus of this chapter. Nevertheless, we should understand some of the beginnings of what we have today. In crude and basic form, the Egyptians knew most of our modes of administration by 1500 BC. With the exception of parenteral drugs, they used gargles, snuffs, inhalations, suppositories, fumigations, enemas, poultices, decoctions, infusions, pills, troches, lotions, ointments, and plasters. In the Ebers Papyrus, various forms of more than 700 drugs have been mentioned amounting to more than 800 prescriptions (1). These drugs came from plant, animal, and mineral sources. But the botanical ones predominated for internal use. Examples were acacia, castor bean, wormwood, dates, fennel, figs, garlic, and poppy seeds to name a few. Mineral substances included alum, iron oxide, limestone, sodium carbonate, salt, and sulfur. The most popular vehicles were beer, milk, wine, and honey. In fact, honey and wax generally served as the binding agent for solid dosage forms.

By 1000 BC, in Egypt and in many other areas of the Middle East and Orient, prescription formulas were handed down from practitioner to practitioner oftentimes by scribes. Medicinal plants also were cultured by this time for therapeutic uses. The pharmacist of this time was considered to be an assistant or individual in the employment of a physician, who compounded medications under the supervision of the physician. The job included going into the fields to gather the appropriate plants, minerals, and other ingredients. Pharmacy in ancient Greece and Rome showed few differences because the Romans adopted most of their customs from the Greeks and especially their ideas regarding medication. The tradition of rational medicine may be traced back to the writings of Hippocrates, approximately 400 BC. It was believed that the four humors (blood, phlegm, yellow bile, and black bile) needed to exist in harmony, and disease was caused by problems with these humors. Drugs then were classified according to their qualities—actions on the humors. The accepted leader of pharmacy was Galen, who led his disciples to polypharmacy, using as many as 25 different ingredients in a prescription. His system of humoral pathology and the therapy based upon it dominated Western medicine for nearly 1500 years.

After the breakup of the Roman empire in the fourth and fifth centuries AD, the culture remained intact in the Byzantine Empire while Western Europe was filled with small kingdoms of barbarian tribes. Greek science and medicine, though, were assimilated by the Islamic civilization as it expanded under Mohammed and his successors in the conquest of lands near the Middle East during the seventh century. The works of the various Greek scientists were translated into Syrian and Persian and later into Arabic. The Arabs contributed enormously by bringing together the drug lore of Greece, Egypt, Mesopotamia, India, China, Persia, and other nearby areas. It was during this period and in the Islamic culture that pharmacy apparently first emerged as a separate profession. Evidence indicates that in the ninth century in Baghdad, pharmacy was an independent, well-defined profession (2).

The next major event comes from Paracelsus, born in Switzerland in 1493. He vigorously attacked the humoral system, arguing that qualities such as hot and cold were only effects of a disease rather than the cause. His own theory of disease stressed the localized nature of the disequilibrium of the body as a whole. He also emphasized that remedies were specific for given diseases. At the beginning of the 18th century, the philosophies of Para-

celsus were gaining but the humoral theories still had their followers. There were no dominant or agreed upon definitions in therapeutics. Most physicians were eclectic and empirical
in their approaches, drawing upon the remedies from the traditional galenicals, newer synthesized drugs, and others popular in various regions. During the period of the Enlightenment, some of the magical and medicaphysical remedies were discarded as well as were
ineffective empirical therapies. Modifications of the Arabic knowledge began emerging dif-
ferentially in the various European areas that were now becoming nations. These practices,
which accompanied the settlers to North America, are responsible for pharmacy practice in
the United States today.

Most of what was seen in the United States in the 19th century can be traced back to
two predominant imported forces: the practices of the German pharmacists and the practices of the English pharmacists.

The practice of pharmacy is different in most parts of the world. It would be difficult, if
not impossible, to indicate that any one system is superior over others, as in actual fact, the
practice characteristics in each nation have evolved as a response to the environments in that
nation. The practice of pharmacy is directed and guided by the political system, economic
system, geography, wealth, level of industrial development, religious and cultural traditions, and numerous other factors. The major similarities that do occur throughout the
world are remnants of colonial history. For example, many former British colonies have,
upon gaining independence, made only minor revisions and modifications to their previous
pharmacy statutes and practices rules. Therefore, there are some similarities among the
various commonwealth nations and past commonwealth nations. Many of these countries
accept the British Pharmacopoeia (BP) as their official compendia. Similarly, Francophone
nations, usually previous colonies of France, have continued the French traditions and patterns of practice. In fact, there are strong ties because the practitioners of many of these
nations continue to be educated in France, purchase French-labeled and -supplied reference works, equipment, and pharmaceuticals.

Before examining specific areas of the world or regions, it is necessary to discuss several
other matters. We can, as a means of better understanding international differences in
pharmacy, choose to look at the world along several parameters. If we look at the world
according to the level of industrial development (generally parallel to wealth), we would find
that pharmacy practices in most of Western Europe, Canada and the United States, Australia, New Zealand, and several other nations have certain major similarities and common
features. The other side of this spectrum would be that the nations having the lowest per
capita income and being the least developed, principally in Africa and several other areas of
the world as well, use a pharmacy system in which the public sector provides virtually all
health care through government-owned and -operated clinics.

One might also choose to look at the world along political lines. In this case, we would
find that in the capitalist societies and in most social democracies, we have two parallel,
interacting, and yet quite separate pharmacy delivery systems. One would find a govern-
ment- or state-operated system generally available to persons receiving low-income assistance, pensioners, the military, and veterans, among others, and a privately operated system in which patients are expected to pay for services themselves or receive assistance
through a private insurance scheme of some sort. In the socialist/communist nations, we
generally find the absence of the private sector pharmacy system. Taking its place is an
integrated state-operated system for the dispensing of drugs, usually in a coordinated and
regionalized system, whereby drugs and services are abundant in a wide variety of metropolitan or regional capital universities and teaching facilities and are found to increasingly

lesser degrees as one moves into remote agricultural villages and rural enclaves. We must, keep in mind, though, that pharmacy is only one component of the health care delivery system in which it operates. The proportion of resources spent on pharmaceutical services and drugs ranges from 5% in some of the most developed, western countries, to more than 50% of the total health budget in some third world countries. It would be difficult, there-fore, to consider pharmacy practice alone without having an understanding of the overall health care delivery system of which pharmacy is only one component. Although little is written about conformity with pharmaceutical laws and regulations, it is a reasonable rule of thumb, which is accepted in general terms by most individuals, that in the more industri-ally developed nations with a higher proportion of physicians and other well-trained health care providers, the pharmacist fulfills a role of dispenser of prescribed medications for the most part. On the other hand, in nations and areas where physician resources are scarce and perhaps unavailable, we find that the role of the pharmacist becomes one with greater em-phasis on advisor, diagnostician, and prescriber. Drugs that require a prescription by a duly licensed prescriber/physician in many of the western countries are routinely sold by the pharmacist after a brief conversation and the use of his/her expert opinion about the best course of therapy for a patient. This role is probably reluctantly assumed in many countries but is undertaken in an attempt to fill the enormous vacuum present where there are few alternatives other than the pharmacist.

Figures can be interpreted many ways but the information in Figure 12.1 indicates that the lesser quantity (and perhaps quality) of drugs used in the developing countries cost a greater share of the overall budgets of those nations. In other words, the respective products are basically more expensive or are more expensive in relation to other goods and services purchased.

The World Bank prepared an annual development report that lists health spending by central governments. A recent report of this information is depicted in Figure 12.2.

Although the data are somewhat dated, it is nevertheless interesting to examine the differences in expenditures on health in various, related countries. Let us look at some 1974 data showing health spending as a percentage of gross national product in 17 countries in Europe as seen in Figure 12.3. Differential statistics regarding life expectancy, infant mor-tality, and death rates associated with certain diseases can be seen to vary and be very much related to industrial development and national wealth. Much more in-depth information is available from the annual statistical reports of the World Health Organization (4).

Before looking at the individual regions and then the individual countries within each region, it is appropriate to examine some international comparisons regarding health man-power and health resources. From an examination of these data, it becomes easier for us to make projections, estimate needs and demands, and construct assumptions regarding

Region	%
World	0.73
Developed countries	0.74
Developing countries	0.70
Latin America	0.83
Africa	0.79
Asia	0.78

Figure 12.1. Drug consumption in the world economy: percentage of gross national product, 1979. Adapted from the Sixth Report on the World Health Situation, Part 1, Global Analysis, World Health Organization, Geneva, 1980 p 23.

GNP $ per Capita	%Government Spending on Health	Regions
Under $400	1–1.5	India, China, parts of Southeast Asia, most of Sub-Saharan Africa
$400–4000	1.5	Latin America, some of Africa and Asia
Over $4000	3.0	Western Europe, Japan, Australia, New Zealand, Canada, United States

Figure 12.2.   Health spending by central governments. Adapted from the World Bank Development Report, Statistical Yearbook, 1981, United Nations, New York, NY, 1983 p 314.

trends. The reader is cautioned also that reporting methods vary widely among different nations and that the numbers, although indicative, may not always be completely accurate. Sometimes this is because of insufficiencies or insensitivities in a national reporting system and it also can be the case that nations do not want to look bad to their neighbors and other nations and therefore submit numbers that are less than 100% accurate. Table 12.1 (5) presents a fascinating comparison of health manpower and resource ratios to a population reported to the World Health Organization. The numbers of health care practitioners per 100,000 population are so diverse between developed and developing countries that procedures and protocols obviously must differ in the developing countries if they are to provide care to the vast populations depending on them for service.

For more specific information regarding the actual resources and types of health care personnel and facilities available, see Table 12.2. It is evident that massive differences occur in the resources available in the various countries around the world. This situation remains even today, but the reasons for it have never been agreed upon. Although it is said that everything comes down to the ability to afford more resources, there are other factors at work such as competing traditional and local healing systems, national priorities with the state budgets, wars, and other intertribal and regional altercations that sap the resources of a nation.

Ranking by GNP per Capita	% GNP Spent on Health	% Private
1 Switzerland	5.0	30
2 Sweden	7.3	8
3 Denmark	7.0	7
4 West Germany	6.7	22
5 Norway	5.6	5
6 Belgium	5.0	16
7 Netherlands	7.3	30
8 France	6.9	23
9 Austria	5.7	35
10 Finland	5.8	5
11 UK	5.2	11
12 Czechoslovakia	5.1	11
13 Italy	6.0	13
14 Poland	4.8	—
15 Spain	4.8	37
16 Ireland	6.2	13
17 Greece	3.5	34

Figure 12.3.   Percentage GNP spent on health. Adapted from Tucker D. The World Health Market. Bicester UK: Facts on File Publications, 1984, p 80.

Table 12.1 Health Manpower by Occupation and Rate per 100,000 Population around 1975, Availability of Date and Population Covered by the Data

Health occupation	World*					Developed countries					Developing countries				
	Number	Rate per 100 000 population	Availability of data			Number	Rate per 100 000 population	Availability of data			Number	Rate per 100 000 population	Availability of data		
			Number of countries or areas	Population covered (in thousands)	% of world population			Number of countries or areas	Population covered (in thousands)	% of world population			Number of countries or areas	Population covered (in thousands)	% of world population
Physicians	3 037 674	76.86	193	3 952 295	99	2 089 319	190.65	39	1 095 899	100	948 355	33.18	154	2 858 307	99
Medical assistant	676 016	82.00	56	824 436	21	624 609	168.96	8	369 687	34	51 407	11.31	48	454 699	16
Multipurpose health auxiliaries	1 820 134	160.24	20	1 135 911	29	—	—	—	—	—	1 820 134	160.24	20	1 135 911	40
Midwives and assistant midwives	790 145	29.31	161	2 695 448	68	484 579	59.87	33	809 400	74	305 566	16.87	128	1 811 667	63
Nurses and assistant nurses	6 904 613	174.75	193	3 951 132	99	5 035 582	459.52	39	1 095 841	100	1 869 031	65.46	154	2 855 291	99
Traditional medical practitioners	596 967	33.61	14	1 776 308	45	3 715	6.01	1	61 832	6	593 252	34.60	13	1 714 476	60
Dentists	551 211	18.64	188	2 957 702	75	437 372	42.09	38	1 039 153	95	113 839	5.93	150	1 918 349	67
Dental operating auxiliaries and dental hygienists	55 398	5.30	61	1 045 448	26	51 363	11.64	15	441 145	40	4 036	0.67	46	604 310	21
Dental laboratory technicians	95 886	9.04	79	1 060 908	27	91 553	13.92	16	657 838	60	3 284	0.81	63	403 070	14
Pharmacists	691 873	23.39	178	2 958 038	75	518 439	47.97	37	1 080 706	99	173 434	9.24	141	1 877 330	65
Pharmaceutical assistants	297 045	20.42	114	1 454 452	37	240 364	40.36	25	595 564	55	56 681	6.60	89	858 888	30
Laboratory technicians and assistant technicians	476 622	16.81	176	2 835 121	71	418 385	47.31	31	884 307	81	58 237	2.99	145	1 950 814	68
X-ray technicians and assistant technicians	211 226	7.95	162	2 658 210	67	174 968	19.88	28	879 902	81	36 258	2.04	134	1 778 308	62
Sanitarians and assistant sanitarians	153 527	6.80	156	2 256 924	57	73 474	12.41	25	591 906	54	80 053	4.81	131	1 665 018	58

Sources: WHO questionnaires; United Nations Demographic Yearbook

*Excluding Bhutan and Democratic People's Republic of Korea. Data for China were provided by the State Statistical Bureau and the Ministry of Public Health, Bejing, and relate to 1978.

Table 12.2   Hospital Establishments and Health Personnel: Latest Available Year

	Hospital establishments and beds Establissements hospitaliers et lits				Health personnel Personnel de sante						Midwifery personnel Sages—femmes et asso-milees
Country or area Pays ou zone	Year Annee	Establish-ments Establisse-ments	Beds Lits	Population per bed Population par lit	Year Annee	Physicians Medecins	Population per physician Population par medecin	Dentists Dentistes	Pharma-cists Pharma-ciens	Nursing personnel Personnel infirmier	
AFRICA—AFRIQUE											
Algeria—Algerie	1978	183	45168	389	1979	6881	2643	1483	1058	16927	2335
Angola—Angola	1972	347	18011	322	1973	383	15404	...	87	3115	284
Benin—Benin	1978	371	4968	680	1979	204	17009	13	55	1294	312
Botswana—Botswana	1976	21	2137	328	1975	72	8750	6	10	544	...
Burundi—Burundi	1975	...	4489	857	1974	81	45432	6	11	590	89
Cape Verde—Cape Vert	1978	23	575	539	1978	51	6078	2	6	123	223
Central African Republic— Republique centrafricaine	1978	63	3104	...	1979	84	26666	4	15	1113	315
Chad—Tchad	1978	...	3373	...	1978	90	...	4	9	933	96
Comoros—Comores	1978	6	698	...	1978	20	16500	1	2	124	35
Congo—Congo	1978	473	6876	212	1978	274	5328	2	28	1915	413
Djibouti—Djibouti	1977	11	1050	...	1977	64	...	4	5	256	17
Egypt—Egypte	1978	1473	81254	490	1980	43547	...	5764	14729	26162	21785
Equatorial Guinea— Guinee equatoriale	1977	65	3577	95	1975	5	62000	...	...	248	2
Ethiopia—Ethiopie	1978	83	9850	3016	1978	515	57689	15	101	1667	...
Gabon—Gabon	1975	41	4046	...	1977	207	2560	20	28	...	...
Gambia—Gambie	1978	16	699	815	1978	49	11632	6	2	179	91
Ghana—Ghana	1978	269	16533	662	1979	1482	...	80	579	13800	3026
Guinea—Guinee	1976	314	7650	...	1977	300	15467	...	150	2000	...
Guinea-Bissau— Guinee-Bissau	1978	10	910	...	1979	88	6363	6	1	474	59
Ivory Coast—Côte d'Ivore	1975	...	8346	589	1975	321	15234	21	45	2859	453
Kenya—Kenya	1978	...	24708	601	1978	1466	...	230	245	14296	...
Lesotho—Lesotho	1977	88	2564	488	1977	67	18657	3	4	...	...
Liberia—Liberia	1973	41	2527	652	1975	170	9235	19	25	542	488
Libyan Arab Jamahi-riya—Jamahiriya arabe libyenne	1979	64	13897	197	1980	4057	734	340	443	7419	1472
Madagascar— Madagascar	1978	749	16401	...	1978	811	10221	88	86	2309	1227
Malawi—Malawi	1978	294	9531	594	1977	116	...	15	6	1437	...
Mali—Mali	1977	192	3512	1743	1978	287	23135	14	24	2117	532
Mauritania— Mauritanie	1977	12	545	...	1976	76	...	4	5	560	20
AFRICA (cont.)— AFRIQUE (suite)											
Mauritius—Maurice	1979	34	3215	293	1978	433	2078	46	59	1443	424
Morocco—Moroc	1977	132	23669	771	1978	978	...	155	136	...	...
Mozambique— Mozambique	1980	321	13180	794	1980	323	32414	96	8	2156	457
Namibia—Namibie	1973	66	6905	97	...	...	...	...	...	...	...
Niger—Niger	1978	...	3165	1576	1978	134	37238	10	12	1080	2006
Nigeria—Nigeria	1979	9270	69750	1069	1979	6584	11330	269	2780	29515	25730
Réunion—Réunion	1977	11	2642	...	1977	367	1335	89	144	1721	78
Rwanda—Rwanda	1980	248	7889	640	1980	164	30792	1	10	525	464
St. Helena—Sainte-Hélène	1979	1	54	92	1979	3	1666	1	...	30	7
Sao Tome and Principe—Sao Tomé-et-Principe	1978	16	665	120	1978	43	1860	1	2	147	15
Senegal—Sénégal	1977	44	5827	...	1978	391	13759	50	116	3193	550

Table 12.2   Continued

Country or area Pays ou zone	Year Annee	Establish-ments Establisse-ments	Beds Lits	Population per bed Population par lit	Year Annee	Physicians Medecins	Population per physician Population par medecin	Dentists Dentistes	Pharma-cists Pharma-ciens	Nursing personnel Personnel infirmier	Midwifery personnel Sages—femmes et asso-milees
Seychelles—Seychelles	1975	7	300	. . .	1979	27	2222	4	3	191	131
Sierra Leone—Sierra Leone	1979	112	3939	858	1979	185	18270	14	7	1587	. . .
Somalia—Somalie	1972	. . .	5163	569	1980	279	16630	2	. . .	1834	556
South Africa—Afrique du Sud	1973	788	156245	152	1973	12060	2016	1767	4761	53835	28399
Sudan—Soudan	1978	154	17015	1020	1979	2165	8249	318	538	12762	7580
Swaziland—Swaziland	1976	33	1717	294	1978	75	7200	7	10	131	731
Togo—Togo	1979	. . .	3346	738	1979	139	17769	7	38	1763	586
Tunisia—Tunise	1978	. . .	13923	436	1980	1728	3686	329	794	7168	784
Uganda—Ouganda	1975	420	18156	636	1977	436	24700	38	14	2800	2379
United Republic of Cameroon—Republique-Unie du Cameraun	1977	1003	21271	372	1979	603	13681	75	107	4320	2266
United Republic of Tanzania—Republique-Unie de Tanzanie Tanganyika—Tanganyiko	1977	2407	33714	. . .	1977	960	. . .	45	25	5658	1400
Zanzibar—Zanzibar	1967	15	875	400	1967	43	8140	2	3	217	394
Upper Volta—Haute-Volta	1977	44	3627	1762	1980	127	54409	9	23	1245	222
Western Sahara—Sahara occidental	1972	5	262	344	1971	53	943	3	4	39	8
Zaire—Zaire	1979	942	79244	322	1979	1900	13452	58	414	14661	3043
Zambia—Zambie	1979	782	26599	212	1979	714	7913	17	47	3161	1545
Zimbabwe—Zimbabwe	1976	. . .	17393	374	1979	1016	. . .	143	332	6719	2150
NORTH AMERICA—AMERIQUE DU NORD											
Antigua and Barbuda—Antigua-et Barbuda	1978	6	617	113	1978	32	2187	4	17	62	163
Bahamas—Bahamas	1978	6	879	261	1980	197	1218	31	37	673	120
Barbados—Barbade	1978	13	2187	123	1979	201	1293	24	. . .	680	425
Belize—Belize	1977	. . .	665	226	1977	46	3261	6	1	211	115
Bermuda—Bermudes	1978	3	477	104	1978	58	. . .	24	2	. . .	. . .
British Virgin Islands—Iles Vierges britanniques	1978	1	34	382	1978	10	1300	2	2	42	1
Canada—Canada	1977	1371	207666	112	1979	43192	548	10000	16052	. . .	. . .
Cayman Islands—Iles Caimanes	1978	2	40	400	1979	16	1042	4	3	39	14
Costa Rica—Costa Rica	1979	40	7506	289	1979	1506	. . .	239	. . .	1192	. . .
Cuba—Cuba	1979	. . .	44004	222	1979	13531	722	2953	773	26457	. . .
Dominica—Dominique	1973	6	312	. . .	1978	10	8000	2	. . .	89	47
Dominican Repub-lic—Republique Dominicaine	1973	339	12618	351	1973	2374	1866	516	1065	3332	89
ElSalvador—ElSalvador	1978	67	7668	567	1980	1491	3179	560	. . .	. . .	. . .
Greenland—Groenland	1970	18	666	75	1980	57	877	25	. . .	463	. . .
Grenada—Grenade	1978	. . .	639	172	1978	25	4400	4	1	37	107
Guadaloupe—Guadeloupe	1978	10	2314	138	19078	313	1022	71	108	821	55

Table 12.2 Continued

Country or area Pays ou zone	Year Annee	Establishments Establisse-ments	Beds Lits	Population per bed Population par lit	Year Annee	Physicians Medecins	Population per physician Population par medecin	Dentists Dentistes	Pharma-cists Pharma-ciens	Nursing personnel Personnel infirmier	Midwifery personnel Sages—femmes et asso-milees
Guatemala—Guatemala	1973	159	12115	457	1979	819	...	...	...	4345	...
Haiti—Haiti	1978	57	3896	1239	1979	600	...	73	...	1486	2425
Honduras—Honduras	1978	43	4634	742	1979	1141	3120	183	392	5126	3791
Jamaica—Jamaque	1974	34	7780	...	1979	759	2845	87	151	3430	485
Martinique—Martinique	1977	13	3392	94	1979	364	879	101	138	876	102
Mexico—Mexique	1974	1575	67363	863	1974	31571	...	1879	112	40998	634
Montserrat—Montserrat	1970	2	86	116	1978	7	1428	1	2	65	32
Netherlands Antilles—Antilles neerlan-daises	1968	8	1969	109	1968	120	1783	29	18	...	28
Nicaragua—Nicaragua	1976	67	4697	474	1980	1212	...	190	...	4687	...
Panama—Panama	1978	67	6954	251	1978	1550	1129	250	157	1337	...
Former Canal Zone—Ancienne Zone du Canal	1975	...	...	...	1975	153	287	8	13	265	...
Puerto Rico—Porto Rico	1978	129	13172	252	1980	4057	907	741	1436	14392	199
St. Kitts-Nevis—Saint-Christophe-et-Niéves	1978	7	380	131	1980	16	...	5	1	227	123
NORTH AMERICA (cont.)—AMERIQUE DU NORD (suite)											
Saint Luca—Sante-Lucie	1975	7	545	202	1977	40	2750	5	21	160	66
St. Pierre and Miquelon—Saint-Piere-et-Miquelon	1977	2	82	...	1977	6	833	2	...	20	1
Saint Vinc. and the Gren.—Saint-Vinc.et-Gren	1972	...	529	170	1974	19	...	2	...	147	2
Trinidad and Tobago—Trinité-et-Tobago	1975	25	4815	224	1980	786	1488	69	...	2837	...
Turks and Baicos Islands—Iles Turques et Coques	1977	1	20	...	1979	3	2000	1	0	12	11
United States—Etatis-Unis	1978	7159	1350097	164	1978	424000	524	117000	136000	1514000	...
United States Virgin Islands—Iles Vierges américanes	1970	...	248	271	1974	96	...	...	...	352	...
SOUTH AMERICA—AMERIQUE DU SUD											
Argentina—Argentine	1971	2864	133847	176	1975	521	...	...	...	...	...
Bolivia—Bolivie	1975	345	10722	526	1974	2583	2117	1182	1902	1552	...
Brazil—Bréso;	1976	5426	445818	245	1974	62743	...	...	...	42985	...
Chile—Chili	1978	293	38622	277	1979	5671	...	1477	290	24066	1962
Colombia—Colombie	1978	809	43098	594	1977	12720	1969	4407	...	19971	...
Ecuador—Equateur	1973	221	13594	495	1977	4660	1622	1370	...	1225	...
Falkland Islands (Malvings)—Iles Falkland (Malvinas)	1977	1	27	66	1980	3	618	1	...	8	5

Table 12.2   Continued

Country or area / Pays ou zone	Hospital establishments and beds / Establissements hospitaliers et lits				Health personnel / Personnel de sante						
	Year / Annee	Establishments / Establissements	Beds / Lits	Population per bed / Population par lit	Year / Annee	Physicians / Medecins	Population per physician Population par medecin	Dentists / Dentistes	Pharmacists / Pharmaciens	Nursing personnel / Personnel infirmier	Midwifery personnel Sages—femmes et assomilees
French Guiana—Guyane française	1978	7	724	82	1979	59	1016	14	18	287	11
Guyana—Guyana	1978	55	3906	209	1979	85	...	12	32	881	546
Paraguay—Paraguay	1975	143	3816	694	1979	1700	1747	855	860	2636	783
Peru—Perou	1977	437	29934	547	1979	11682	1480	3477	3309	16696	2147
Suriname—Suriname	1978	17	2073	178	1978	214	1728	21	13	1035	88
Uruguay—Uruguay	1976	64	11946	...	1979	5400	533	2300	...	15200	1206
Venezuela—Venezuela	1978	444	41386	317	1978	14771	888	4342	3187	38061	...
ASIA—ASIE											
Afghanistan—Afghanistan	1977	58	3084	4020	1978	906	...	97	187	583	484
Bahrain—Bahrein	1978	10	1028	340	1980	363	991	26	48	1025	113
ASIA (cont.)—ASIE (suite)											
Bangladesh—Bangladesh	1978	519	19925	4248	1979	7909	10954	164	197	2461	1167
Brunei—Brunéi	1978	4	553	361	1980	84	2738	16	3	464	100
Burma—Birmanie	1977	488	28454	...	1979	6996	...	376	80	6272	14851
China—Chine	1979	65009	1932083	508	1980	447000	2225	...	25241	697532	70843
Cyprus—Chypre	1978	117	3198	193	1980	560	1125	182	264	1519	199
Dem Kampuchea—Kampuchea dem	1971	94	7500	893	1971	438	15297	71	79	3639	1426
Democratic Yemen—Yemen democratique	1978	45	2622	707	1980	258	7634	9	16	2250	329
East Timor—Timor oriental	1971	74	1590	373	1973	20	32000	...	2	23	2
Hong Kong—Hong Kong	1978	77	19624	234	1980	3836	...	763	335	390	6910
India—Inde	1978	...	508907	1254	1978	178000	3586	...	...	113455	57650
Indonesia—Indonesie	1979	998	83101	1751	1979	12400	11740	2500	1800	62200	76499
Iran—Iran	1976	...	55500	606	1979	16200	2282	2367	528	8364	638
Iraq—Iraq	1978	201	24717	498	1980	7323	1784	1293	2022	6121	2267
Israel—Israél	1978	84	20387	180	1979	10200	371	2600	2000	28400	...
Japan—Japan	1977	8470	1207003	94	1979	148580	779	49577	90480	475945	26267
Jordan—Jordanie	1978	31	2568	1172	1980	1715	1889	351	550	2477	207
Korea, Democratic People's Republic of / Rep. pop dem. de Corée	1979	...	210000	83	...	...	...	...	...	...	...
Korea, Republic of—Coree, Republique de	1978	...	58052	636	1980	22564	...	3620	24366	101445	4833
Kuwait—Koweit	1977	26	4401	257	1980	2335	784	214	486	7607	714
Lao People's Democratic Republic Republique democratique lao populaire lao	1975	38	3232	401	1976	156	21667	15	16	1028	352
Lebanon—Liban	1970	143	10727	260	1979	5030	260	730	1002	3681	614
Macau—Macap	1977	4	1708	158	1980	269	1078	62	...	749	1320
Malaysia—Malaisie Peninsular—Peninsulaire	1973	220	35150	273	1977	1438	...	350	81	9745	2746
Sabah—Sabah	1977	17	2589	...	1977	110	8435	15	16	1423	...
Sarawal—Sarawak	1978	...	2666	448	1979	154	...	122	...	959	1242
Maldives—Maldives	1977	1	40	3500	1977	9	15555	1	1	34	177

Table 12.2 Continued

Country or area Pays ou zone	Hospital establishments and beds Etablissements hospitaliers et lits				Health personnel Personnel de sante						
	Year Annee	Establish-ments Etablisse-ments	Beds Lits	Population per bed Population par lit	Year Annee	Physicians Medecins	Population per physician Population par medecin	Dentists Dentistes	Pharma-cists Pharma-ciens	Nursing personnel Personnel infirmier	Midwifery personnel Sages—femmes et asso-milees
Mongolia—Mongolie	1979	1607	17220	94	1980	3686	453	146	237	6836	909
Nepal—Nepal	1978	67	2427	5529	1980	487	28767	17	1	438	1443
Oman—Oman	1979	28	1428	...	1980	514	1731	23	47	1070	23
Pakistan—Pakistan	1979	...	50936	1567	1980	23594	...	1018	1673	9943	9932
Philippines—Philippines	1978	1168	76101	597	1980	6063	...	897	475	804	7495
Qatar—Qatar	1978	...	563	...	1978	186	1129	12	5	...	79
Saudi Arabia—Arabie saoudite	1978	92	12140	680	1978	5029	1642	262	229	7180	...
Singapore—Singapour	1978	20	9583	243	1980	2096	1140	485	368	7545	779
Sri Lanka—Sri Lanka	1978	469	41513	341	1980	2055	...	218	472	6481	3350
Syrian Arab Republic—Republique arabe synenne	1978	130	8732	953	1980	3880	2314	1344	1744	6250	1638
Thailand—Thailande	1976	349	52178	823	1979	6395	7215	1122	1266	16332	21567
Turkey—Turquie	1978	776	86526	498	1980	27241	1648	7077	12059	31883	16036
United Arab Emirates—Emirats arabes unis	1977	...	682	342	1980	1114	...	146	69	2293	...
Viet Nam—Viet Nam	1978	11015	192449	266	1980	12936	4154	770	10367	9363	14009
Yemen—Yemen	1978	23	2799	1993	1979	513	11091	22	72	1371	69
.EUROPE—EUROPE											
Albania—Albanie	1977	928	16313	156	1977	2641	966	637	532	6801	5098
Austria—Autriche	1979	...	85204	88	1980	18888	397	1145	3192	32165	1100
Belgium—Belgique	1978	502	90291	108	1980	24536	401	4353	9682	83833	4400
Bulgaria—Bulgarie	1978	...	95691	92	1980	21796	406	4839	3648	45449	7897
Channel Islands—Iles Anglo-Normandes	1978	12	1352	...	1980	188	691	59	38	1240	57
Czechoslovakia—Tchécoslovaquie	1977	557	184779	81	1980	42210	362	7746	6846	100947	6676
Denmark—Danemark	1978	132	42535	119	1978	10572	482	4664	1364	24023	694
Foeroe Islands—Iles Faroe	1975	3	296	135	1979	55	727	28	8	341	15
Finland—Finlande	1978	...	73700	64	1980	9016	...	3938	5033	48701	887
France—France	1977	3548	644118	82	1977	91442	580	27683	33510	341526	8899
German Dem. Rep.—Rep. dem. allemande	1978	...	177386	94	1978	32397	517	8864	3481	...	...
Germany, Fed. Rep. of—Allemagne, Rep. of	1978	3328	714879	85	1979	135711	452	32950	32368	260253	5493
Gibraltar—Gibraltar	1976	3	253	100	1977	21	1429	7	13	254	12
Greece—Grèce	1978	701	58994	158	1979	22337	423	7177	...	...	...
Hungary—Hongrie	1978	...	93942	113	1980	26768	...	3303	43281	63998	2601
EUROPE (cont.)—EUROPE (suite)											
Iceland—Islande	1978	45	3775	58	1977	424	518	155	134	1791	156
Ireland—Irlande	1978	219	34625	95	1979	4174	807	963	2017	23866	...
Isle of Man—Ile de Man	1977	2	619	97	1979	80	750	20	32	780	59
Italy—Italie	1977	1893	573923	98	1979	164555	345	...	43500	...	...
Luxembourg—Luxembourg	1979	...	4539	79	1979	505	712	117	202	...	89
Malta—Malte	1971	9	3431	96	1975	382	864	44	293	2178	95
Monaco—Monaco	1978	1	390	76	1979	59	508	30	52	386	6
Netherlands—Pays-Bas	1978	309	98933	...	1978	24878	560	5052	1382	53750	874
Norway—Norvège	1978	907	61006	66	1979	7813	520	4000	2404	47450	829

Table 12.2   Continued

Country or area / Pays ou zone	Year / Annee	Establishments / Establissements	Beds / Lits	Population per bed / Population par lit	Year / Annee	Physicians / Medecins	Population per physician / Population par medecin	Dentists / Dentistes	Pharmacists / Pharmaciens	Nursing personnel / Personnel infirmier	Midwifery personnel Sages—femmes et asso-milees
Poland—Pologne	1978	1103	265646	131	1979	61460	573	16527	15274	149415	15287
Portugal—Portugal	1978	502	52327	187	1979	18088	...	484	4327	...	...
Romania—Romanie	1978	...	195019	112	1979	31285	704	6790	6205	...	12269
Spain—Espagne	1976	1226	192864	186	1979	81658	...	3532	21986	...	4620
Sweden—Suéde	1977	701	122478	67	1978	16340	506	7810	3830	66880	3290
Switzerland—Suisse	1976	474	72438	87	1979	14843	428	3700	...	40000	1650
United Kingdom—Royaume—Uni											
England and Wales—Angleterre et Galles	1977	...	409796	119	1978	75000	654	...	13018	189063	21142
Northern Ireland—Irlande du Nord	1978	...	17315	88	1979	2410	641	503	1060	9837	1362
Scotland—Ecosse	1978	342	58674	88	1979	9353	...	1818	...	62443	3896
Yugoslavia—Yougoslavie	1977	...	129393	169	1978	29980	732	5964	5131	63243	6962
OCEANIA—OCEANIE											
American Samoa—Samoa américaines	1978	...	187	160	1979	26	1153	7	1	169	...
Australia—Australie	1977	2369	175017	80	1980	26140	559	6200	5400	119900	5930
Cook Islands—Iles Cook	1976	8	161	124	1979	22	909	8	2	60	6
Fiji—Fidji	1977	30	1573	381	1979	294	2108	47	57	1235	...
French Polynesia—Polynesia française	1978	30	890	157	1979	125	1120	46	19	408	15
Guam—Guam	1979	4	223	448	1978	70	...	29	29	333	...
Kirbati—Kirbati	1978	23	460	130	1979	19	...	2	2	98	142
Nauru—Nauru	1971	2	207	34	1971	10	700	2	1	61	...
New Caladonia—Nouvelle Caládonie	1978	34	1541	90	1979	164	853	41	39	408	16
New Zealand—Nouvelle Zelande	1977	333	31758	97	1980	4880	635	1145	2510	19200	...
OCEANIA (cont.)—OCEANIE (suite)											
Niue—Nioue	1977	1	42	...	1979	4	...	4	...	32	2
Pacific Islands (Trust Territory)—Isle du Pacifique (Territoire sous tutelle)	1978	7	462	281	1978	48	2708	22	1	345	24
Papua New Guinea—Papouasie—Nouv. Guin	1978	185	11316	264	1978	212	14103	35	16	1780	215
Samoa—Samoa	1978	16	674	222	1979	60	2500	12	6	139	48
Solomon Islands—Iles Salomon	1979	146	1446	152	1977	32	6666	3	2	248	...
Tokelau—Tokelaou	1978	3	39	...	1979	4	...	...	...	11	11
Tonga—Tonga	1978	8	300	300	1979	30	3333	10	3	197	25
Tuvolu—Tuvolu	1977	8	64	...	1977	3	...	1	1	19	...
Vanuatu—Vanuatu	1977	...	700	...	1977	28	3571	...	...	240	...
Wallis and Futuna Islands—Isles Wallis et Futuna	1972	5	108	...	1974	3	3333	...	...	16	10
USSR—URSS	1980	23100	3324000	80	1980	995600	...	...	239900	2790000	...
Ukrainian SSR—RSS d'Ukraine	1980	(3800)	(627100)	80	1980	(182500)	274	(...)	(...)	(511000)	(...)

PHARMACIST IN SELF-MEDICATION AND INFORMATION PROVISION

The pharmacist is in an unusual situation in the United States compared to most of the rest of the world with regard to self-medication and information provision. In nearly every country in the world, the sale of medicines is restricted to properly licensed pharmacies. Therefore, it is assumed that the general public has an impression that drugs are important, potentially toxic, and medically oriented. Contrast this with the availability of over-the-counter drugs in North America in grocery stores, supermarkets, vending machines, door-to-door sales, and general variety stores, gas stations, etc. It would not be surprising for the typical consumer to consider drugs to be innocuous substances of a general commodity nature because they are so freely available via self-service in the United States. This is not the case elsewhere where persons must make a conscious effort to visit a pharmacy and purchase an over-the-counter drug from an individual wearing a white jacket. Perhaps this relationship and setting enable the pharmacist to play a more central and important role in the provision of information and control of self-medication. This large difference between practice seen in the United States and elsewhere also relates to a common source of difficulty regarding clinical pharmacy and one of its principal components, the drug history/patient profile. American pharmacists are quick to criticize their foreign colleagues for the abrogation of this responsibility. Foreign pharmacists argue that this record kept in the pharmacy is superfluous and completely unnecessary, verging on wasteful. They argue that in most health care systems, a patient must enter the system through a gatekeeper who is the patient's assigned primary care physician. This individual would have a complete record of the medications as well as tests and other therapies at a single place. When a therapy has been prescribed by a referred consultant, the record goes back to the general practitioner so a complete record is always maintained. Many foreign pharmacy practitioners think that the activities of which American pharmacists are so proud are merely self-serving and of little or no consequence to the patient.

The role of information provider is enhanced in many countries because rigid legislation prevents the advertising of nearly all types of over-the-counter drugs. It is believed by health care professionals throughout much of the world that the advertising of drug products creates or expands demand, causing increased sales to persons who might not actually need a product but who are convinced of a perceived need due to advertising. As we know, there are few restrictions about truthful product claims for drugs in the United States. In fact, it is virtually impossible to watch a television news program or turn through the pages of a woman's magazine without finding over-the-counter drug advertisements. This fundamental difference in the role as information provider very much relates to the position held by the pharmacist in his/her respective societies.

Although a Gallup Poll found that the pharmacist is trusted near the top of a list of professions and occupations, numerous studies indicate that the pharmacist is not a first choice for therapeutic consultation or information when other providers such as physicians are accessible. This is not the case in Europe, Africa, and most of Asia where the pharmacist is more accessible and is consulted more freely and frequently than in North America.

It also should be pointed out that the converse of the regulations regarding limitation of medicine sales to pharmacy holds true in most countries. These same or related laws prohibit the sale of merchandise that is not therapeutically or medically appropriate in a licensed pharmacy. So, we see some very limited cosmetics, baby foods and supplies, and perhaps some limited other items for the sick room, but toys, furniture, garden supplies, magazines, etc. are not found in pharmacies, further contributing to the orientation of a professional source. Most of these rules are public information and have been reprinted at one time or another in the *International Digest of Health Legislation,* a quarterly publication from the World Health Organization in Geneva, Switzerland. This publication addressed topical matters as well as reporting major changes in legislation in all health-related areas in each issue.

REGULATIONS REGARDING PHARMACY PRACTICE

We will discuss individual regulations in a country-by-country review, but certain characteristics are found in common throughout many nations and the most important of these deserve comment at this point.

Location

The locations of pharmacies are regulated in many developed countries and to a lesser extent in developing countries with little or no regulation in the United Kingdom, the United States, Canada, and many of the more advanced English-speaking nations. Because the community pharmacy is considered to be a public health resource for the community, and because it is recognized as a scarce resource, legislation exists, principally in Western Europe where even though there may be private ownership of pharmacies, a potential owner must request permission to locate a pharmacy at a given venue. The pharmacy regulatory authorities evaluate the location and make a recommendation to the local health authorities or to the ministry of health, depending on how this is organized. The reason for these regulations is to prevent a misallocation of such resources. If pharmacies are too close together, the fixed costs of doing business will remain the same, but both pharmacies have the potential of losing money or having to increase their prices because of revenue difficulties. Therefore, if pharmacies are located far enough apart from one another, this provides a reasonable likelihood that a pharmacy will be economically viable to serve the individuals proximate to it with continuity. Such rules also ensure that persons in nearly all neighborhoods, regions, and areas will have some access to pharmacy services because they cannot all be located in the most heavily traveled street corners in the capitol city. The most common legislation requires that pharmacies be no closer than 500 meters in densely populated cities or that a pharmacy must be able to demonstrate that there are 5000 unserved persons in order to be granted an operating license. This would then ensure that pharmacies are constructed in newly developing suburban and rural areas as populations shift or as the number of persons in the older parts of cities increases. The rules for operation of pharmacies and licensure have recently been coordinated and codified within the European Economic Community (EEC) where policies are now consistent for 20 nations.

Drug Schedules

Again, the United States is probably in a minority situation. In this country, we have two major categories of drugs. These are those available without a prescription, called over-the-counter drugs, intended for unsupervised self-medication, and a second category referred to as prescription-legend drugs requiring a written or oral order from a medical care practitioner, usually a physician or dentist. Within the prescription-legend category, the United States complies with the 1971 International Convention on Narcotic Drugs and limits the production through quotas provided to manufacturers for these addictive substances as well as requires prescription status, etc. for these agents. But overall, there are still only two categories of drugs. This is not the case in much of the world where there are anywhere from three to nine different categories. It is typical to have a list of drugs that may be available in pharmacies for over-the-counter sale even on a self-service basis without the participation of a pharmacist. In many places, there is a second category in which the pharmacist may sell an over-the-counter drug personally after ascertaining that it is an appropriate drug and the patient knows how to use it properly. There are yet other categories for drugs with a high potential of toxicity, and such poisons must be sold over the counter by a pharmacist who records the purchaser's name and address. It is in cases such as this one that the pharmacist is obliged to make certain that the individual knows how to handle the product and the pharmacist should be convinced, using his/her best professional judgment, that the purchase is for legitimate intentions. There are additional schedules found in some countries where drugs may be dispensed with no refills permitted and additional schedules that require a written prescription with no possible refills. There are other categories in which the prescription may be refilled by the patient for a specified period of time. Other categories limit the site for the use of drugs. Certain programs permit some drugs to be used only in hospitals that have certain resuscitation or other apparatus needed in the event that an emergency reaction might occur. Some other drugs are available only to persons who are experienced in some medical specialty areas working in certain types of approved institutions, etc.

There is a movement in the United States that has been ongoing for close to 20 years to have a third category of drugs that could be sold only by the pharmacist. It would be comprised of some of the more problematic drugs presently available over the counter and some drugs that have been on the prescription-legend list and used safely for many, many years. This issue continues to be rejected by the Food and Drug Administration, which maintains that once labeling is prepared that enables one to use a drug under unsupervised conditions, there is no necessity for the pharmacist's involvement and therefore two categories of drugs are considered sufficient. The National Association of Retail Druggists proposed that there be four categories of drugs in the United States and as long as the Food and Drug Administration remains adamant, and as long as the major organizations in American pharmacy do not join behind a common banner, it is unlikely that this situation will change from the present one in the United States. There appears to be a high level of satisfaction with the numerous systems of drug schedules in other countries, so it would be difficult to say that there is any trend or motion in one specific direction. It appears that the numerous configurations of schedules will remain for the time being and probably for the intermediate future as well.

Merchandise Variety

This issue was briefly discussed earlier. The pharmacy laws in nearly every country are very specific about what can or cannot be sold in a pharmacy. Because a pharmacy is intended to be a place where drug services, pharmaceuticals, and information services are transferred, it would seem to be incompatible to have itmes of a less serious nature. This thinking has continued more than 150 years in some countries and appears to be a solid practice in virtually all of Europe and in selected portions of the world elsewhere. Just as precluding pharmacies from stocking and selling toys, food, and hardware items creates or enhances an image, so does the prohibition of the sale of drugs and drug-related products in general merchandise stores. This should convey a meaning or message to consumers that drugs, items that are purchased in a very specialized outlet, should be treated carefully and unlike most of the other products purchased by these individuals.

One other facet of this matter also merits inclusion in the treatment of this subject. Pharmaceutical societies in some countries form cooperative or jointly-owned ventures and prepare products that are sold and made available only in pharmacies. These products, such as soaps, skin cleansers, creams, and toothpastes, are promoted only through pharmacies and sold only through pharmacies. One could only assume that this endeavor is an attempt to create an image of certain products unavailable in ordinary health and beauty aids stores. Moreover, since the product is only available through registered pharmacies, one might infer that these products are of a higher standard and, perhaps, more potent.

Hours of Operation

The regulation of community pharmacies is generally more complete in Europe than in North America and much less so in Africa, the Middle East, and Asia. In Europe, the ministries of health at various times and due to varying reasons have delegated some of the responsibilities for oversight of pharmacies to the national pharmaceutical associations. Some of these responsibilities have been delegated to local governments as well and, in some cases, jointly administered. The hours of operation of pharmacies, although not strictly a component of the law, are standardized and agreed upon by local pharmaceutical authorities with the approval of local health authorities. In nearly all instances, the hours of pharmacies within countries, or at least within states or providences, are identical. Because the hours are somewhat abbreviated over what an American pharmacist or consumer is familiar with, a rotation system is generally in place. It is always interesting to see the reaction and expression of American pharmacists visiting pharmacies in France or elsewhere on the continent where a small sign in the window announces which pharmacy and its location will be opened late that evening or during the weekend. Yes, pharmacies cooperate in taking turns at covering patient needs during less than peak times.

The actual hours of operation are dictated in Scandinavia and especially so in Sweden where all of the community pharmacies are owned by a government-controlled organization. Another area in which wide variation exists is the requirement so familiar in the United States that a properly and currently registered pharmacist must be available and in the pharmacy during all of its time of operation. In many places, such as in Africa and the Far East, a pharmacist sells the use of his/her diploma to the use of a nonpharmacist shop owner and the pharmacist visits the store once a day, once weekly, or in some cases only when there is a problem. This is commonplace in many countries. The rules differ widely in this area with some requiring that the pharmacist be present a minimal number of hours per day, others specifying a minimal percentage of the number of hours open, and numerous configurations upon these general policies. It can be said, though, that most countries permit the pharmacy to operate without the physical presence of the pharmacist during all of its opening hours.

To introduce another concept, in nearly all countries it is a requirement that a community pharmacy be owned by an individual. This person becomes the responsible party for that pharmacy and, therefore, cannot own or be responsible for any other pharmacies. In effect, this eliminates the phenomenon we know in the United States as the chain pharmacy. In fact, the only places other than the United States where chains exist to any considerable degree are Canada and the United Kingdom and there, the Boots and Underwood chains are still minorities compared to the enormous number of independently owned chemists' shops. Typical hours of community pharmacies outside the United States are generally from 8:00 AM until 6:00 or 7:00 PM 4 days a week, with late hours until 8:00 or 9:00 PM 1 evening per week, with abbreviated hours on Saturday, perhaps until 2:00 PM, and no service on Sundays or holidays.

Laboratory and Other Services

As was pointed out in the beginning of the chapter, pharmacies developed in each country based upon individual traditions and historical events, thereby offering a differing range of services. Pharmacies in Eastern Europe and in some portions of Southern and Western Europe offer some clinical laboratory services. The most common of these is pregnancy testing. Although dying out as something from the past, pharmacies in England and some other portions of the continent also provided examinations and fittings for spectacles or prescription eye glasses. Some pharmacies such as those in Japan are responsible for regional or area hygiene. The pharmacist goes to schools, swimming pools, and other locations to perform air, water, or food purity or contamination tests. Extemporaneously made preparations are done perhaps 20% of the time in Eastern Europe, and perhaps 10% of prescriptions are categorized this way in West Africa. In the United States, the proportion of extemporaneously prepared or compounded prescriptions continues below 1% of all prescriptions dispensed as the industry has increased its share with prefabricated drug products. Pharmacies in Asia and in Northern Europe have intricate analytical laboratories on the premises where the purity of incoming raw materials and ingredients from manufacturers and wholesalers are tested for purity, strength of active ingredients, and contamination. In addition, because these pharmacies also produce a considerably greater proportion of products made at the pharmacy, such as their own tablets, solutions, and ointments, this same analytical laboratory serves as a quality control laboratory for testing and culturing their own products. Of course, such laboratories are not to be found in North America and herein lies a very basic difference in the orientation of pharmacy education in the two respective areas as well. It is unlikely that a pharmacist in North America would know very much about how to undertake such tests while conversely, his/her European colleague would have a much lesser educational background about pathophysiology and the biomedical side of practice.

PAYING FOR PHARMACY SERVICES

Developed Nations of the West

Most of the developed nations of the West have a two-tiered pharmacy system. There are private and public sectors that operate simultaneously and coexist peacefully. In this model, such as would be found in most of Africa and Central and South America, there would be a large proportion of the population that would be considered indigent or of the lower socioeconomic strata attending clinics or hospitals for their primary care. These clinics or hospitals are generally owned and operated by the state through either the national or regional government and provide health services at little or no cost. For those individuals who are able to pay for their care and choose to receive the care in less crowded conditions and perhaps with less time spent in the waiting room, there are privately operated pharmacies. The single major difference beyond the cosmetic ones lie in the range of pharmaceuticals carried. The private sector pharmacy would generally have in stock most of the common, modern, and new branded products from the large multinational pharmaceutical houses. The clinic or public sector pharmacy would tend to have a somewhat more limited formulary with an emphasis upon generic products available through bid procedures in the international marketplace. In the developing country, these small numbers of pharmacists who are in practice would be salaried by the health authorities and found at clinic pharmacies or pharmacies in hospitals or regional health centers. If privately owned pharmacies exist, they would be in small numbers in most cases and oftentimes owned by pharmacists in partnership with others who had the capital for such a venture. These private pharmacies are generally located in the larger cities where members of the middle or upper class might reside. The ownership is rewarded through profits and if there were employee pharmacists in a privately owned pharmacy, he/she would be paid an agreed-upon salary. In the developed nations in the West, pharmacists are paid an hourly salary or an agreed-upon weekly salary. When the owner also works at the pharmacy, he/she receives a salary but is also entitled to the after-tax profits, if any, at the end of the year.

Eastern Europe

In Eastern Europe, the state owns all of the health facilities and employs all health workers. In addition to pharmacists having employment in polyclinics, health centers, and hospitals, there are community pharmacies that are owned and operated by the state. In all of these situations, the pharmacist receives a salary that is generally the same for all workers with a similar number of tenure years within the organization. In the state-owned pharmacies, there is generally a fixed copayment for prescription drugs paid by most individuals. The exceptions are for elderly persons, some disabled veterans, and others who have certain pathologies for which a certain list of drugs would be provided without copayment to these individuals. It is the intention in such schemes that the drug is cheaper than having relapses or acute phases of a disease in which hospitalization, with its intendent expense—family separation—is required.

Other Schemes

Most nations pay for their pharmaceutical services as has already been mentioned. There are some unusual configurations of service and payment that are worthy of at least mention. The Dutch have a program in which citizens are assigned to a specific pharmacy. The pharmacy is then responsible for the care of these persons and is paid accordingly. Pharmacy services in Japan have always been an enigma since the end of World War II. Physicians receive very low fees for office visits but receive additional sums for each injection, diagnostic test, procedure, and sale of prescription drugs. Therefore, it has been estimated that only about 3% of all drugs are obtained through community pharmacies in Japan, because physicians bill the patients or the insurance companies for drugs in order to increase their incomes.

PHARMACY IN DEVELOPING COUNTRIES

Most developing countries continue with some modified and amended revisions of the drug regulations and pharmacy practice acts that were in place while colonial powers were present. The problems with pharmacy in developing countries could be the subject of an entire book. It is difficult for pharmacists to practice because transportation and communication systems as well as large parts of the infrastructure sometimes leave something to be desired. Oftentimes drugs arrive late or close to the expiration date of the item, journals and educational materials sometimes arrive very late or never at all, and some orders cannot be filled because there are limits to how much foreign exchange can be released or obtained through the central financial authorities to purchase imported drugs. In most countries in the developing world, foreign exchange is extremely scarce and can only be obtained from the sale and export of domestically made products or services. In addition, there are considerable pressures on the part of pharmacists who have to "make do" with shortages of drugs and complete outages of some products that could be the drug of choice for certain pathologies. Given the serious shortage of medical manpower, additional responsibilities sometimes are on the shoulders of the pharmacist who is asked to sell products that would otherwise require a prescription but, because there is no medical practitioner around, is indeed sold by the pharmacist.

Heat and humidity in some areas, especially the tropics, work against having an adequate and assured inventory. The drugs deteriorate rapidly in these circumstances. Besides the shortages of foreign exchange, delivery problems, and infrastructure limitations, the pharmacist practicing in developing countries sometimes faces rivalries with native healers or practitioners of some local healing system. If that were not enough, it is sometimes necessary to make payments to some officials for permits or to facilitate shipments, transportation needs, etc. Because the regulations about pharmaceutical products oftentimes are more rigorous on paper than is the actual regulatory environment, pharmacists practicing in some developing countries have an additional responsibility or burden in determining which products of local manufacture are efficacious and safe so that they may be recommended and sold.

WORLD HEALTH ORGANIZATION AND PHARMACY

There are several major initiatives supported by the World Health Organization that are of direct applicability to pharmacy practice. The first of these is the establishment and operation of the standard International Nomenclature system. The World Health Organization publishes a book, the *INN,* which assigns generic names to new, pharmacologically active compounds. It is only through such international standards that we are able to communicate with each other in the scientific literature and to have international commerce because penicillin G, for example, means the same thing to any health care practitioner, the pharmaceutical industry, governments, and insurance companies all around the world. In addition to this standardization of nomenclature, the World Health Organization (WHO) also publishes the *International Pharmacopeia.* This publication is different from other regional, national, or international pharmacopeias in that the tests for active ingredients and purity are designed to be conducted without the necessity of having sophisticated, expensive, and delicate high-tech apparatus. Most of the tests can be done with a few drops of commonly available and relatively inexpensive chemical reagents, and perhaps the most complex tests require thin-layer chromatography, a technique that is performed virtually anywhere. The *International Pharmacopeia,* therefore, enables importers all over the world, but especially in the least developed countries, to be able to test materials received by them. The other major initiative of the WHO are the sponsorship and facilitation of the Essential Drugs concept. This program encourages and assists nations in adopting the use of a list of approximately 250 products. These products are generally available through international tenders in generic form and are known to be safe and effective from many years of successful use. The Essential Drugs Program has as its goals the increase in the quality of therapeutics with a simultaneous objective of lowering the cost of pharmaceuticals for nations who can ill afford to pay for some of the fancier and newed branded products. There are numerous other programs that are directly or only tangentially related to pharmacy such as the International Convention on the Quality of Drugs in International Commerce, which requires laboratory assay certificates and certifications of meeting tests in the country of origin, the various narcotic conventions, and controlled substance agreements. WHO, in cooperation with a number of other United Nations agencies, fosters the transfer of technology and the support of industrialization such as with local production and repackaging of pharmaceuticals. There are also efforts underway to foster immunization activities and to assist in cleaning water and providing oral rehydration salts and training to communities, as well as massive efforts regarding family planning and research on tropical diseases.

SOME COMPARATIVE STATISTICS

It is interesting to look at some of the unique, individual features involved with the practice of pharmacy in different countries. Let us begin with Western Europe and look at a system in the **United Kingdom** where there is a national health insurance program supported by salary deductions from workers. More than 95% of health facilities are owned by the national government, and general practice physicians receive virtually all of their salaries from the national government as well. Patients sign up with a physician who is paid a fixed amount of money for each person on his/her panel, irrespective of their health status. Obviously, it would behoove the physician to try to keep people well so they do not bother him nights, weekends, and even during regular hours, but consult as infrequently as possible. In England the pharmacies are individually owned by pharmacy practitioners who receive about 95% of their revenues from the prescriptions that are filled on behalf of National Health Service (NHS) patients. All of the pharmacies have a representative negotiating committee that negotiates to establish prices with the Department of Health and Social Services (DHSS). The pharmacy shops complete an inventory survey in which they compute their cost of dispensing prescriptions and the inclusion of certain other services. From this, individualized dispensing fee for each pharmacy is computed. That fee is paid to that pharmacy for each prescription dispensed. At the end of the month, the pharmacy sends the filled written prescriptions to one of nearly two dozen pricing bureau offices that compute the cost of ingredients for the prescription and add the agreed-upon dispensing fee to each, thereafter mailing a check to the pharmacy. The pharmacist oftentimes keeps no record of these prescriptions once they are dispensed because refills are a rarity and also because a great deal of trust is evident. For example, if a shipment of prescriptions is lost, the pricing bureau would pay the pharmacy the expected amount given the monthly fees trends from the previous months. Patients covered by the national health insurance pay a small copayment that is modified periodically by the different parties in office and because of needs due to inflation, etc. Some persons exempted from the copayment are the extremely needy, mothers with children less than 1 year of age, persons with one of a specified list of chronic conditions, certain pensioners, and others.

There is a small but growing market in the private sector in England because private health insurance is a very much sought-after fringe benefit and at the moment is only accorded to higher level business executives and some wealthier professionals. The same physicians and pharmacies provide services through the private sector, for the most part, but having private insurance generally decreases the waiting time and permits people to be seen and treated more rapidly. Recently, in an effort to decrease costs, the DHSS established a list of generic drugs that would be paid for and thereby refused payment for the more expensive varieties of these products.

In **France,** as in most of the European community, graduation from an accredited college of pharmacy is the only necessity for licensure in addition to some possible internship. There is no board examination as we know it in the United States. France has its own pharmacopeia but now recognizes the European Pharmacopeia. As is the case in England, prices are fixed so that all pharmacies pay the same prices for drugs from their wholesalers, and they sell the products at fixed prices listed in a tariff book, again as in England. This negates the need for any comparative shopping as the prescription would cost the same amount in any pharmacy. France does limit the number of pharmacies by distance from each other as discussed in a previous section. Also, the variety of items that may be sold in a community pharmacy is limited to health-related products. Virtually all persons in France are eligible for the social security system benefits, and products are accredited after they are approved for marketing into one of several social security reimbursement schedules. The 70% reimbursement rate is the typical category requiring the patient to pay only 30% of the cost of the drug. The French government uses this category placement as a bargaining lever in order to help keep the cost of drugs down because the products are not approved for the social security list until the authorities agree on their official, standard prices.

Sweden has an unusual situation for Western Europe because in 1970, all of the nearly 700 pharmacies in the country were purchased by the government. The Swedish government established a quasigovernmental organization, Apoteksbolaget, which operates what might be called a government-owned pharmacy chain corporation. The stores have standardized services, product lines, prices, hours, etc. Some of the more interesting features regarding the Swedish pharmacy system include the three levels of employees: the fully qualified pharmacists, the prescriptionists with 2 years of college, and the pharmacy technicians who obtained their education in specialized secondary schools. Although the prescriptionist category is due to be phased out in the near future, these are the persons who operate the remote, rural pharmacies in many parts of the north. Sweden, as do nearly all of its neighbors, uses standard trade packages for dispensing. Although in the United States one would count out 37 tablets and place this amount of medicine in a bottle, in Scandinavia and in most of Europe, the preparations are packaged at the factories in quantities that are intended to cover one episode of care. For example, if an antibiotic is to be used 4 times a day for 5 days, it would come in packages of 20 already prepared from the manufacturer. Similarly, if a drug was to be used daily for 1 month, it would be in a package of 30 capsules or tablets. This is called unit of use packaging and is extremely common.

Prices are fixed in Sweden and the other interesting feature is the use of single line wholesalers. Wholesalers bid for the business of manufacturers and, therefore, one would order the products of one company or manufacturer from one wholesaler and the products of other companies from other wholesalers. In this way, it is necessary to have accounts with both of the major, national wholesaling corporations.

In **Norway,** pharmacy practice is slightly different again. The most interesting feature of Norwegian pharmacy lies in something called the "need clause." When a product is submitted to their food and drug administration, not only does the manufacturer have to show evidence of safety and efficacy and a proposed selling price, but also the authorities examine the need for the product. If there are already several related products in the same therapeutic category or even several brands of a specific chemical entity already available, the authorities would not approve an additional item unless it was more effective, safer, or cheaper. This enables the Norwegians to maintain a prescription drug list of only about 25,000 products, and this includes all strengths and sizes. It is estimated that the market in the United States has nearly 4 times as many items available. In addition to the "need clause," the pharmacies in Norway also have some other unique features. They are individually owned, but there is an extremely high tax on pharmacy profits after a specified amount. The reason for this tax is that the very prosperous stores located in the city centers of the major urban areas in effect subsidize the pharmacies in the north beyond the Arctic Circle. In this way, pharmacists earn the same incomes irrespective of where their pharmacy is located. Prices are standardized so that persons in remote areas are not penalized with higher prices. Another unique feature of the Norwegian system is its wholesaling operation. Although there is private ownership of manufacturing and community pharmacies, there is only one wholesaling corporation, the Nordsk Medicinal Depot. This corporation has several branch offices and is charged with maintaining adequate supplies of drugs in case of emergencies or national need. It is felt by the Norwegian authorities that it is unfair to ask wholesalers in the private sector to maintain enough drugs to enable the country to operate for 30 days because this ties up an enormous amount of capital. They undertake this endeavor themselves.

Denmark has independently owned pharmacies, but these pharmacies cannot be sold to anyone by the existing owner. When the owner dies or retires, the pharmacy reverts back to the pharmaceutical society, which selects the most worthy candidate for pharmacy ownership. This is generally someone who has a good record of professionalism and has been on a waiting list for the longest time to purchase a pharmacy. The pharmacy is then sold through the cooperation of the society to this new individual and oftentimes the society arranges financing for the new owner. Drug prices are fixed and a great deal of manufacturing goes on in a laboratory owned by the pharmaceutical society as well as at pharmacies themselves. At the governmental level, all of the drugs marketed in the country are in one of several schedules based upon percentage of reimbursement to the patient. For example, most drugs for acute conditions such as infections are reimbursed at 75%, requiring the patient to pay only 25%. Other drugs that may have slightly less medical value may be reimbursed at 50% and drugs that are for purely cosmetic purposes, have unproven efficacy, or are considered obsolete may have no reimbursement attached to them. This is a strong motivation for patients to ask their physicians for drugs in the highest reimbursement category.

In **West Germany,** there is a great deal more outside the private sector with privately owned pharmacies dealing with generally nonprofit but nongovernmental insurance funds or sickness funds. Many of these are extensions of the old guild system in previous centuries wherein employees paid money into a fund through their union or trade association, which purchased health insurance on their behalf. There is a combination of government and private hospitals although government-owned facilities predominate. Given the very strong pharmaceutical industry in the Federal Republic of Germany and its political power, there have not been great pressures seen in this country regarding the use of generic products or, for that matter, even pricing pressures. It is speculated that one reason for this is the fact that importing nations sometimes require that the price in their country can be no greater than the price that the product sells for in its country of manufacture.

Italy and **Spain** both are similar to the other European countries previously mentioned with private ownership of pharmacies and national health services that care for a large proportion of the population. There are fixed drug-price schedules in these countries and both have rules regarding the location of community pharmacies to minimal distances or to unserved numbers of patients. In recent years, the situation has been improved but previously, the regulations were not rigidly enforced, enabling persons to ask for and purchase prescription-legend products by asking for advice from the pharmacist or by asking for a product by name on an over-the-counter basis.

The **Netherlands** is perhaps one of the more interesting examples of pharmacy in Europe. The government delegated to the Royal Dutch Pharmaceutical Society the authority to approve new licenses for pharmacies. This has resulted in the lowest ratio of pharmacies to population in any country in Europe with one pharmacy serving approximately 13,000 people. This would compare with one pharmacy for about 4500 persons in the United States. With these large numbers of persons per pharmacy, the income of Dutch pharmacists is the highest in Europe. In fact, it is oftentimes higher than physicians and dentists and during recent years has been the highest of all health professions in Holland. The strength of the ability of society to enforce these limitations has been declining and new, smaller pharmacies have been opening up. Also, the standardization of the health regulations within the European community has permitted pharmacists from surplus areas such as Belgium to move to the Netherlands where there is higher pay because of an artificial scarcity of pharmacists. In Holland, at least until recently, as the government is considering changing this policy, people are assigned to a specific pharmacy where they receive all of their care and where they are known by the pharmacist. The government then pays the pharmacy for the pharmaceutical care and responsibility for these individuals.

Leaving Europe, let us look at two previously British territories. In **Canada,** pharmacy practice is very similar to that of the United States with chain pharmacies and private ownership, but the similarity ends because there is a universal health insurance program in Canada. The pharmacies dispense drugs to patients and are reimbursed by the provincial governments. The plans differ in each of the provinces with Manitoba, Saskatchewan, and Quebec having very complete coverage with varying degrees of lesser but still basically comprehensive coverage and all of the other provinces and territories. In Canada, the number of schedules of drugs is increased, there are different regulations, and the British Pharmacopeia is the official compendium.

One of the more interesting features in Canada occurred in the Province of Ontario where a PARCOST program was introduced in the early 1970s. PARCOST stands for prescriptions at reasonable cost. Cooperating pharmacies receive a decal for their shop windows if they promised to dispense drugs with a maximal dispensing fee which is changed periodically but known to be somewhat less than what might be charged in some pharmacies. In addition, the PARCOST pharmacies may dispense generic products from a list of approved sources and be indemnified should any problems arise from this practice. In essence, then, PARCOST pharmacies guarantee a dispensing fee and highlight the use of approved generic products.

Australia is one of the more unusual nations with regard to pharmacy services that are probably regulated to a greater extent here than in any other country. The price of the pharmaceutical is considered when the government approves a product for marketing, and the postmarketing surveillance and utilization review policies of the country are well beyond that found in most of the other western nations. In addition, a book entitled *Pharmaceutical Benefits* is published quarterly. This is a listing of all of the drugs that are reimbursable in the national health services scheme of the country. For each drug in the listing it specifies who may prescribe the drug (such as only certain specialists), the site (for example, only in long-term care facilities or certain specially-equipped hospitals), maximal quantities, and in some cases a requirement that the drug be used only for certain very limited, specified diagnoses. This is an extremely rigid program and has pharmaceutical prices among the lowest in the world.

New Zealand has a program somewhere between that found in the United Kingdom and in Australia with a national databank for drug interactions that, interestingly enough, is not by drug interaction but by patient. Because the population is so limited, it is possible to keep track of the allergies and other reactions to drugs for each person in the nation. This information is, of course, accessible by practitioners and is used for a rather impressive research program. Generic drugs are featured and branded products are sold at very low prices following rigid negotiations with manufacturers. The pharmacies are independently, privately owned but there are rules regarding hours of operation, merchandise that must not be sold, etc.

Another nation that has interesting features worthy of consideration is **Japan.** As previously mentioned, in Japan, virtually no prescriptions find their way to the community pharmacist because they are dispensed or administered in the physician's office. Pharmacies in Japan look very much like American pharmacies with a host of souvenirs, cameras, cosmetics, toiletries, and many other non-health-related products. This is done of necessity to enable these shops to have sufficient revenues given their very low prescription drug income. There is a huge and thriving over-the-counter market in Japan, which is principally served by community pharmacies.

An interesting feature of the Japanese drug regulatory system is the limited period of a new drug approval. In the United States and much of Western Europe, once a drug is approved for marketing, it is able to stay on the market indefinitely unless some horrible catastrophe associated with it is discovered, and then there are legal means to remove the product from market. In Japan, after 6 years, it is necessary for the manufacturer to reapply for an additional license for an additional 6 years. This continues for the market life of the product. The Japanese have been able to keep the number of products on the market down since it is not cost-effective for a firm to go through the application process for a product that is either obsolete, has been supplanted by better drugs, or whose sales have fallen to such a low level that it is not a wise investment. Also, when a product is not considered to be as efficacious as originally thought, this is a acceptable way to remove the product from the market without having to make excuses about the decision to cancel it. This 6-year policy is used then by the government and the manufacturers.

The **People's Republic of China** has two simultaneous systems. One is a system of pharmacies providing western medicines. All of these are owned by the state with most pharmacy items being dispensed at clinics at the factories, colleges, hospitals, and health centers. Larger cities have a few community pharmacies where one may walk in and purchase such products. In addition, there is also a system for the dispensing of Chinese traditional remedies, many of which are herbal in nature. The state continues to fund almost an equal number of pharmacy schools, training practitioners for the western and traditional methods. Payment is made by the patient only for a very small extent with the remainder of the cost being absorbed by the state. In remote rural areas, the barefoot doctor makes his/her rounds with a bag containing about 25 different drug products, intended to assist patients with trivial conditions and aid patients who need to be taken to areas for more intensive care. The government intends to increase the number of qualified practitioners and decrease its dependence on barefoot doctors over time.

In the socialist nations of **Eastern Europe,** we find a pharmacy system that appears on the surface to be the same as what one might see in Western Europe with the difference that all of the shops are owned by the state pharmaceutical authorities. The payment systems differ slightly between the nations as to the percentage of reimbursement and the limits of the number of products available, yet the services are similar if not equivalent and very similar to what would be seen in most other developed areas in the world. The major problem in the socialist bloc is with shortages of products. This is a result of an administered economy in which multiyear plans determine how much of various chemical substances are to be produced so that if there is a medical problem in which a drug need far exceeds the amounts used in previous years, there may not be enough product available. In addition, it is a dilemma when a new product is made available, yet it is not promoted by the manufacturers who are stuck with inventory of the raw materials of the previous product. The only way they are able to buy the new raw materials is by selling the materials on hand. There have been experimental efforts to do something about making the system more flexible.

Czechoslovakia and **Bulgaria** have been able to limit the products on the market to approximately 1000 by removing some of the more expensive and obsolete ones. People are generally assigned to a source of care, either at a school, their place of work, or a local clinic where their records are maintained and where they would receive primary care and pharmaceutical services, in most cases. Pharmacies in **Hungary** and **Poland** have begun carrying expanded lines of over-the-counter drugs and there even have been some experiments with self-service.

Pharmacy services in other parts of the world have some unique features, but, again, generally have developed in response to the traditions and economic and political policies of those nations. Pharmacy services in most of the developing countries are at a less advanced state with minimal record keeping and a good deal of compromises having to be made to use drugs that are available as opposed to what might be the drug of choice, were it available. Some nations that have only two, three, or four pharmacists use persons without formal training to be dispensers, sometimes under the supervision beyond the limited amount of training. The WHO publishes several splendid manuals to assist in the training of health workers (6).

CONCLUSIONS

Pharmacy practice around the world contains similar functions, but these are done by different persons having different levels of training and being called different names in most countries. Additionally, these individuals are paid in differing fashions for dispensing under different systems and circumstances to patients who pay nothing, something, or all of the product depending on the drug, the system, and the country. Nevertheless, drugs are transferred from source to patients with need throughout the world. This system has been going on for no less than 2000 years with major modifications as technology and resources have permitted. It would not be accurate to indicate that practice is more advanced in one place or another even though the standards of purity and government inspections, etc. may be more advanced in one place or another. Pharmacy practice in Kenya, for example, may be more rewarding and more involved in primary care activities than might be possible even in New York City.

Nevertheless, it must be kept in mind that numerous systems for the dispensing and control of drugs are available and should be considered when decisions and policies are to be made.

SOME USEFUL ADDRESSES AND REFERENCE SOURCES

There is an international organization that is the umbrella organization for all national pharmaceutical associations. This is the Federation Internationale Pharmaceutique located at 11 Alexanderstraat, 2514 JL, The Hague, Netherlands. The international activities mentioned previously are coordinated by the World Health organization. There are two most relevant divisions: the Pharmaceuticals Division and the Essential Drugs Program. Both are located at the World Health Organization, CH1211, Geneva 27, Switzerland. The International Narcotic Conventions, dealing with quotas and regulations regarding abusable substances, are coordinated through the International Narcotic Control Office at the United Nations, Vienna, Austria. An organization that coordinates the activities of the Pharmaceutical Manufacturers Associations around the world is the International Federation of Pharmaceutical Manufacturers Associations, 67 Rue de St. Jean, CH1201, Geneva, Switzerland. The International Red Cross also is located in Geneva, Switzerland as is the World Council of Churches main office for health activities. The United Nations, New York, NY 10017 is able to assist persons interested in the lists maintained by the United Nations such as banned substances and drugs removed from the market in member nations.

The general activities of the World Health Organization stem from their regional offices. For Africa, the office is at P.O. Box 6, Brazzaville, Republic of Congo. For North and South America and the Caribbean areas, the office is the Pan American Health Organization (PAHO) at 525 23rd Street N.W., Washington, DC 20037. For the Eastern Mediterranean area, the regional office of the World Health Organization is at Box 1517, Alexandria, Egypt. For Europe, the European regional office of the WHO is located at 8 Scherfigsvej, Copenhagen, Denmark. The Southeast Asia office is located at Indraprastha Estate, Ring Road, New Delhi, One, India; and the office for the Western Pacific is located on Taft Avenue, P.O. Box 2932, Manila, Philippines.

REFERENCES

1. Sonnedecker G, ed. Kramers and Urdang's History of Pharmacy. 3rd ed. Philadelphia: Lippincott, 1963, pp 7.
2. Parascandola J. A brief history of drug use. In Wertheimer AI, Bush PJ, eds. Perspectives on medicines in society. Hamilton IL: Drug Intelligence. 1977, pp 10.
3. Tucker D. The World Health Market, Bicester UK: Facts on File Publications, 1984.
4. World Health Statistics. Annuals. Geneva: World Health Organization. 1986.
5. Sixth Report on the World Health Situation, Part 1, Global Analysis, Geneva: World Health Organization. 1980.
6. World Health Organization. Expanded Program on Immunization, Training for Mid-level Managers. Geneva: World Health Organization. 1981. (There are a large number of publications in this series.)

SUGGESTED READINGS

1. Maxwell RJ. Health and wealth, an international study of health care spending. Lexington MA: Lexington Books, 1981.
2. The use of essential drugs: a report of a WHO expert committee. Technical Report No. 685. Geneva: World Health Organization, 1983.
3. A barefoot doctor's manual. Philadelphia: Running Press, 1977.
4. Fry J, Farndale W. International medical care. Wallingford PA: Washington Square East Publishers, 1972.
5. Kohn R, White K. Health care: an international study. New York: Oxford University Press, 1976.
6. Roemer M. Health care systems in world perspective. Ann Arbor MI: Health Administration Press, 1976.
7. Raffel M. Comparative Health Systems: Descriptive analyses of 14 national health systems. University Park, PA: Pennsylvania State University Press, 1984.
8. Quick J, ed. Managing drug supply. Boston: Management Sciences for Health, 1982.
9. Quick J. The Institute of Pharmacy Management international reference book, London: Milbank Publications, 1985.
10. Golladay F. Health problems and policies in the developing countries. The World Bank, August 1980.

11. Golladay F. Pharmaceuticals and developing countries: a dialog for constructive action. Washington DC: National Council for International Health, August 1982.

12. Golladay F. An updated list of publications produced by national drug regulatory authorities and other agencies. Geneva: World Health Organization, June 1986.

13. Golladay F. Policies for the production and marketing of essential drugs. Washington, DC: Pan American Health Organization, 1984.

14. Golladay F. Health information for international travel. US Department of Health and Human Services, Atlanta: Centers for Disease Control, June 1986.

15. Golladay F. British national formulary. London: British Medical Association and the Pharmaceutical Society of Great Britain. No. 10, 1985.

16. Nordic statistics on medicine, 1981-1983. Uppsala: Nordic Council on Medicines, 1986.

17. Facts: Medicine and health care in Denmark. (Assn.) of the Danish Pharmaceutical Industry) Foreningen of danske Medicinfabrikker, Copenhagen: 1986.

18. Silverman M, Lee P, Lydecker M. Prescriptions for death. Berkeley: University of California Press, 1982.

19. Silverman M, Lee P, Lydecker M. Pills and the public purse, Berkeley: University of California Press, 1981.

20. Ingle JI, Blair P. International dental care delivery systems, Cambridge MA: Ballinger, 1978.

21. Harris MF. Pharmacy education in the Eastern Commonwealth Caribbean. Pharm Int. 1982;3:280-284.

22. Kvĕtina J. Solich J. Clinical pharmacy education and rational drug therapy in Czechoslovakia. Pharm Int. 1982;3:277-278.

23. Johansen HE. Danish pharmacy. Pharm Int. 1982;3:245-248.

24. Allison A, Froese E, Hall J, et al. A drug information service for a developing country: Zimbabwe. Pharm Int. 1982;3:280-184.

25. Acheampong YB. Drug information for patients in the third world. Pharm Int. 1982;3:129-31.

26. Summers RS, Froese EH. The clinical pharmacy programme in Zimbabwe. Pharm Int. 1982;3:52-53.

27. Krówczyński L. Postgraduate education of pharmacists in Poland. Pharm Int. 1982;3:44-5.

28. Endresen E, Andrew E. Continuing education for pharmacists in Norway. Pharm Int. 1981;2:241-244.

29. Wolf E. Pharmaceutical continuing education in the FRG. Pharm Int. 1981;2:125-127.

30. Bonal J, Altimiras J, Serra J. Clinical pharmacy in Spain. Pharm Int. 1981;2:4-5.

31. Wolf E. Pharmacy in Austria. Pharm Int. 1981;2:4-5.

32. Harron DWG. Pharmaceutical education in the Sudan. Pharm Int. 1980;1:9-11.

33. York P. Ujamaa for pharmacy in Tanzania. Pharm Int. 1980;1:8-11.

34. McLeon C. Contrast in pharmacy manpower planning between the United States and northern European countries. Drug Intell Clin Pharm. 1986;20:210-212.

35. McCreedy C. Swiss community pharmacy—some lessons for the UK. Pharm J. 1985;235:784-786.

36. Dunn WR, Hamilton DD, Lilja J. Education in Sweden. Pharm J. 1985;235:561-562.

37. Pharmacy in the third world: seminar on professional and management aspects. Commonwealth Pharmaceutical Association. 11-16, Pharm J. 1985;235:299-316.

38. Griffin JP, Taylor DG, Weber JPC. Regional differences in medicine usage in the UK. Pharm Int. 1986;7:243-245.

39. Ginjaume EC. New ideas for the control of extemporaneous compounding: the Spanish Professional Formulary. Pharm Int. 1985; 6:84.

40. Thakur RS. Enough pharmacists available to man pharmacies in rural areas. Ind J Hosp Pharm. 1984;83:6-7.

41. Jain L, Saxena S. A study on purchase for drugs without regular prescriptions. Ind J Hosp Pharm. 1984;83:201-202.

42. Penn RG. The review of medicines in the UK. Pharm Int. 1983;4:205-210.

43. Sharpe D. A national advertising campaign on behalf of British community pharmacists. Pharm Int. 1983;4:155-157.

44. D'Arcy PF. Action programmes: FIP Third World Project. Pharm Int. 1983;4:157-158.

45. Appelbe GE. Professional responsibility and the law. Pharm Int. 1983;4:159-162.

46. Cox RGB, Griffin JP, Allen P. The free movement of medicines in Europe: a survey. Pharm Int. 1983;4:80–82.
47. ten Ham M. The Netherlands board for the evaluation of medicines (1971–1980). Part 1: Organization and Procedures. Pharm Int. 1984;5:46–50.
48. ten Ham M. The Netherlands board for the evaluation of medicines (1971–1980). Part 2: Quantitative aspects of drug registration. Pharm Int. 1984; 5:66–69.
49. Richards RME. Pharmacy in China. Pharm Int. 1984;5:167.

13
Public Health Role of the Pharmacist

PATRICIA J. BUSH
KEITH W. JOHNSON

INTRODUCTION

Before dealing with the specific role of the pharmacist in public health, public health should be defined and distinguished from its logical alternative, private health. In 1976, a high-level commission inquiring into higher education for public health said that public health is "the effort organized by society to protect, promote, and restore the public's health. The programs, services, and institutions involved emphasize the prevention of disease and the health needs of the population as a whole" (1). This definition suggests that the scope of public health is broad, and population based rather than individually based. The common themes in public health are organized and collective. Public health problems are not health problems or diseases as they are presented by a series of individuals to a health care provider for cure, alleviation, or prevention, but they are considered in the context of the community. It is a private health problem to diagnose and treat a specific disease in a patient. It is a public health problem to determine the prevalence of that disease in a community, compare that prevalence with rates of the disease in prior years, and plan health services to reduce the prevalence of the disease. Public health professionals ask questions like, "How frequently does this disease occur, and to whom does it occur? What is the impact of this disease in the community? How is this disease transmitted? Can it be prevented? How important is it compared with other health problems existing in the community? What can the community do to lessen the impact of the disease?" This does not mean that public health is limited to enumeration, analyzing, and planning. Public health also includes the specific actions that are taken on behalf of individuals after enumerating, analyzing, and planning. Whether a practitioner is paid by the public or private sector does not determine whether the practitioner is engaged in public health activities. What determines whether the practitioner is engaged in public health activities is whether the activities address a community problem.

TWO PUBLIC HEALTH LEVELS

From the perspective of a person doing public health, public health exists on two levels, the micro and the macro (2). At the micro level, public health services are relatively direct as compared with the macro level. For example, the director of a public health clinic is functioning at the micro level, whereas the person who evaluated the need for the public health

379

clinic, planned it, and allocated resources to it functioned at the macro level. Viewed in terms of these levels, the public health role for particular categories of health professionals such as pharmacists can be seen from two perspectives: (a) at the micro level, from the perspective of a health professional whose primary role is not public health but who is performing some public health function, and (b) at the macro level, from the perspective of a health professional whose primary role is in public health.

WHO DOES PUBLIC HEALTH?

With the discovery of the "miracle" antibiotics in the 1940s, medicine began to turn away from the traditional doctor-patient relationships and take an increasingly technological or disease orientation toward patients. In the 1970s, this disease orientation began reverting to a patient orientation. The parallel situation in pharmacy has existed with recent emphasis on patient and interprofessional relationships. Conventionally, health professional students study basic sciences and then learn by "practicing" those skills believed necessary to perform their professional role under the tutelage of role models. For pharmacy students, this traditionally has meant learning about the drug, its source, formulation, and biopharmaceutics, and how to translate a physician's order into a therapeutic product. When pharmacy students "practiced," there was not necessarily any interaction between a student and patients (or customers), or between the student and other health professionals. However, paralleling medicine, as pharmacy became more patient oriented, students began to "practice" in clinical settings, and role models began to include community and hospital pharmacists, some of whom were practicing micro level public health activities, many of which are discussed below. In this respect, pharmacy began to resemble medicine, nursing, and dentistry, i.e., health professional students interacting with patients under the guidance of practitioners. However, these other professions, unlike pharmacy, long ago recognized that their training, whether disease or patient oriented, failed in terms of teaching public health because it did not take a population perspective. These other professions now have their special schools and departments of public health and community medicine that teach public health and train public health professionals. Because pharmacy education does not offer a distinct public health tract, any training relating to public health must be gleaned by the student from other components of the curriculum or pursued through a formalized program in a school of public health (3, 4).

Schools of public health do not produce one type of health professional as contrasted with schools of medicine or pharmacy. Instead, they produce persons from a variety of backgrounds who have adapted their knowledge and skills to the field. As well as practitioners, these include biostatisticians, epidemiologists, environmental specialists, nutritionists, and health educators, whose training focuses them on public health problems. Some of these find employment at the macro level of public health; others, most often practitioners and health educators, integrate public health concepts into their practices at the micro level. However, it is not necessary to obtain a degree in public health to perform public health activities. Increasingly, health professionals, including pharmacists, are recognizing their important roles in the health of their communities (5).

PHARMACISTS' RESPONSIBILITIES IN PUBLIC HEALTH

Because of the variation in pharmacy practice, the responsibilities of pharmacists in public health are more apparent to some pharmacists than others. For those pharmacists whose primary position is at the macro level of public health, their public health responsibilities are clear. However, to others such as pharmacists employed by the public sector but who work at the micro level, for example, in public health clinics, their responsibilities in public health may not be as clear. Community pharmacists may have no idea of their responsibilities in public health (6, 7).

The activities of community pharmacists in public health derive from two characteristics. First, they consider themselves to be professionals, and second, they are citizens with high visibility and high accessibility who enjoy an unusual amount of respect from the public. To fulfill the definition of a professional (8), pharmacists have a duty, an obligation, to place the welfare of patients above their own individual, and especially economic, interests. The obligation of pharmacists as citizens derives from an assumption that responsibilities accrue to privileged positions. Because public funds are used to educate pharmacists, and because pharmacists are allowed special rights such as the right to determine who shall practice pharmacy and how it shall be practiced, the public expects pharmacists to use their expertise on its behalf and to contribute to the public welfare. It is perhaps the greatest challenge of pharmacy to meet the public's increasing expectations. In perhaps no other health profession is the conflict between economic interest and public welfare more apparent than in community pharmacy practice today. The risk of not accommodating the public interest is that pharmacy may lose the public trust that it now holds.

Types of pharmacist public health activity vary from policy formulation to individual patient counseling. On the one hand, there are pharmacists who are involved in policy formulation that is, of course, a macro level public health function (2). Some of these individuals are involved in drug policy and some are involved in other types of health policy. In general, health policy, whether drug oriented or not, includes formulation, implementation, monitoring, and possibly regulation, each of which has subcategories of activities such as priority setting and health planning. On the other hand, at the individual micro level, community pharmacists respond to perceived individual patient needs that meet public health goals (e.g., drug education), but these activities are not necessarily part of an organized community initiative that has arisen from policy formulation procedures.

Community public health planning should take into account drug-related activities and may be performed by both the public and private sectors. Pharmacists are well qualified, by their expertise and by their accessibility and position of trust in the community, to participate at both of these levels.

It is these important macro and micro public health roles of the pharmacist (policy formulation, public and community activities, individual patient activities) that are addressed in the remainder of this chapter.

POLICY FORMULATION

One of the most important public health-related functions of the pharmacist (and probably one of the least exercised) relates to policy formulation. The establishment of overall system parameters favorable to addressing drug- and/or pharmacy-related concerns would go far in addressing public health concerns related to the use of medications. Some might argue that once a pharmacist crosses the line into policy formulation, he or she is no longer practicing pharmacy. Using standard practice definitions, this may be true. However, whether the traditional role of the pharmacist is being met is not the issue. Rather, the issue is one of the training and expertise held by the person engaged in the work. In defining and resolving public health issues that relate to the delivery of pharmaceutical services, individuals knowledgeable about the profession and the issues confronting the profession are in a place to contribute significantly. If the profession of pharmacy is not represented at these decision-making levels, the full potential of the pharmacist's role may not be realized and the public's health will not be well served.

Health policy formulation activities can take place at the organization, local, state, national, or international levels. Involvement can range from salaried full-time positions to voluntary temporary advisory positions. The types of issues that may involve pharmacists include the following:

- Identification of health-related public/community problems.   In the broadest sense, this is based on epidemiologic principles and includes the collection of the data necessary to make decisions as to cause, effect, and remedy. Problems may include prevalence and incidence of disease states, extent and severity of adverse reactions to medications, rates of compliance in the taking of medications, drug costs and the resulting effects on use of medications, prescribing characteristics of physicians and other prescribers, rates of error in the dispensing of medications, promotional activities of drug manufacturers, and self-medication. Pharmacists trained in epidemiology and related research disciplines can contribute significantly to this identification process.
- Setting health priorities.   In any society with limited resources, priorities must be set as to which programs need the greatest and most immediate attention. This setting of priorities often falls under the legislative/regulatory process because more often than not, it is tax money that is being allocated. In other instances, the private sector will be allocating dollars and will be defining priorities for the users of services. In either instance, however, an unbiased analysis of the assessment of needs is necessary to make rational decisions. This is part of setting the agenda for health care delivery (9).
- Health planning.   After priorities have been established, it is necessary to determine how programs can best be set up to meet the defined needs. Part of this process involves resource allocation and definition of roles (10).
- Program evaluation.   Integral to any program is its evaluation. It is critical to generate data to feed back into the planning process. By including an evaluative component, the policy formulation process is alive and not stagnant.
- Reimbursement/economics.   Costs are critical in all aspects of health care, from new drug development to the actual delivery of services. Effective and fair allocation of resources is essential. Accessibility and payment for needed services, including drug coverage, must be addressed.
- Legislative/regulatory programs.   Many legislative and regulatory actions deal with drug availability, pharmacy services, and related programs. At the national level, the work of the Food and Drug Administration (FDA) in approving new medications and controlling the availability, manufacture, and promotion of such is crucial to the public's health. The work of other federal regulatory agencies such as the Drug Enforcement Agency, the Consumer Product Safety Commission, and the Federal Trade Commission, as well as the work of the United States Pharmacopeia in the establishment of standards for strength, quality, purity, packaging, and labeling also relate to the public's health. In addition, the United States Congress and the various state legislatures offer similar opportunities for involvement.
- Increasing access to health services.   Although in actuality a health planning issue,

the importance of increasing access to health services merits special attention. Pharmacists are among the most available and accessible of all health care providers. Maximizing their potential would go a long way in increasing access to health services.

PUBLIC/COMMUNITY ACTIVITIES

At the local level, there is an abundance of public health activities in which the pharmacist can become involved. Many of these are organized by local health departments and are based at sites other than the community pharmacy. Other activities that are general public health functions legitimately can be centered in the pharmacy itself, even though the effects of the program extend into the community being served (11).

In discussing public/community public health activities, it is important to differentiate between true community activities and individual patient care. Although some of the same approaches and programs can be used in providing community and individual services, the difference lies in the focus of the intervention. A true public/community public health focus is aimed at the community at large, whether taking the form of simple awareness generation as found in educational programs or the form of broad scale diagnosis/intervention attempts as found in screening programs. In either case, the aim is the community-at-large, not service to the individual patient. The ideal outcome of public/community public health activities would be either preventing a negative health event from happening in the first place or ensuring adequate early treatment of a negative health event that is in the process of occurring. By allocating resources to prevention/early treatment programs the hope is that fewer resources in the long run would be required for individual patient care.

Some prime examples of public/community public health activities of the pharmacist would include the following:

- Immunization. Assist in organizing and implementing public immunization programs. Although pharmacists may not in most instances actually be administering the immunizations, logistical support is essential. More importantly, the pharmacist is in a key position to educate the community about the importance of immunization and thereby to encourage widespread participation.
- Substance abuse. Substance abuse includes illicit drugs, the inappropriate use of licit drugs, the inappropriate use of certain solvents, smoking or chewing tobacco, and alcohol. Again, education is central. But in this area, actions may speak louder than words. Pharmacists should not sell alcohol or tobacco products. And this should be publicly proclaimed. The community should know why these products are not available at their community pharmacy. In relation to the inappropriate use of licit drugs, patients should be warned about abuse potential; and for those over-the-counter products that may be misused, strict controls as to access should be instituted (12).
- Sexually transmitted disease. With the spread of acquired immune deficiency syndrome (AIDS), this public health activity takes on critical dimensions. Although important for the other sexually transmitted diseases, the life-threatening nature of AIDS takes precedence. Educational programs promoting safe sexual practices especially as related to the use of condoms are essential. In addition, the prominent display and ready accessibility of condoms for sale are important in minimizing barriers to their purchase and use (13).

- Family planning.   Providing information on the alternatives available for contraception is an important public health role of the pharmacist. Although this activity can take the form of individual patient care, the dissemination of information relating to comparative effectiveness, safety, and price of contraceptive measures is also appropriate for a broader audience.
- Health promotion.   Transferring to the community at large information relating to diet, exercise, and other health promotion concepts can be an important part of the public health role of the pharmacist.
- Fluoridation.   The positive effects of fluoride on caries prevention are well documented. The pharmacist who is aware of the fluoride content of local water supplies and who actively advises community members to seek out additional supplementation, if necessary, is providing a valuable public health function. This role has taken on added importance in a least one state. As of 1986, the pharmacy practice act in Florida authorizes pharmacists to actually prescribe fluoride supplementation in certain situations.
- Poison prevention.   When it comes to poisonings, time and knowledge are crucial. Pharmacists have a responsibility not only to provide advice on a one-on-one basis but to instill in the community at large the importance of quick action in case of poisoning and what to do if a poisoning occurs. This is a prime example of how a pharmacist can educate to protect the public's health. The community pharmacist also can serve as a link to various poison control centers.
- Quackery.   Billions of dollars are spent each year on remedies that do not work, some of which can be dangerous. And promotional efforts for these products tend to prey on those most vulnerable—the terminally ill and individuals who feel that they are not socially acceptable because of certain characteristics (e.g., obesity). Providing objective information about such unproven (and possibly unsafe) remedies can have a positive impact on the public's health. The pharmacy can appropriately serve as the center for the collection of information on substances/techniques being promoted in the community. And closer to home, the pharmacist should not promote or sell products of questionable efficacy.
- Disaster preparedness and aversion.   The potential for natural disasters such as floods, earthquakes, and tornados varies with the pharmacist's community. Every community has the potential for manmade disasters such as chemical spills, gas leaks, and plane crashes. Here the pharmacist combines his or her special health expertise with the duty of a citizen to join others in the community to develop disaster preparedness plans. The pharmacist can dispense emergency preparedness information and be prepared to provide first aid and medication. In the event of a nuclear accident of the sort that occurred at Three Mile Island and Chernobyl, the pharmacist should be able to provide potassium iodide to those exposed to radioactivity.

  Stocking potassium iodide is, of course, no defense against the ultimate public health threat, nuclear war. The pharmacist's response to this threat should be to join with other health professionals to create awareness of the dangers of nuclear disasters and what steps can be taken to avert them.
- Environmental protection.   Chemicals, including drugs, industrial solvents, and pesticides, have a tremendous potential for polluting our environment and negatively impacting public health. As the health care professional having the most direct link to chemistry, the pharmacist is in a position to educate the public about hazards of chemicals and their appropriate disposal.

- Work place safety.   The community pharmacist is in a position to monitor work place safety by establishing a good ongoing dialogue with patrons and being alert to the implications of requests for self-medication. In addition, community education as to the importance of reporting incidents so that remedial actions can be taken to prevent recurrence can have an overall positive impact.
- Peer review.   A potentially important public health role of the pharmacist relates to the assessment of the quality of care delivered by colleagues (physicians and other prescribers as well as pharmacists). Most generally completed under the auspices of third party payers or regulatory bodies, the assessment of the appropriateness of prescribing practices of individual prescribers can have a profound effect on the quality of care delivered.
- Data collection.   In policy formulation activities, data are needed on which to base decisions. There are two ways in which the pharmacist can participate in this data collection. First, the pharmacist should report problems with drug preparations, medical devices, labeling, nomenclature, and drug promotion to the Drug Product Problem Reporting Program that is funded by the FDA and operated by the United States Pharmacopeia. Such reporting ensures that the problems will be brought to the attention of both the FDA and the manufacturer and that trends will be studied because the data are computerized for long-term analysis. Second, adverse drug reactions should be reported directly to the Drug Experience Branch of the FDA. By reporting perceived problems, the pool of data used in making decisions will be enhanced for the public's welfare (14).

Public/community health activities are generally tied directly in with educational efforts. In the pharmacy curriculum, the lack of a component on how to effectively teach can be a tremendous hinderance in carrying out this role. Not only must the pharmacist know how to communicate, but he or she needs to know how to teach.

The educational role can be group focused or individually focused. Both are important. In the group approach, presentations to schools, clubs, health care provider personnel, church groups, etc. allow the opportunity to address a larger audience with an important general message. This general message should, however, be tied to individual counseling.

INDIVIDUAL PATIENT ACTIVITIES

Individual patient activities are those most difficult to think of as being public health in nature. But they are. Convincing a patient with strep throat to complete the full course of antibiotic therapy is of benefit not only to the patient but to the community he or she might infect. In addition, the example taught to one individual regarding appropriate care will be transferred to others by that individual. People are interested in their health and the health care experiences of their friends and neighbors. And in the long run, with the high cost of health care and the impact this has on all of us, improving safety and efficacy of therapy will help to minimize costs for the community as a whole.

- Individual patient education.   The pharmacist should really be able to shine when it comes to patient education. He or she is the last person in the chain of health care delivery to have access to the patient (either directly or by proxy). It is at this point that some of the most effective education can take place. Education can cover proper use of prescribed medications, self-medication, compliance, side effects monitoring, nutrition, and/or disease prevention.

- Screening and referral.   As one of the most accessible individuals in the health care delivery system and as a ready and reliable source of information for a consumer concerned about his or her health, the pharmacist can serve in a simple triage capacity. This can be done through regular screenings (as for high blood pressure) or through individual advice provided on request (13).

The community pharmacist also can serve an important function by providing knowledgeable referrals for persons seeking information about health clinics, social services, and benefits eligibility. As the most accessible health contact in a neighborhood, the pharmacist is a natural to seek out for such information. Almost every person has a need for this type of counseling for themselves or others at some point in their lives. People want to know how they can find out about Medicaid or Medicare benefits; how to sign up for government programs such as Women, Infants, and Children Care (WIC); who can use public health clinics; who is eligible for home health care services. Although the diverse nature of this information means that it will take the public-minded pharmacist some time to acquire, once assembled, it is not difficult to keep up to date. Moreover, such a collection of data could be a project taken on by the local pharmaceutical association in a community and made available for all pharmacists so that they could provide public health information to their neighborhoods.

- Medication maintenance.   Court-ordered deinstitutionalization of mentally ill but not dangerous persons has increased the number of "street" people who are in need of a regular supply of psychotropic medications. Frequently, these persons are required to travel considerable distances for their medications, and often they are not capable of this. The urban pharmacist is ideally suited to serve as a distribution point for medications for these persons and monitor compliance, effectiveness, and side effects, reporting to the appropriate authorities when problems are evident.
- Compliance counseling.   To maximize the positive effects of a medication, it must be taken as directed. This is an extremely difficult thing for the average patient to do. The pharmacist is in a position to enhance the likelihood of compliance whether it be by patient education, follow-up calls, or the construction of simple compliance-aiding devices (13).
- Patient monitoring.   The pharmacist is in a position to help monitor the effectiveness of therapy. Simple questions asked of the patient when a prescription is refilled can help zero in on inappropriate or ineffective therapy.
- Family counseling.   As is the case with patient education in general, the pharmacist who has developed a good continuing dialogue and knowledge about his or her patients will be in a position to provide advice on a variety of subjects affecting the patient and his or her family. Counseling may relate to medical, economic, or other needs.

HOW TO PARTICIPATE IN PUBLIC HEALTH ACTIVITIES

It should be stated that many pharmacists have in the past been involved in public health activities, particularly those at the micro level, without thinking about the activities in terms of public health. The work being done simply had to be done for the community. In fact, many public health activities are common sense activities that are a part of traditional pharmacy practice. The intensity of such activities probably was greater in the past, before discounting, large-volume operations, mail order, and the like. In one sense, price competition has decreased public health-type activities in the community pharmacy (15).

A pharmacist's participation in public health activities is partially dependent on one very important factor, "state of mind." He or she has to want to provide these services. He or she has to put the patient/customer's needs at the top of everything else. It is a mission. It is a commitment.

At the macro level of public health activities, there are obviously full-time positions that can be appropriately filled by pharmacists. The bulk of the involvement is, however, voluntary in nature. Public health departments, voluntary health agencies, health provider groups, and other organizations need individuals to serve on advisory panels, review committees, and other ad hoc bodies providing support and advice. This may cover drug abuse programs, immunization programs, or any of the functions previously identified.

Contact the local chapters of various voluntary agencies such as the Red Cross, the American Cancer Society, or any other similar organization. Check with your local health department. Identify public health-related programs based in professional societies, such as the American Pharmaceutical Association. Volunteer your services, share your ideas, and be available. The more you become involved, the greater will be the potential for your future involvement.

At the micro level, establish public health programs as part of your pharmacy practice. Provide literature relating to public health concerns such as family planning, sexually transmitted disease prevention, smoking, drug abuse, and nutrition. Back up these literature services by being available for consultation. And most important, serve as a role model. Do not sell cigarettes. Do not push questionable over-the-counter remedies. Practice what you preach.

One of the most prominent threads that ties public health activities together is education. Learn how to communicate; learn how to teach or persuade; learn how to motivate. The most difficult person to teach is the person who does not care about his or her health. And this is exactly the person who needs the most help.

For many community pharmacists who want to participate in patient-directed public health education activities, the bottom line is "Who is going to pay?" And this is a legitimate question. Our policies for pharmacist reimbursement traditionally have been based on payment for goods delivered—not payment for services rendered. Thus, advice without delivery of actual medication most often will not generate income for the pharmacist providing that advice. Schools, clubs, and nursing homes in most cases will not have funds to pay for presentations/programs by pharmacists. Voluntary health organizations will not routinely pay for the input of pharmacists serving on boards, committees, or other advisory bodies.

Many pharmacist public health activities will remain as voluntary services. Direct patient care, however, even without delivery of medication, can have a positive effect on pharmacy income and overall health care costs. Ideally, because patient services are part of the professional responsibility of the pharmacist, the salary received by the pharmacist and the charges made for prescription and nonprescription medications take into account the costs of the delivery of those services. In the real world of competition, this is difficult. The positive effect on income may have to come from public relations/promotion and the resulting effect on building more business. Good works are generally rewarded. Let the public know about your public health activities. Do not underestimate the effects of counseling and compliance promotion. People like the personal interest shown and will let their friends and neighbors know about positive experiences (and negative ones too, so be careful).

The most important income may be "psychic income." You are helping people. And that is just about the most significant and rewarding thing you can do. That's why you became a pharmacist, isn't it?

REFERENCES

1. Higher Education for Public Health. A Report of the Milbank Memorial Fund Commission, 1976.
2. Bush PJ, Johnson KW. Where is the public health pharmacist? Am J Pharm Educ 1979;43:249–252.
3. Gibson MR. Public health education in colleges of pharmacy: I. The background and problem; II. A survey of instruction; III. The testing, analysis of tests, conclusions and recommendations. Am J Pharm Educ 1972;36:189–200; 1972;36:561–570; 1973;37:1–21.
4. Beardsley RS, Bootman JL, Christensen DB, et al. Report of the Ad Hoc Committee on Public Health. Pharmacy in Public Health: Roles and Curricular Considerations. Am J Pharm Educ 1985;49:413–418.
5. Policy statement 8024(PP) of the American Public Health Association. The role of the pharmacist in public health. Am J Public Health 1981;71:213–216.
6. Bush PJ, ed. The Pharmacist Role in Disease Prevention and Health Promotion. Bethesda: American Society of Hospital Pharmacists Research and Education Foundation Inc, 1983.
7. Rappoport HM, Freeman RA, Smith MC, Garner DD. Assessment of realistic public health roles for pharmacists. J Soc Admin Pharm 1984;2:57–66.
8. Freidson E. Profession of Medicine. New York: Harper & Row, 1970.
9. Wertheimer AI. Public health priorities for the USA. Pharm Int 1984;5:(Oct):240–243.
10. Penna RP. Pharmacists as health planners—they're already involved. Am Pharm 1979;19(4):23–24.
11. Forno JJ. The pharmacist and the community: the role outside the prescription department. In Proc Fifth Annual Pharmacy Practice Institute, Albany College of Pharmacy, Oct 2–3, 1982, pp 60–68.
12. Anthony J. The drug use control function and the pharmacist role in drug abuse prevention. Pharmacopa 1973;12:10.
13. Mayer FS. The pharmacist: gatekeeper of the community's health. Hosp Formul 1976;11(2):84–86.
14. Kilwein JH. The pharmacist and public health. US Pharmacist 1978;3:(March):61–66.
15. Wertheimer AI, Johnson KW. Health advisory opportunities for RPh's grow as medical science progresses. Am Drug 1984;192:102.

SELECTED READINGS

THE PHARMACIST AND PUBLIC HEALTH [a]

John H. Kilwein

Public health is of importance to all health professionals. Certain basic concepts and perspectives discussed in this article will enable pharmacists to better understand public health and its relevance to the practice of pharmacy, and, perhaps, motivate some pharmacists to become more involved in specific public health programs.

Professionals trained in clinical sciences commonly encounter some initial difficulty understanding the manner in which public health and the clinical sciences differ from each other. Public health is often contrasted to clinical medicine, for example, in that (a) the focus of public health is on human population groups rather than individual cases; (b) attributes of healthy as well as ill members of population groups are studied; and (c) there is a strong emphasis on the prevention of disease.

Because the clinician typically treats individual patients who are already ill and who come from relatively narrow segments of the population, it is very difficult, if not impossible, for the clinician to generalize about the health of the larger community from observations made on these patients. For example, a health professional whose practice is all white and middle-class cannot, from this practice alone, comment with a high degree of certainty on the way race and social class might be related to the problem of high blood pressure. To do so would require making observations on representative samples of various racial and socioeconomic groups, i.e., adopting the public health focus.

Public health is also broader in scope than most health professions, drawing not only from the health sciences but also from disciplines normally considered outside the health care field, e.g., engineering, law, anthropology, etc. This is so because the health status of a community is determined by much more than the medical activities that take place in that community. The point is dramatically illustrated by the fact that overall mortality in the United States began a sharp decline at the beginning of this century, decades before the miracles of modern medicine. This reduction is largely attributed to better nutrition, improved sanitation, and a declining birth rate.

In their efforts to improve the health status of communities, public health thinkers have traditionally conceptualized disease (and injury) as resulting from an unfavorable interaction of agent, host, and environment. Most simply stated, an agent is a factor whose presence or absence causes disease (e.g., tubercle bacillus, vitamin B deficiency). Host factors refer to those physical and psychological attributes of a person that predispose or protect from disease (e.g., advanced age, antibody levels). Finally, the physical, biological, and social environments in which the host and agent are enmeshed can obviously do much to foster or suppress the development of disease. Public health efforts are usually directed toward one or a combination of the above factors. For example, water filtration and chlorina-

---

[a]Edited and reprinted with permission from Kilwein JH. The pharmacist and public health. US Pharmacist 1978;3:61–66.

tion constitute a direct attack on several of the enteric disease agents. In a polio immunization program an attempt is made to stimulate host resistance to the disease. Malaria control programs often involve a modification of the environment, as when marshes are drained in order to eliminate breeding grounds of the vector of the disease.

Three levels of disease prevention are said to exist in public health. *Primary* prevention consists of the efforts undertaken to prevent the development of disease in susceptible populations. These include measures to promote general health (e.g., providing adequate nutrition), and specific measures (e.g., providing immunizations). *Secondary* prevention involves the early detection and quick treatment of disease in order to reverse, halt, or slow its progression. *Tertiary* prevention consists of those efforts that limit disability from disease and promote rehabilitation where disease has already inflicted damage. Physiotherapy is a prime example of tertiary prevention.

It is not to be implied from the foregoing that there is a basic antagonism between public health and the clinical sciences, or that one is more important than the other. This is not the case, for in many ways the two areas overlap, and in other ways they complement each other. To make a correct diagnosis a clinician is aided by knowledge of how a disease is distributed in various subgroups of the population. This data is, of course, derived from epidemiological studies, which will be discussed later. On the other hand, health examination surveys, done on population groups, require that those making the diagnoses possess sound clinical skills. In addition, individual clinical practitioners, when viewed in the aggregate, comprise a major part of the health care system—itself a very important public health concept.

SOURCES OF DATA

Although pharmacists come across morbidity and mortality statistics in their professional readings, few probably have clear notions regarding the sources of health data. Listed below are some of the more important sources of data, sources from which many mortality and morbidity rates are derived.

The Vital Registration System

In this country individual states have the responsibility for officially recording birth, death, marriage, and divorce. Certificates of vital events are completed at the city or county level and then sent to the state health department. Each state forwards copies of these certificates to the National Center for Health Statistics (NCHS), a branch of the United States Public Health Service (USPHS), where they are compiled and analyzed. The results are published monthly in the *Monthly Vital Statistics Report,* and cummulated annually in *Vital Statistics of the United States.*

The System of Notifiable Disease Reports

All 50 states require the reporting of specified communicable diseases. The number of notifiable diseases varies from 40, in some states, to 70 in others. Included in these lists are diseases that may result in serious epidemic outbreaks (polio, rabies, cholera, smallpox, etc.). Physicians are legally required to report cases of notifiable disease to local health departments which, in turn, transmit this data to the state health department. The states send weekly reports on these diseases to the Center for Disease Control in Atlanta. This agency publishes *Morbidity and Mortality Weekly Report,* a summary of the incidence of about 25 notifiable diseases. A major weakness of the system of notifiable disease reports is the fail-ure of many physicians to report these diseases.

The National Health Survey

One of the most comprehensive programs designed to generate health data is the continuous National Health Survey, conducted by the USPHS. This program actually consists of several distinct surveys involving national samples of the population and samples of health care institutions. The National Health Survey develops statistics on acute and chronic disease, injury, disability, nutritional status, fertility trends, and the distribution of certain physio-logical characteristics (e.g., serum cholesterol and blood pressure levels). In addition, infor-mation is collected from hospitals, nursing homes, and clinics to develop statistics on the institutions themselves and the people they serve. Findings from these surveys are periodi-cally published by the NCHS in *Monthly Vital Statistics Reports* and in a series of monographs.

Other Sources of Data

Besides the aforementioned major sources of health statistics, there are many individual efforts at data collection by local and state health departments, health centers, and volun-teer agencies. The National Institutes of Health also conduct important morbidity surveys on specific diseases such as cancer. Records from industry, the military, schools, insurance companies, and voluntary health plans are often utilized for generating health data; how-ever, when they are so utilized caution must be exercised in generalizing findings from these specific groups to the larger population. Finally, the U.S. census provides much of the pop-ulation data necessary for the calculation of morbidity, mortality, and other rates.

EPIDEMIOLOGY

Public health and other health professionals frequently resort to the methods and strategies of epidemiology in their efforts to describe and explain the occurrence of disease in human populations. Epidemiologic studies are usually divided into several major classes: descrip-tive, analytic, and experimental. Descriptive epidemiology describes the *amount* and *distri-bution* of disease, injury, and death in population groups. Descriptive epidemiology permits a breakdown of morbidity and mortality rates by characteristics of person (e.g., sex, race), place (e.g., urban, rural), and time (e.g., spring fall). Thus descriptive data indicate *who* is most likely to be affected by a certain condition, *where,* and *when*. These data also aid in the rational planning of health services, and they provide clues to disease etiology. For example, the association between tooth decay and the amount of flouride ions in drinking water was suggested by descriptive studies showing variation in the rates of dental caries by geographic regions.[5]

Analytic epidemiology goes beyond description, attempting to explain disease in terms of cause and effect. There are two classes of analytic studies, case-control studies and cohort studies, both involving the testing of specific hypotheses.* In case-control studies the re-searcher selects a group of patients with a disease (cases) and a group free of the disease (controls). The groups are matched on important variables such as age, sex, and race. The researcher then goes back in time to determine if the groups differ in past exposure to some

---

*Case-control studies are also referred to as retrospective studies, cohort studies as prospective studies.

suspected causal variable (Table 2). One such study has shown, for example, that women between the ages of 15 and 44, with thromboembolic disease, were more likely than controls to have been users of oral contraceptives.[6]

The cohort study, on the other hand, begins with a sample of people free of the disease under investigation. Individuals in the sample are classified according to their exposure to a suspected casual factor (e.g., users of oral contraceptives vs. nonusers). The subjects are then followed over a certain time period in which we compare the incidence rates of the disease (e.g., thromboembolic disease) in the exposed and nonexposed groups. The case-control study tells us what proportion of a diseased and nondiseased group experienced past exposure to a suspected cause. The cohort study tells us what proportion of an exposed and non-exposed group will develop the disease. The latter is generally considered more valuable health information.

Experimental epidemiology also involves the formulation of an hypothesis. Subjects in this type of research are randomly assigned to an experimental or control group by the research. Where randomization cannot be carried out matching may be employed. The two procedures have the same goal: to assure the similarity of subjects in both groups. The researcher then exposes the experimental group to the experimental (casual) variable, while the control group is typically given a placebo. Differences in outcome between groups may then be attributed, with varying degrees of probability, to differences in exposure to the experimental variable. The Salk field trials of polio vaccine, in which thousands of children were given either the vaccine or a placebo, constitute a major example of experimental epidemiology.[7] Although experimentation is considered the best test of cause-effect relationships, ethical and practical considerations frequently preclude its use on human population groups. In such cases the researcher must resort to one of the other research methods that, to a greater or lesseer extent, approximate true experimentation.

PUBLIC HEALTH AND THE PHARMACIST

This section deals with some of the ways pharmacy and public health interrelate. To begin with, because of its depth and scope, the undergraduate education offered by most pharmacy schools provides an excellent background for the pharmacist who would like to pursue graduate work in the field of public health. Programs in public health schools usually fall into two broad areas: administrative (e.g., hospital administration) and scientific (e.g., epidemiology). In short, the B.S. degree in pharmacy should allow the holder of that degree to enter one of a number of programs in these areas. Furthermore, a pharmacist with a public health degree need not necessarily leave the field of pharmacy. Training in health planning, for example, could readily lend itself to the planning of pharmaceutical facilities, manpower, and services. In the like manner, a pharmacist-epidemiologist could apply the methods of epidemiology to the study of drug use and abuse. Conversely, since drugs play such an important part in the overall health care system, some public health students could benefit by taking relevant courses in schools of pharmacy.

In the employment area we again see the interaction of pharmacy and public health. Pharmacists currently function in public health agencies at all levels of government. On the federal level the USPHS employs pharmacists both as career officers and as Civil Service employees. In fact, the Indian Health Service, a branch of the USPHS, has probably gone farther than any other agency in using pharmacists as providers of a wide range of primary care services.[1] In the author's own County of Allegheny, Pa., a pharmacist is now the health officer for one of the Health Department's most active districts. Skolaut has provided a very good summary of employment opportunities for pharmacists in the government.[2]

In Public Health and Community Medicine, by Burton and Smith, there is considerable comment on the public health role of the practicing pharmacist.[3] Much of that role is actually an elaboration on the behavior expected in good pharmacy practice. For example, the pharmacist is cited as an important community resource person on drug related matters. Familiarity with the local people also enables the pharmacist to function as a valuable resource person to researchers conducting epidemiologic studies in the community. Health education is cited as another activity common to both public health and pharmacy. When counseling patients on their medication regimen the pharmacist is actually engaging in health education. Furthermore, pharmacies themselves can be used for the distribution of printed material on health related matters.

Burton and Smith feel the pharmacist could provide an additional needed service by explaining to patients what benefits they might be entitled to under current health legislation. This is especially important with elderly and poor patients. Today some pharmacists are even using the pharmacy as a screening center for conditions such as high blood pressure and diabetes. Screeming, of course, has long been an important public health tool. On the organizational level the American Public Health Association and the American Pharmaceutical Association are addressing themselves to issues of common concern. Finally, it is suggested that pharmacists participate more in the activities of local health groups and official health agencies, perhaps by serving on various committees and boards.

These, then, are a few ways in which pharmacists can contribute—and are contributing—to the health and welfare of their patients and the community. In the final analysis, public health is as much an attitude as it is a concept.

REFERENCES

1. Matiella A, Nease KO, and Caplan MF: Portrait of a pharmacy primary care program. JAPhA NS16:455, 1976
2. Skolaut MW: Pharmacists in government. In: Remington's Pharmaceutical Sciences. Ed 15. Easton, PA, 1975, pp 47–53
3. Burton LE, and Smith HH: Public Health and Community Medicine for the Allied Medical Professions. Baltimore, The Williams & Wilkins Co., 1975

THE ROLE OF THE PHARMACIST IN PUBLIC HEALTH[b]

Policy Statement 8024(PP) of the American Public Health Association

I. STATEMENT OF THE PROBLEM

Currently, the pharmacist's role is expanding beyond the traditional product-oriented functions of dispensing and distributing medicines and health supplies. It is generally recognized that those patients who have had medicines prescribed for them have benefited, directly or indirectly, from the services of the pharmacist. However, the pharmacist's services

[b]Reprinted with permission from Am J Public Health 1981;71:213–215.

of today include more patient-oriented, administrative and, in some cases public health functions as well. The general public, public health agencies, health planning bodies, and other health institutions involved with public health give small consideration to these types of pharmacists' services. When consideration is given, it is usually to the product, rather than the patient-oriented or public health aspect of the role.

II. PURPOSE

Because of these factors, and the need to maximize the use of existing health care professionals and facilities, a need has developed to define the role of the pharmacist in public health and to assure productive interchanges between pharmacists and other public health professionals.

III. POSITIONS AND RECOMMENDATIONS

To provide leadership and guidance in identifying and promoting the pharmacist's role in public health, the American Public Health Association, as an initial step, developed this document to: 1) identify the current and future roles for pharmacists in public health; 2) provide essential background information about these roles; and 3) describe means of implementing or maximizing these functions.

A. Role Recognition

There is no formal group known as public health pharmacists as there are public health physicians and nurses. Nevertheless, there are some pharmacists engaged in public health activities. Many of these pharmacists do not recognize they are doing public health work.

It is the position taken here that the public will be better served if pharmacists take a greater role in public health, and that this is more likely to come about if the public health role of the pharmacist is clearly defined, recognized, and encouraged by public health agencies and pharmacy educators. Although the pharmacist has the basic health knowledge on which to build and is often uniquely sited in the community to provide public health services, there are historic reasons why the pharmacist rarely thinks of him or herself, or is thought of by others, in association with public health.

B. Public Health Education of Pharmacists

In the past, medicine was disease-oriented, turning in recent years to a patient-orientation. A parallel situation in pharmacy has been an historic drug product orientation with a recent emphasis on patient and interprofessional relationships. However, unlike pharmacy, some medicine and nursing educators long ago recognized that the traditional health model, whether disease- or patient-oriented, failed in terms of public health because of its inherent inability to take a population perspective. Their solution was to develop the special schools and departments which teach public courses and train public health professionals.

Pharmacy educators have failed to teach public health and to provide role models for pharmacy students in public health at either the macro or the micro level. There are few courses devoted solely to public health in pharmacy, and no textbook emphasizing the role of pharmacy in public health. Neither the American Council on Pharmaceutical Education Guidelines, nor the 1978 Report of the Committee for Establishing Standards for Undergraduate Education in Pharmacy Administration of the American Association of Colleges of Pharmacy have sections specifically devoted to public health.

C. Levels of Pharmacist Public Health Activity

At a micro level, public health service is relatively direct as compared to the macro or planning, evaluating, and administrative level. For example, a community pharmacist who speaks to community groups about drug abuse and provides hypertension screening in his or her pharmacy is providing public health services at the micro level, whereas a pharmacist who is the drug program administrator at a state Medicaid program is providing services at the macro level. At the micro level, public health activities may be considered as a role among a pharmacist's set of roles. Because the low expectation among the public that a community pharmacist's role should include public health activities, a pharmacist is still viewed as a pharmacist despite failure to perform public health activities. When a pharmacist works on the macro level of health planning, evaluation, and administration, then his/her identity as a pharmacist may be lost.

It is primarily the macro level of public health that has been ignored by pharmacy educators in their attempt to expose students to public health. Moreover, the community pharmacist who is involved in public health activities is so rare that relatively few pharmacists are available as public health role models.

The failure at the macro level may be the most damaging for the public, for having pharmacists at the macro level may be critical for having them perform public health activities at the micro level. At the macro level they can address the problem of incentives for pharmacists to perform micro level public health activities. Macro level public health pharmacists who are knowledgeable about the training and abilities of pharmacists, and who understand the health care systems, interprofessional relationships, health economics, and the public's needs, can plan system level changes to provide incentives to community pharmacists to perform public health activities, particularly alternatives to the traditional fee-for-product system. Moreover, at the macro level, there are many functions of health agencies that can benefit directly from pharmacists' unique expertise.

D. Public Health Agency Mission

As defined in 1976 by the Milbank Memorial Fund Commission on Higher Education for Public Health, "Public Health is the effort organized by society to protect, promote, and restore the people's health. The programs, services, and institutions involved emphasize the prevention of disease and the health needs of the population as a whole." A public health agency carries out this mission on four fronts:

1. *Public health service delivery,* filling the most critical gaps in the community's health service delivery system;
2. *The environment,* protecting the community against environmental health hazards;
3. *The community health care provider system,* assisting and reinforcing that system in responding to the health needs of the people; and
4. *The consumer,* assisting individuals to achieve optimal health status through more ef-

fective use of the provider system and activation of medical self-help principles in daily life.

Furthermore, the agency must be capable of program evaluation to assure that its mission is attained, and that each service component contributes in a cost beneficial manner.

Opportunity exists on each of the "fronts" for inclusion of most health care provider types. The inclusion of a particular profession depends on demonstrating that the profession's potential contribution is unique, on target and cost beneficial in performing the agency's mission.

E. Public Health and Pharmacists' Services

Public health as interpreted today may be viewed broadly as a set of functions:

1. Planning for health care for wide geographic areas or communities;
2. Managing, administering, and evaluating health care programs, systems, and facilities;
3. Providing direct personal health care service (including health education, maternal and child health, etc.) and environmental health;
4. Developing and promoting legislation, and deriving regulations pertaining to the public's health, and
5. Training health care workers needed to carry out these functions.

These broad functions may be carried out by individuals, systems, and facilities organized by governmental agencies, by private individuals, and communities, and encompass both macro and micro level activities.

There is little to suggest there has been public health encouragement of the pharmacist's full expertise in these areas. In a few instances, pharmacists have asserted themselves and have established a functional capacity in public health, but these are the exceptions rather than the rule.

Health Planning and the Pharmacist

Component

In divising plans to meet the health care needs of specific geographic areas or communities, health planners and planning organizations must address issues such as:

- expenditures for drugs and payment sources,
- location and use of health care facilities and providers,
- strategies for health improvement, and
- health problems of the community.

Community pharmacists are an underutilized source of factual and anecdotal health data which could assist health planners as they seek to meet the needs uncovered by each issue.

Implementation

Pharmacists, along with other health practitioners, can join with health planning bodies to seek answers to these needs, as was recently demonstrated successfully in North Carolina.

Health planning bodies can also initiate relationships with local pharmacy organizations to provide epidemiological data on prescribing patterns, patterns of illness, and various socio-economic factors related to prevalent disease states. A community pharmacist can be strategic in assisting health surveys, and in advising people about and referring them to public health services.

Health Care Management and Pharmacists

Component

Health Care system managers, administrators, and evaluators are intimately involved on a day-to-day basis with assuring appropriate organization of services to meet patient needs and demands. The distribution of drugs and supplies is only part of a pharmacist service that should be included in the health care system management program. The day-to-day needs of patients and health team members for drug related information and consultation must also be considered in the organization of health care services.

At present, most health care organizations only encompass the product-oriented aspect of the pharmacist's role and define his/her services as an administrative function. This organizational structure ignores the needs of the health team to benefit from the drug knowledge of the pharmacist and forces a pharmacist who provides such knowledge to burden the intra-organization communications system. Inclusion of pharmacist services in the clinical services subsystem permits full interaction and use of his or her expertise. In this manner, pharmacists may contribute to the system's management function by providing appropriate management information (e.g., the number and cost of prescriptions dispensed), and to the needs of the system to provide health care.

Pharmacists may manage as well as work in health programs, as is the case in Allegheny County, Pennsylvania, where a pharmacist is the Health Officer for one of the Health Department's most active districts. The pharmacist with the MPH degree is particularly well qualified to manage, administer, and evaluate public health programs, particularly those involving abusable substances and medicines, and those requiring the cooperation of community pharmacists.

Implementation

Public health agencies providing personal health services should be encouraged to include patient care activities of the pharmacist as part of their medical care organizational subsystems to permit greater interaction with patients and participation with other health professionals in providing clinical services.

Personal and Environmental Health Care Services and the Pharmacist

Component

In the personal health services component of public health, drugs are used as the most frequent therapeutic modality. Consequently, there is a need for prescribers and those who administer medicines to maintain up-to-date information on drugs and therapeutics. There is also a need to provide counseling to patients to assist in increasing compliance with therapeutic regimens, and to assure that medicines are taken properly. These needs, coupled with the need for primary care practitioners in underserved areas, point to the greater use of the pharmacist.

A pharmacist currently contributes to personal health services as part of an organized system or from a freestanding support base—a community pharmacy. Many inpatient and ambulatory care programs have added a clinical pharmacy segment to the traditional distribution function. Pharmacists now function in medical screening clinics, in the medical management of chronic disease states, and in minor disease diagnosis and treatment, often to protocols and after additional training. In the community pharmacy, pharmacists provide rehabilitation support to individuals and organizations by giving advice on the use and selection of ostomy and other surgical appliances and equipment. The literature is replete with examples of the pharmacist functioning in hypertensive and colorectal screening, venereal disease control and contraception programs, and providing health education, not to mention the role in over-the-counter (OTC) drug choice and use. In rural areas, the pharmacists have supported environmental programs such as water pollution control, sanitation, and waste disposal.

Implementation

Health planning agencies, public health education programs, and health departments need to give greater recognition and provide greater liaison to these activities performed for the public's good. Two public health agencies—Sacremento County, California and Multnomah County, Oregon—are known to use pharmacists in these areas.

Health Legislation, Regulation and the Pharmacist

Component

The promulgation of public health legislation and subsequent regulation is not a field generally associated with the pharmacist's public health role. But there are myriad concerns which legislators and those in regulatory agencies address relating to the pharmacist's role in public health and the products they dispense. However, legislators and those who form the regulations need testimony, data, and feedback on pending and implemented laws and regulations. Through professional associations and, at times, through individual professionals, pharmacists provide background data, legislative content and exposition to local, state and federal governments.

Many local, state and federal agencies have begun to recognize the need for pharmacist input. At the federal level, pharmacists are employed in such agencies as the National Center for Health Services Research (NCHSR), the Health Care Financing Administration (HCFA), the Food and Drug Administration (FDA), Veterans Administration, US Public Health Service, Office of Technology Assessment, and the Bureau of Health Manpower. Pharmacists at the state and local levels are employed in administering the drug component of Medicaid programs, as well as regulating the practice of pharmacy.

Implementation

Local, state and federal agencies should recognize the role of the pharmacist at the macro and micro levels in contributing to the public's health, and should identify mechanisms to include pharmacist's participation in legislation and regulation.

Pharmacists and the Training of Public Health Workers

Component

Because of the roles of drugs in modern medical care, most health professionals are trained in methods and issues related to their role and its relationship to drugs. Nurses, physicians, physician assistants, nurse practitioners, dentists, nutritionists, and other health workers need varying degrees of information related to drug therapy and pharmacists need information about the public health role of each of these disciplines. Pharmacists of today are actively teaching physician assistants, nurses, and physicians techniques of prescribing and issues related to the drug use process. Information about drugs is taught through the mechanisms of in-service training, newsletters, seminars, courses in nursing and medical schools, and continuing education.

Implementation

As schools of public health update curricula, they should be encouraged to expose their students to the contribution pharmacists make to public health and the training of public health workers, and to encourage pharmacists to obtain the MPH and the DrPH degrees in Schools of Public Health.

IV. DESIRED ACTION

As discussed in this paper, the pharmacist's role is expanding to include more patient-oriented and public health functions. In order to facilitate further development in this area, the APHA is urged to take the following desired action:

1. To support the inclusion of pharmacists in the composition of the team of primary care practitioners;
2. To support the inclusion of pharmacists in the definition of public health practitioners:
3. To encourage the inclusion of public health concepts in the curricula of schools of pharmacy; and
4. In its communication with health planning agencies, schools of public health, schools of pharmacy, and public health agencies, disseminate the important information discussed in this position paper.

14
Unresolved Issues

CHARLES D. HEPLER

> God, give us grace to accept with serenity the things that cannot be changed, courage to change the
> things which should be changed, and the wisdom to distinguish the one from the other.
>
> Reinhold Niebuhr

Although people sometimes think of time as a single line leading to a single future, it is perhaps more useful to think of alternative futures, for the future depends on many forces. Many of these forces are beyond the control of even large groups of people, for example, a professional association, or, for that matter, the population of a nation. One must accept and adapt to changes wrought by such forces. Some forces can be shaped but not controlled, and a few can perhaps actually be controlled.

The present is but a freeze frame from an endless interplay of complex forces. The hottest unresolved issues of pharmacy (for example, in 1988, expansion of hospitals into ambulatory care, mail order and "deep discount" prescription services, physician dispensing, the entry-level Pharm. D.) are simply dimensions and details within those still pictures. Every individual may understand the unfolding story and respond to those forces as he/she chooses, but the future will turn out a little bit differently for each, depending on those choices. Some may see the story as a chaotic rock video filled with related but unconnected impressions. Careful examination may, however, dimly reveal an underlying structure. To the extent that structures can be seen, wisdom and courageous action can change the future, not necessarily by changing the forces themselves but by changing the effect of those forces.

Our society is now entering a great transformation, the "information revolution," the like of which has not been seen in our lifetimes. The last such social and economic shift was the industrialization of America. Over a mere 100 years, America changed from a rural, agricultural nation to an urban, industrial nation. During this period, an entire agricultural way of life was replaced by an industrial way of life: new social institutions like the central banking system, the professions, and labor unions arose, and new concepts of finance (commercial paper), society (the consumer), organizing (bureaucracy), and commerce (merchandising) were invented. These changes were accompanied by conflict, as represented in this country by the American Civil War and resistance to organized labor. Elsewhere—in France, Russia, Japan, and China—governments were overthrown to allow industrialization.

Industrialization did not burst on the American scene in 1800 in full flower. It had begun in England many years earlier and penetrated America gradually. Likewise, the shift to an information-based economy may have begun some years ago. Naisbitt (1) would mark the "turning point" in 1956–1957, when the number of white collar (information) workers first outnumbered blue collar workers. "Now more than 60% of us work with information . . . ," and "only 13 percent of our labor force is engaged in manufacturing . . ." (1). In

1981, AT&T grossed $58 billion, some on information hardware, some on services. In 1984, revenues of IBM were 50% greater than those of the entire United States steel industry (2).

Steelworkers, automobile workers, and others employed in traditional industrial jobs already are being laid off despite periods of general economic growth. A major point of contention between the United Automobile Workers and the "big three" automobile manufacturers in their 1987 contract negotiations was job security in the face of automation. The "sunbelt" is growing and the industrial North is becoming the "rustbelt," perhaps on its way to a rebirth in computer manufacturing and information-related occupations. According to a 1987 story in the *Chronicle of Higher Education,* the United States Department of Labor estimates that 6 million new executive, professional, and technical jobs will open up in the next decade, compared to 1 million in unskilled and laborer categories (3).

The Pharmacy in the 21st Century Conference (P21C) (4) considered four alternative socioeconomic scenarios of which the future of pharmacy will be a part. They were called the "continued growth," "decline and stagnation," "disciplined society," and "transformation" scenarios. Almost half of the participants at P21C chose the "continued growth" scenario as most likely. "Disciplined society," "transformation," and mixed scenarios each got about 15%, while "decline and stagnation" got about 8% (5). This essay assumes a mixture of two of them, the "continued growth" and "transformed society" scenarios. It will assume that the United States economy will continue to grow and prosper over the next quarter century, leading to material plenty (some would say overabundance). In addition, some people will choose, in the midst of plenty, to simplify their lives and will seek spiritual, emotional, and intellectual growth as much as or more than additional material things.

The major forces shaping the future of pharmacy can be classified into three groups: technology, economics, and social values and institutions. The following analysis of the effect of those forces on pharmacy will suggest that pharmacy can best respond to these forces by expanding the informational component of pharmacy practice and by returning to its fundamental relationship with society—that is, by accepting responsibility for what Brodie has called drug use control (6). In order to do that, pharmacy must go through a process of occupational reconstruction (7) and self-renewal.

TECHNOLOGICAL FORCES

There are three types of technology shaping medical care in general and pharmacy practice in particular: computers and robots, communications, and therapy. Computers have already increased pharmacists' productivity per man-hour. Hospitals are adopting computerized medical records, including drug records. Microcomputers like the personal computer and minicomputers for small offices are moving into more and more medical practices.

Once prescription information exists in electronic form in the doctor's office, it can be communicated electronically. The paper prescription becomes, if not actually obsolete, just one alternative means of communicating. Once prescriptions can be communicated to the pharmacy electronically, they can be communicated to another computer, which can further process that prescription. This would be feasible today, for example, for typing prescription labels. Further prescription processing may be possible in the future.

The last major technological barrier to an actual robotic drug dispenser was the capacity of a machine to "see" the identity of the drug being dispensed. Practical optical input devices like bar code readers have removed that barrier. Pharmacy robots are in use in Japan, and prototypes are being tested in the United States. Automated prescription fillers or hospital drug cart fillers will tend to further increase pharmacy productivity and would reduce demand for pharmacists unless offset by increased numbers of prescriptions.

Communications technology (either computer links or magnetic cards like the debit cards in use now) can eliminate the information barriers that seem to block some important parts of clinical pharmacy (specifically, evaluation of drug appropriateness) in the usual drugstore setting. Major personal privacy issues surely will be raised by proposals to put medical records on pocket cards or to routinely transmit them over telephone lines. The resolution of those issues may be crucial for pharmacy. If pharmacists are seen chiefly as drug merchants, then their access to diagnostic and other information may be limited or denied, thus institutionalizing the pharmacist in that role, i.e., as a supervisor of robots. Public officials have not always seen pharmacy as more than a drug business. The most famous example was Warren Burger's comparison of the dispensing pharmacist to a clerk selling books. Just as the clerk need not have read the books he sells, he said, the pharmacist can sell drugs even if he knows little about them (8).

The specific unresolved issues related to computing and communications technology are, then, as follows: (a) whether pharmacists can add value to the medical care process beyond drug dispensing, more specifically whether they add value beyond the capacity of computerized decision making; and (b) whether they will gain access to the patient information needed to add that value. Resolution of the second issue depends on the opinion of the public and its policy makers about the value of pharmacy as related to the pharmacist's "need to know" full information about the conditions for which the drug is prescribed. Each of these has related economic and social issues and will come up again in later sections.

The third technologic subgroup is therapeutics. Smith has written of a "second pharmacological revolution" based on intracellular chemistry, genetics, and immunology (9). Check (9) has summarized major new drug groups that may arise from new understanding of prostaglandins, hormones, monoclonal antibodies, immunomodulators, and neurotransmitters. There may be new vaccines. New drug delivery systems or dosage forms are being developed, for example, implantable sustained release polymers and pumps. Specialized carrier molecules and liposomes will carry drug agents to their site of action before releasing and activating them. Many of these new drugs and dosage forms will replace traditional drug therapy. Many will require new expertise and new services.

The issue here is quite fundamental: whether pharmacy will be asked to distribute these new technologies to end users. It is not safe to assume that pharmacists will automatically be given this responsibility. Radiopharmaceuticals are an example of a technology that seems obviously a part of pharmacy to some pharmacists but which is often managed in hospitals by nonpharmacists, often through departments of nuclear medicine. Monoclonal antibodies, for example, might well enter the hospital through a hematology department rather than through the pharmacy.

This issue obviously depends on the education of pharmacists in the sciences of immunology, immunopharmacology, and genetics and their expertise in providing professional services for new therapies. Pharmaceutical education (faculty and students) should seriously address the educational preparation necessary for controlling the use of new-tech therapies. In particular, it seems necessary to avoid mislabeling proposals for *new* basic science teaching, which, for example, may reduce emphasis on older disciplines in favor of newer ones like genetics or immunology, as antiscience proposals.

Education, although necessary, may not be sufficient by itself to ensure a major role for pharmacy in new-tech therapies. The issue also may depend on the relationship between pharmacy and the originators of new therapeutic agents. The originators may seek a channel through which to introduce a new product. Because the new product might fail if not used correctly, they would want a channel that could provide services to ensure the proper use of the product. Pharmacy should consider offering its services to the high-tech companies that are developing these new treatment modalities.

A somewhat less fundamental issue is the effect of new dosage forms and delivery systems on "prescription volume." Many new delivery systems allow infrequent dosing, e.g., monthly. This may combine with robotics to reduce the demand for traditional prescription services.

ECONOMICS

Medical care has traditionally been considered a special commodity in this country, one outside the normal business environment. Medical care decisions have traditionally been between the professional and his/her patient (with, perhaps, limited suggestions from any third party who might have to pay the bill). This has been seriously reconsidered in light of the increasing proportion of the national wealth that has been flowing to the health professions, especially since passage of Medicare and Medicaid in 1965.

In a macro view, health and medical care expenditures in the United States during 1985 reached $425 billion, up 9% from 1984, and up 71% in 5 years. In 1983, such expenditures represented 10.5% of the Gross National Product (GNP) (the value of all of the goods and services produced in the United States) and the proportion is rising. (In comparison, construction represented only 4% of GNP in 1983.) The United States spends more on health care than it does on defense. Individual Americans spend more annually on health care than they do on automobiles and gasoline (10). The consumer price index—a measure of inflation—increased by 3.8% in 1983 for all consumer items, by 6.3% for all medical care, and by 9.2% for a hospital room. Some of this is hidden in the costs of other goods and services. For example, a new car may be said to contain more health care than steel, for automobile manufacturers spend more for the fringe benefit of employee health care than they spend for steel. Some have focused on the supply side, asking if drug manufacturers, physicians, and other health professionals really should receive as much of the national treasure as they do.

Health economists, sociologists, businessmen, and professionals have analyzed the system and found it deficient in many regards (11, 12). Two deficiencies pertinent to this discussion are fee-for-service payment and direct purchase of medical services by patients. Two important changes are aimed at these deficiencies.

First, employers, labor unions, and government are experimenting with ways to shift medical care purchase decisions away from the doctor, the patient, or a relative. A simple example is the preadmission approval or "second opinion" required by many medical care plans. A more extensive idea is called "managed care," in which a representative of the individual who will actually pay the bill has a right to participate in medical decisions. This can extend to "third party purchase" (distinguished from third party payment, in which the payer is more passive) in which the program will authorize care only from providers who have agreed to specific prices or conditions such as care management. Third party purchase lends itself well to competitive bidding by would-be providers.

The other major idea is to pay for results (outcomes) instead of efforts (inputs). The familiar cost-plus (fee-for-service) method pays for inputs (hospital days, laboratory tests, office visits, prescriptions). A provider can increase income by selling more units of service, e.g., hospital days. Under output-based payment, the provider gets an amount that does not depend on how much it spent. The most familiar example is the system of Diagnosis Related Group (DRG) payments to hospitals under Medicare. In this system, the hospital gets paid a specific amount based on the patient's diagnosis, complexity, and so on, but not based on how much the hospital spent. In other words, the DRG system pays for outcomes, not inputs.

Another version of payment for outputs is capitation, in which a provider is paid a fixed amount per time period (usually a month) for providing specified goods and services to a patient. This combines the concept of a contract for care, described above, with the concept of paying a fixed dollar amount. Fixed-dollar payment puts the contractor at financial risk and requires that he or she limit the cost of providing care in a way that is the opposite of our familiar fee-for-service or cost-plus reimbursement system.

The combination of provider contracts and fixed-dollar payment may cause a consolidation of service providers. First, some hospitals, clinics, doctors, pharmacists, etc. may be unable to compete. In a market with excess capacity (e.g., too many pharmacies), providers may simply disappear. In markets without excess capacity, the providers probably will become employees or otherwise become part of larger organizations. Second, for efficiency, large purchasers might prefer to negotiate contracts with large, comprehensive providers rather than with hundreds of solo practitioners. Third, certain cost-shifting tactics are possible under capitation if different providers have responsibility for different stages of care. For example, a hospital paid under DRGs or capitation might be tempted to discharge a patient a bit too early if discharge makes the patient somebody else's responsibility. A comprehensive provider who has contracted for almost all aspects of care (inpatient, outpatient, and preventive) would have less to gain from such tactics.

These two cost reduction strategies raise a number of issues for pharmacy. The fundamental question is, of course, how far and how fast they will spread. This is unpredictable, especially because they can be implemented locally, e.g., by a labor union or large employer. Any large or small segment of the American health care market, even a community or individual market, can develop its own structure and reimbursement methods in its own time.

Given that a particular market does restructure along the general lines described above, the crucial economic issue for pharmacists in that market will be whether the managers of comprehensive health care corporations, e.g., health maintenance organizations (HMOs), see pharmacy as a part of the overhead cost of doing business (e.g., housekeeping expense) or as part of the production of medical care. In one possible scenario, pharmacy is seen merely as part of overhead, perhaps as a primarily legal requirement of doing business. In this view, the management of a comprehensive health care provider would wish to include only minimal amounts of pharmaceutical services. Existing pharmaceutical services would be cut to the bone to lower costs and meet competition. This scenario is one of continued decline for pharmacy. Present trends toward mass production prescription filling (as symbolized today by discount drugstores and mail-order prescription service) would continue to increase market share. Later, dispensing robots might be used. One economic disadvantage of robots is that they require organized information and large volumes to be efficient, but if providers will be consolidating anyway, for the reasons outlined above, there may be sufficient volume. Obviously, in this scenario of the future, technicians and robots will displace pharmacists from their jobs.

In a second scenario, pharmacy is understood to be part of the production of medical services, i.e., to be able to influence patient outcome in some significant way. In this scenario, pharmaceutical services would not be endlessly chiseled away, although they might become more efficient. Medical care program managers, convinced that drug use control ("clinical") services can reduce length of stay, number of hospital admissions, or number of physician visits, would not focus on the cost of pharmaceutical service but rather on its consequences. They would understand that simple dispensing services without adequate clinical services would be penny wise and pound foolish. They might want to expand such services, to help the health care corporation compete. In this scenario, technicians and robots would liberate pharmacists from routine mechanical tasks, giving them more time for judgmental and creative drug use control tasks.

A series of relatively specific issues arise from these scenarios. The first major issue for pharmacy is its ability to market itself as a valuable part of medical care. This seems to be the central issue of pharmacy's future. First, and most importantly, marketing to health care managers and corporate benefits managers will require objective evidence[a] that adding pharmaceutical services to the medical care process results in lowered total cost at equivalent or better levels of care. There is already significant evidence of program effectiveness for inpatient pharmacy services, although not all is in economic terms. There is less evidence for organized outpatient services and virtually none for drugstore practice (13, 14). More evidence is needed, especially cost-effectiveness evidence for ambulatory care pharmacy. In addition, this information needs to be better communicated, not only to medical care program managers, but to pharmacy managers as well.

A second part of such marketing is a clear description of the product: what services are part of "clinical pharmacy" or "drug use control." Third, an independent pharmacist seeking a contract for care with a capitation-paid provider would need to develop a payment method that included financial risk sharing, not fee-for-service. In other words, pharmacy should be ready to accept responsibility for the consequences of its services, not merely to market a group of functions called "clinical pharmacy."

A second major issue arising from the economic scenarios presented above concerns interprofessional relationships. Other occupations, especially nursing and physicians' assistants, probably will be seeking larger roles in the new health care system. Some of their objectives may overlap with some of the objectives of pharmacy, for example, treatment of minor medical conditions and drug prescribing. At the same time, medicine seems to be experiencing shrinking autonomy along with increasing numbers. It may resist attempts by other occupations to expand into its "turf." First, pharmacy should realistically assess the strength of its evidence for efficacy in drug use control. Second, pharmacy should try to identify the new gatekeepers in medicine, for there is no reason to suppose that medicine will be allowed to decide on everyone else's functions. Third, pharmacy should seek alliances with other occupations, especially nursing, in pursuit of common long-term goals. It should most certainly avoid petty or short-term disputes, as have occurred in some states (e.g., Virginia) where pharmacy fought prescribing by clinical nurses instead of asking to be included.

A third issue for pharmacy in the comprehensive health care corporation is ethical. Professions traditionally give their primary loyalty to the client or patient, and secondarily to their professional colleagues. The business ethic demands loyalty to the corporation, ultimately to its owners (stockholders), but often in practice to its managers. As health and medical care become more "businesslike," more employed professionals may experience

---

[a]Objective evidence does not necessitate absolute proof. Few professions can actually prove the value of their services.

ethical dilemmas. Many of these may be expressed as questions of professional autonomy ("Don't I have a right to decide what is best for my patient?"), professional self-regulation ("Can a nonpharmacist judge my work?") or collegiality ("Do I have to keep 'trade secrets' when I talk to my colleagues?"). There is evidence that occupations like pharmacy can continue to professionalize in large bureaucratic organizations if the professionals are insulated from some aspects of the bureaucracy (15, 16). At the same time, there is hope that the concept of bureaucratic organization may change as corporate managers and scholars come to terms with the information revolution (17).

A fourth issue concerns the structural integrity of pharmacy. It has two parts: (*a*) whether pharmacy can avoid serious internal divisions (civil war) resulting from economic hardship, and (*b*) whether it can produce enough competent clinical pharmacists to make an impact on the market. If the market for medical care services in a community reorganizes according to the economic scenario described above, some drugstores will lose patients to HMOs, hospital outpatient clinics, etc. In microscopic business-oriented terms, this might appear as cutthroat competition rather than the result of major economic forces. Drugstore owners might be tempted to fight rather than switch, diverting essential time and effort into political lobbying or destructive battles within the profession. The second aspect is actually closely related: the issue of whether there are enough clinically competent pharmacists in a community to effectively deliver on the promise of pharmacy's cost effectiveness. The future of pharmacy depends to a large extent on devising ways to organize subprofessionals (technicians) and pharmacists at different skill levels into effective patient care teams and how to rapidly retrain existing pharmacists to sharpen their clinical skills. This may require new partnerships between practitioners and educators. A set of educational issues has been addressed elsewhere (18).

SOCIAL FORCES

First, and most obviously, the population characteristics of the United States are changing. The proportion of elderly in the population is increasing from approximately 11% in 1980 to perhaps 25% by 2020. The female proportion of the population increases with increasing age.

If the baby boom started in 1945, then the first baby boomers will become "senior citizens" in 2010. This group, which has been described as a bulge moving through American history ["a pig passing through a python" (19)], made society feel its wants in its infancy (Dr. Spock), its childhood (GI Joe and Barbie dolls), its adolescence (lowering the drinking age), and its young adulthood (raising the drinking age). When they retire, they will again make their presence known to the rest of the nation.

One specific issue for pharmacy is whether the drug therapy of the elderly, which is usually more difficult than for younger patients, will be translated into increased demand for pharmaceutical services. It is tempting to suppose that this will occur, until one realizes that the American Association of Retired Persons has led campaigns promoting the use of generic equivalent drugs and operates a mail-order prescription service. These two issues, one opposed initially by many pharmacists, the other still opposed by most pharmacy organizations, demonstrate not only the obvious divergence of views but also, more importantly, the inability of pharmacy to meet the needs of many elderly patients. The poor quality of much drug therapy in nursing homes, a condition that is widely accepted although difficult to prove, raises the additional issue of the capacity and commitment of pharmacy to care for the elderly.

Second, priorities seem to be shifting, especially the balance between social cost and social benefit. Our society has begun to ask whether it really benefits more than it loses from some relatively new technological possibilities (e.g., genetic engineering, life-support technology, in vitro fertilization, surrogate motherhood) and is struggling with new ethical dilemmas. How, for example, do we continue to express reverence for life when we can technologically maintain both meaningful life and a hollow mockery of life? Is amniocentesis ethical if it may allow parents to abort a fetus for trivial causes, e.g., undesired gender?

Third, this country of rugged individualists is beginning to seriously consider rebalancing individual freedoms with group rights, for example in the areas of civil rights, pollution, and gun control. One medical example is the concept of health care as an individual right, which really entered with the Great Society. It has so far survived contemporary economic changes but has been limited in the name of public financial interest (see above). Another example is limitations of the treatments (e.g., transplants) that some institutions may provide. Government health programs will pay for some organ transplants only in approved hospitals, in effect asserting a public right to limit the freedom of hospitals to sell whichever services they wish.

A fourth area of important social change is the gradual weakening of rules and procedures as a means of influencing the behavior of individuals, especially at work (17, 20). Rules and procedures are typical of industrialization, and as our society moves into the postindustrial information era, it seems inevitable that some rules will not work as well anymore. We may not be able to invent new rules fast enough to keep up with change. Callahan has suggested that we will return to reliance on "good character" and intelligence, as preindustrial societies did (20).

A fifth social trend is the weakening of the relationship between the consulting professions and society. According to Larsen, the professions were created in response to the social and economic upheavals caused by the industrial revolution (21).[b] Services with three characteristics presented serious marketing problems both to providers and to prospective patients. Those characteristics were:

1. Closeness to fundamental values like health, property, spiritual grace;
2. Complexity beyond a layman's skill to evaluate, especially before the fact;
3. Inherent individualization, personalization.

Buying and selling valued, complex, and specific services requires trust between strangers. May sees the relationship between a professional and his/her client as a covenant, defined as the exchange of a gift and a promise, whereby the exchange alters the basic relationship between the parties (22). In a professional covenant, the professional promises competence (knowledge, skill, and appropriate attitudes of caring for the patient's welfare). In exchange, the patient grants the professional authority.

Starr writes that the patient can give two kinds of authority to the professional. First, the patient can follow the professional's directions. Second, and more importantly, the patient can accept the professional's interpretation of signs, symptoms, and circumstances. This in effect allows professions and professionals to create demand for their own services, something that businessmen are rarely if ever allowed to do, and only against significant public resistance.

The professional is expected to use this authority to make his or her living but must use it primarily to further the patient's valued interests, not his or her own. Covenants are volun-

---

[b]This discussion is developed in more detail in Ref. 15.

tary and fragile. If a patient begins to suspect that the professional is not bringing sufficient competence (including attitudes) to the exchange, he or she may begin to withdraw authority. This might at first be expressed as reduced compliance with the professional's instructions, which might in turn reduce the efficacy of the professional's regimen. Later, the patient might begin to resist accepting the professional's interpretations of signs and symptoms, for example, by requesting a second opinion.

An analogous process seems to occur in whole societies of patients and professionals, except that on a societal level, competence includes the additional requirement of sufficient numbers to make a meaningful impact on society's needs. Society can increase or decrease the amount of authority it grants to a profession, for example, through protective legislation like professional practice acts, based on how well that profession seems to protect society's interests.

Examples of this process are plentiful today. Medicine went through a period of very rapid increase in authority, justified by scientific progress, but is now well into a period in which society has been taking back authority, such as medicine's one-time absolute control over medical school admissions, licensure, and hospital privileges. The advent of "self-help" (home birthing, hospice, nonprescription drugs, etc.) was a stronger sign. *Medical Nemesis* (23), a book alleging that medicine was changing from a profession into an industry and misusing its authority, was just one of many scholarly warnings. Some in society today seem thoroughly disillusioned with the health professions, to the extent that they seem willing to replace them with business corporations and the market (see "Economics," p. 404).

There are two important applications to pharmacy. First, pharmacy has allowed itself to become a somewhat passive conduit for drug technology, adding too few valued, complex, and specific services. (Call this the issue of the professional standing of pharmacy.) Second, pharmacy has long been a confusing hybrid of business and profession. (Call this the issue of the occupational purpose of pharmacy.) Confusion about professional standing was addressed above, and it is sufficient here to say that public opinion eventually seems to find expression in free societies. The restructured market for health care, addressed above, may be a lens through which public opinion can be focused. The issue of the standing of pharmacy in the eyes of the public may indeed be more important than its prestige among health care managers.

Confusion about the purpose of pharmacy is more troublesome because the business and professional systems are theoretically incompatible, and there seems to be little discussion, let alone consensus, on this issue. The Dichter report found, years ago, that most of the people who viewed the pharmacist as a professional were elderly, and that the young tended to view pharmacy as a business (24). Pharmacy has seemed to make few or no substantive changes in response to that information. In fact, the image (and probably the reality) of pharmacist as businessman may have grown tremendously in recent years. The very reason for the existence of any profession is to serve the public interest, under a covenant (i.e., within moral bounds). In contrast, a business is expected to pursue its own interest, under contracts (i.e., within primarily legal bounds.) The trend in other professions toward reducing the professional covenant to a set of business contracts does not legitimize the hybrid status of pharmacy. Rather, it erodes the authority of other professions just as it has eroded that of pharmacy.

The issues for pharmacy and the other professions are how to renew their covenants in order to regain professional authority. It is necessary to convince the public that pharmacists accept a commitment to the welfare of individual patients. It is possible on the one hand that the reductionist trend has created irreversible cynicism among the public. On the other hand, it is possible that other social changes will create a strong, perceived need for protection and reassurance. The many social trends described so far might suggest a future somewhat along the following lines:

> Care includes awesome high-tech medical procedures. Many patients are elderly people whose families live elsewhere. Health professionals are employed by business corporations whose financial interest under capitation is to limit the amount of care provided. This care is given in a climate of confusion about individual rights, in which the old rules of behavior are not always observed.

This scenario points clearly to public demand for a technically competent occupation that is committed to patient advocacy. That is, of course, the original purpose for which the health professions were created. There is no compelling reason why pharmacy must accept this role, for other occupations, e.g., nursing, may be more developed in that direction. The alternatives for pharmacy, however, seem much less attractive.

The sixth social trend involves corporate responsibility for professional actions. Through the Darling decision and similar judicial decisions, hospitals and other health care corporations have been held responsible in part for the actions of professionals working within them as employees or even as "guests" (25, 26). A logical consequence of this may be some increase in corporate authority to determine who may perform certain professional duties, ranging beyond "credentialling" (ubiquitous today) to such things as corporate authorization of activities beyond usual limits (e.g., pharmacist prescribing by protocol).

The public issue is, of course, the need to increase flexibility in moving functions among occupations, balanced against the risks of allowing health care corporations to have a role in the process. The issue for pharmacy is the opportunity to expand its function through corporate mandate as well as legislation, balanced against the ethical problems of being employed by financially motivated corporations.

A final trend involves the reasons that people work. Naisbitt and Aburdene predict that the supply of adequately educated and skilled workers for information processing and personal service jobs will become more important than the supply of venture capital. There may be serious shortages of workers in many industries. In the "continued growth" and "transformed society" scenarios, these people will not necessarily be attracted by higher salaries alone. They may expect a greater voice in the organizations that employ them, and may choose jobs as much for their intrinsic worth as for their pay. Miller points to the competitive need to capture such workers' "discretionary time," time that management cannot overtly control. This may require quite dramatic changes in the structure and management of health care institutions. Within pharmacy, as robotics liberate many people from a preoccupation with repetitive, task-oriented jobs, the proportion of skilled knowledge workers will increase. A whole new management style may be needed (27).

CONVERGING FORCES

Having outlined some major forces and issues, it may be helpful to summarize and to consider how they may interact.

Computers and robots may displace rote procedural activities (e.g., cart filling, prescription filling) and predictable recall (e.g., basic drug dosages, drug interactions). They will not displace judgment, creative problem solving, or interpersonal skills. Communications technology may eliminate the information gap that separates "clinical" and "distributive" pharmacists. Drug distribution may eventually go largely to robots, but drug use control will remain a professional activity for a long time.

Changing therapeutic technology will require professional competence at the point of use to provide creative problem solving and interpersonal services.

The changing market will push many free-standing physicians, pharmacists, and other professionals into larger organizations, either as employees or contractors. It will make drug use control mandatory, because the provider who cannot control drug use may be unable to prevent drug-related morbidity and consequently be unable to control total costs. In a capitation-paid comprehensive care environment, economic survival will depend on the ability to make inexpensive care work, e.g., to keep people out of the hospital. The net effect may be the irresistible combination of pharmacy ideology (the philosophy of pharmaceutical care) with economic necessity.

Changing social structures, especially regarding allocation of scarce resources, exacerbated by a market-regulated health industry paid by capitation, where the old rules do not apply, will place a premium on interpersonal skills, not only in problem solving but in communicating with patients. There is no reason to believe that patients will trust large provider corporations in the future any more than they trust General Motors today. It seems important for the health professions to renew their commitment to the professional covenant.

The big issue for pharmacy in each of these is, of course, what part pharmacy will play. In the open, rapidly evolving early postindustrial society, new occupations will arise and old occupations will decline or die. It seems clear that traditional drugstore and drug distributive pharmacy cannot survive in that society.

PHARMACEUTICAL CARE: REPROFESSIONALIZATION OF PHARMACY

Given that American society is going though a major change in its economic and social structure, at least equal in magnitude to the industrial revolution, it should not be surprising that the health professions, which were born in the industrial revolution, may need to grow up to meet the needs of the postindustrial age. Pharmacy will inevitably be buffeted by forces beyond its control; without a plan, it may have little hope that the outcome will suit either its needs or the needs of society.

The reprofessionalization of pharmacy may involve the following four major issues: (*a*) the central activity of pharmacy; (*b*) the goal of reprofessionalization (whether to focus inward on philosophical issues or outward on the contribution of pharmacy to society); (*c*) the organizational structure for pharmacy, especially whether to construct the strongest possible core activity or to arrange strong specialties around a relatively weak core; and (*d*) marketing the new profession.

First, pharmacy should address the issue of its "social object," i.e., its central function in society. This issue has at least two dimensions. The first dimension concerns the type of activity that pharmacists perform for patients. Traditionally, that activity was dispensing pharmacy, principally emphasizing the providing of drug products. This was once a complex activity but has degenerated to a largely mechanical one. A second core activity arose in the late 1960s, as an antithesis to dispensing pharmacy. This activity, which I will call *clinical pharmacy* for want of a better term, emphasizes the providing of therapeutic drug information relevant to specific patients, but separate and distinct from drug products themselves.[c] Finally, there is the concept of *pharmaceutical care*. Pharmaceutical care is the

---

[c]This use of "clinical pharmacy" to denote professional services that are purely or predominantly informational is narrower than some uses of the term. This usage is consistent, however, with the usage of "clinical" as distinguished from "distributive," a common distinction nowadays. The term clinical pharmacy is also sometimes used to denote services that are here being called *pharmaceutical care* services.

synthesis of the two activities that historically preceded it. Pharmaceutical care is defined as a relationship between a patient and a pharmacist in which the pharmacist accepts responsibility for drug use control functions (6) and provides those services governed by awareness of, and commitment to, the patient's interests. In other words, pharmaceutical care marries the product and the information in a package of goods and services designed to suit the needs of individual patients. Its long-term goal is to reduce fragmentation between prescriber, advisor, and dispenser. Perhaps most would agree that pharmaceutical care is the most professional of the three alternatives, in the sense described above: it has the greatest value to society, requires the greatest complexity, and is inherently most personalized of the three activities. At issue is the process through which pharmacy will consider its purpose and what consensus it will reach. Hospital pharmacists have begun the process through a series of national, regional, state, and local conferences on the clinical role of pharmacy beginning in 1985 with the American Society of Hospital Pharmacists invitational conference at Hilton Head Island, SC.[d]

The second dimension of the "social object" issue involves the scope of pharmaceutical services. Society will be deciding how to gain access to new therapeutic modalities and new drug delivery systems, for example, monoclonal antibodies, immunomodulators, implantable pumps, while minimizing money costs and other risks. (Society's decisions here seem very similar to its historical relationship with the existing professions.) Correspondingly, the sponsors of this new technology will have to choose a channel of distribution that will optimize penetration into its potential market. Pharmacy has two decisions to make for each new technology. First, can pharmacy increase its value to society by controlling the use of that particular new technology, or will trying to control the new technology have too high an opportunity cost? Will the new technology simply distract pharmacy from more important duties? Second, if pharmacy decides that it wants to control a technology, how can it gain control of that technology? Pharmacy should expect competition, as shown by decisions to control radioactive drugs through nuclear medicine departments in hospitals.

The second task of reprofessionalization is to choose the focus and fundamental goal of the reprofessionalization (28). Two choices (there may be more) are to focus internally, to achieve ideological purity, or to focus on the relationship of pharmacy to society, to pursue authority. If pharmacy chooses to focus on itself, it will emphasize shared knowledge, belief, assumptions, values, and practices among clinical pharmacists (i.e., the culture of clinical pharmacy). Pharmacy tends to splinter into subcultures of pharmacists who feel comfortable about one another's values, assumptions, and practices. In this focus, the "clinical" pharmacist functions on a level separate from other pharmacists, perhaps as a "specialist."

In contrast, pharmacy can focus on the impact that it has on society's problems, as described earlier. The external objective of reprofessionalization is, therefore, to maximize the contribution of pharmacy to society's drug-related needs. Because manpower is one prerequisite, pharmacy must provide enough competent pharmacists to make an impact. The annual Pharm. D. output (200–300 postbaccalaureate and 600 first professional degree students) (29) may not suffice to make that impact. In this focus, all pharmacists would strive to practice clinically; indeed, professional competence for a pharmacist would be defined in terms of pharmaceutical care. The issue is whether pharmacy should seek ideological goals in separate professional educational programs and professional associations or seek a common, probably diverse culture that will allow it to make the greatest possible contribution to society, thereby securing authority.

---

[d]See the June 1985 issue of the *American Journal of Hospital Pharmacy.*

Because any group with legal objectives may associate freely in the United States, the real issue is not for one organization to dominate the others or to convince the public that it speaks for the others. Rather, the issue is the capacity of the existing organizations of pharmacy to enter a common "authority project," to focus power, and to accommodate differences toward that end.

The decision made in the second step leads immediately to four interrelated issues about how pharmacy should constitute its components and how they should relate to each other and to society. This is the issue of general practice versus specialization.

Definition of Specialty Practice

One choice is the rapid formation of specialties around a limited—perhaps hollow—core of general practice. There is, in 1988, some movement in that direction, built on the idea that "clinical pharmacy" (as an informative service) composes a specialty practice, while "distributive pharmacy" makes up the core general practice. That core may turn out to be hollow unless technicians and robots are to be accepted as the general practitioners of the future.

Another choice is the construction of the strongest possible general practice based on a common ideology of pharmaceutical care. This issue is related to the issue of ideology versus authority, for the clinical pharmacy specialty movement apparently seeks ideological purity, while the pharmaceutical care movement seeks authority.

Establishment of Educational Standards

The distinction between general practice and specialty practice implies that entry level education prepare the noviced for general practice, while specialized postgraduate education or training be used for entry to the specialty. If pharmaceutical care becomes the central activity of pharmacy, then educational standards will have to be revised accordingly. Conversely, if clinical pharmacy is a specialty practice, relatively little expansion in basic educational standards will be needed, although continued development of postbaccalaureate education and training would be necessary.

The question of the B.S. versus the Pharm. D. as the first professional degree of pharmacy therefore rests upon a decision regarding the general practice of pharmacy. If pharmacy decides that its central activity is pharmaceutical care, then comes the question of the appropriate curriculum. The two issues here seem to be (a) how much curricular reform is politically possible in schools of pharmacy (18) and (b) the maximal length of entry-level curricula that will be supported by society (in terms of public support and ability to recruit students). Therefore, the issue of education is connected to public opinion about the value of pharmacy, as addressed repeatedly above. Finally, whether the degree should be doctoral depends on the standards in the larger society. Clearly, 5 years of postsecondary education has not justified the doctorate, while 7 years has. It seems that the appropriate degree for a 6-year curriculum would depend on the special requirements for the degree, e.g., thesis, comprehensive examination, or unusual practical experience requirements. A professional master's degree after 6 years is a logical but (to many) unpalatable compromise.

Recruitment, Reeducation, Resocialization

The basic identity of pharmacy and its definition of general practice will influence who is recruited to pharmacy. If pharmacy decides that its core practice will remain a business-oriented distributive activity, then it should expect to attract a majority of young people who desire a business-oriented distributive career. The relatively few "specialists" in clinical pharmacy or pharmaceutical care can then be recruited from that pool, as at present. Conversely, if the core activity of pharmacy is pharmaceutical care, then it may attract more students with interests, aptitudes, and personal goals more consistent with patient care.

One often overlooked issue in this process is the amount and type of motivation felt by present practitioners to retrain and to resocialize, i.e., to adopt new beliefs and values about their practices. If pharmacy defines pharmaceutical care as its core activity, then competence in pharmaceutical care can reasonably be expected of all practitioners. Those who lacked such competence would feel moral as well as economic pressure to retrain and resocialize, in other words, to become competent for the new practice. If, on the other hand, pharmacy isolates clinical practice as a specialty, then clinical competence would be optional. Practitioners would feel no more moral pressure to change than would a general practitioner of medicine or dentistry feel moral pressure to become a cardiologist or orthodontist.

The economic forces described above seem to point toward pharmaceutical care as the core activity of general practitioners. The economic scenario described earlier suggests strong divisive forces at work within pharmacy. One important strategy to counter such forces is to retrain and resocialize dislocated midcareer practitioners. Depending on how widely and how fast the economic scenario plays out, this may amount to tens of thousands of practitioners. A project of this magnitude will surely require consensus among educators, political leaders, and practitioners. If pharmacy remains a set of isolated subcultures, it may be unable either to maintain internal cohesion or to retrain enough pharmacists to make an impact on society.

Marketing Pharmaceutical Care

The fourth and last step in the reprofessionalization of pharmacy returns us to an earlier topic. Pharmacy must create a market mechanism for pharmaceutical care. Some of the issues (21) are:

1. Choice of client. Shall pharmacy market itself directly to the public? to the health care corporation? to both equally? Whose interests will pharmacy promise to protect? To whom will it offer its first loyalty?
2. Creation of perceived exclusiveness. The customer must recognize something special in the services of pharmacy. How can pharmacy express the concept of pharmaceutical care most effectively to its target audience?
3. Establishment and maintenance of minimal standards of performance. Society will ultimately accept or reject the claim of pharmacy to provide special and valuable services based on actual performance. Pharmacy will need a quality control mechanism that is more effective than the current customary professional self-regulation.
4. Control of supply. Pharmacy will initially need to provide large numbers of practitioners competent in drug use control, or its impact on society will not be large enough to succeed.

In conclusion, pharmacy faces multiple futures. That is, there is not one pharmacy: there are as many "pharmacies" as there are practice sites, communities, and individuals, and as many futures as there are combinations of forces. The magnitude of this challenge for pharmacy should inspire awe, especially because each of these forces interacts with the others. For example, pharmacy may not be able to recruit enough students motivated toward patient care until it changes its professional standing with the public, but it may be unable to change its professional standing until it agrees on its social object, and so on.

In seeking a structure in this confusing jumble of individuals and forces, it is necessary to consider the philosophical principle that the people will eventually have their way in a free society. Although this principle is hard to prove, the landscape of history is littered with examples of businesses, industries, or occupations that died because they failed to serve the public interest. The occupation called pharmacy, and each individual within it, should return to its preindustrial origins in valued, complex, specific, and committed public service if it wishes a happy postindustrial future. Pharmacy can prosper in the future no more than the extent to which it serves the public.

> Don't fight forces; use them.
>
> R. Buckminster Fuller

REFERENCES

1. Naisbitt J. Megatrends. New York: Warner Books, 1982, pp 13-14.
2. Samuelson RJ. Our computerized society. Newsweek, September 9, 1985.
3. Chronicle of higher education. September 17, 1986, p 1.
4. Bezold C, Halperin JA, Binkley HL, Ashbaugh RR, eds. Pharmacy in the 21'st century: planning for an uncertain future. Alexandria, VA: Institute for Alternative Futures and Project Hope, 1984.
5. Check WA. Summary of the discussion and small group exercise on the future of pharmacy. In Bezold C, Halperin JA, Binkley HL, Ashbaugh RR, eds. Pharmacy in the 21'st Century, Alexandria, VA: Institute for Alternative Futures and Project Hope, 1984, p 218.
6. Brodie DC. Drug use control: keystone to pharmaceutical service. Drug Intell 1967;1:63-5.
7. Manasse HR, Jr. The twenty-first century hospital: where is the pharmacist? Hosp Pharm 1987;22:16-26.
8. Burger W. Concurring Opinion, Virginia State Board of Pharmacy, et al. v Virginia Citizens Consumer Council Inc. Permanent (archival) Reference 25 425 U.S. 748. See also quotation in Francke DE. Am J Pharm Educ 1976;40:448-52.
9. Check WA. New drugs and drug delivery systems in the year 2000. In Bezold C, Halperin JA, Binkley HL, Ashbaugh RR, eds. Pharmacy in the 21'st Century, Alexandria, VA: Institute for Alternative Futures and Project Hope, 1984, pp 135-160.
10. Easterbrook G. The revolution in medicine. Newsweek, January 26, 1987.
11. Jeffers JR. Conflicting economic pressures in health care. Hosp Admin 1971;284:1180-5.
12. Goldsmith J. Death of a paradigm: the challenge of competition. Health Affairs 1984;3:5-19.
13. Black BL, ed. Resource book on progressive pharmaceutical services. Bethesda MD: American Society of Hospital Pharmacists, 1986.
14. Hatoum HT, Catizone C, Hutchinson RA, et al. An eleven-year review of the pharmacy literature: documentation of the value and acceptance of clinical pharmacy. Drug Intell Clin Pharm 1986;20:33-48.
15. Hepler CD. Pharmacy as a clinical profession. Am J Hosp Pharm 1985;42:1298-1306.
16. Hall RH. Some organizational considerations in the professional-organizational relationship. Admin Sci Q 1967;12:461-78.
17. Naisbitt J, Aburdene P. Re-inventing the corporation: transforming your job and your company for the new information society. New York: Warner Books, 1985, pp 79-118.
18. Hepler CD. The third wave in pharmaceutical education: the clinical movement. Am J Pharm Educ 1987;51:369-85.
19. Dychtwald K. Consumer behavior: speculations on the future of aging, wellness, and self-care. In Bezold C, Halperin JA, Binkley HL, Ashbaugh RR, eds. Pharmacy in the 21'st Century. Alexandria VA: Institute for Alternative Futures and Project Hope, 1984, pp 67-78.

20. Callahan D. Ethics and health care: the next twenty years. In Bezold C, Halperin JA, Binkley HL, Ashbaugh RR, eds. Pharmacy in the 21'st Century. Alexandria VA: Institute for Alternative Futures and Project Hope, 1984, pp 79–86.

21. Larsen MS. The Rise of Professionalism. Berkeley CA: University of California Press, 1977.

22. May WF. Code and covenant or philanthropy and contract? Hastings Center Rep 1975;5:29–38.

23. Illich I. Medical Nemesis. New York: Random House, 1976.

24. Dichter Institute for Motivational Research. Communicating the value of comprehensive pharmaceutical services to the consumer: an analysis of public regard for the pharmacist and for comprehensive pharmaceutical services: final report of the Dichter Institute for Motivational Research, Inc. Washington, D.C. American Pharmaceutical Association, 1973.

25. Steeves RF, Patterson FT. Legal responsibility of the hospital pharmacist for rational drug therapy. Am J Hosp Pharm 1969;26:404–7.

26. Southwick AF. The Law of Hospital and Health Care Administration. Ann Arbor, MI: Health Administration Press, 1978, pp 409–11.

27. Miller L. American spirit: visions of a new corporate culture, New York: William Morrow and Co., 1984.

28. Birenbaum A. Reprofessionalization in pharmacy. Soc Sci Med 1982;16:871–8.

29. Penna RP, Sherman MS. Enrollments in schools and colleges of pharmacy, 1985–86. Am J Pharm Educ 1986;50:411–434.

15
Pharmacists of the Future

JEROME A. HALPERIN

In attempting to determine what the future holds for pharmacists, it is first important to define the time frame being considered. We know only one thing about the future: the future is uncertain. The years 1990 and 2190 are both in the future, but how pharmacists may fare may be substantially different in the 2 centuries between them. The more distant into the future the greater its uncertainty. The year 1990 is so close there is little uncertainty about it, i.e., there are few major changes likely to affect pharmacy and pharmacists in 1990 that are unknown or unexpected now. Two hundred years from now, 2190, is so uncertain that speculation about it is not relevant for pharmacists today. This chapter focuses on the period 2010–2025, far enough away so that events that may affect the profession and its practitioners are not well known now, but close enough so that many of the readers of this text will be in the prime of their professional lives and events affecting pharmacy during that period will have direct relevance to them and the way they practice their profession.

The years 2010–2025 were also the time frame on which the Conference on Pharmacy in the 21st Century, a strategic planning project of the pharmacy profession held March 1984, focused. The Conference grew out of a recognition that because the future of pharmacy is uncertain, a thoughtful, structured process of considering pharmacy's future is required. Cosponsored and funded by major professional and trade organizations, nine pharmaceutical manufacturers, The Institute for Alternative Futures, the Institute for Health Policy of Project Hope, and a Washington, D.C., law firm, the Conference was attended by over 50 people representing pharmacy and other sectors of the health care delivery system. The Conference considered the forces that may affect health care delivery and pharmacy in the early part of the 21st century. This chapter draws heavily from the discussions and predictions of that Conference.

THE FUTURE—WHAT MIGHT IT BE LIKE?

The future will be shaped by global sociopolitical, environmental, and economic forces. The changes that the bases can be about can yield profound differences. The Institute for Alternative Futures (IAF) has developed scenarios that describe four Alternative Futures representing different results of change: Continued Growth, Decline and Stagnation, Disciplined Society, and Transformation.

Continued Growth

The Continued Growth scenario represents an optimistic extension of the current system of technological sophistication and economic expansion. The scenario predicts full employment, new technologies abounding with sophisticated communication, widespread computer use, and rapid mobility. Large multinational corporations will expand into partner-ships with governments ensuring economic development and making a wealth of technology, expertise, and new markets available in the United States. Information that will change education will be instantly accessible to households in the United States. The envi-ronment will be stressed, but not unduly.

Health care expenditures will increase to 13% of the Gross National Product (GNP) by 2020. Health care technologies will be more complex and more effective. New vaccines will prevent many diseases and new drugs will cure many diseases not possible before, including heart disease and most cancers. Life extension will be achieved in part through organ and tissue transplants, which will become more available. Physician jobs will be aided signifi-cantly by biomedical advisors.

Decline and Stagnation

Economic hard times with deepening recessions, social unrest, and serious resource short-ages mark the Decline and Stagnation scenario. Pollution of the environment will bring about the "greenhouse effect," seriously affecting the climate of the earth, leading to food shortages and damage to the water supply. Government will become increasingly unable to cope with, much less correct, the major societal problems.

Disease outbreaks will occur, but the health care system will attempt to deal with them through isolating the infected persons rather than curing the disease. The poor and the elderly will suffer disproportionately under a two-tiered health care system, with the tier serving the poor and middle classes being severely underfunded. Only 6% of the GNP will be spent on health. Health status will decline, largely due to food shortages and increases in infectious diseases. Innovation will slow and although drugs will be greatly sought, the older, reliable, cost-effective technologies and therapies will predominate. Alternative ther-apies and providers will grow in number.

Disciplined Society

The scenario for the Disciplined Society represents an Orwellian reaction to hard times oc-curring throughout the end of the 20th century. American Society will abandon its tradi-tional freedoms for the sake of a tightly controlled, disciplined society in which security, comfort, and material successes are gained through rational management, enforced conser-vation, and efficiency. Centralized management systems and behavioral control ("Big Brother is Watching You") will be achieved through effective communication and informa-tion-processing technologies. Business and government will ally in symbiotic relationships to regulate socioeconomic activity. Health will be achieved through order and order through health. Health will be regulated and destructive personal behavior will not be tolerated. Health care will represent 8% of the GNP and public health programs will be very success-ful. Elderly persons will not be provided with opportunity for life extension but will be af-forded the opportunity to die comfortably.

A national health care system will evolve with clear standards for evaluating and apply-ing cost-effective therapies for use by physicians and other health care personnel. Expensive therapies will rarely be used for any except the very affluent or influential.

Transformation

Western industrialized society will adopt some of the cultural values of the East and will undergo transformation into a more decentralized, participatory society whose values emphasize personal growth and cooperation as envisioned by Naisbitt and Toffler. Society will become more globally oriented but locally based, i.e., managing the business of the world through cottage industries. Overproduction, once the driving force of American industry, will be eroded by a value change to voluntary simplicity and ecological balance. Technology will continue to be an important aspect of economic well-being but will be less important than the drive for inner (spiritual) growth.

Advanced technologies will emerge from cooperative arrangements between decentralized governments and organizations. Opulent lifestyles will become less popular and less sought as society puts a high value on frugal material and rich spiritual lives.

Health care will become highly competitive and change dramatically as less reductionist, more holistic approaches recognize the power of personal "body wisdom." Nonconventional health providers will compete successfully with physicians to replace the licensure systems that currently provide physicians with, essentially, government-endorsed monopolies. The move toward self-care and toward the nonconventional providers, away from traditional medicine, will act to help reduce health expenditures to 6% of the GNP.

SHAPING THE FUTURE—KEY TRENDS

On a less macro scale, key societal and health care trends occurring today will continue. They will exert profound changes on the health care system of the 21st century and pharmacy. These trends can be classified in any number of ways, but they are divided here into four categories: demographic, social, technological, and economic.

Demographic Trends

Aging of America

Global population continues to grow at record rates and will reach 7.8 billion by 2020. The United States population will increase by 15% over the next 20 years and will change dramatically in its ethnic composition. Hispanics will account for 25–30% and the proportion of blacks and Asians will increase as whites decrease; however, the single most profound demographic change occurring today is the rapid aging of the population. The "baby boomers" of the post-World War II era, who represent about $1/3$ of all living Americans, are entering their 40s. By the year 2000, the youngest of this group will be in their 30s while the oldest will be in their 50s. From a health standpoint, the baby boomers will exert their greatest economic effect between the years 2010 and 2025. The United States population over 65, now about 11%, will exceed 20% by their time. As the baby boom generation reaches the stage of degenerative illness, the health care system will experience an unprecedented wave of health care cost pressure for acute and chronic care.

The elderly present specialized problems of health and medical care. This sector accounts for 30% of the total health care spending. Their spending power, greater than that of any other group, is 1.5 times the United States average and twice that of the under-35 population. Many of the problems are associated with compliance with medical regimens, especially in the cases of "polypharmacy" in which patients consume many drugs at varying times throughout the day and night for a variety of conditions, often under unsupervised or poorly supervised conditions. Confusion, noncompliance, and interactions can and do occur with alarming frequency and represent for the pharmacist a continuing and growing challenge to provide pharmaceutical products and services, especially information, in accessible reliable ways.

Life Enhancement and Life Extension

Life enhancing and life extending are two ways by which life expectancy may be improved. The concepts affect life span differently by increasing its length or improving its quality. Life extension, increasing the number of years in the human life span, has not achieved significant progress in increasing the upper limit of human life, 120–140 years for an individual, but it has been remarkably successful in lengthening the mean life span by reducing early mortality. Life enhancement, improving the quality of life, is also known as compressing morbidity or "squaring the life cycle curve." The concept here is to keep people living healthy productive lives longer and then dying abruptly without long, debilitating illnesses. Science has not yet discovered the secrets to life extension, but life enhancement can be made possible through improved health care, organ transplantation, genetic engineering, use of bionics and prosthetics, and new and better drugs.

Social Trends

Self-Care and Self-Help

The latter half of the 20th century has seen a dramatic return to individualism, stemming in part from the "me" generation ideas of the 1960s and 1970s. People are committed to getting control of their own lives and evaluating the impact of their behavior on their health. This movement has given rise to self-care and self-help in which people are becoming more responsible for their own care and being more selective in seeking professional help. Home health care, an element of this trend, is emerging as a more popular, cost-effective alternative to institutional care. In addition to being less expensive, patients do better at home and are happier.

The startling fact is that increasingly, people are unwilling simply to follow orders in matters concerning their health. Recent data from the United Kingdom reveal that the public is prepared to take medical advice but is less willing to follow doctors' orders, preferring to make their own health decisions. As more people decide to assume more responsibility for their own lives they reject authority, looking less to the physician for guidance, preferring exchange and dialogue to orders and instructions. In a 1984 study, 42% of the people expressed less faith in doctors than they used to have. Compared with 22% in 1979, this is a remarkable shift of attitudes in 5 years.

The fascinating aspect of this change is that it comes from a country where social welfare programs have been the major sources of health care and a National Health Service insurance program has been in effect for many years.

Increased Consumer Confidence

Going hand-in-hand with the self-help and self-care movement is the trend for consumers to be sufficiently competent to make better informal decisions about the health products they purchase. They are asking more questions, seeking more information, and taking a more active role in their health care. Speakers at the 1986 Annual meeting of the European Proprietary Drug Association (AESGP) stressed the need for consumer information in the context of observable changes in attitudes that have a bearing not only on the manner in which treatment is available, but in the programs for the prevention of illness as well. The role of the individual in the decision-making process in health care is emerging as a critical factor in the implementation of such programs.

An offshoot of increased consumer confidence is disintermediation, i.e., elimination of the middle man. Examples include self-service gasoline stations, direct wholesale buying through home computers, and other developments making various levels and kinds of management unnecessary. Disintermediation like this translates to convenience shopping, convenience in buying and packaging. Baby boomers tend to be fairly wealthy and sophisticated shoppers who favor convenience over tradition in choosing their shopping outlets. They prefer supermarkets and mass merchandising outlets to the traditional drugstore outlets. The growing trend toward self-medication, including new drugs for nonprescription (OTC) use and Rx to OTC switches, is a health care example of disintermediation of direct intent to pharmacists.

Wellness and Health Promotion

Better diet, exercise, and elimination of smoking and alcohol are among the manifestations of a trend toward being healthy. Publications on wellness, including a new journal of health promotion, are becoming more widespread, and there is growing recognition that the ultimate role of health care systems is to keep healthy people healthy.

There is considerable demand for more and different health care products and services particularly from healthier, younger groups (those under 45). It indicates a largely unfulfilled demand for preventative health care products and services.

HEALTHY CORPORATION

This corporate manifestation of the health promotion and wellness movement spans from dramatic growth of industrial/occupational health programs featuring such things as health prevention programs, nutrition programs in company cafeterias, gymnasiums and health clubs, child care programs, etc. Wellness programs are becoming important benefit programs that firms are beginning to advertise in their recruitment program while wellness programs are among the fastest growing corporate benefits. An underlying motivation, of course, may be fewer sick days and higher productivity, happier and healthier work forces. Yet to be seen is whether these programs can survive periods of economic slowdown.

Holism

The approach to health is becoming more "holistic" and less reductionist. Rather than treating individual symptoms or organs (reductionist approach), there is a new and growing movement to consider the whole person. As nutrition is recognized as a more important component of health care, pharmacists will become part of the holistic approach by providing products, information, and counseling on nutrition and nutritional products as well as drugs.

Technology Trends

Food and Nutrition Revolution

Knowledge of the importance of nutrition to human health, manifesting itself in concerns about cholesterol and saturated fats in the diet, the need for fiber, calcium, and trace elements, and the growing consumption of a variety of vitamin and mineral supplements as well as sources of omega 3 fatty acids (fish oils) etc. demonstrate the validity of the notion, "You are what you eat." Recent studies by the National Cancer Institute and the National

Heart, Blood, and Lung Institute reflect changes in federal policy about the importance of nutrition in the onset of disease and enhancement of health.

Biochemical Individualism

Recognition of the incorrect notion that human beings are essentially the same biochemically is coming from new knowledge about immunology, genetics, biochemistry, etc. This trend will lead to new "custom-made" drugs for individuals and afford a new technological challenge to pharmacy providing new meaning to compounding by the pharmacist.

Computers and Telematics

Computers plus telecommunications technologies, including cable television, satellites, videotext, etc., will provide an array of high quality information in all areas, especially health for improved delivery of health services. Improved computers and communications technology will facilitate direct two-way communication between patients and physicians. The physician may be able to monitor the patient's status without the patient coming into the physician's office. Once properly programmed, computers may allow patients to prescribe for themselves as well as providing them the opportunity to monitor their therapies themselves. Physicians also may choose to request that pharmacists monitor drug therapies by this technology once physicians have initiated it.

High Tech—High Touch

In his book, *Megatrends,* John Naisbitt describes the reactions of people to the impersonality of high technology as "High Tech—High Touch". Health care examples of the human compensation to high tech medical care are the birthing and hospice movements.

Pharmacists are in unique positions to provide high touch to the increasingly high-tech new drugs and delivery systems available today and the even greater specificity and technology of those in the future.

Changing Patterns of Disease

Medical science has produced a shift from acute infectious diseases to chronic diseases and psychosocial diseases including chemical dependencies, stress-related disorders, and bioenvironmental diseases (e.g., reactions to environmental chemicals, cigarette smoke, etc.). Some of these may be the result of another trend, the toxification of the environment from environmental pollution.

Economic Trends

The Corporation as the Conscious Buyer of Medical Care

Employers are becoming active in trying to moderate/reduce the costs of medical care. Medical care will be purchased like any other product or service, based upon bids that must meet quality specifications while competing on price and service. The goal of corporations is to achieve substantial cost savings while maintaining quality health services programs, but to "corporationalize" it is generally not in their interest. Corporate interest is not served by duplicating community services, thus it is unlikely that corporations will routinely find themselves in competition with community pharmacy by operating their own drug dispensing centers, however, economics will likely be the driving force that will determine whether the corporation is better served through support of community-based pharmaceutical services or internal programs.

Increased Pressure for Cost-Effectiveness

New medical care technologies and drug therapies will become increasingly expensive, and growing concern over health care expenditures and rationing of health care services will force careful examination of the cost effectiveness of these new products and services. Diagnosis related groups (DRGs) and pharmaceutical reimbursement schemes such as the Competitive Incentive Plan (CIP) are current examples of the trend.

Government efforts to hold down health care costs will not be very successful in the long run; people will not trade cost for quality and access. Technology growth in health care delivery continues to force confrontations with the question of cost effectiveness. The issue, however, is not whether health care costs can be controlled, but rather what impact such controls will have on the health care system if technology is limited. The operative assumption is that if new technologies really contribute to improved health care, they will be cost effective.

Changing Role of the Hospital

As treatment advances permit greater opportunity for non-hospital-based care and home care, the hospitalized population will shrink to about one-half its current size. The hospital of the future will be transformed into the critical care source but of a widely dispersed network of small clinics, physician's offices, and remote health locations with a radius extending about 200 miles and connected by air and group critical care transportation systems and computer/telematic-based information and monitoring systems.

Hospital-based pharmacists in the environment of the superspecialized hospital will give new meaning to the notion that pharmacy is a clinically based practice and provide opportunity for the Millis Commission's concept of the clinical pharmaceutical scientist to become established.

Pharmaceutical Industry Demographics

Significant changes now underway will change the demographics of the pharmaceutical industry substantially. A favorable economic environment in the 1980s has fueled unparallel growth in the industry, marked by record stock prices, acquisitions, and an influx of new companies to the American market. Not since pre-World War II days have as many European pharmaceutical manufacturers including Bayer, Berlex, E. Merck, Boehringer-Mannheim, Boots, Glaxo, Fisons, and others recognized the need to participate in the single largest drug market of the world. Domestically, new entries into the market are coming from large chemical companies (e.g., DuPont, Monsanto, and Kodak) and small biotechnology companies are leading the therapeutic revolution from synthetic chemical to recombinant deoxyribonucleic acid (DNA)-based drugs (e.g., Genentech, Cetus, Amgen, and others). Finally, the growth of the generic pharmaceutical market, fueled by changes in the United States regulatory system, has brought a whole new segment of non-research-based companies (as far as new molecule development) into the sector.

NEW DRUGS AND DELIVERY SYSTEMS

Pharmacists in the 21st century will have to be comfortable with significantly advanced drug and drug delivery systems that will treat and cure diseases and conditions that are not now treatable by drugs. The only human illnesses that can be reliably cured with drugs in 1986 are infectious diseases; they are the only ones for which cause is known.

George Teeling-Smith, in "The Second Pharmacological Revolution," describes the evolution of drug therapy from the 1860s to the present. Beginning with elucidation of the DNA structure in the 1950s, Smith says that we have entered a period in which therapies are based upon an understanding of intracellular chemistry. The most likely achievements will be in the areas of viral diseases, cancer, and autoimmune diseases.

New therapeutic entities will have the following properties: Drugs will be more specific; they will be based upon natural substances including proteins and peptides; and an approach to understanding how natural body substances interact with their receptors will be facilitated through computer modeling, as was used in the development of the renin inhibitors.

New Drugs and Drug Classes

Immunomodulators. Drugs to maintain proper functioning of the immune system will be synthesized in large quantities through genetic engineering, such as interferon and interleukin 2.

Neurotransmitters. Peptides to transmit nerve cell impulses will be developed for treatment of Parkinson's disease, Alzheimer's disease, amyotrophiclateralsclerosis (ALS) (Lou Gehrig's disease), and schizophrenia.

Neurotrophic hormones. This new class of agents will stimulate regrowth of nerves in degenerative nerve disease. Experimental treatment of ALS with thyrotropic releasing hormone is already being tried.

Genetic engineering. Medical applications of recombinant DNA technologies already postulated for products of this technology include production of large amounts of medically useful materials, e.g., human growth hormone, factor VIII, correction of inherited diseases, i.e., those diseases due to a single, identified mutant gene that are susceptible to correction by insertion of functional gene; and oncogene suppression for prevention of cancer by synthesis and insertion of antioncogenes to prevent expression of the oncogene.

Prostaglandins. These nonpeptides cannot be easily synthesized by microorganisms and will be synthesized in the laboratory. Their applications include: anticlotting agents—prostacylins to prevent heart attacks or clot formation in ischemic leg ulcers; treatment of asthma by inhibiting leukotrienes; and prevention of ulcers and healing of gastrointestinal bleeding.

Vaccines. New vaccines will be developed for prevention of diseases, especially viral diseases not previously preventable, including acquired immune deficiency syndrome (AIDS) and herpesvirus diseases.

New Delivery Systems

New delivery systems of all types will become commonplace. They will include the following:

Controlled release technologies oral and transdermal systems that release drugs into the body at predetermined and carefully controlled rates. Current examples include the OROS (Oral Release Osmotic System) tablets (e.g., Acutrim—CIBA Consumer Pharmaceuticals: transdermal scopolamine, nitroglycerin, and estradiol—CIBA-GEIGY; and Clonidine—Boehringer-Ingelheim).

Magnetic systems involve drugs bound to beads of porous polymer combined with magnetic molecules, also bound to beads. When implanted, the system releases the drug at the site of action through application of a mild magnetic field. This technology will be useful for pulsed drug delivery.

Monoclonal antibodies will reduce side effects from current anticancer drugs by targeting them to specific antigens on cell membranes. They also will reduce rejection bone marrow grafts by killing donor cells that cause graft versus host condition and will and treat infectious diseases.

Respiratory delivery is a system in which particle size controls the site of action in the respiratory tract. The technology will be especially useful to deliver peptides, including gonadotrophin hormone releasing hormone (male contraceptive) and vasopressin (memory enhancer) insulin and vaccines.

Liposomes are lipid water emulsions containing trapped drug that is released when the liposome is taken into the cell and degraded. They can encapsulate drugs for liver or lung disease and treat parasitic diseases by invading the parasite while sparing the host.

Neurotransmitters are a class of natural peptides that will deliver drugs directly to the brain.

Erodable polymer implants represent a technology that will find application in delivering drugs that require pulsed dosage delivery and enzyme response release systems. They also will be used in computer-assisted drug dosing systems to fine-tune dosing of drugs with narrow therapeutic windows and correct for physiologic responses, e.g., diurnal variations, by controlling drug release from implanted polymers or pump.

Implications for Pharmacy

The pharmacist of the future will have to understand different kinds of drugs and drug delivery systems including pumps, patches, controlled release oral systems, liposomes, implants, and specific monoclonal antibodies. Pharmacists will handle gene-splicing enzymes and nucleic acid precursors for individualized gene therapy. These drugs of the future will be more specific, more complicated, more potent, and more related to individual biochemical needs of patient.

To practice in this high tech environment, the pharmacist must:

- Be comfortable with the high-tech aspects by understanding the biology of the condition and the biochemistry of the drugs as well as dosage schedules;
- Be competent in the high-tech aspects as an information giver. Even if a patient's initial orientation to his/her drug regimen is from the physician as via computerized instruction, detailed human explanation will be more important than ever. Patient counseling, long claimed by pharmacy as one of its strongholds, will be tested here.

PHARMACY WORLD FORCE

Subsidy programs of the 1970s will yield an excess number of professionally trained health personnel extending into the early 21st century. Although the population will grow by more than 10%, the total supply of health professionals will grow by 32% by 1990 continuing the decline of the "seller's market" for physicians' services that began in the late 1940s. As we enter the 21st century, there will be an underemployed cadre of physician specialists. The ratio of health professionals in the population will increase from 1:12.5 to 1:10 by 1990.

Incentives to practice will be important. The level of participation will be determined by sex distribution of physicians and method of reimbursement, i.e., fee for service, capitation, or diagnostic related group based. The overwhelming change that is likely is the growth of group practice. Only 40,000 physicians practiced in group settings in 1969. By 1984 this number had more than tripled to 140,000 and shows signs of continuing.

For pharmacy the increase in ratio over the past 3 decades has been modest and related to population growth from 56.6 per 100,000 in 1950 to 62.4 per 100,000 in 1979. This trend is likely to continue. The most profound change in pharmacy during this period is a demographic one: whereas less than 4% of pharmacists were female in 1950, 19% were female by 1980, and now greater than 50% of pharmacy students are female. The realization is that the majority of practicing United States pharmacists will be female by the end of the 20th century. Women now make up the majority in several European countries. An international conference on women in pharmacy (1987) has been convened to consider the impact of this change on the profession.

Earlier, female pharmacists worked shorter work weeks, left the profession earlier, and did not return. That trend is changing. Currently female pharmacists are working longer hours and are less likely to leave the labor force than are men. Moreover, many of those who do leave anticipate returning within a few years. Therefore, pharmacy cannot expect attrition among women to limit its work force.

The second major trend affecting pharmacists is their site of employment or practice setting. As late as 1966, 68.5% of pharmacists owned their own pharmacies or worked for independent owners. In 1980 that figure had dropped to 38%. In 1984 30% of pharmacists worked for chain stores and 20% for hospitals. By the early 21st century the transformation of pharmacy from a profession of independent store owners to employees of large organizations will be virtually complete. Although Alvin Toffler, in *The Third Wave*, sees an eventual return to small service-oriented retail outlets, this change, if it comes about, will likely be later than the early part of the 21st century and will likely represent a part of a larger more significant societal transformation.

Large organizations, in their goal to become more cost efficient, will seek to substitute technicians and machines for professionally trained pharmacists whenever possible.

INTERFACES AND TURF BATTLES

A 1978 study of what pharmacists do, sponsored by the American Pharmaceutical Association (APhA) and American Association of Colleges of Pharmacy (AACP) revealed that pharmacists' time could be allocated to four major functions:

- Processing prescription orders—48%.
  Verifying the prescription, filling, labeling, and delivering the completed medication to the patient are some of these functions. This role can be eroded by pharmacy technicians, nurses, physicians' assistants, nurses, physicians, and technology itself (through prepackaging and automated dispensing).

- Management and administration—33%.

  Budgeting, inventory control, ordering, pricing, hiring and firing of pharmacy personnel, etc. Make up those areas of responsibility. These functions are much more important in the independently owned pharmacy but are frequently delegated to nonpharmacists in chain stores, hospitals, HMOs, etc.

- Patient care—12%.

  Activities relating to gathering patient-related information, looking for potential interactions or problems in the therapeutic regimens, and monitoring drug therapy are included here. Newer surveys might add pharmacist prescribing and dosage adjustment. These activities interact and conflict, in part, with the roles of physicians, nurses, physicians' assistants, and nurse practitioners.

- Educating health care providers and patients—7%.

  This function required, or occupied, the least amount of the pharmacist's time in 1978 but is currently becoming a far more important function. It includes teaching health providers of all kinds about drugs and their applications, providing drug information, consulting on drug therapy, and establishing and implementing quality assurance procedures over the whole range of drug dispensing distribution and use. Physicians, nurses, pharmaceutical and biomedical scientists, and computers can encroach on this pharmacist role.

Current trends show the patient care and education functions increasing while the prescription processing and management activities are declining. The trend on prescription processing is likely to reverse again. Pharmacy began with compounding individual prescriptions for individual patients. Centralized pharmaceutical manufacturing changed the pharmacist's role to dispensing premade drug products. New, more sophisticated drugs tailored to individual patients' needs will require the pharmacist to spend more time in compounding and dispensing. Even this role, however, can be eroded by nonpharmacist pharmaceutical scientists, highly trained pharmacy technicians, or physicians.

Alternatively, as drug therapy becomes more sophisticated and complex, more of the individual tasks of compounding and delivering tailor-made high-tech drug products will be conducted by a team of lesser trained pharmacists, technicians, and aides under the supervision of a highly trained, advanced degree pharmacist.

Physicians can do many functions now performed by pharmacists and as the number of physicians as well as their ratio to pharmacists increase, there is greater likelihood of them doing so. The most likely area for physicians to exert their political and professional muscle will be in the newly emerging role of pharmacist prescribing. As the oversupply of physicians continues to expand, they will be less likely to tolerate any encroachment on one of their most closely guarded prerogatives by pharmacists.

The supply growth of the 1980s and 1990s will afford physicians more time to spend with their patients, enhancing and extending the physician-patient relationship, balancing the high-tech aspect of medical care with a high touch personalism that will provide information (including drug information—a role that pharmacists have cut out for themselves) and a more holistic approach to medical care.

Pharmacists, especially those with advanced training and degrees, have become increasingly successful in becoming pharmacokinetic consultants to physicians. In some institutions, physicians have, after prescribing the drug, left the determination of the dose, dosage regimen, and monitoring of drug therapy through assays, etc. to pharmacists. As the physician supply expands and with the availability of easy-to-use computer software, physicians may elect to do more of the pharmacokinetics themselves.

Physician dispensing, always an anathema to pharmacy, has reemerged in the mid-1980s and has gained momentum to the point where the Federal Trade Commission has supported the practice in a proceeding before the Maryland State Board of Medical Examiners on the basis of its beneficial effects on competition. A serious risk of physician oversupply is that physicians may on a wide scale start selling drugs again in their offices and clinics, taking both business and opportunity for professional service from pharmacists while defending the practice as being good medicine by reducing the percentage of unfilled prescriptions and being economically better for their patients.

Nurse practitioners and physicians' assistants both are seeking to share with the pharmacist any expansion of the non-physician-prescribing authority, and in a few states they may have such authority where pharmacists do not. The limited success of pharmacist prescribing now suggests a difficult uphill battle to extend the authority beyond limited success of the 1980s.

The physical acts of verifying and filling prescriptions are already heavily delegated by pharmacists to technicians and pharmacy aides. This will likely continue and widen to include automated dispensing under the pharmacist's supervision.

Pharmacists can expect to be displaced from many traditional roles as the increased use of computerized patient records and data bases, use of in-home diagnostic and therapeutic materials and equipment, and automated dispensing become available.

PHARMACY EDUCATION

After several years of decreasing enrollment, 1986 brought an increase in enrollment and a new (the 73rd) college of pharmacy, Campbell University in North Carolina, the first since the University of Arizona in the 1950s. The 74th college of pharmacy, Southeast College of Pharmaceutical Sciences (Florida) began enrolling its first class in the fall of 1987. The percentage of women continues to outnumber men: the sex ratio of pharmacy students at enrollment is 56% female: 44% male. In speculating about the sex ratio shift, one pharmacy educator speculated that the outstanding men have gone to business and engineering schools, but data are unavailable to support this hypothesis.

Pharmacists, before the 1960s, had been trained in the synthesis and analysis of the physical and chemical properties of drugs, as well as the design of dosage forms. Pharmacology education was classical textbook and did not relate to the understanding of disease, drug therapy, or dosing. Knowledge in the clinical use of drugs was not considered necessary for a pharmacist. Pharmacists operated businesses and considered themselves entrepreneurs. People who entered pharmacies were thought of as customers. A resolution before the 1987 APhA House of Delegates sought to change that image by endorsing programs that encourage innovations in the practice of pharmacy in a changing health care environment.

Pharmacy education in the late 1980s continues to be a didactic process of teaching a series of facts. Pharmacy students do not benefit from a practitioner-based process of integrating facts and applying the integrated knowledge base to real life situations involving patients until late in their education.

Clinical pharmacy, the first (but still incompletely established) practice specialty, emerged in the late 1960s. It marked the first time that the pharmacist played a direct role in advising physicians in the selection and management of drug therapy for patients and the first time pharmacists developed clinical skills associated with direct patient management. Today, there are three differing levels of clinical skills among pharmacists: none, little, and advanced skills. Pharmacy and medicine have yet to agree on the integration of roles of the clinical pharmacist in the patient care setting, although progress continues.

In 1965 no college of pharmacy taught clinical pharmacy and now all pharmacy schools teach it to some degree. Of the 72 pharmacy schools, only 10 currently offer the Pharm. D. degree, 27 offer both the B.S. and Pharm. D., and 35 the B.S. only. In the 1982–1983 academic year, 2605 of 19,350 pharmacy students were enrolled in Pharm. D. programs. The move is clear: By the 21st century all pharmacy schools will offer the Pharm. D. degree, either as an option or as the sole degree.

With few exceptions undergraduate curricula in the 5-year programs continue to be oriented toward the generalist. The Pharm. D. curricula afford more opportunity for differentiation, and three themes for these programs are common: clinical pharmacy, biopharmaceutics, and drug information (itself a generalization). It is only at the graduate Ph.D. level, however, that real differentiation occurs and pharmacists specialize in industrial pharmacy, pharmaceutical chemistry, medicinal chemistry, pharmaceutics, etc. The danger to pharmacy here is that graduates from these programs are not identified as pharmacists per se, but as scientists belonging to a larger community, not readily identified with the profession.

The pharmacy curriculum will soon become too short to permit the accumulation of the knowledge required for practice in the 21st century. The amount of new biomedical, pharmaceutical, computer, and communications sciences as well as the production of new drugs and dosage forms, including tailor-made drugs for individual patients using nucleic acids, enzymes, and fermentation processes, i.e., "designer gene machines," will require longer periods of study. Pharmacy education will become more individual and less structured with 6–9 years required for the average student. Demonstration of proficiency in the required areas will determine the time required for graduation.

Pharmacy has been attempting to institute specialties, i.e., practices wherein the practitioner is identified as a pharmacist but is perceived to be different from the traditional retail or hospital pharmacist. Although clinical pharmacy has been attempting longest to organize as a specialty, its lack of acceptance as an essential component of health care delivery by the medical community has prevented recognition as an accepted specialty. Nuclear pharmacy has fared better and, for almost a decade, was the only true specialty of pharmacy, with its own certification program and acceptance by the medical system, until the recent establishment of certification in geriatric pharmacy. Although some pharmacists choose to limit their practices to certain areas, e.g., consulting pharmacy, poison control, biopharmaceutics, drug information, etc., none of these areas is crystallized sufficiently to define a true pharmaceutical specialty.

Pharmacists speak of emerging new roles and authorities in areas such as drug monitoring, dosage adjustment, and prescribing, but, with the exception of some limited prescribing authority in Florida, these new roles are yet to be achieved and face strong opposition from physicians. Several reasons for this resistance are obvious, e.g., encroachment on the physician's professional and economic turf, but others are more subtle and more substantive. As one physician observed, it is unlikely for physicians to prescribe and pharmacists to treat because it breaks up the "cycle of therapeutics," i.e., the need for one "case manager" to see whether a disease improves or not. Although this argument may have some validity for hospitalized patients under continual observation by a physician, the argument breaks down for ambulatory patients and outpatients who may see a physician only infrequently after a drug has been prescribed, especially if the prescription authorizes refills. Even in group practices and clinics, patients may not see the same physician at each visit. The argument is frequently made that physicians are not monitoring drugs now. For most prescriptions written today, the physician does not see the patient again because he/she does not return for follow-up visits.

Advances in pharmacy education can overcome some of the resistance and fears surrounding pharmacist prescribing, adjusting dosages, etc. One key is biology. Although pharmacy education is strong in chemistry and in understanding the drug and its behavior in the body from the chemical and kinetic perspectives, physicians do not perceive pharmacy education to be strong enough in biology, particularly human pathophysiology. Pharmacists must understand more about the disease process, the body's mechanisms to cope with it, and how physiology and pharmacy must come together in an integrated approach to patient management. Physicians will always be able to object to pharmacists prescribing drugs and manipulating their dosage until pharmacists demonstrate a greater understanding of that process.

Changing the educational system from one that teaches facts to one that requires an integrated approach to patient management must occur. Pharmacists will need to know more about diseases and their effects on the body as well as more knowledge of immunology, biochemistry, microbiology, physiology, etc. to wisely compound and dispense the high tech drugs and dosage forms of the 21st century. Of course, once they have this knowledge, the interface problems with physicians will be exacerbated and turf battles will be common, and specialization in recognized specialty practices with established entry requirements and certification will be the key to survival.

Another aspect of pharmacy education that deserves more attention now and will demand even greater priority in the future is communication. As much as pharmacy boasts about the amount of patient education and consultation it provides to patients now, it is still inadequate and far less pervasive than some pharmacy educators and spokespersons will believe. Pharmacists are still too reluctant to emerge from their prescription departments and speak with patients and consumers (although one drug chain reports that it stations a pharmacist in the OTC department to advise consumers on products, which, if true, is a laudable exception). Patients and consumers need accurate, clear, concise information about their drugs and responsive, clear answers to their questions now. As drugs become more sophisticated and communications become more automated with computers and telematics, the high touch of human conversation with knowledgeable, sensitive, and understanding pharmacists to assure that they understand and accept the information and directions about their drugs and how they must be used is essential. Pharmacy education must be better at teaching pharmacists what to communicate as well as the need to speak to their patients and consumers directly, instead of through intermediaries (clerks and technicians), and they must be better at training pharmacists in communication skills to do it right. Jere Goyan often observes, "I am tired of people who communicate bad information clearly."

CERTIFICATION

Public and peer acceptance of a profession is enhanced through certification of its members. The certification process affords a visible stamp of approval that the practitioner has completed a recognized educational program and has successfully achieved a level of proficiency or competency through examination according to a rigorous standard.

Pharmacists are certified now through examinations by state boards of pharmacy (or their equivalent) in the same way that other health practitioners are certified or licensed to practice their professions under the public health laws or policy powers of the state. With the current exception of nuclear and geriatric pharmacy, however, pharmacists are not certified to practice in specialties. The certification issue has been clouded in recent years by efforts to recognize professional stature. In an attempt to improve the public and perhaps professional perception of B.S. and M.S. pharmacists, several states have adopted the P.D.

(Doctor of Pharmacy) title. The title has been awarded without a requirement to qualify or pass any proficiency or competency standards, thus its acceptance has generally been poor and it has not served its intended purposes. It is unlikely that it will survive into the 21st century.

Other specialty practices will rise to the level where they will formalize and establish their own standards for certification as pharmaceutical sciences become more sophisticated and specialized. Pharmacy should embrace the notion of specialties for, in the words of Louis Rossiter, Ph.D., of the Medical College of Virginia, "Certification will give you a brand name practice" and make you more secure.

PREDICTIONS

Perhaps because of the logic of the associations of current issues and trends with society as we know it today, or the alien nature of the other scenarios, the Conference on Pharmacy in the 21st Century predicted that the future of pharmacy lies in the Continued Growth scenario.

In the continued growth scenario, pharmacy will fare well. Pharmacy personnel in the year 2010 will increase 5% to 280,000, of whom 40–50% will be technicians and aides. Of the graduate pharmacists, Pharm. D. and B.S. degrees will be equally common. The primary role of pharmacists will be advising patients on their drugs and monitoring their therapy.

High technology dosage forms will represent a significant part of the market and will not be held closely accountable for cost effectiveness. OTC drugs will increase to 50% of total drug sales, up from about 33%, and a "third class" of pharmacist-dispensed drugs will emerge in face of opposition from pharmaceutical manufacturers. The total market will increase sigificantly with expenditures for drugs reaching $100 billion in 1980 dollars.

Self-care will increase, but so will the demand for more professional care. Improved technology and health information data will improve the quality of health care, which will be provided at multiple sites including short stay, critical care hospitals; extended care facilities; and large multiservice, ambulatory sites—"medical supermarkets." Many pharmacies, especially those in large shopping centers, will evolve into health centers, employing a full cadre of health care professionals. This concept is already being realized in a few large mass merchandisers where the pharmacy departments have been expanded into health centers. Academic medical centers will continue, but their major problem will be finding financial support for research while continuing to provide quality health care. Hospitals too will feel the effects of growth, increased cost, and the impact of the self-care trend. They will risk evolving to centralized critical care facilities serving a broad geographic area or places where people come to die, although the terminally ill could choose death at home or in a hospice.

Corporations will provide on-site health care to reduce lost time associated with doctors' visits. Although critics may argue that on-site health care will limit freedom of choice, if the employer pays the bill, the employee-consumer is less likely to opt out of the program to undertake his own health care. Physician dispensing in corporate health programs will exacerbate the conflict between corporate health programs and community-based pharmacy services. Cost containment will continue to be a national priority. The majority of pharmacists will be employed and unionized. Independently owned pharmacies will be replaced almost completely by chain outlets or nationally franchised outlets.

Prescription departments will shrink substantially and will change dramatically to accommodate compounding high-tech new drugs in individualized prescriptions. Some prescription departments will have been eliminated entirely in some pharmacies to make room for the expanded number of OTC products resulting from increased Rx to OTC switches. The growth in the OTC industry will pressure nondrug outlets more than pharmacies as food and mass merchandisers do a higher proportion of OTC drug sales.

Prescriptions will be filled more by technicians and machines than by pharmacists, and prescriptions will routinely be telecommunicated to pharmacies by computers or on magnetic cards given to patients. Information about drugs and drug effects is readily available, provided by pharmacists and computers, but despite this abundance of information, adverse events are not uncommon because of inappropriate self-therapy. Pharmacist's influences on the purchase of OTC drugs will decline as more sales of these products proportionately move to nondrug outlets.

Drug research will lead to the development of specialized therapeutic agents and dosage forms that target a specific organ system or create a narrow range of pharmacodynamic effects in order to minimize adverse events. Moreover, drugs will be specifically tailored to meet the biology of children, adults, and geriatric patients. Still others will be designed to meet the needs of persons whose individual biological/biochemical make-up differ from the norm, e.g., people with enzyme deficiencies, certain inborn errors of metabolism, etc. Drugs will be very expensive due to their high cost.

Selection, maintenance, and monitoring of drug therapy will be largely delegated to clinical pharmacists whose malpractice insurance premiums will nearly match those of physicians. The oversupply of physicians feared in the 1980s will not materialize. The demand for medical services will increase for continuous and preventive care, just as the large numbers of physicians trained entered practice. The borders between health professionals continue to blur. Pharmacists will continue to take over some physicians' roles, especially in pharmacokinetic profiling, dosing, and monitoring, while physicians' compounding and dispensing will grow.

Home health care for chronic debilitating and terminal diseases will continue to be encouraged as a cost containment effort and because sophisticated home therapeutic management equipment will be readily available and trained health care professionals will stay in constant contact through telemetry. The "right to die" issue will become of greater significance as many people will choose to end their own lives instead of being maintained through life support systems.

Virtually all of the colleges of pharmacy will continue and will offer the Pharm. D. degree—almost exclusively. Teaching facilities will remain about the same size, but research facilities will double. The number of volunteer facilities will outnumber the paid facility 20:1. Enrollments will increase about 10%, but the curriculum will become self-paced and competency oriented. Most studies will require 6–9 years to complete the program, which will no longer be one curriculum but a wide variety of courses and educational options leading to a choice of specialties. Significant expansion of the physical and biological sciences will take place in recognition of their importance to understanding disease and drug therapy.

Lectures will be all but eliminated (an event likely to be welcomed with enthusiasm) and students will educate themselves through self-discipline using user-friendly computers with a wide variety of stimulating, intensive, instructional programs designed to impart knowledge and discover, early, those students who are neither academically nor attitudinally committed to the profession. Clinical clerkships will take up 25% of the curriculum, and laboratories will have been essentially replaced by computer graphics, media simulations, etc.

Tables 15.1 to 15.3 provide summaries of the outcomes of each of the four alternative futures scenarios.

Table 15.1. Alternative Futures for Health Care in 2010 ᵃ

Scenario Element	Continued Growth	Decline and Stagnation	Disciplined Society	Transformation
Population (in 2010)	283 million	275 million	270 million	283 million
65 and over	14%	13%	14%	14%
Medical system Goal	"Conquer disease" and extend life	Ameliorate disease	Order through health and health through order	Aid individuals to promote their health and self-care
Approaches	Provider-mediated diagnosis and therapy of specific diseases using high technology	Triage, care dependent upon economic status; low to medium technology for most, high technology for wealthy	System-coordinated health promotion and treatment	Knowledge development for effective self care and treatment; variety of physical, spiritual, and behavioral approaches and various levels of providers
Key to Health	Better medicine lifestyles	Better medicine and employment/income increased out of necessity	Diet, nutrition, exercise, medical care increased because of cost effectiveness	Faith, family, friends, diet, exercise, nutrition, some medical care increased because of individual preference, better information technologies and medical support
Nature/capacity for self-care	Developed as adjunct to physician care			
Compression of morbidity (CM) and Life extension (LE)	Some CM, LE for many through transplants, etc.	Limited CM or LE; CM for affluent and healthy poor; LE for most wealthy	CM, but LE only for elite	CM and some "natural" LE; relatively few transplants
Health care personnel Right to practice	Licensure of allopathic physicians and others approved to practice at physician direction	Licensure of allopathic physicians; more illegal practitioners of various schools	Institutional credentialling	Credentialling of providers by schools of therapy; free market; reliance on tort law and consumer policing

Table 15.1. (Continued).

Scenario Element	Continued Growth	Decline and Stagnation	Disciplined Society	Transformation
Artificial intelligence	Miniaturized computers and very expert systems aid physicians in all aspects of care; good consumer AI products available; hospital on the wrist	Expert systems available to some physicians and care facilities; good consumer AI available but not widely distributed	Wide use of computers and expert systems by consumers and providers; big brother-on-the-wrist	Diverse software for computer and expert systems, widely used by consumers and providers
Care for aging	Life extension sought through organ transplants, etc. Extensive care provided for most elderly	Care varies depending on income Inadequate care for many	Expensive care for aged deemphasized; otherwise, good care	Health promotion emphasized; treatment for aged; greater acceptance of death
Care for children	Sophisticated care for virtually all children Mainstreaming of problem children Bionic disability enhancers common genetic screening, counseling locates defects	Care varies depending on income, poverty leads to greater childhood disease Epidemics common	Expensive care for children warranted if cost-effective genetic counseling and engineering reduce birth defects	Sophisticated care, as noninvasive as possible Bionic disability enhancers Instruction in immune system self-enhancement Greater acceptance of death (less heroic measures) Genetic counseling, prenatal care, leads to fewer birth defects

Research and technology	Vaccines and cures for heart disease and some cancers Effective bionics	Few breakthroughs as research underfunded Focus on cures for epidemics	Effective health care system; behavior and attitude modification common	Self-regulation of mind/body relationship proven as an effective disease detection, prevention tool vaccines, and cures for disease and cancers
Apex of technology	Hospital-on-the-wrist	Telemedicine	Individual health monitoring; early warning; community-based	Hospital-on-the-wrist as well as nonmechanical self-diagnosis/self-regulation
Common procedures/technology	High technology care Organ/limb transplants Sophisticated imaging Bioelectric therapies	Modest proven technologies	Cost-effective, proven technologies	High technology Self-regulation therapies Food as drugs
Expenditures (% of GNP for health care)	13%	6%	8%	6%

aEdited and reprinted with permission from Bezold C, Halperin J, Binkley H, Ashbaugh R, eds. Pharmacy in the 21st century. Alexandria VA: Institute for Alternative Futures and Project Hope, 1985, pp 26–28. Copyright, American Association of Colleges of Pharmacy.

Table 15.2.   Research and Technology in the Four Futures [a]

	Continued Growth (CD)	Decline and Stagnation	Disciplined Society	Transformational Society
Climate for R & D	Strong	Poor; little basic research	Good	Strong
Health R & D as % of GNP (0.3 in 1980)	0.5%	0.2%	0.4%	0.5%
Government-public vs. industry R & D ratio (2:1 in 1980)	1:3	1:3	2.3:1	1:1.5
NIH budget (0.12% of GNP in 1975)	$5.6 billion (0.10% GNP)	$.78 billion (0.06% GNP)	$3.0 billion (0.08% GNP)	$3.7 billion (0.10% GNP)
% of grants approved	60%	50%	80%	
University/industry relationship	Separate but equal	Retrenchment	Nationalization of universities and close industry link	Decentralized; healthy relationship
Research advances				
Diagnostics	Three dimensions of any part of body to 2 mm	Some advances; available only to the wealthy	Same as CG although appreciation of expensive high technology is more limited	Three dimensions of any part of body to 2 mm
Gene therapies	Common		Substance abuse controlled by "libido suppressing factor"	Common
Screening/abortion	Widely used			Widely used

Heart disease	Eliminated	Substantially reduced		Eliminated with vaccines and "eclectic vitalism"
Cancer	Eliminated	Substantially reduced		Eliminated with vaccines and "eclectic vitalism"
Life expectancy	82 men 85 women	Same as 1980–1985		Same as 1980–1985
Health professionals	Superspecialists	High-tech medicine with fewer customers	Highly specialized	Specialized by task, including "soft technologies"
Pharmacy schools/education	Pharm. D.s exclusively after 2005; for complex cellular, immunological, and genetic therapies Little drug dispensing or patient counseling	Oversupply and unemployment among pharmacists Chain store and hospital pharmacy managers		Greater counseling roles, especially with substance abusers
Unresolved health problems	Degenerative diseases, especially arthritis, blindness and hearing loss Senility Mental illness Drug abuse	Cirrhosis Substance abuse Homicide Suicide Despair that "puzzles of diseases will be solved"	Degenerative diseases Neurological handicaps Mental illness	
Health care system	Retirement age now 72	Two tier: low quality National Health Service for most	Highly efficient Prenatal genetic screening Little spent to sustain elderly after 70 (retirement age)	
GNP for health care	13%	6%	8%	16% until epidemic of 2018, then 6%

[a]Edited and reprinted with permission from Bezold C, Halperin J, Binkley H, Ashbaugh R, eds. Pharmacy in the 21st century. Alexandria VA: Institute for Alternative Futures and Project Hope, 1985, pp 131–133. Copyright, American Association of Colleges of Pharmacy.

Table 15.3.   Alternative Futures for Pharmacy Practice and Education in the United States [a]

	Continued Growth (CG)	Decline and Stagnation (D&S)	Disciplined Society	Transformation
Professional environment				
Cost-containment measures	High priority	High priority	High priority	Low priority
Unionized professionals	Highly likely	Likely	Prohibited	Unlikely
Technicians or automated dispensing machines	Common	Common but drug usage down	Common	Machines only (no prescription drugs)
Locus of practice	"One-stop" health centers	Primary chain	Chain and HMO-like outlets severely regulated	Some independent pharmacies remain
Ratio of OTC/RX drugs in numbers	Increased	Somewhat increased	Somewhat increased	Greatly increased
Demand for clinical services	Increased	About the same	Increased but tightly controlled	Increased but changed toward holistic concepts of practice
Demand for distributive services by pharmacists	Decreased	Decreased greatly	Decreased	About the same demand but different services
Ratio of new drugs (developed since 1984) to total number of drugs	Large fraction	Small fraction	Large fraction	Small fraction
Cost of drugs	Expensive but effective	Same as CG	Same as CG	Expensive but less so than CG

Vaccine usage	Increased drastically	Increased	Same as CG	Increased but less than CG
Physical environment	Degenerated	Greatly degenerated	Improving	Staying about the same
Home health care	Increased	Greatly increased	Increased	Primary mode of care
Education				
Number of schools	About the same	Decreased to about ½ of present numbers	Same as D&S	Fewer than D&S
Number of students	Increased by 10%	Decreased by 30%	Increased by 20%	Decreased by 70%
Degree	All Pharm. D.	Predominantly Pharm. D.	All Pharm. D.	All Pharm. D.
Length of curriculum	Varies by student 6-9 years	Six years	Same as D&S	Students progress at own rate up
Curriculum structure	Many tracks	Very standardized	Nationally standardized	Wildly varied
Basic science component	Significantly expanded	Same as CG	Same as CG	Similar to CG but new areas such as "herbalogy" added
Teaching methodology	Lectures decreased, media increased, including simulation for both basic science and clinical teaching	Lectures greatly decreased, media use greatly increased	As in D&S but media educational modules supplied by government	As in CG but with some "guru"-type instruction
Instructional emphasis	Emphasis on skills development, problem-solving, and self-evaluation	Similar to CG	Similar to CG	More self-instructional
Specialization	Highly specialized	Specialized	Same as D&S	According to student desires
Computer use in instruction	Every student owns at least one computer and uses it daily	As CG but with fewer instructors available	As CG but use dictated by government	As CG but used differently

aEdited and reprinted with permission from Bezold C, Halperin J, Binkley H, Ashbaugh R, eds. Pharmacy in the 21st century. Alexandria VA: Institute for Alternative Futures and Project Hope, 1985, pp 199–201. Copyright, American Association of Colleges of Pharmacy.

SUMMARY

The future of pharmacy over the next 4 decades will be shaped by a series of societal trends and economic forces that are occurring today. The future holds both promise and risk for the vitality of pharmacy in the health care system of the 21st century. Evolutionary changes in pharmacy education and practice to keep pace with the environmental changes that are driving the health care system must be planned now, put into action, and monitored continually to assure they are keeping up with the changes.

With thoughtful attention to planning, the future of pharmacy should be secured. Inattentiveness presents serious risks to the profession and its place in the 21st century. Current students, the readers of this text, will reap the rewards or bear the brunt of successes or failures by contemporary leaders and educators to secure their futures.

SUGGESTED READINGS

1. American Journal of Health Promotion. Syracuse, NY.
2. Baker KN. Pharmacy practice and the future. Am Pharm 1984;24(1):38.
3. Bezold C, ed. Pharmaceuticals in the year 2000. Alexandria, VA: Institute for Alternative Futures, 1983.
4. Brodie DC, Smith WE. Implications of new technology for pharmacy education and practice. Am J Hosp Pharm 1985;42:81.
5. Bullock BB. Another look at pharmacy's future. Am Pharm 1983;23(4):4.
6. Codling MD. The over-the-counter drug industry: a quiet revolution. Spectrum, Pharmaceuticals Products and Technologies. Boston: Arthur D. Little Decision Resources, 1987.
7. Dickinson JG. What's wrong with APhA? Am Pharm 1985;25(6):334.
8. Dickinson JG. Pharmacists Fighting Back. Address to the Missouri Pharmaceutical Association Convention, Osage Beach, MO, May 15, 1986.
9. Eckian AG. The frontiers of Rx to OTC switch. Presented to the 1986 Research and Scientific Development Conference. The Proprietary Association, New York, December 10, 1986, in press.
10. Finston M. J & J Prescribes "Wellness." The Start Ledger, January 22, 1987, p 44.
11. Franke DE. Pharmacy in the year 2000. Drug Intell Clin Pharm 1975;42:454.
12. Goldsmith JC. The U.S. health care system in the year 2000. JAMA 1986;256(24).
13. Gosselin R. Pharmacy's potential. The Apothecary June/July/August, 1984, p 19.
14. Hayes AH Jr. Keynote Address. Washington DC: 8th General Assembly of World Federation of Proprietary Medicine Manufacturers, September 22, 1986.
15. Health care practices and perceptions, A consumer survey of self-medication. Prepared for the Proprietary Association by Harry Heller Research Corp. HHR 72792, 1984.
16. Hetherington M. Seniors and self medication: synergistic input of pharmacy in the 80's and 90's. Can Pharm J 1984;377.
17. Hirschorn MW. . . . While pharmacists seek bigger role in health care. New York: The Wall Street Journal.
18. James B. The future of the multinational pharmaceutical industry to 1990. London: Halsted Press, 1977.
19. Johnson RC. Malpractice (letter to the editor). Am Druggist, 1987;195:116.
20. Kanig JL. The frontiers of the professional/OTC interface. Presented to the 1986 Research and Scientific Development Conference. The Proprietary Association, New York, December 10, 1986, in press.
21. Kline CH. Non-prescription drugs: from folk remedy to high tech. Presented at First General Session of the 8th General Assembly of the World Federation of Proprietary Medicine Manufacturers, Washington DC, September 22, 1986.
22. Levy G. Preparing for pharmacy's future. Am J Pharm Educ 1983;49:332.
23. Diener CH, ed. Lilly digest. Indianapolis: Eli Lilly & Company, Pharmaceutical Division, 1986.
24. Lunan HN. New developments in pharmacy—how does the institution meet this need? Drug Intell Clin Pharm 1975;9:453.

25. Manell S, Johannson S. The impact of computer technology on drug information. North Holland: Elsevier, 1982.
26. Diner CH, ed. Lilly digest. Indianapolis: Eli Lilly & Company, Lilly Corporate Center, 1986.
27. Naisbitt J. Megatrends. New York: Warner Books Inc, 1984.
28. New study of pharmacists reveals top interest in Rx and OTC products. Pharmacy Times, November 1986, p 63.
29. Oddis JA. Pharmacy in the health-care environment. Am J Hosp Pharm 1986;43:1435.
30. Oddis JA. Frontiers of change in pharmacy practice. Illinois Pharmacist, January 1985, p 9.
31. Parachini A. Centenarian population on the rise. Los Angeles Times, January 20, 1987, Part V, p 1.
32. Pharmacists for the future. The Report of the Study Commission on Pharmacy, The American Association of Colleges of Pharmacy, Health Administration Press, Ann Arbor, MI, 1975.
33. Pharmacy in the twenty-first century: results of a strategic-planning conference. Am J Hosp Pharm 1985;42:71.
34. Bezold C, Halperin J, Binkley H, Ashbaugh R, eds. Pharmacy in the 21st Century. Alexandria VA: Institute for Alternative Futures and Project Hope, 1985. Copies of this book examining alternative approaches for the delivery of health care in the future can be obtained from the American Association of Colleges of Pharmacy, 4720 Montgomery Avenue, Suite 602, Bethesda, MD 20814 ($18.50 per copy, prepaid). Copyright, American Association of Colleges of Pharmacy, used with permission.
35. Pinco RG. How OTC's can be marketed in the 21st century. Presented to the 1986 Research and Scientific Development Conference, The Proprietary Association, New York, December 10, 1986. Proceedings in press.
36. MD Rx dispensing should be encouraged, FTC Bureaus say. PMA Newsletter. Pharmaceutical Manufacturers Association, Washington DC, January 12, 1987, p 5.
37. Schwartz MA. Educational needs for pharmacy practice in the year 2000. Drug Intell Clin Pharm 1975;9:447.
38. The Kiplinger Washington Letter, The Kiplinger Washington Editions, Washington DC, December 26, 1986.
39. The Sunday Star Ledger. November 2, 1986, p 51.
40. Toffler A. The third wave. New York: Morrow, 1980.
41. Vickery DM. Life plan for your health. Reading MA: Addison-Wesley Publishing Co, 1978.
42. Vital Statistics. American Association of Colleges of Pharmacy, Bethesda, MD, Revised August 1986.
43. Wertheimer AI. A look ahead. Pharm Practice. p 411.
44. West CM. Back to school. American Druggist, January 1987, p 116.
45. Whitney HAK Jr. The education and utilization of pharmacy supportive personnel. Drug Intell Clin Pharm 1975;9:452.
46. Young P. A terrifying scenario for year 2050. Sunday Star-Ledger, Newark, NJ, November 23, 1986, sect 3, p 1.
47. Zellmer WA. Can pharmacy control its destiny? Am J Hosp Pharm 1985;42:69.

Index

Page numbers in *italics* indicate figures; those followed by *t* indicate tables.